Telehealth Networks for Hospital Services:

New Methodologies

Vincenzo Gullà
ADITech, Italy

Angelo Rossi Mori
National Research Council, Italy

Francesco Gabbrielli
Rome General Hospital Umberto 1, Italy

Pietro Lanzafame
Centro Neurolesi, Bonino Pulejo, Italy

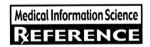

Medical Information Science
REFERENCE

Managing Director:	Lindsay Johnston
Editorial Director:	Joel Gamon
Book Production Manager:	Jennifer Yoder
Publishing Systems Analyst:	Adrienne Freeland
Development Editor:	Austin DeMarco
Assistant Acquisitions Editor:	Kayla Wolfe
Typesetter:	Erin O'Dea
Cover Design:	Jason Mull

Published in the United States of America by
Medical Information Science Reference (an imprint of IGI Global)
701 E. Chocolate Avenue
Hershey PA 17033
Tel: 717-533-8845
Fax: 717-533-8661
E-mail: cust@igi-global.com
Web site: http://www.igi-global.com

Library of Congress Cataloging-in-Publication Data

Telehealth networks for hospital services : new methodologies / Vincenzo Gulla and Angelo Rossi Mori, editors.
     pages cm
 Includes bibliographical references and index.
 Summary: "This book carefully focuses on and describes different networks that link hospitals and their services to patients outside their territory, focusing on the technology, users and collaboration necessary that are integral to the function of a telehealth network"-- Provided by publisher.
  ISBN 978-1-4666-2979-0 (hardcover) -- ISBN 978-1-4666-2980-6 (ebook) -- ISBN 978-1-4666-2981-3 (print & perpetual access) 1. Telecommunication in medicine. 2. Medicine--Computer network resources. I. Gulla, Vincenzo, 1955- II. Mori, Angelo Rossi, 1949-
  R119.9.T4454 2013
  610.285--dc23
                                        2012037524

British Cataloguing in Publication Data
A Cataloguing in Publication record for this book is available from the British Library.

All work contributed to this book is new, previously-unpublished material. The views expressed in this book are those of the authors, but not necessarily of the publisher.

Table of Contents

Detailed Table of Contents

Section 1

This section collects 8 chapters where concepts are deeply analysed, compared to the population longevity and chronicling disease requirements experienced worldwide, in environments with completely different living conditions and rules. The reader will have the chance to learn from the beginning and make treasure of the experiences and ideas that have made these applications successful.

Chapter 1

> *Angelo Rossi Mori, Institute of Biomedical Technologies (CNR), Italy*
> *Mariangela Contenti, Institute of Biomedical Technologies (CNR), Italy*
> *Rita Verbicaro, Institute of Biomedical Technologies (CNR), Italy*

Modern telemedicine is one component of the pervasive eHealth solutions being deployed in several countries. Differently from the past, telemedicine has no longer to be considered with a strictly technology-driven perspective, but rather as an enhancing factor and a resource for the design and enactment of innovative organizational models that a region is introducing to cope with the sustainability of the healthcare system. In order to achieve its maturity in clinical working practice and widespread diffusion, telemedicine should be carefully planned by policy makers as a component of the healthcare action lines that drives the innovation of the organisational models and delivery channels in the healthcare provision. The attention should be put on the care processes improvement and governance, to the collaboration among professionals and to the patient engagement, not only on technological implementation issues.

Chapter 2

> *S A Davis, University of California Merced, USA*

This chapter addresses an eHealth definition for review, thoughts on eHealth systems, resistance to change issues to be considered, the CVS Minute Clinic's introduction of innovation and disruptive eHealth care models and systems, a systems engineering management proof of concept project with the Kansas Department of Corrections, and globally-oriented conclusions and recommendations.

Telemedicine is an innovative healthcare system capable of ensuring both higher efficiency and better cost-effectiveness. In the first part, the chapter discusses the demographic changes of the society and their impact on family organization and on Ancient rule. In the middle part, the chapter focuses on the eHealth and Telemedicine concepts, on the recognition of their potential roles in the National Health Services. The last part of the Chapter is dedicated to the Italian situation.

Chapter 4

Paediatric cardiology is a subspecialty ideally suited to telemedicine. A small number of experts cover large geographical areas and the diagnosis of congenital heart defects is largely dependent on the interpretation of medical imaging. Telemedicine has been applied to a number of areas within paediatric cardiology. In this chapter, the authors examine the current evidence pertaining to telemedicine applied to paediatric cardiology including their own experience, the importance of research and, in particular, economic evaluations.

The European Space Agency (ESA) is, since 1996, active in telecommunications field and has initiated various projects which have demonstrated that satellite communications are a powerful technology for enlarging the reach of Telemedicine services toward geographically isolated regions, especially those with a high burden of diseases, such as many areas in Sub-Saharan Africa. In 2006 the Telemedicine Task Force (TTF) with the mandate to explore the potential of Telemedicine via Satellite for this region has been established on initiative of ESA and the European Commission, with representatives of African stakeholders and the World Health Organization (WHO). The projects should and will be presented in China for finding bilateral cooperation between Italian and Chinese Civilian and Military technologies and opportunities present already in the field.

DREAM (Drug Resource Enhancement against AIDS and Malnutrition) is a programme made from the Community of S.Egidio started in 2002 in Mozambique and now spread in 10 countries of sub-Saharan Africa (Mozambique, Malawi, Tanzania; Kenia, Rep. Guinea; Guinea Bissau, Nigeria, Angola; Cameroon, Congo). It is a holistic programme to fight HIV and Malnutrition. To date, DREAM has 33 centres already operational and 13 molecular biology laboratories that guarantee constant monitoring to DREAM patients. More than 95,000 patients are under assistance, and 55,000 of them are in HAART treatment. This chapter gives a detailed description of the authors' experience.

Chapter 7

There is increasing uptake of telehealth for long-term conditions (LTCs). However, evidence of their effectiveness remains largely inconclusive. The objectives of this chapter are to determine the effectiveness of telehealth and to update existing checklist on key success factors for implementation of telehealth.

Chapter 8

This study examines the relationship between telemedicine utilization, the availability of physicians, the level of urbanity of a locality, and the physical distance between a locality and an urban health facility at the county level within a rural state in the United States. The results are useful for practitioners and may motivate further studies.

Section 2

This section drives the reader to explore the following subjects: How communication technologies are changing medical practice; The practical role of telemedicine in patient data management systems and services provisioning; Technology innovation for healthcare professional networks; Telemedicine networks service delivery organization models; Providing the main technical guidelines to the reader willing to implement telemedicine networks and services. The chapters included in this section drive the readers throughout a number of very impressive telemedicine application experienced by hospitals worldwide, addressing different pathologies, using different technologies and methods. For each chapter, the authors highlight the lesson learned delivering their experience to the readers.

The adoption of Telematics medicine or Telemedicine marks an important structural change in the mode in which deployment of medical care is being routinely provided. It is not a matter of using more or less developed technologies but mainly a deep change to the way in which countries and governments decide to provide and manage their national healthcare system. There is definitely a new paradigm taking place. Thus, the telemedicine approach implies deeply changing the way healthcare is provided. The authors are aware that this will take time, as any cultural revolution, but for the time being we need to start adapting our mentality and our networks to integrate and allow the two methods to cohabit together. Technology is one of the leading tools to allow this to happen, and it is necessary to understand what requirements are needed to get the maximum success. Years of experience have dictated the main rules and guidelines exploited in detail in this chapter.

Chapter 10

Telemedicine service has dramatically increased in San Giovanni-Addolorata hospital in Rome in the last two years. Stated as an experimental service in 2005, telemedicine has gained the status of usual service in 2008 and now has reached a good functional level since the creation of a dedicated department within the hospital in late 2009. This chapter shows the results obtained and gives a brief description of the operational workflow.

The authors introduce some concepts about the remote follow-up of Implantable Cardioverter Defibrillators (ICD). Even if this type of remote monitoring system is relatively new, literature has demonstrated the utilization in clinical practice and during the last few years medical industry has provided different devices. Starting from the background, some models of utilizations are presented, focusing on the description of the main functions provided by some devices offered on the market. Next are explored the motivations for which remote follow-up is needed: a better management of the patient is described in several studies and the integration of clinical information from monitoring devices in Electronic Medical Records is presented as the important step in order to provide comprehensive clinical information about the patient, also economic issues are shown. Then some experiences realized in U.S. are explored and at last are proposed to the discussion a number of questions as contribution to the next research. Some Italian recent experiences in the field of remote monitoring and home care of patients with heart failure with and without implantable devices are reported.

In this chapter the main aspects of Telemonitoring are described and discussed within the field of chronic respiratory diseases. The authors describe the various challenges they faced, in the order in which they did. First they face the problem of effectiveness of the method, then the problems related to the economic viability, and finally the problems related to the operating method. They conclude that remote monitoring is a promising method in terms of effectiveness of follow-up that must be performed under well controlled conditions. They still require further validation studies to improve the effectiveness and reduce the effects of new issues that arise.

The focus of this chapter is to asses a new model of care in dementia, particularly Alzheimer's Disease (AD). According with sociotechnical approaches, the authors describe a proof of concept, Information and Communication Technologies (ICT) intervention as technical and organizational model of robust, reliable, and efficient clinical practice to meet the medical, psychological, and social needs of AD people and their family. The authors also propose the "Identification-Recognition-Evaluation-Application Model" as process methodology in a telemedicine project. In their perspective, the technology has to be analyzed as technology-in-use, a process coming out from an ecology of specific actions and actors. Finally, the authors describe their experience with a longitudinal study in which ICT networking technologies are used to implement coping strategies, in order to improve the quality of life of AD families.

The author defines a scenario for providing Health Services through the Digital Terrestrial Television (DTT), both for patients (monitoring health parameters) and healthy citizens. A number of services will be provided over DTT, not only by means of informative or interactive applications broadcast and installed on the set-top box, but also as transactional services through the secure return channel. However, much effort has to be spent to guarantee the usability of that new TV-based interface, which is quite different from that of a PC-based Web application.

Over recent years, informatics and computer sciences have changed dramatically the practice of clinical cytopathology. New types of cameras and microscopes connected to computers made image capture and transmission possible (telecytology). The wide implementation of telemedical systems in the field of cytopathology became a necessity dictated by the need of real-time results for therapeutic decisions. A telemedical application is a valuable tool for cytopathologists in order to manage and promote inter-laboratory collaboration. The result is better cytological data management and sharing. ISO 15189:2007 for medical laboratories requires successful participation in proficiency testing programs. This chapter emphasizes on the necessity of developing a proficiency test for cytopathology labs wishing to be accredited according to ISO 15189:2007, and examines the feasibility of using low cost telemedical applications and solutions for this purpose. Furthermore, the authors give clear and comprehensive guidance concerning various financial, legal, professional, and ethical problems in this field.

Chapter 16

Emergency events are always very critical to manage as in most cases there is a human life risk. Such events could become even more serious when occurring in remote areas not equipped with adequate healthcare facilities, able to manage life risk. This is the case in many rural geographical areas. In such scenarios telemedicine can play a very important and determinant role. This chapter describes the basis of the experience about telemedicine application in a small hospital located in the town of Branca, near Gubbio, Italy. The experience has shown how the use of videocommunication-based telemedicine systems has improved the service and what procedural impact the adoption of such technology has required.

Section 3

This section provides a deep analysis of Telemedicine or Telematic medicine projects' main critical issues, driving the reader to understand healthcare needs and how to match them with technologies. The role of R&D and how new incoming technologies may influence the telemedicine market is exploited as well. The section gives the reader a critical analysis about the organization models and the rules that should be followed to implement in-hospital tele-healthcare making the point between traditional resistances and telemedicine innovations. The section includes a number of chapters introducing innovative technologies and methods into the hospital telemedicine deployments services including wellness, health prevention and digital imaging distribution.

Chapter 17

In modern Medicine and Surgery, innovations arise from interdisciplinary work. Therefore, to analyse how Telemedicine R&D is influencing strategies and organizational models in healthcare systems, we have to study how ICT and Robotics innovations can interact with structured healthcare services on a large scale. The problem is interdisciplinary, and the answer has to be on different levels: economical, technological, and organizational. Overall, change needs two paradigms: from Telemedicine to Telematic Medicine and Surgery and from financial strategies for saving to Lean Thinking for innovations. The innovation of value can be obtained when healthcare organizations combine innovative Telematic Medicine and Surgery services with utility, prices, and costs. To work on these innovations without rearranging the whole organizational flow around the future e-health service means inducing the healthcare organization to generate wastes and face unnecessary expenses attached to future healthcare processes with such high and probably unsustainable costs.

Chapter 18

Giovanni Saggio, University of Rome "Tor Vergata," Italy
Valentina Sabato, University of Rome "Tor Vergata," Italy
Roberto Mugavero, University of Rome "Tor Vergata," Italy

Every day, all around the world, millions of people request postural and/or motor rehabilitation. The rehabilitation process, also known as Tertiary Prevention, intends to be a sort of therapy to restore functionality and self-sufficiency of the patient, and regards not only millions of patients daily, but involves also a huge number of professionals in medical staffs, i.e. specialists, nurses, physiotherapists and therapists, social workers, psychologists, physiatrists. The care is given in hospitals, clinics, geriatric facilities, and with territorial home care. Due to the large number of patients, the medical staff and facilities necessary to support the appropriate postural and motor training, as well as the monetary costs of rehabilitation, is so huge, it is very difficult to estimate. Thus, every effort towards a simplification of the rehabilitation route is really desirable and welcome, and this chapter intends to cover this aspect.

Chapter 19

Aldo Franco Dragoni, Università Politecnica delle Marche, Italy

In view of the rapidly progressive increase in the average population age, "Ambient Assisted Living" (AAL) European program defines the actions and policies needed to promote the improvement of living conditions within domestic spaces to foster autonomy, safety, and social inclusion for the elderly or disabled. The idea is to design an innovative and comprehensive information system for AAL, an ICT-based "Virtual Caregiver," which is informed, intelligent, and friendly, and which constantly monitors the health warning, informing and advising the elderly while controlling the environment and then asking for help when needed. The system will have the ability to establish interactive communication with the person but also extend it automatically outside the house in times of need. Virtual Caregiver will be able to enable the software protocols that activate the emergency phone calls to the family, medics, or even first aid in emergencies.

Chapter 20

Chitsutha Soomlek, University of Regina, Canada
Luigi Benedicenti, University of Regina, Canada

An agent-based wellness indicator is an information visualization system designed to present wellness and decision-support information to individuals and their caregivers by elaborating the data provided by measuring devices utilizing the unique characteristics of software agents. The authors' wellness indicator is constructed from an operational wellness model they developed. The model allows an automatic measuring system to calculate the wellness level for a number of indicators resulting in an overall wellness level. These results can be presented in a simple graphical format. The software has been evaluated by following the steps provided in the framework for testing a wellness visualization system. The evaluation is carried out by both general users and healthcare professionals. The results show positive feedback on various aspects of the indicator, and confirm that the wellness indicator can assist people to have a better understanding of their personal state of well-being and can support caregivers in delivering their services.

The assessment of the Spontaneous Motor Activity (SMA) of the life style LS) is fundamental to establish the daily Physical Activity (PA) dose as therapy. The recent employment the accelerometer (AiperMotion 440 PC –Aipermon GmBH – Germany), can immediately distinguish "active" from "sedentary" subjects providing a larger adhesion to the exercise program. The study aims to verify the role of the accelerometer evaluating the effects with obese-hypertensive patients. After three months of regular physical exercise the body composes parameters, investigated principally resulted to be improved. The accelerometer determines a real and objective visualization of the LS expressed as PAL resulting in a direct, early improvement of the parameters strongly related with the cardiovascular risk. The results support the educational role of the employ of the accelerometer.

The field of eHealth is rapidly evolving. The new models and protocols of application of info-communication technologies for healthcare purposes are developed. Despite of obvious advantages and benefits practical application of eHealth and its possibilities in everyday practice is slow. Much progress has been made around the world in the field of digital imaging and virtual slides. But in Georgia telecytology is still in evolving stages. It revolves around static telecytology. It has been revealed, that the application of easy available and adaptable technology together with the improvement of the infrastructure conditions is the essential basis for telecytology. This is a very useful and applicable tool for consulting on difficult cases. Telecytology has significantly increased knowledge exchange and thereby ensured a better medical service. The chapter aims description of practical application of telecytology under conditions of Georgia.

Preface

INTRODUCTION

The real innovative cultural step for medicine is the overcoming of current generic conceptualization of the field (involving together medical, ICT technical, administrative, and legal problems) towards a new model of Telematic-Medicine and Surgery and a new health organization, Tele-Health. The provisioning of healthcare in homes, de- hospitalization, specialist medical care in remote areas, and so on, needs new rules and management models in addition to other technologies.

Furthermore, tele-health, as an organizational process, doesn't lend itself to existing medical activities but it contributes to work share-out and collaboration within a hospital context and between hospitals and territories. Hospitals can extend into a patient's house, and, conversely, then patient is made virtually present in hospitals. So represented, the relationship between professionals, patients, and information is transformed.

WHY THIS BOOK?

Many times we have asked ourselves about telemedicine and its applications. We are surrounded by models, proposals, projects, solutions that industries, research institutes, and governments have attempt to put in act, sometimes with very good results some others failing to meet the milestones and the gaols to put together a sustainable and replicable model. Our intention is to discuss about the positive results and experience in this field and draw simple and understandable guidelines that can support decision makers to identify the most suitable and implementable solutions in their local environment.

The method followed is simply to highlight some aspects we believe to be very important and to describe models of general understanding, showing concrete implementation examples supporting these choices. We will give an overview of the most developed and cutting edge technologies and how these can effect improvements in remote healthcare delivery systems, design delivery scenarios and feasible business models.

The book has been implemented thanks to the active and very appreciated cooperation with worldwide experts and researchers that have shown a great level of competence and experience. We will not take into considerations important and well know subjects such as:

- The ageing of the population, which leads to an aggravation of chronic conditions (>70% of healthcare costs),
- Patients information in monitoring their own health,

- Healthcare costs control,
- The lack of availability of qualified personnel and specialist in remote areas.

These topics are well developed and deeply exploited in many literature studies, but we focus on applicable solutions with the aim to draw a set of reference guidelines .

WHO DO WE ADDRESS?

The authors have worked in close cooperation to put together their knowledge, acquired in years of industry, research, and medical practise with the aim to send a message of feasible support to industries, governments and decision makers. Nevertheless these ideas and elaborations can be the basic for future studies aiming to improve even better solutions for the implementation of more suitable quality of life and health care models.

We address health care stakeholders willing to deploy or plan a territory healthcare service networks, or provisioning model, including all the players inside centralized structures and remote or dense populated areas, GPs, specialist, remote ambulatories or small hospitals.

We believe that the results of this work will be useful to service providers willing to pursue new business models provisioning healthcare, governmental bodies planning telematics medicine tools and to understand better the challenges the procedural and structure changes needed to design a telemedicine network.

AIM OF THE BOOK

The purpose of this book is to provide evidence of how researchers and practitioners understand the health market and to describe key points to health professionals (or health organizations) that should know when planning and implementing new tele-health services or improving existing telemedicine systems to provide value-added medical services. It will underline the methodologies needed to optimize resources and to manage telemedicine projects. Tele-health and its applications are considered as a "socio-technical" or "relational" system, one that doesn't ponder devices, users, and usage context separately, but evaluates them in their mutual interaction. A brief survey about "technology-in-use", a term that identifies technology and its potentiality when they are employed, modalities in which they are actually used on-the-field by users and their community in connection with other devices, techniques, and practices already in use. Studying tele-health as a technology-in-use (i.e. as a sociological problem) will make it possible to bring to light all the hidden work done by users to make the technology usable and reveal the work done by technology to incorporate user needs. Experiences and case studies reported using this approach—that technologies are not born usable and reliable but only become so with their users and their usage in real environments. The exploitation of telemedicine models is a challenging task which this book attempts to explore. In doing so, many models and country experiences have been collected in order to allow the readers to analyse the main features of the design and identify its own applicable model. It is not intended here to give a unique solution but guidelines, rules, and elements which should be addressed to cope with the lack of resources coordination to provide cost effective health management tools, meeting the expectation of an integrated efficient healthcare system available anywhere anytime.

Among all we aim to give better understanding to:

- The direct economic factors, as the suitability to attract resources to activate and maintain the programs, the economic benefits with respect to the investment, the timeliness of return, the impact on the efficiency of the care system;
- The systemic benefits about quality of care, as the citizens' satisfaction, the ability to promote new organizational models, the contribution for a sustainable evolution of the health system, the impact on the jurisdiction as a whole;
- The technological feasibility, relying on the existence of previous success stories and know-how, the scalability and the critical mass of the program, the intrinsic modularity of the problems faced by the tele-health program, the issues of a possible co-existence of the paper flows with the electronic flows, the advantages from the availability of enabling infrastructures;
- The cultural feasibility, considering the predisposition of involving the users from a cultural and an organizational point of view, the degree of independence from incentives, regulations and agreements, the awareness of managers and professionals, the degree of support from public debate and from the consensus of public opinion.

The reader will have the opportunity to learn from the multiple experiences reported in the chapters:

- The models for telemedicine development in hospital services,
- The roles how to manage and harmonize telemedicine projects for hospital e-care,
- The benefits,
- Models and draw guidelines that may fit into each ones reality.

Vincenzo Gulla
Aditech SRL, Ancona Italy

Angelo Rossi Mori
Institute of Biomedical Technologies (CNR), Italy

Francesco Gabbrielli
General Hospital Umberto I Department of Surgical Science P.Stefanini, Italy

Pietro Lanzafame
Neurology Research Center "IRCCS Centro Neurolesi Bonino-Pulejo," Italy

Acknowledgment

The editors are very proud of the work performed with exceptional diligence of the authors and want to thank all for the high level of professionalism provided in their contributions. Each author has contributed with his experiences and skills to suggest methods, solutions, and recommendations that the editors find of enormous relevance and absolutely helpful to any reader willing to have a clear picture of how, where and when a telemedicine solution may be implemented. A special thanks to the Advisory Board for its high level support and to the reviewers that have made this work possible. Thanks to the great team work of all the participants, the editors envisage this book to become a guideline for telemedicine hospital networks and provide a positive influence to improve telemedicine services deployment.

Section 1

Chapter 1
Policies on Telemedicine–Enhanced Hospital Services:
Prioritization Criteria for the Interventions at Regional Level

Angelo Rossi Mori
Institute of Biomedical Technologies (CNR), Italy

Mariangela Contenti
Institute of Biomedical Technologies (CNR), Italy

Rita Verbicaro
Institute of Biomedical Technologies (CNR), Italy

ABSTRACT

Modern telemedicine offers to hospitals a whole range of opportunities to improve the appropriateness of their care provision, to offer new services to primary care and to contribute to patient engagement. In this chapter, the authors briefly discuss their approach to facilitate the collaborative production of region-wide telemedicine roadmaps involving the hospitals, explicitly based on national and regional healthcare strategic priorities. In addition, as an operational contribution to support their approach, they introduce a conceptual frame for evaluating and prioritizing multiple ICT-enhanced innovation interventions, within an all-inclusive plan. The proposed frame captures relevant evaluation criteria belonging to four broad categories: the systemic benefits related to the quality of care; direct economic factors; the cultural viability; and the technological feasibility. As an example, the authors simulate an application of our conceptual frame to the comparative assessment of three kinds of telemedicine-enhanced interventions: (i) to improve the care processes driven by the hospital, (ii) to support health professionals, and (iii) to promote citizen's engagement.

DOI: 10.4018/978-1-4666-2979-0.ch001

1 INTRODUCTION

The use of computer technology in medicine began with the rise of electronic digital computers in the early 1950s (Perednia et al., 1995). The story started with "Medical Informatics", or better "informatics applied to medicine" (Greenes et al., 1990). Then evolved into "Healthcare informatics" or "Healthcare information systems" to take into account the needs of the healthcare facilities and the changes in focus from few isolated applications to increasingly more complex integrated solutions (Siau, 2003).

Next came the time of "ICT for healthcare", where the "Communication" assumed an increasing role (Detmer, 2003).

Later the term "eHealth" was introduced, where the change of perspective was particularly significant: the main soul is now "health" (instead of "healthcare"), and ICT takes a secondary role, becoming the prefix "e-" only to remember that in the information society also health can no longer be the same (Oh et al., 2005; Pagliari et al., 2005). At this stage several national and regional authorities started to issue their eHealth roadmaps, working to develop the necessary infrastructures, such as secure networks, the electronic signature, the digital health card, as well as the longitudinal Electronic Health Record (EHR) for every citizen (eHealth Era, 2007).

The traditional distinction between *healthcare informatics* and *telemedicine* (and telehealth, telecare) was fading out, into a comprehensive sector about *the meaningful use of information and communication technologies to support the improvement of quality and effectiveness of the care systems* (Blumenthal, 2010).

Eventually in the Anglo-Saxon countries another term is taking over: e.g. *"Connecting for Health"* in England (Cross, 2006); "Health Connect" in Australia (DoHA, 2009) and for Kaiser Permanente (Raymond, 2005), a large American Health Maintenance Organization. The emphasis

is no longer on technological solutions, but on health and connection (among people), with the patient at the center.

Indeed, even the European Commission has recently modified the name of its Directorate General on "Information Society and Media": as of 1st July 2012, the Digital Agenda of the EU is managed by the European Commission Directorate General for "Communications Networks, Content and Technology", shortly "DG Connect".

At the same time, countries and regions are increasingly looking for novel and more effective organization model for the health care delivery system, in order to address the burden of chronic diseases and to achieve sustainability and continuity of care (WHO, 2005). In the reorganization of the welfare system as a whole, eHealth and telemedicine applications represent an enabler for the flexible set up of "virtual healthcare facility", where autonomous but collaborative entities, among which the patient's home is included, can effectively interact to overcome the constraints of space and time (Camarinha-Matos, 2002).

In this perspective also the role of hospitals change, by providing specialized care services in collaboration with the community resources, through agreements on shared care processes (e.g. DoH, 2004) enhanced by a modern approach to telemedicine (Joint Commission, 2008). Actually modern telemedicine offers to hospitals a whole range of opportunities to improve the appropriateness of their care provision, to offer new services to primary care and to contribute to patient engagement.

Nevertheless, even if the fundamental components for the modernization of the healthcare enhanced by the technologies seem to be so close at hand, still an overall systemic vision is not yet set-up (European Commission, 2008; European Files, 2010).

Actually, the systemic uptake of eHealth and telemedicine solutions into the ongoing routine operation of healthcare depends on appropriate interventions, enacted with the aim to support more general strategic goals of the healthcare systems (e.g. Scottish Centre for Telehealth, 2010)). The innovation process implies a deep understanding on the implications and impacts of different technologies to different objectives (e.g. Zanaboni et al. 2012)); at a national or regional level it also requires evaluation criteria for comparing and prioritizing different competing intervention areas.

In this chapter we briefly discuss our approach to facilitate the collaborative production of region-wide telemedicine roadmaps involving the hospitals, explicitly based on national and regional healthcare strategic priorities, which will be introduced in section 2.

In addition, as an operational contribution to support our approach, we introduce a conceptual frame for evaluating and prioritizing multiple ICT-enhanced innovation interventions, within an all-inclusive plan. The proposed frame captures relevant evaluation criteria belonging to four broad categories: the *systemic benefits* related to the quality of care; direct *economic factors*; the *cultural viability*; and the *technological feasibility*. In section 3 we outline the four broad dimensions to assess the main features of each intervention, then in section 4 we present a set of potential action lines and section 5 we show a simulated application of the frame.

2 THE NATIONAL AND REGIONAL POLICIES ON THE HEALTHCARE SYSTEMS

National and regional authorities, as well as healthcare organizations, should put special attention to the phenomenon of Connected Health, in order to take advantage of the opportunity offered by the ICT as an enabling factor for innovative organization models and healthcare process improvements

and to develop optimal eHealth and telemedicine roadmaps respondent to the healthcare planning priorities (Rossi Mori et al., 2009).

Today many technological solutions are available to support a sustainable development of the healthcare system and to take advantage of the opportunities opened up by the advanced management of information and knowledge. Nevertheless, the bottom-up, technology-driven introduction of telemedicine was very rarely able to become a massive and pervasive success story. As a matter of fact large scale adoption of eHealth and telemedicine solutions should be pursued in a wider size of the decision contexts, with systemic, long-term goals and precise intermediate objectives (OECD-NSF,2011).

For this reason we expect that a top-down systemic approach to telemedicine modalities, conceptualized as organizational and service modules to be integrated into the ongoing transformation of healthcare delivery, could be successful, effective and sustainable in the long period.

In this new perspective national, regional and local healthcare action plans should be considered with the purpose of identifying the possible role of technologies in the achievements of the intended general goals of change management and quality improvement in different intervention areas (Rossi Mori et al, 2005).

Then, in every region multiple initiatives should be carefully planned in a balanced way according to local resources, capabilities and needs, with a coherent strategy of pilot studies, transfer of know-how, implementations on limited areas or to specific targets (childhood, chronic diseases, elderly, …), predicting since the beginning a stepwise extension to the whole territory.

In other words, in order to define optimal and successful roadmaps on eHealth and specifically on telemedicine, before dealing with technological implementation issues, it is necessary to concentrate the analysis on the healthcare policies and on the derived concrete action plans at all decisional levels.

Actually, the approach and the strategic targets of the healthcare world are focused on the sustainability and on the improvement of quality of the care provision, to be achieved with innovative organizational models and the diffusion of evidence-based clinical pathways.

Priorities of the healthcare world include the need to move resources from the acute care in the hospitals to proactive prevention and continuity of care in the community (e.g. elderly, chronic diseases, newborns, …), to effectively valorize competences and skills of the most specialized professionals, to integrate the social and healthcare aspects, to encourage the active empowerment of the citizen-patient, and to promote clinical governance and quality throughout all the level of services.

These targets imply structural decisions for the system setting, and it is from these decisions that the context for a coherent set of appropriate solutions on ICT and telemedicine should eventually originate: i.e. as a part of the normative, organizational, logistic, trade-union, cultural, educational issues that need to be faced for an economically sustainable evolution of the healthcare sector.

According to this approach, telemedicine-enhanced care services assume the role of one of the component within a comprehensive strategy and a coherent action plan.

It is clear that it is difficult to separate the plans for the telemedicine modules from the plans about other technological solutions and, more important, about the innovative organizational models that are being deployed.

However, if the policy makers are more aware on the potentialities of telemedicine solutions, with respect to each particular organizational model, then they can take more informed decisions about the allocation of resources for innovation. At the same time, if the telemedicine services are embedded within precise healthcare action plans, they could perhaps be recognized as enabling

components and result as more sustainable in the long period.

3 THE CRITERIA TO BALANCE THE DECISIONS AMONG TELEMEDICINE INTERVENTIONS

Regional healthcare planning involves global and inclusive programs, which set priorities and objectives for all the healthcare sectors: from prevention to emergency care, from primary to hospital and community care. In this context innovative organization models and eHealth and telemedicine roadmaps should undertake long term synergic actions for all the different settings of care delivery.

Several actions lines need to be initiated at the same time, with a precise evolution plan in mind, starting with small-scale pilots to provoke a public debate and a progressive cultural growth.

Policy makers should attract and optimally allocate resources among the various action lines, and drive the change management. As a decision support tool for them, we developed a conceptual frame for evaluating eHealth and telemedicine interventions. The frame should allow to perform an assessment of telemedicine interventions across very different kinds of action lines and to systematically evaluate benefits, obstacles and risks for their deployments, so that harmonized and balanced action plans are eventually produced.

The four dimension of our conceptual framework are the following:

- Systemic benefits for which evaluation criteria are related to the effects on the internal quality of care programs; they look at: the level of innovation in the healthcare system intended as the capability to promote new organizational models and service delivery channels for a sustainable care; the citizens' satisfaction; the effect on the national/regional context as a whole (reduction on working days lost due to sickness related absence, new business and jobs opportunities, ...);

- The direct economic factors, clustering criteria like: the capability to attract resources to activate and maintain the interventions; the level of return on investment; the timeliness to achieve economic benefits; the capability of improving the efficiency of the care processes (included the chance of resources re-allocation);
- Cultural viability of the solutions in respect to the easiness of engaging users from a cultural and organizational perspective: the awareness among managers and operators, the presence of innovators and the availability of adequate ICT skills; the level of dependency from incentives, regulations and agreements; the influence of ongoing level of the public debate and of the consensus of public opinion;
- The technological readiness about the telemedicine solutions, considering: the existence of success stories and know-how, either on ICT in general or on specific solutions; the size of the minimum critical mass for a significant pilot and the progressive scalability of the infrastructure; the inherent modularity of the scenario and the flexibility of non-disruptive approach (e.g. the coexistence with paper-based modality); the technological adequacy of existing or planned infrastructure required and the pre-existence of interoperable operational components; the adequacy of awareness and technical skills of operators.

In our view the relative relevance of each criteria is intrinsically subjective and it is not possible to merge the above dimensions into a comprehensive indicator to rank the action lines in a unique and robust way. The frame should be used as a conceptual map on the basis of which a

group of stakeholders perform systematic assessments about the contribution of technology to the various conceivable interventions. Differences in the individual assessments can trigger systematic discussions on the possible perspectives, in order to explore the different points of view, leading to a more accurate revision of the assessments. Actually even if the dimensions are general, the values assigned to each criteria deeply depend on the peculiarities of each local situation and every group of stakeholders should adapt the assessments to its local context.

The final goal is to let the group of stakeholders reach a consensus on the priorities to design a regional roadmap, and especially to compare the intermediate objectives of every concrete action line within an all-inclusive plan. To this aim empirical principles should be developed to make the final decisions about the allocation of resources and the time schedule among the different action lines.

4 POLICY-DRIVEN HEALTHCARE INTERVENTIONS AND TELEMEDICINE IMPACTS

In order to show a practical example about the intended usage of the conceptual frame, in this section we introduce a sample of policy-driven interventions, for which a relevant impact of telemedicine could be expected.

According to a top-down approach we have first identified three main intervention areas; for each of them we have then described different intervention scenarios.

In the following of this section the first cluster of interventions (care processes) is focused on the routine care provision, the other two are related on novel services for different specific end users (i.e. to support health professionals and to encourage the citizen involvement).

4.1 Expanding the Role of the Hospital in the Care Processes

At present, the most widespread usage of ICT in the healthcare field regards the administrative management of the facilities, the organization within the diagnostic services and the reimbursement of the activities, as well as the ancillary processes related to orders and reports.

However the core processes in this sector are related to the clinical aspects of the care provision as a response to the patient's problems and for prevention purposes. Therefore it is reasonable that the maximum impact – both in terms of quality and optimization of resources – will be obtained by the proper support to care, by using the technologies to enhance new types of organizational models. The availability of routine data, captured in appropriate formats during the evolution of the care processes, could also facilitate the processing of timely indicators for governance, benchmarking and self-audit.

The hospitals could keep the opportunity of using telemedicine solutions to offer enhanced care services, by improving the internal coordination and efficiency of different departments as well as by opening their walls towards a systematic collaboration with primary care resources or by promoting more appropriate admissions.

Also inter-organizational models of care delivery are typically disease-oriented networks, as for instance hub-and-spoke networks between reference hospitals and local emergency departments for trauma-care services; or the managed care networks for chronic diseases recommended in the Chronic Care Model, in which a clear and scheduled collaboration among general practitioners and specialist physicians is needed for the active prevention of exacerbation of chronic diseases.

Actually any disease-oriented network is first and foremost a rational reorganization of services, with a clear definition of roles for the different point of care at different levels of specialization. The requests (and sharing) of information between operators of different healthcare facilities can be reasonably modeled and formalized, and then supported by advanced ICT and telemedicine solutions (clinical document sharing, teleconsultations, management of home devices, …).

Table 1 contains a non-exhaustive list of possible telemedicine-enhanced interventions oriented to care processes improvements in an inter-organizational collaborative environment driven by hospitals.

Table 1. Examples of possible telemedicine-enhanced interventions oriented to the improvement of care processes, driven by the hospital

• **Collaborative pre-hospitalization and follow-up involving a reference hospital and local facilities:** To manage preliminary activities by exchanging of data and teleconsultations in a systematic way according to an explicit agreement between a hospital and remote local facility, finalized to the admission to the hospital.
• **Early discharge from hospital, with follow-up at home:** To monitor the follow-up of a patient after an early discharge from hospital, maintaining a high level of quality and safety. It may involve capturing and sending data or signals from home devices.
• **Tele-triage for urgency/emergency transportation:** A remote consultation about transportation, in case of severe trauma or other life-threatening situations, to assess its need, its urgency, and the most appropriate facility. For example: (i) a paramedic or a physician sends a signal from ambulance; (ii) a trained person sends data from an isolated location; (iii) a radiologist sends images to a neurosurgeon.
• **Urgent tele-consultation with a specialized center:** To define critical conditions and perform first aid before (e.g. in remote areas) or during (e.g., ambulance) any transportation, e.g. for stroke, myocardial infarction, severe trauma. It may involve capturing and sending data or signals, as well as video-communication.
• **Chronic Disease Management:** To apply a model that involves a collaboration between GPs, specialists, healthcare district, hospital specialists and patient/informal caregiver. It includes the patient-physician interaction and the use of remote sensors and biomedical devices. It is applicable for example at different stages of diabetes, heart failure, COPD (providing also for their interactions with other concurrent conditions). It may involve the systematic sharing of relevant documentation (disease registry, disease-specific network, Electronic Health Record).

4.2 Support for Healthcare Professionals

Interventions in this area are intended to help professionals in their daily work activities. In the present context of high specialized and fragmented care suitable telemedicine solutions may be oriented to assist specialist physicians in the hospital to be more effective and to play a new role within the primary care processes. Main goals are to support more informed medical decisions, the coordination among virtual teams and the prevention of medical errors.

From the point of view of the management of the health care facilities, this approach may lead to a targeted spending to achieve faster and consistent benefits.

A number of useful solutions, primarily based on the timely availability of information and knowledge, are already available, even if not yet fully exploited. In fact, safe and effective approaches to manage clinical information,

complemented by telemedicine procedures, are nowadays technically possible at reasonable cost. However, their wide adoption in the working practice requires an extensive debate to establish the general principles of large scale deployment, working out its limits and capabilities. A change suddenly imposed on all the professionals and on the entire population could meet strong resistance. It would seem more reasonable that an intervention targeted towards some categories such as the major chronic diseases, frail elderly people and/ or early childhood, may instead better meet the acceptance of clinicians and patients.

A non-exhaustive list of possible telemedicine-enhanced measures in support of health professional is presented in Table 2.

4.3 Citizen's Engagement

This set of actions is aimed at supporting the citizens, together with their informal caregivers, to have a closer interaction with the health system

Table 2. Examples of possible telemedicine-enhanced interventions in support to health professionals, involving also the hospitals

• **A registry with the notifications of the contacts of the patient with the care professionals:** The clinicians involved in the care provision to a given patient – specially for chronic diseases and frail elderly people, at home or in residential facilities, with frequent hospital admissions – actually should behave as a kind of a particular 'functional care team', i.e. as an ad hoc 'virtual facility' different for each patient, because it depends on the (multiple) health issues and the social situation within the specific ecosystem of that patient. The registry could be the basic platform to facilitate their interaction through a set of additional services.
• **Problem-specific Patient Profiles:** For the patients in a stable chronic state, the clinicians could generate and maintain a profile, including a predefined data set, specific for each problem. The sharing of these documents among the professionals involved in the care process allows for a better coordination among the "virtual team" around each patient.
• **Teleconsultation:** It is the typical application of telemedicine, to allow a professional to receive advice on complex cases from an expert colleague. With the modern web-based solutions, the basic video connection is easily available everywhere, even from smartphones, together with the sharing of the relevant documentation about the patient. More sophisticated equipments could be needed for particular scenarios; however they are no more the main bottleneck for the diffusion of this approach.
• **Interaction between social services and health services:** Still using the basic infrastructure for sharing documents and reports from routine care events, the experience can be extended beyond the health care system, to also include social services. Major difficulties are not technological, but of political and organizational nature.
• **Lifelong Electronic Health Record – EHR System:** An online collection of "all" the clinical documents on an individual, made securely accessible to authorized operators. In practice, initially one or more of the following types of documents will be shared: discharge letters, patient summaries produced by the GP, diagnostic reports. If the documents are stored in a proper standard format (e.g. by ANSI-HL7 CDA), with a suitable header, then it is possible to organize the collection and to filter the documents according to predefined parameters. In particular, if the header contains an explicit reference to the health issue(s) related to the document, then the collection could be arranged into problem-specific folders.
• **Increase the usability of authoritative clinical knowledge, legislation and practical information:** The Internet can facilitate the timely dissemination of information, constantly updated (including e.g. care paths reference, Evidence Based Medicine, …).

and to share the responsibility towards their own health. The goal is to promote transparency of healthcare delivery organizations, ensure citizens' awareness about their rights, increase the appropriate access to the services, as well as to positively influence patients' lifestyles (proactive prevention) and compliance to treatment.

The hospital here has usually a subordinate involvement, except in very peculiar situations of very close collaboration with community services.

In this kind of interventions the direct economic return of investment is important, but not its main purpose: in fact, a sensible impact both on resources used by the system and on the health of the population may be expected in the medium to long term as a consequence of the increase in the user satisfaction, in their involvement and awareness on the process of care, in the overall quality of care processes. Also, the greater efforts for their take up are not on financial or technical issues but more on political and organizational ones.

A non-exhaustive list of possible telemedicine-enhanced measures to improve citizen's engagement is presented in Table 3.

5 A SIMULATED COMPARISON AMONG THE THREE SCENARIOS

On the basis of the three action lines introduced in section 4, in this section we describe a simulated application of the frame to assess the main features of each intervention.

In Section section 5.1 we provide a short introduction about the envisaged process to elicit and compare the assessments among broad clusters of interventions or among more elementary actions; in Section 5.2 we present the conceptual frame, which consists of 16 criteria organized into 4 dimensions, and show a simulation of its usage.

Table 3. Examples of measures to promote citizen's engagement

• **Collaborative engagement in the care process:** The availability of an explicit, dynamic agenda (with reminders), which specifies the objectives, the roles and the planned activities of each actor, including the patient, could improve the awareness and the proactive engagement of the patient.
• **Management of home-based devices:** Most chronic patient may be able to manage the increasingly smarter and cheaper devices, to perform measures and to send them to a remote server. A skilled operator could monitor the incoming data and generate alarms for the most appropriate clinician. Where suitable, the remote operator could offer an interactive support to perform the measures.
• **Yellow pages:** Description of names, addresses, opening hours and services of healthcare facilities in the territory of a local healthcare authority, or in a hospital. If the data are structured according to an agreed format, they could be shared among different portals and presented in a uniform manner, both across providers in the same region and in neighboring areas of different regions; the information could be filtered and adapted to the patient's specific needs, in a patient's portal.
• **Simplification of administrative procedures:** This service is targeted at the citizens and enables them to carry out autonomously some procedures, such as the choice of GP, the request for exemptions, prosthetic assistance and so on. It pursues the administrative simplification, which is one of the major demands by the citizens, and eliminates or reduces travelling needs.
• **Children's Record:** The electronic version of the pediatric health booklet, fed with information from the parents and the pediatrician. It may include several components: periodic health assessment, factsheets on key issues encountered during growth, managing appointments and deadlines, annotations, effective mail management.
• **Access to selected clinical information knowledge:** Clinical information is not always guaranteed by independent organizations and therefore cannot be always considered reliable. Knowledge can relate to: poison aid-centers, access to decision-making flow-charts, management of individual diseases or procedures. The knowledge can be made accessible via web sites, call centers, interactive television or tele-text. Part can be offered in different languages, in support of minority languages relevant in the country.
• **Regular interaction between professionals and patients:** The aim is to facilitate the regular interaction between individual healthcare professionals or points of care and their chronically ill and/or fragile patients, perhaps with the use of biomedical devices and sensors. It may be mediated by non-medical staff in a point of care or in a dedicated service center. Applicable for example at different stages of diabetes, heart failure, COPD (perhaps with other concurrent conditions) and for frail patients. The professionals could use mobile devices (i.e. laptop, tablet, smart-phone).

5.1 A Cyclic Process of Comparative Assessments to Reach Consensus

In our simulation we suppose that an imaginary team of policy makers, as representatives of different stakeholders, adopts an iterative collaborative process, in order to achieve a shared evaluation of the main features of the three lines of action.

Each expert starts individually evaluating each intervention by assigning a value ranging from 1 star (non significant) to 4 stars (highly relevant) to each criterion in the framework. Average for each dimension and for each action line is then calculated and represented in a diagrammatic way by using radar charts.

The individual evaluations are then refined in an iterative process with cycles made of an individual assessment, followed by a comparison and then by discussion on similarities and differences, until a consensus agreement within the team of policy makers is reached.

5.2 Simulated Results and Visual Rendering of the Assessments Process

In Table 4 we present the possible result of an evaluation of the criteria for each intervention by a single expert, during one of the various cycles of refinement. Please note that the assigned values are intended here for demonstration only; in a real case, each stakeholder should assess the various components according to the local context and the individual point of view.

The qualitative assessments can then be transformed into numerical value, calculating the average for each dimension and for each cluster as shown in Table 5.

In order to quickly grasp strengths and weakness of each line of actions with respect to the different criteria, the average for each cluster could also be graphically represented with radar charts as presented in Figure 1.

In our simulation, this imaginary expert evaluated that:

- The optimization of care processes outside the hospital walls through ICT and telemedicine can lead to long-term incalculable benefits to the healthcare system and the health of the citizens, but it still requires a significant progress in the cultural aspects and it presents obstacles in large-scale implementation;
- The activities in support of health professionals and their decision-making processes, for the timely access to individual information and the maximum usability of clinical knowledge, can have good economic and systemic returns in the medium term, but require an assumption of political responsibility and organizational commitments to overcome the resistance of the professionals to change established routine habits. In addition, advanced clinical applications should still evolve to achieve an unanimously acceptable level of efficiency and friendliness;
- The action line for the involvement of citizens in a proactive role does not have strong direct economic advantages; however the patient's satisfaction would bring to a widespread acceptance and the long term benefits, especially on the active prevention of the consequences of chronic diseases, can have a persuasive impact on healthcare.

CONCLUSION

The modern telemedicine, as one component of the pervasive eHealth solutions being deployed in several countries, should be intended as an enhancing factor for the innovative organizational models that a region is introducing to cope with the sustainability of the healthcare system.

Table 4. A simulated example of the detailed assessments by an individual expert

Systemic Benefits	Citizen's Engagement	Support to Professionals	Care Processes
effects on the internal quality of care programs	+++	++++	++++
level of innovation in the healthcare system (capability to promote novel and more sustainable organizational models and service delivery channels)	+++	+++	++++
impacts on citizens' satisfaction	++++	++	+++
effects on the country as a whole (less absences from workplace, new jobs, opportunities for industry, etc)	+++	++	++++
Direct Economic Factors			
capability to attract resources to activate and maintain the programs	+++	++	+
return on investment	++	+++	++++
timeliness for direct and indirect economic benefits	+	++	+
Impacts on the efficiency of the care system	++	++	++++
Cultural Viability			
level of predisposition of involving users (from a cultural and an organizational point of view)	+++	++	++
awareness of managers and professionals and availability of innovators and suitable ICT specialists	+++	+	++
degree of independence from incentives, regulations and agreements	++	++	+
influence of public debate and consensus of public opinion	++	+++	+++
Technological Readiness			
availability of success stories and know-how (both on ICT in general and on specific solutions)	++	+	+
size of minimum critical mass, intrinsic scalability and modularity, and flexibility	+++	++	+
availability of enabling infrastructures, pre-existence of interoperable components	+++	+++	++
professionals awareness and adequacy of technical skills	++	+	+

Table 5. Summary of the simulated assessments for an individual expert

	Citizen's Engagement	Support for Professionals
systemic benefits	3,3	3,0
direct economic factors	2,0	2,3
cultural viability	3,3	1,8
technological readiness	2,8	1,8

We argue that the failures of the bottom-up approach adopted in the past could be avoided by a strong top-down policy to control the phenomenon of a widespread diffusion of the technologies related to the information and the communication in the healthcare field.

In order to achieve its sustainability, telemedicine should be carefully planned by policy makers as a component of the healthcare action lines that manage the revision of the organizational models in the healthcare provision, with an attention to

Figure 1. Visual representation to compare the simulated assessments on three scenarios

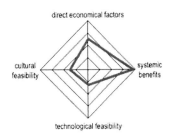

a. Care processes

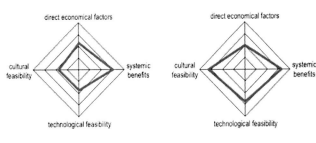

b. Support to healthcare professionals   c. Citizens' engagement

patient engagement, collaboration among the professionals and governance of the care processes.

In the last decades the academy and the industry were able to conceive and bring into the market a very large number of effective telemedicine solutions. Now it is the time to rationalize the demand side, i.e. to develop the toolkits for the policy makers to take the optimal decisions for a widespread diffusion of telemedicine-enabled care services.

As a contribution in this direction, we developed a grid to facilitate a systematic discussion among stakeholders to figure out the deployment of innovative organizational models, balanced across different action lines.

We claim that with the aid of the proposed framework the policy makers could be able to systematically discuss in details about their agreements and disagreements on each criteria and to amalgamate the subjective bias of the different experts into a comprehensive outline, in order

to reach a common vision of the advantages and difficulties of each action line.

This analysis could lead to a more balanced decision about the overall objectives of their plans and about the optimal distribution of resources among short term and long term actions.

The same approach can be also applied more in detail, e.g. to each individual component within the scenarios, in order to appreciate their ability to fit with the overall healthcare objectives.

ACKNOWLEDGMENT

This work was partially supported by the European Project ANCIEN - Assessing Needs of Care In European Nations (FP7 HEALTH-2007-3.2-2, Project #223483). The authors had the opportunity to discuss this topic and develop new visions within the Task Force Sustainable Telemedicine & Chronic Disease Management of the European Health Telematics Association (EHTEL) and within the IGEA Project (by the Italian Ministry of Health) about Disease Management for Diabetes.

REFERENCES

Blumenthal, D., & Tavenner, M. (2010). The "meaningful use" regulation for electronic health records. *The New England Journal of Medicine*, *363*, 501–504. doi:10.1056/NEJMp1006114

Camarinha-Matos, L. M., & Afsarmanesh, H. (2002). Design of a virtual community infrastructure for elderly care. In Camarinha-Matos, I. M. (Ed.), *Collaborative business ecosystems and virtual enterprises.*

Canada Health Infoway. (2011). Welcome to infoway's resource centre. Retrieved October 24, 2011, from https://www.infoway-inforoute.ca/lang-en/working-with-ehr/resource-centre

Continua Health Alliance. (2009). *Connected health vision, personal telehealth overview.* Retrieved October 24, 2011, from http://www.continuaalliance.org/connected-health-vision.html

Cross, M. (2006). Will connecting for health deliver its promises? *British Medical Journal*, *332*(7541), 599–601. doi:10.1136/bmj.332.7541.599

Department of Health. UK. (2004). *Improving chronic disease management.* Retrieved October 24, 2011, from http://www.dh.gov.uk/en/PublicationsandstatisticsPublications/PublicationsPolicyAndGuidance/DH_4075214

Department of Health and Ageing. AU. (2009). *HealthConnect evaluation.* Retrieved October 24, 2011, from http://www.health.gov.au/internet/main/Publishing.nsf/Content/B466CED6B6B1D799CA2577F30017668A/$File/HealthConnect.pdf

Detmer, D. E. (2003). Building the national health information infrastructure for personal health, health care services, public health, and research. *BMC Medical Informatics and Decision Making, 3*(1).

eHealth ERA - Towards the Establishment of a European eHealth Research Area. (2007). *Report eHealth priorities and strategies in European countries.* Retrieved October 24, 2011, from http://www.ehealth-era.org/index.htm

European Commission. (2007). *Accelerating the development of the eHealth market in Europe: eHealth Taskforce report 2007.* Retrieved October 24, 2011, from http://ec.europa.eu/enterprise/policies/innovation/policy/lead-market-initiative/ehealth/index_en.htm

European Commission. (2008). *Telemedicine for the benefit of patients, healthcare systems and society.* COM(2008) 689.

European Commission. (2011). Ageing well in the information society action plan. Retrieved October 24, 2011 from http://ec.europa.eu/information_society/activities/einclusion/policy/ageing/action_plan/index_en.htm

European Science Foundation. (2010). *A holistic citizen-centric vision for information and communication technologies to support personal health.* Declaration by the members of the European Science Foundation Exploratory Workshop on Social Care Informatics and Holistic Health Care, Keele University, UK, July 2010. Social Care Informatics meets Health Care Informatics. Retrieved October 24, 2011, from http://iig.umit.at/dokumente/n29.pdf

Gartner. (2009). *eHealth for a healthier Europe! – Opportunities for a better use of healthcare resources.* Swedish Presidency of the European Union. Retrieved October 24, 2011, from http://www.regeringen.se/sb/d/574/a/129815

Greenes, R. A., & Shortliffe, E. H. (1990). Medical informatics: An emerging academic discipline and institutional priority. *Journal of the American Medical Association, 263*(8), 1114–1120. doi:10.1001/jama.1990.03440080092030

Hägglund, M., Chen, R., & Koch, S. (2011). Modeling shared care plans using CONTsys and openEHR to support shared home care of elderly. *Journal of the American Medical Informatics Association, 18*(1), 66–69. doi:10.1136/jamia.2009.000216

Hägglund, M., Henkel, M., Zdravkovic, J., Johannesson, P., Rising, I., Krakau, I., & Koch, S. (2010). A new approach for goal-oriented analysis of healthcare processes. *Studies in Health Technology and Informatics, 160*, 1251–1255.

Hägglund, M., Scandurra, I., & Koch, S. (2010). Scenarios to capture work processes in shared homecare - From analysis to application. *International Journal of Medical Informatics, 79*(6), e126–e134. doi:10.1016/j.ijmedinf.2008.07.007

Nace, D. K., & Gartland, J. (2011). *Providing accountability: Accountable care concepts for providers*. Relay Health. Retrieved October 24, 2011 from http://healthsystemcio.com/white-papers/providing-accountability-aco-concepts-for-providers/

OECD-NSF. (2011). *Building a smarter health and wellness future*. Summary of main workshop messages, Washington, 15-16 February 2011. Retrieved October 24, 2011 from http://www.oecd.org/sti/smarterhealth

Oh, H., Rizo, C., Enkin, M., Jadad, A., Powell, J., & Pagliari, C. (2005). What is eHealth (3): A systematic review of published definitions. *Journal of Medical Internet Research, 7*(e1). doi:10.2196/jmir.7.1.e1

Pagliari, C., Sloan, D., Gregor, P., Sullivan, F., Detmer, D., & Kahan, J. (2005). What is eHealth (4): A scoping exercise to map the field. *Journal of Medical Internet Research, 7*(e9). doi:10.2196/jmir.7.1.e9

Perednia, D. A., & Allen, A. (1995). Telemedicine technology and clinical applications. *Journal of the American Medical Association, 273*(6), 483–488. doi:10.1001/jama.1995.03520300057037

Raymond, B. (2005). The Kaiser Permanente IT transformation. *Healthcare Financial Management, 59*(1), 62–66.

Rigby, M., Hill, P., Koch, S., & Keeling, D. (2011). Social care informatics as an essential part of holistic health care: A call for action. *International Journal of Medical Informatics, 80*(8), 544–554. doi:10.1016/j.ijmedinf.2011.06.001

Rossi Mori, A., & Freriks, G. (2005). A European perspective on the cultural and political context for EHR deployment. In Kolodner, R. M., Demetriades, J. E., & Christopherson, G. A. (Eds.), *Health-e-people: Transformation to person-centered health systems*. Springer Verlag.

Rossi Mori, A., Mazzeo, M., & D'Auria, S. (2009). deploying connected health among the actors on chronic conditions. *European Journal of ePractice, 8*(1). Retrieved October 24, 2011, from http://www.epractice.eu/files/European%20Journal%20epractice%20Volume%208_1.pdf

Scottish Centre for Telehealth and Telecare. (2010). *Scottish Centre for Telehealth strategic framework 2010 – 2012*. Retrieved October 24, 2011, from http://www.sctt.scot.nhs.uk/strategy.html

Siau, K. (2003). Health care informatics. *IEEE Transactions on Information Technology in Biomedicine, 7*(1), 1–7. doi:10.1109/TITB.2002.805449

Steventon, A., & Bardsley, M. (2012). Effect of telehealth on use of secondary care and mortality: Findings from the Whole System Demonstrator cluster randomised trial. *British Medical Journal, 344*, e3874. doi:10.1136/bmj.e3874

The European Files. (2010). *The telemedicine challenge in Europe*. The European Files.

The Joint Commission. (2008). *Guiding principles for the development of the hospital of the future*. Retrieved October 24, 2011, from http://www.jointcommission.org/topics/default.aspx?k=750

World Health Organization. (2005). *Global report preventing chronic diseases: A vital investment*. Retrieved October 24, 2011, from http://www.who.int/entity/chp/chronic_disease_report/full_report.pdf

Zanaboni, P., & Wootton, R. (2012). Adoption of telemedicine: From pilot stage to routine delivery. *BMC Medical Informatics and Decision Making*, *12*(1). doi:10.1186/1472-6947-12-1

Chapter 2
Global Telemedicine and eHealth:
Advances for Future Healthcare-Using a Systems Approach to Integrate Healthcare Functions

S. A. Davis
University of California Merced, USA

ABSTRACT

This chapter is about the intersections taking place globally in the delivery of healthcare. In today's world, quality health is about access: access to transportation to the hospital, access to the right people, doctors, nurses, and specialists, and the doctor's access to the latest lab tests and equipment. But in our future, all of this goes away. You do not need transportation, as medical ecosystems are becoming ubiquitous. Access to the best medical care available means access to the hospital system living in the cloud. The best labs are built into our phones whereby today's array of sensors can be focused on prevention and delivery systems designed for keeping people healthy. Behind this is the driving vision that medicine will be transformed from reactive and generic to predictive and personalized, reaching patients from the cloud through their telephones in their own homes, making up for a coming shortage in doctors and nurses. Where this brings us is that there is an abundance of confusion as to what Telehealth and eHealth is or what it will be. This chapter addresses an eHealth definition for review, thoughts on eHealth systems, resistance to change issues to be considered, the CVS Minute Clinic's introduction of innovation and disruptive eHealth care models and systems, a Systems Engineering Management proof of concept project with the Kansas Department of Corrections, and globally oriented conclusions and recommendations. (Diamandis & Kotler, 2012).

DOI: 10.4018/978-1-4666-2979-0.ch002

INTRODUCTION

For the last 50 years, different to other industries, technological advancements in medicine have increased abundantly, rather than decreased costs in the delivery of healthcare. However, recent developments in mobile health technology, addressed here as Telehealth and eHealth, gives hope that the technology tide is turning and that these trends will cause technology to improve care (which it has successfully done for years) and drive costs down. Resistance to change will hopefully be overcome by behaviorally designed mobile application technology user interfaces. So, where does this hope come from? A study by a recent Information Week article has hit the nail on the head. 70% of polled hospitals and/or healthcare organizations plan to deploy the iPad by the end of 2012. This matched with market research indicating that 81% of physicians (In the United States alone) will own a smart phone or tablet by the end of 2012. Of those, more than 50% will use Telehealth and eHealth applications daily in 2012. Globally it is predicted that 500 million people will be using mobile Telehealth and eHealth applications by 2015. The world and Telehealth and eHealth personnel will turn these applications into Trojan Horses. Competition has driven down the overall costs of powerful 'pocket' computers to the point that they are becoming as ubiquitous as cell phones were just five years ago. What this will mean is that developing nations will not have to build the healthcare infrastructure that has been developed over the past fifty to sixty years in the industrialized world. The objective of this chapter is to provide you with a vision and perspective of the future of eHealth and the behavioral and systemic challenges to be overcome.

BACKGROUND: THE GLOBAL EHEALTH DEFINITION FOR THE FUTURE

Telemedicine healthcare delivery systems are currently using advanced communications technology based on connectivity, interactions, transactions, information, and intervention. It started with National Aeronautics and Space Administration, NASA, as human astronauts were flying in space. NASA's advanced communication satellites and the ability to monitor the health of the astronauts was the tipping point for the delivery of healthcare digitally. The revolutionary and potential effect on the digital delivery of healthcare globally provides the capability to: bridge interactions between clinicians and patients, overcome barriers of distance and time, build virtual communities that will interact and share knowledge and expertise, enhance the continuity of care and greatly improve access to healthcare in remote and isolated areas. (Bowonder, Bansal, & Giridhar, 2005)

Our definition for Telemedicine - eHealth is seen as:

e-Health is an emerging field in the intersection of geo-medical informatics, public health and business, referring to health services and information delivered or enhanced through the Internet cloud and related technologies. In a broader sense, the term characterizes not only a technical development, but also a state-of-mind, a way of thinking, an attitude, and a commitment for networked, global thinking, to improve health care locally, regionally, and worldwide by using information and communication technology.(J. M. Eisenberg)

Telemedicine - eHealth (referred to as eHealth in this chapter) will act as the center piece for responsive healthcare delivery by providing: delivery of healthcare where patients and providers are not at the same location at the same time, a new mechanism for providing networked medical knowledge through relational and cloud computing technologies. (Currier & Kshetri, 2011)

Using a different approach to delivering global eHealth care, a 'System of Systems' approach will require looking at traditional medical practices and developing new models to integrate medical, healthcare and communication functionality. This approach will be used to combine the skills of various healthcare and system engineering professionals with emerging and advanced computer and telecommunication technology. The healthcare functionality that exists today in health care delivery environments is obsolete and not integrated therefore the delivery of healthcare is more complicated and cost-ineffective. System of Systems is a collection of task-oriented or dedicated systems that pool their resources and capabilities together to obtain a new, more complex 'meta-system' which offers more functionality and performance than simply the sum of the constituent systems. The methodology for defining, abstracting, modeling, and analyzing system of system problems is typically referred to as system of system engineering. System of systems education and problem solving involves the integration of systems into a system of systems engineering process that ultimately will contribute to the evolution of a healthcare 'social infrastructure.' (System of Systems, Wikipedia, July 11, 2011) The following table identifies requirements that are particularly critical to be addressed by senior members of the eHealth stakeholder community as they engage in defining and applying an eHealth system of systems engineering approach toward a wider acceptance of eHealth (A System of Systems Engineering requirements analysis primer is shown in Table 1).

Table 1. Selection of requirements to be addressed as part of the eHealth system of systems analysis and approach

• The influence and rise of Generation Y who have spent their lives 'wired'
• The role of the user interface to ensure interactivity and credibility
• The eHealth legislation required for change
• The roles of and endorsement by the Centers for Medicare and Medicaid (CMS)
• The roles of states in supporting cross-practice/licensing to enable the growth of eHealth
• The design of a business model for getting parties and providers engaged
• From 'where' will eHealth leadership emerge, corporations, government, coalitions
• Other countries currently developing eHealth centers of excellence
• Cultural differences as medical staff and patients endorse greater numbers of remote patient monitoring
• Privacy, liability and security issues across the globe. This will be made possible on a large scale by the rise of cloud computing
• Technology, infrastructure and broadband availability to include the role of geo-location systems
• Accessibility to best-practice and neutral information based on sound science, anytime and anywhere
• The power of 'gamification' of products and services
• The role of artificial intelligence as it is used to filter data and diagnose some conditions
• How companies will respond in the future to the burden of healthcare costs
• The legal credentials and licensing required for providers, from a global perspective
• The fact that the patient does not have to see the doctor and that they will have the ability to 'shop' for the best/least expensive medical products and services
• Reimbursement policies and procedures regarding eHealth and how costs will be reimbursed
• The sophistication of sensor technology, reliability and sensitivity
• The shortage of trained staff and the rate at which eHealth is integrated into healthcare educational systems, to include training systems that need to be developed and disseminated (Monitor Group and the Financial Times., 2011)

The health consumer will become a self-administering user of knowledge-based patient care. Knowledge-based systems will be more responsive as patients are able to explore the web world, learning about their condition, diagnosis and treatments available to them, often before the first interaction with their medical care provider. Innovative and Disruptive Health portals, available to both medical professionals and patients, will proliferate through health information systems, genomics, biotechnology, professional development, nanotechnology, drug treatment, mental treatment, diagnostic and robotic portals.

MAIN FOCUS OF THE CHAPTER

Information Technology Models for Health Delivery Systems

In the past healthcare institutions, medical practices, medical devices and electronic health record systems (EHR) have been traditionally designed to operate independently. Institutions and private practices struggle with the financial resources to transition from paper to EHR or to integrate several systems previously hosting laboratory values, scanned records or the potential of eHealth information. With the increasing complexity of the global healthcare environment, stand alone and proprietary devices and systems are no longer an acceptable solution for delivery of cost effective and sustainable medical care. Electronic health records, medical devices and remote telemedicine information systems *must* have the capability to integrate with other vendors' equipment and software systems in order to improve the delivery of the quality of healthcare, reduce global healthcare costs, and provide for more comprehensive and secure delivery of healthcare information.

The importance of applying modern systems engineering solutions, such as delivery systems and interoperability, to be used to improve patient care, safety and to reduce costs (i.e., combining

of functions, elimination of redundant costs and replication of efforts) is key to moving the integration of medical delivery systems forward (Pema, G. 2010). At the highest level, the obstacles to be dealt with are:

- Just in the United States alone, the healthcare delivery system is investing annually over a $1.7 Trillion in healthcare. Healthcare delivery systems are plagued with inefficiency and poor quality. Most healthcare providers lack the information delivery systems necessary to coordinate a patient's care with other providers, to share needed patient information, to monitor and adhere to evidence-based practice guidelines or have the ability to measure and improve performance. According to studies conducted by Rand Health, Efficiency savings result when the same work is performed by fewer resources. The potential efficiency savings for both inpatient and outpatient care could be over $77 Billion a year. The largest savings come from reduced hospital stays (as a result of increased patient safety and better scheduling and coordination), reduced nurses' administrative time and more efficient drug utilization (as a result of more efficient decision support and medical expert systems). Sharing patient information in a coordinated way is the key to improving the quality of healthcare. Electronic sharing is less costly than transporting clinical information from facility to facility or healthcare personnel to healthcare personnel (Hillestad, R, Bigelow, J, 2011).
- Across countries and multiple clinical studies, there are two kinds of intervention that require investment and intervention to enhance healthcare globally. They are 1) chronic disease management and 2) disease prevention which must be managed by health information technology and

the associated functional delivery systems (Hillestad, & Bigelow, 2011). In the case of chronic disease management, healthcare delivery systems can help to identify patients in need of tests or other services and it can ensure the integrated recording of results. Patients using REMOTE monitoring systems will have the ability to transmit their vital signs directly from their homes to their healthcare providers, allowing prompt interventions to *potential* problems. Effective chronic disease management can reduce the need for and costs of hospitalization, thereby improving quality of life and reducing *costs*. In the case of disease prevention, vaccination and screening measures facilitated by health information systems designed to integrate patient's medical records, flag risk factors and recommend the appropriate preventive services (i.e., vaccinations, mammograms, colonoscopies and other key tests).

- Adoption of cross-vendor standards-based interoperability for medical device integration and comprehensive, population based, real time standardized EHR delivery systems. This is currently hindered by device interfaces that have to be customized over and over again which results in long development times, increased costs and often incomplete integration of medical device and systems functionality.

- Medical device integration is critical and often an overlooked function of *EHR planning. To be successful Health Level 7 Standard(HL7) feeds into the EHR* system is critical (http://www.hl7.org/). Multiple stakeholders must be engaged and involved in EHR development, planning and integration to include physicians, nurses, clinical and biomedical engineering. Additionally, negotiations across hospital channels, in-depth understandings of point-of-care workflows, medical device connectivity capabilities, standardized vendor device

offerings and product and functional integration strategies must be developed as well as maintained to achieve sustainable operations.

- The benefits of integrated automatic data collection systems have yet to be broadly realized or broadly deployed. Healthcare data collection systems need to include, heart rate, non-invasive blood pressure, respiration rate, weight, oxygen saturation, blood glucose, etc. and are received from acute and chronic care monitoring devices. This data has become so important that healthcare institutions (in the United States)are requiring that their Clinical Information Systems, Anesthesia information management systems, Electronic Health Record Systems, Electronic patient monitoring systems and hospital/healthcare information systems provide interoperability so that key vital signs are stored in a central repository to track patient progress over time. (Vaz, C, 2007). Guidelines and measurable standards need to be designed and met in the development of eHealth applications and websites, thereby helping to move eHealth forward. See Table 2.

- Relatively few health care providers have access to Health Information Management Technology (Hillestad & Bigelow, 2011). Only about twenty five percent of hospitals and twenty percent of physicians' offices have Health Information Management *Technology* Systems (HIMT). Hospitals and physicians having fifty percent or more of their patients on Medicare do not have HIMT systems.

- The capability to share information from system to system is greatly lacking. Implementation of HIMT systems is growing *but* System Engineering Management (System of Systems Management) protocols and training are not uniformly in place and their greater impact is not understood. There are challenges being encountered by healthcare providers and health information technology (IT) in developing strategies for systems to fully integrate (i.e. institutions systems with out-patient clinics, laboratory, radiology and remote data with the EHRs. And worse, there is no current market pressure to develop HIMT systems that talk to each other. A primary method of approach to overcome the challenge and the barriers between systems engineering and healthcare providers to ensure that the design, development and integration of healthcare delivery systems span all security, physical, cultural, physical, amid regulatory boundaries. Attempting to implement multiple aged systems into new EHR's currently in play simply cannot enable effective and efficient healthcare delivery. This current approach will most likely create additional barriers to future standardized healthcare delivery systems because of the high costs of replacing or converting EHRs compliant with Health Level 7 Standard (HL7). There is even more of 'catch twenty two' as the question of who pays for HIMT systems and who profits. Patients benefit from gaining an improved quality of health, payors benefit from lower costs but providers will incur the costs to implement a HIMT system and will have lower revenues after implementation. For example, if HIMT systems are used to reduce drug events, then bed days are reduced, and voila, reduced bed days means reduced hospital income! Yet another consideration is the pending Centers of Medicare and Medicaid (CMS) penalty to healthcare practices and institutions for a 30-day readmission (i.e., Congestive Heart Failure patients).

- One of the larger barriers to adoption of eHealth is the disconnect between medical research and medical product developers. Researchers are not trained to translate

their findings for use in the marketplace and product developers often do not integrate evidence-based research into product design. The translation of 'evidence based' research into product design is critical to support the evolution of eHealth technologies. Healthcare Management Information Technology and Behavioral Health Scientist experts need to be integrated at the research and development (R&D) level with product developers to create integrated solutions. If guided properly, medical researchers can also assist in understanding what functions need to be included and integrated in order to improve the quality of eHealth applications. Another significant factor for consideration is that eHealth technology is moving light speed ahead of research in health most academic institutions. Frequently researchers in academic institutions are driven by grant dollars, not in commercialization, because they believe their capability to compete for grant dollars is based upon the proprietary nature of the work they are engaged in, it is a method of securing salaries and positions (i.e., a requirement of an academic position) and that other researchers would have access to the work they are engaged in to obtain grant funding. Translation is not part of the existing paradigm (Emont, & Emont, 2007).

- Resistance to a complete 'systems' solution that meets regulatory, security, safety and clinical requirements for patient care. So far a systems engineering management effort has not appeared to address the 'research-to-practice' gap. Commercialization will need to be driven by factors such as cost and time to development, rates of acceptance, significance of need, relative market strengths, etc. Additionally, demographics and psychosocial factors or access to technology to enable consumer engagement is very limited. System studies across cultures for addressing issues such as literacy and health literacy are limited. The importance of studying how interactive health communications in reaching underserved populations needs to be addressed. How can this population are better served if there are low levels of literacy much less capabilities for addressing and using the internet (Emont & Emont, 2007).

- The issue of system 'usability' is critical and needs to be tailored to the user who has low literacy and is considered of low cultural relevance, literally, coupled with language issues. Standardized man-machine interfaces to include a foundation for the look and feel of the hardware device structure needs to be addressed. A systems study of how this population can gain access and connect to technology is necessary.

- Resistance to modeling interoperable clinical use cases, or lack of documented use cases, and engineering requirements for a systems engineering management approach to medical delivery (MD PnP, 2009*).*

By now you should be getting the picture of *why* we are at a point in our fast paced society that delivery of integrated healthcare systems is vital. In summary, the benefits of data and information delivery models for interoperable healthcare devices and services are visited in Table 2 (Vaz, C, 2007).

Solutions and Recommendations

The key teams that need to participate in this disruption of healthcare delivery systems include:
Patients who can participate in the use cases as well as contributing to the development of more

Table 2. Benefits of standardized health care delivery systems

For the Patient	To increase patient safety by decreasing entry errors and allow healthcare professions, with secure access, to document live and review the patient record remotely To provide more physician/patient contact time, resulting in a higher quality of patient care. The higher quality of information provided to the healthcare professional by the patient or clinical information feeds, providing a significantly decreased change of medical errors and increased quality of health care
For the Nurse	To decrease documentation time allowing increases in productivity. A user interface is provided that allows the nurse to validate information in 'real time' and to add live data as assessments or telephonic medical information changes. To support quality data and information collection (radiology results, vital signs or remote EHR access) providing increased surveillance for patients, even when not at the bedside. At the same time, relieving the pressure of routine, automatable vital signs and other sensory tasks. This provides immediate access to current patients records to expedite collaboration with the physician
For the Physician/ Physician's Assistant (PA)/Nurse Practitioner (NP)	To prevent errors in diagnosis, prescribing, and testing medications, by basing decisions on the *entire* patient history thus providing the capability to make educated decisions based on evidence-based practice guidelines, making the care provider more time efficient
For the Patient, Physician, PA/NP, and the Nurse	To provide complete and comprehensive data and information on the patient health records To securely and quickly share assessment, diagnosis, treatment and patient progress across healthcare institutions, regions, states and countries, which enable the patient to be provided the highest level of healthcare To enhance the overall healthcare professional and patient experience To reduce stress related to legal liability
For Decision Support Systems, Best Practice Systems, EMR Systems	To provide comprehensive and secure digital files to include historical patients healthcare information. 'Cloud' access to and integration of patient records will allow both interchange, review and audit of patient progress and quality of care To enable future functional devices to seamlessly connect with the systems To increase security and prevent tampering of Patient Records and Comprehensive Medical Systems information

competent user interfaces ranging from the home, healthcare clinics or institutions, medical offices, to the computer or cellular systems.

Managers and Engineers who can analyze clinical use cases to generate functional specifications, access current standards to perform 'gap analyses,' and to evaluate proposed (open and standardized) technologies. Diverse management and engineering expertise is essential.

Healthcare and delivery organizations who can specify performance requirements, require adherence to medical device interoperability and standards adherence in vendor contracts. Consumer demand and increased responsibility of regulatory agencies that support new regulatory paradigms can tip interoperable healthcare delivery systems forward. Again, on a global basis.

Medical device manufacturers who will participate in the development and adoption of interoperability standards who will participate in use case development and functional prototypes and testing. How to motivate device manufacturers in the development of standards will be a behavioral challenge.

Conclusion: The current healthcare delivery systems have many problems, but the problems can be overcome with interaction of the stakeholders in the healthcare industry, using a system of systems engineering approach to eHealth complexities (Truscott, Rande, McQueen, & Parston, 2011).

Resistance to Change

Why? In ancient Greece, Sisyphus was cursed for all eternity to roll a boulder up the mountain top, only to have the boulder fall back down again and again. Introducing change in healthcare seems like a task worthy of Sisyphus. There are countless obstacles to implementing change in modern healthcare. Inside every healthcare institution and practitioners office there are multiple organizations to be dealt with, federal and state regulations, accreditations, competitive pressures as well as constant changes in technology, administrative

processes and medical practices. All this happens within the critical care, often life and death, 24/7 environments of healthcare.

Technological changes such as the use of bar codes to allow nurses and physicians to check the accuracy of the medications before administration to patients, which then connects to the patient's electronic health record, and verifies their medication history. Statistics note that 1 in every 6.4 administration of medicines contains errors. This technology has proven to eliminate up to thirty three percent of 'reported' errors. At the same time the system makes the healthcare environment safer for the patient but on the other hand may be more time consuming for the healthcare practitioners (Hanan & Cronin, 2011; Hook, Pearlstein, Samarth, & Cusack, 2009; Clinfowiki, 2010).

Leadership in healthcare institutions must have the skills to lead and mentor the organization through the change and the clinical practitioners need to have buy-in regarding the technology to be purchased and integrated as well as the learning curve associated with new technology. Too often resistance to change is the result of Senior Management calling a meeting and announcing the changes that are going to take place without consulting the healthcare 'delivery' team. This team must be involved during the planning, training, implementation and evaluation of the change process. A systems engineering management approach is key to implementing this sustainable change. In most situations leaders lack the practical tools that help them to structure, plan and execute engagement strategies.

Physician's resistance to change continues to be a barrier in implementing and delivering interoperable eHealth systems. Implementation of Electronic Health Record Systems which contain Computer Physician Order Entry Systems and Clinical Decision Support Systems through 2010 has been very slow and more problematic than anticipated. The issues of self-evidenced malpractice or threat of such litigation drives physician resistance to endorse self-documenting systems related to their patient care. The systems have been poorly integrated and interfere with the user's established work flow. Only 15% of United States hospitals have implemented these systems. However, 2010 proved to be the year that many hospitals ramped up their approach to meet the first stage of meaningful use criteria. The data shows significant adoption levels of EMR-c applications increased from 2009 to 2010. The numbers of hospitals reaching Stage 6 of the HIMSS Analytics EMR Adoption Model SM doubled last year, John P Hoyt, FACHE. FHMSS, Executive Vice President, Organizational Services, HIMSS (Clinfowiki, 2010). Several key barriers to resistance are the high costs, challenges of multiple systems integration and the healthcare practitioner's resistance. Drivers to be considered in addressing healthcare practitioner's resistance are:

- Before the pre-implementation stage physicians will have a set of expectations about what the 'new' system will do for them. If the expected functions are not delivered, resistance behaviors will result. Two critical aspects are systems design, to include userability, and implementation MUST be factored into the process. Involving physicians in the systems design is critical and financial reimbursement for participants, physicians, nurses and clinical personnel, is an expectation to ensure successful implementation. Information Technology (IT) professionals should not lead the project, it is critical that a diverse team of healthcare practitioners that are the leaders and champions which will prove to be invaluable in overcoming resistance by the staff. A lowering of productivity should also be factored into the levels of expectation during the first six months to reach maximum system productivity. Key to success is TRAINING and round the clock technical support.

- Physicians have a culture in which they operate. They have taken an oath in which their profession is centered on the patient, especially to do no harm. Physicians are a brotherhood and sisterhood and medical practice is not just another 'business as usual!' The quote helps to put in perspective the battlefront that pervades the delivery of cost effective healthcare globally: "Current healthcare efforts have gone astray because the health system's movers and shakers fail to take into account the physician culture." Richard Reece, MD. Physicians live in a world where patients often take the doctor's word as ultimate, co-operating with first dollar coverage without discussion of money, they are free to order what they please based on clinical judgment, place trust in the physician's superior knowledge along with the physician culture based in autonomy. Bottom line, Physicians pride themselves on being able to treat patients their way. With Computerized Physician Oriented systems, they know they will be forced to use system ordered medications along with protocol restrictions. Physicians feel they will be losing their freedoms as the power shifts to Medical Directors, Pharmacy and Therapeutic computerized systems (Reece, 2008).

- The difference between hospital and physician cultures is growing. Hospitals want a more managed, monitored and data-based systems which are fraught with enlarging the gap between physician and hospital. This may take further evolution of the role of the physician rather than the manager of the information system.

- Fear of technology can also be a roadblock to change. Informal leaders, not upper level management, and champions could be the conduit to diminish these fears. Resistance to change is reduced by spending time with those who 'get it,' who are positive about the change and want to lead change. A study by Mirkley and Stein produced some interesting results relating to the 'sources' of resistance and strategies for acceptance for nursing staff. They found that resistance to change takes on a variety of forms and is complex and a multidimensional phenomenon. They found out that the resistance was not related to the functionality of the technology BUT with cultural factors such as lack of time and loyalty to historical models of paper documentation. Experience with computers was not the issue. The nurses stated that there were often fears of the system prior to using it. What they resisted was the addition of just one more item to their workday and that the traditional paper driven systems would take much less time than electronic systems. That for example, on line charting systems were more time consuming. Currently most nurses' schedules are overloaded and they must care for a very large number of patients on any given shift. In critical care units there is an even higher frequency of activities such as taking vital signs every fifteen minutes, not every four hours. They often feed that their patients are more critical than having to deal with their computer. A key point and takeaway is that it is critical that the user interface be designed with the nurse or clinician in mind, not the computer programmer who has designed the interface (Kirkley & Stein, 2004).

- Cultural and societal factors also may play a large role in attitudes toward computers themselves causing resistance for healthcare practitioners willingness to embrace new technology.
- Under communication alone brings about resistance. The effect of lack of communications is that people do not know the plan, goals, timelines, and expectations which creates an atmosphere of frustration and confusion.

- The often perceived costs of implementing medical 'systems' with a sustainable system architecture that will support computerized physician order entry medication delivery, ventilation and fluid delivery, decision support capabilities, monitoring of device performance, comprehensive collection of medical data and patient records, standardized selection of best of breed medical devices, workflow, process improvement and change management for patients throughout the continuum of patient care.
- Medical schools will need to recalibrate their curriculums to include eHealth concepts, practices and eHealth care delivery models.
- Vendors will be resistant to standardized and common protocols and interoperability.

Conclusion: Physicians, Patients, Medical Personnel and Business must develop a new understanding of the potential of eHealth and develop a new medical delivery culture embracing eHealth (Report Linker, 2010).

CVS Pharmacy and Caremark Model for the Future of eHealth Delivery

Just over four years ago CVS Pharmacy and Caremark merged to create a unique healthcare delivery model, referred to as Minute Clinic McDoc in a Box. The model was disruptive as it targeted low-risk patients with specific healthcare needs by offering standardized diagnostics and primary care services such as vaccinations in an affordable, convenient and fast way. They have expanded into chronic care management, addition of physical exams, wider ranges of vaccinations and injections and biometric screening. Minute Clinic McDoc is the intersection of retail principles with healthcare quality to provide better access, convenience, and confidence at a lower cost. From 2005 to 2008 they built the largest geographical healthcare delivery organization in the United

States. The purpose was to integrate high quality low cost healthcare into the consumer's lifestyle. To do this they focused on understanding the motivations of both the patient AND the staff. Their technology extends the range of coverage and reduces the cost of access to such medical care largely through eHealth technology. This is the equivalent to the visiting nurse/practitioner delivering services to remote areas.

They have a network of over 565 clinics in 26 states, including 100 seasonal clinics. One of the critical components of this model was the role that Management Information System Technologies would play in the diffusion process of their Health Delivery Systems. The vision behind the merger was to bring together the touch points in pharmacy driven healthcare which included the drug stores, the retail clinics which provide healthcare for everyday illnesses, the mail-order pharmacy, and their customer care call centers with the intent of providing the most cost effective healthcare delivery solution for the patient.

The Minute Clinic McDoc in a Box, herein referred to as McDoc, is based on the following:

- **The target market:** McDoc's market penetration strategy is clear age-based and socio-economic segmentation — learning that generational values have a very large impact on acceptability. The current healthcare system was built for the Greatest Generation. The Greatest Generation sees their Doctor as the gatekeeper of all information, advice, and access. Boomers come in armed with a wealth of information and have a two way dialogue with their primary care physician (PCP). But for Gen Xers and Millenials – the patient is at center – not the doctor. They want self-sufficiency. The expectations from the consumers are changing. MinuteClinic understood their target audiences were those Gen Xers and the Millennials. So, their market is a younger market, under 45 and Female (known as the seeker for healthcare

for themselves and their families), 40% of the patients seeking healthcare do not have PCP insurance plans. A secondary target market is employed individuals due to services being available after work and on weekends.

- No appointment is necessary and the clinics are open seven days a week. This fast, affordable convenient care was based on reliance upon out-of –pocket payment mechanisms being in place rather than traditional insurance claims based reimbursements. (NOTE: this is evolving and currently over 170 million insureds have access to McDoc in the United States).

- The clinics serve as a one-stop center for fast, cost-effective, convenient and reliable diagnosis and treatment services for common illnesses and vaccinations with costs per treatment ranging from lab tests, to medical exams, to health condition monitoring, to vaccinations with a price range from $15 to $150.

- The clinics position themselves only as a diagnostic and limited care healthcare provider who use a niche demographics penetration strategy to reach and administer to their target market.

- The clinics employee management system is designed to support the low-cost, low-risk, selective services delivery model. The service cost effectiveness is centered upon having certified Nurse Practitioners and Physician Assistants on staff rotating three day twelve hour shifts. The staff is rotated back to community health care 'institutions' to maintain certifications and enable them to practice a broad range of conditions that may not be able to be treated at a Minute Clinic.

- The clinics maintain their own electronic medical records system (MIT (2010; Pearlstein, H, Samarth, J, Cusack, A, 2008).

Proof of Concept: The eHealth Demonstration Project at the Kansas Department of Corrections (KDOC) Correctional Facility

System Engineering Management ("System of Systems Engineering") and eHealth at KDOC

Healthcare is one of the primary social problems in the world. There are many studies that define the problem and potential solutions that have been described in medical journals and the public media.

For many years there has been an attempt to define the solution generally from government agencies, academic institutions and medical device manufacturers that ex amine the healthcare problem from a traditional baseline. Even those pioneers in telemedicine define the starting of the healthcare paradigm that has existed since Hippocrates. The practice of medicine has evolved for centuries under the Socratic Method aided and abetted by advances in technology. Indeed the study of medicine uses similar methods of instruction. This type of instruction leads to specialization and here again the difference is technology.

It was our contention that a different method of analysis should be undertaken using a system engineering management (herein referred to System of Systems Engineering), a technology, developed by Bell Laboratories and utilized by NASA and its contractors on the APOLLO Lunar Landing Program.

A group of NASA engineers and management left the APOLLO program and undertook several projects in various fields of transportation, energy, law and building construction. Others introduced the technology in complex programs such as power plant construction and automotive fabrication.

In 2006, a group of engineering and management personnel were assembled to analyze the telemedicine field and found that similar conditions were present. The field was comprised of academics, device manufacturers, government organizations and a few forward looking physicians, nurses and medical technicians that were interested in applying state of the art technology to perform their functions with additional skills.

The different approach was to combine the skills of various medical professionals with system engineering professionals and emerging and advanced computer and communication technology.

The initial attempt was a "proof of concept" medical system that used off-the-shelf devices integrated into a mobile platform that could be scaled to the environment. The engineering decision and production task was relatively simple but resistance to change from various sectors was encountered and a number of behavioral changes had to be initiated.

Background for the KDOC Proof of Concept

The paradigm of interactive systems engineering management stands behind some of the most impressive accomplishments in engineering, manufacturing and internet technology.

Pioneering use of this approach enabled the success of the dauntingly complex Apollo Lunar Landing Program and has been adopted by virtually every field of human endeavor with one glaring exception – the daily diagnostic work of medical professionals.

The Systems Engineering Management and KDOC teams recently explored the utility of an integrated diagnostic system in the setting of prison health and occupational/sports medicine. Using a system that owes significant lineage to one that NASA flew on the Space Shuttle for remote monitoring of astronaut vital signs, they tested the value of capturing and sharing diagnostic data that included ultrasound, cardiology, spirometry, chronic obstructive pulmonary disease, and diabetes with remote specialist readers in a unique integrated format.

What made this system different? First, it was developed by engineers and practicing physicians who worked from the ground up in close collaboration. Second, it was a user friendly system that ensured that data was rapidly captured and interpreted by a remote network of physicians on an anytime, anywhere basis. Systems engineering management is not a new concept. However, it has been virtually ignored by the medical profession in part because the industry is fractured with each function (medical specialty) or element attempting to optimize their part of the medical profession and protection of their own turf.

NASA developed their integrated system of vital signs functions for application on the Space Shuttle and Space Station with an initial low level of success and adaptation by the astronaut physicians. Meanwhile the discrete providers of diagnostic components such as EKG and Spirometer, attempted to lower the cost and increase the efficacy of their products.

However, these developers ignored the benefits of integration and the development of software algorithms that could replicate expensive hardware and communicate with specialists remotely to increase the efficiency of the total medical system. The System Engineers decided that an integrated medical system would offer a higher level of healthcare at lower cost to medical services providers and could be utilized on a broad range of medical applications such as healthcare institutions, remote medical clinics, correctional institutions, the mining industry and commercial applications such as drugstore clinics linked to medical professionals.

To test this concept, NASA technology was combined with commercial off-the-shelf parts for vital sign testing and an algorithms developed by a pre-eminent German research institute developed under Defense Advanced Research Projects Agency (DARPA) funding. Two different demonstrations were performed under the guidance of professional systems engineering management and skilled medical personnel, from radiologist to license vocational nursing, to test the concepts. These were a three month evaluation in a well-defined medical environment in the Kansas De-

partment of Corrections with 130 study subjects at Lansing Prison, and a one year demonstration in a major sports medical environment at the Golden Gate Fields and Bay Meadows Racetracks, two major racing venues in California's Bay Area.

The team wanted to know if such technology in a clinical medical practice environment compared with the quality of traditional outsourced diagnostics, how it affected the patient outcomes and what further system development was necessary to optimize its value.

PROOF OF CONCEPT: THE PRISON DEMONSTRATION PROJECT

This project was conducted under the approval of the Western Institutional Review Board (WIRB) with the support and cooperation of the Kansas Department of Corrections. The technology chosen for the demonstration was a self-contained medical diagnostic system which incorporated separate medical diagnostic capabilities: Ultrasound, Spirometer, and EKG. The system consisted of a diagnostic based mobile examination system and operator interface to capture diagnostic data and electronically archive it remotely on a secure server. This data was then remotely accessed by a high speed secure internet connection for prison physicians' interpretation.

A series of underlying objectives were established in order to achieve the goals stated above:

1. Evaluate the training necessary for the prison medical staff to demonstrate proficiency.
2. Evaluate the ability to train prison physicians to retrieve secure server based clinical data for interpretation and documentation.
3. Evaluate the ability of the systems engineering management team to learn clinical workflow into the system and respond with agility to end user input, modifying processes and tools to meet end user needs.

4. Evaluate the effect of monthly milestone reviews in capturing feedback, tracking progress and providing needed training for ease of use and more efficient integrated workflow.

5. These processes and technologies were not in use at the prison medical clinic prior to the project.

The main goals of the eHealth Pilot Demonstration Project at the KDOC Lansing Correctional Facility were:

1. To evaluate the potential improvements in medical services delivered to the prison patients

2. To determine the potential cost savings accrued due to the use of the new medical technology, using a patient data set of 130 for credible analysis

3. To evaluate the level of training necessary to effectively use the new medical technology when inserted into a well-defined limited medical environment

4. To determine if better care could be delivered through new in-house diagnostic tools

5. To determine if a better way of evaluating off-hour emergency situations to determine the necessity of an offsite emergency room visit, thus creating the opportunity for less frequent costly emergency transfers

6. To provide more efficient use of physician and nurses' time

7. To facilitate less transfers to the offices of consultants and specialists for advanced diagnostic testing and evaluation

8. To facilitate fewer inter-facility transfers for chronic disease management physicians

9. To determine the impact of potential cost savings

A Summary of the Results of the Demonstration Project

The project demonstrated that the medical services delivered to the prison patients could be significantly improved by the introduction of the new medical technology into the prison medical services. The results are characterized below.

- **Staff leveraging:** Enabling the utilization of physician skills at locations other than the prison where the patient is located. Specialists in the fields of dermatology, ophthalmology, cardiology and pulmonologist can use the remote communications capability of the system with its integrated data base to consult with local physicians across the entire network of prisons.

- **Physician staffing and efficiency:** The centralized nature of the system enabled a single central physician to handle all the routine acute tele-consultations and regular diagnostic data review across the entire prison network.

- The delivery of chronic disease management (with 30%+ of the prison population suffering from chronic disease) utilizing integrated systems and diagnostic tools allows for better management, trending and monitoring of these ailments. This also results in having the capability to initiate preventive measures prior to these disorders spiraling out of control and thus reducing costs.

- Potential cost savings of 25 percent or more were accrued by improved physician and nursing staff utilization, reduced cost for outside medical services and reduced security costs due to fewer trips to outside hospitals and clinics for patient care.

- The training of the physicians and nurses was crucial to the success of the project. The physicians and nurses each received a minimum of training in operation of the system and a level of training to gain an operational familiarity with the operation of the individual medical devices and supplemented with periodic reinforcement training. This level of training proved sufficient for all the physicians and most of the nurses in effectively treating the 180 patients who took part in the project.

The project goals were achieved and the Technology System proved to be valuable in the clinical setting. Nurses were comfortable using the technology, patients were accepting of the technology, and it was demonstrated that there exists potential cost savings as well as improved patient care. The staff felt confident that the technology system could be incorporated into the everyday routine of the nursing staff and physicians. The acquisition of clinical data became easier as the nursing staff gained experience in using the different tool devices and as a direct result of the redesign of the graphic user interface early in the project.

A Summary of Lessons Learned during the Project

Three core impediments were revealed during the project. They were time, space and training. The nurses had limited time for additional work and finding adequate time for the training was a challenge. Training was conducted on site and remotely via web-based technology to overcome time constraints of the staff.

It became increasingly clear that the integrated technology platform provided an excellent tool for baseline setting, monitoring and trending the prison's chronic disease population, specifically in the areas involving cardiac, diabetes and pulmonary issues.

The pilot produced an unexpected result. The image of the clinic in the eyes of the prisoner clientele, as well as providing educational benefits

to the prisoner, resulted in goodwill among the prison population and the healthcare staff.

This limited demonstration project demonstrated the potential value of applying systems of systems engineering principles to medical applications. The different approach was to combine the skills of various medical professionals with system engineering professionals from the ground up with emerging and advanced computer and communication technology based on the real-time use of feedback loops.

CONCLUSION AND RECOMMENDATIONS

- In order to achieve the global changes needed to implement eHealth, the major stakeholders, i.e., hospital organizations, insurance companies, medical device providers, software providers, internet providers, internet security firms, and government agencies need to step forward and exhibit leadership.
- Commercial organizations have market share potential to drive their effort, insurance companies have reduced costs to drive their participation, and government has reduced tax payer funding as motivation. The healthcare industry needs to take the lead to keep the government more involved.
- Major commercial stake holders need to launch a System of Systems Management Initiative including a functional analysis, as developed and applied at MIT and Purdue, funded and supported by intervention with firms such as Humana, General Electric and Philips.
- Using this approach will require forming cross functional design and development teams consisting of physicians, nurses, clinical personnel, the Center for Medical and Medicaid Services, Insurance providers, Hospital providers, security and

privacy regulators, and other and private stakeholders to include patients. This will include support for development of uniform standards, common frameworks, common certification processes, common performance metrics, and common supporting technology structures.

- Such an initiative would enhance and support global interoperability promoting organizations who will support re-visioning of existing standards to meet clinical requirements, collaboration in clinical use case implementations, to empower innovation in the safety and efficiency of healthcare delivery systems. Guidelines and measurable standards are prerequisite to moving eHealth *forward*.
- Enhance and support greater alignment between evidence-based research coming out of academic institutions and the translation of technology-based Health and eHealth solutions into the commercial sector. A focus should be on effectively translating best practices into effective adoption and implementation of communication and functional medical technologies.
- Promote government intervention in the use of Health Information Management Technology (HIMT) systems while incentivizing policy and standards development.
- Expand liability protection for hospitals using HIMT systems.
- Educate healthcare practitioners on lease models for integrated medical systems.
- Promote hospital – doctor connectivity by allowing hospitals to subsidize standardized HIMT systems for private physicians.
- Set up pay-for-use programs for medical providers using interoperable HIMT systems.
- Educate consumers about the value of HIMT systems along with the expected quality of care improvement and reduction in costs, by improving their ability to manage their health.

- Continue to educate and train hospitals and healthcare organizations in the deployment of hand held medical systems. Consistent internet and cloud connectivity and financial support is critical for delivering sustainable eHealth systems.

Telehealth and eHealth are undergoing a sea of change. The prediction is that new innovators and existing players will be quickly drawn to the use of mobile platforms to develop remote healthcare solutions because of new vertical market possibilities. Predictions are that the size of the eHealth market will be put at anywhere between $5B and $35B dollars within this decade.

On March 28, 2008, Nobel laureate economist Paul Krugman happened to be crunching some numbers from the Centers for Medicare & Medicaid Services (CMS) when he came to an alarming conclusion that he published in the New York Times:

Everybody knows that the US spends much more on health care than anyone else, without getting better results. Everyone also knows that health spending has outpaced GDP growth everywhere, thanks to medical progress. What I didn't realize was just how clearly the evidence shows that the rising trend is steepest in the US. We have the biggest increase as well as the highest level. We're No. 1! What this suggests is that a more integrated system wouldn't just achieve a one-time saving, but also flatten the upward trend.

ACKNOWLEDGMENT

Special Acknowledgments for advice and counsel to: Louis L. Davis, Bonne Faberow, John Heibel, Roy G. Helsing, Jim Sullivan, and F. Stephen Wyle.

REFERENCES

A Salud Program. (2011). *Diabetes health, CVS Pharmacy begins free health screenings in communities nationwide.*

Bowonder, B., Bansal, B., & Giridhar, A. (2005). Telemedicine platform: A case study of Apollo Hospitals telemedicine project. *International Journal of Services, Technical and Management, 6*(3-5).

Clinfowiki. (2010). *Physician resistance as a barrier to implement clinical information systems.* Retrieved from clinfowiki.org/wiki/index.php/ Physician_resistance_as_a_barrier_to_implement_clinical_information_systems

Currier, G., & Kshetri, N. (2011). *Baseline mobile, two keys to successful cloud computing, cloud computing in developing economies: Drivers, effects and policy measures. PTC 2010.* Greensboro: University of North Carolina.

Diamandis, P., & Kotler, S. (2012). *Abundance: The future is better than you think.* New York, NY: Free Press, Simon & Schuster, Inc.

Emont, S., & Emont, N. (2007). *Advancing eHealth opportunities and challenges for health e-technologies initiative (HETI) NPO, findings for interviews and surveys of opinion leaders and stakeholders.* Princeton, NJ: Robert Wood Johnson Foundation.

Hanan, J., & Cronin, K. (2011). *Helping nurse managers effectively lead change.* Madison, WI: Howick Associates.

Hillestad, R., & Bigelow, J. (2011). *Can HIT lower costs and raise quality?* Santa Monica, CA: Rand Health, Health Information Technology.

Hook, J., Pearlstein, J., Samarth, A., & Cusack, C. (2009). *AHRQ reports that there are more than a million medical injuries and over 100,000 deaths due the medication errors.* Melbourne, Australia: State Government of Victoria.

Kirkley, D., & Stein, M. (2004). *Nursing economics, nurses and clinical technology sources of resistance and strategies for success.*

Lauterborn, J. (2011). *Technology assessment and requirements analysis helps put medical facilities back on track.* United States Army Online.

MD PnP. (2009). *Advancing the adoption of medical device plug-and-play interoperability to improve patient safety and healthcare efficiency. Center for Integration of Medicine and Innovative Technology, Partners Healthcare.* Massachusetts General Hospital, National Academic Press.

MIT. (2010). *Healthcare business models and operations strategy: A comparative study of Cleveland Clinic and CVS Minute Clinic 15.768: Operations management in the services sector.* Cambridge, MA: MIT.

Monitor Group and the Financial Times. (2011). *Telemedicine market shares, strategies, and forecasts, worldwide, 2010 to 2016.* Cambridge, MA: Author.

Pearlstein, H., Samarth, J., & Cusack, A. (2008). *Using barcode medication to improve quality and safety. Findings from the AHRQ health IT portfolio. Prepared by the AHRQ National Resource Center for Health IT under contract # 290-0023-EF.* Rockville, MD: Agency for Healthcare Research and Quality.

Pema, G. (2010). Telemedicine comes into its own. *International Business Times, 4.*

Reece, R. (2008). *MediaHealth leaders: The physician culture and resistance to change.* Health Leader Media Council.

Report Linker. (2010). *Telemedicine market shares, strategies, and forecasting worldwide*. Report Linker.

System of Systems. (2011). *Wikipedia*. Retrieved from http://en.wikipedia.org/wiki/System_of_systems

The Street. PR Newswire. (2011). *Convenient sports physicals offered at minute clinic walk-in medical clinics inside select CVS/Pharmacy stores for just $39.00*. Woonsacket, RI: Author.

Truscott, A., Rande, G., McQueen, J., & Parston, G. (2011). *Information governance. The Foundation for Effective eHealth*. Accenture Healthcare Systems.

Vaz, C. (2007). *EMR and device integration*. Retrieved from http://charlesconradvaz.wordpress.com/

Walgreen's Newsroom. (2011). *Walgreens take care health systems, forms alliance with core performance to offer employees access to advanced wellness, fitness, and nutrition programs*. Bentonville, AR: Author.

Chapter 3
E–Health and Telemedicine in the Elderly:
State of the Art

Ilaria Mazzanti
Centro di Telemedicina, Italy

Alessandro Maolo
Centro di Telemedicina, Italy

Roberto Antonicelli
Centro di Telemedicina, Italy

ABSTRACT

In the last sixty years, there has been an increase in life expectance especially in females and in industrialized countries. This, along with the reduction of population growth, is leading to a reversal of the population pyramid: a narrow base of adults has to maintain a wide top of elderly people. Old people are often affected by multi-pathologies and comorbidities. Furthermore, the changes in family's structure, particularly the reduction of the central rule of the Ancients, contribute to create the "frail elderly syndrome." Geriatric frailty is found in 20-30% of the elderly population over 75 and increases with advancing age. It was reported to be associated with long-term adverse health-related outcomes such as increased risk of geriatric syndromes, dependency, disability, hospitalization, institutional placement, and mortality. Obviously, it is also associated with an increase in healthcare costs. Telemedicine is an innovative healthcare system capable of ensuring both higher efficiency and better cost-effectiveness. It has wide variety of services, relative simplicity of use and moderate-low costs. Currently there is clinical evidence of telemonitoring impact on management of several clinical conditions such us chronic heart failure, arrhythmias, pacemaker and ICD controls, cardiac rehabilitation programs, and cardiovascular risk factors.

DOI: 10.4018/978-1-4666-2979-0.ch003

INTRODUCTION

It has become clear that Telemedicine, and more generally E-Health, is an area of interest in world circles for research, design and management of healthcare delivery systems for elderly patients. In particular, emphasis on specialized care in areas suffering from a shortage of expertise or where access to healthcare is difficult.

At the present time, more the 11% of the world's population is over 60 years old with the elder population growing faster than the total population in practically all regions of the world. There are significant disparities from nation to nation mainly due to a poor cultural interest in what has been termed as the 'Frail and Elderly.' The scope of importance includes key technologies such as biosensors and communications, multi-disciplinary nets of research in bioinformatics, genomics, neuroinformatics, remote monitoring and diagnostics for the assistance and prevention, diagnosis and treatment of diseases encountered by the frail and elderly. The growing pressures of global demographics, medical advances and patient empowerment are leading to greater and greater demand for more health attention, to the issues of healthcare transformation and to the global societal role of E-Health and Telemedicine.

In the first part the following Chapter will discuss the demographic changes of the society and their impact on family organization and on Ancient rule. It will also explain the meaning of the term "frail elderly" and its importance on management of medical resources.

In the middle part the Chapter will focus on the eHealth and Telemedicine concepts, on the recognition of their potential roles in the National Health Services and the consequent development of national programmes designed to improve their applications in health setting.

The last part of the Chapter is dedicated to the Italian situation; showing, in particular, the important differences, in terms of awareness of the potential role of Telemedicine in management of health problems and subsequent economical investments, between north and south of Italy.

BACKGROUND

At the present time, 1 out of 9 people of the world's population is over 60 years old (see Figure 1), that is to say 740 million elderly people out of a world's population of 6900 million. Most of this elderly population (about 54%) lives in Asia whereas about 21% lives in Europe. In 2050, it is estimated

Figure 1. Percentage of population aged 60 or over

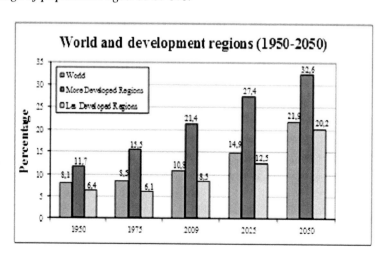

that this proportion will be 1 in 5, that means that the over 60s (2 billion) will represent 20% of the world's population (about 9 billion). This trend towards an ageing population is distributed differently in different countries; particularly, it is more evident in industrialized countries than in developing countries. In fact, at the present time, in Europe, the over 60s are 20% while in Asia, Latin America and the Caribbean these are 10% and 5% in Africa (United Nations, 2009).

Another fundamental aspect of the world's population is the ageing of the elderly. There exists a part of the population called the "oldest old," being 80 or more years old. Now, 14% of the older population (about 103 million people), is oldest old and by 2050 this will rise to 20% which means 400 million people. Among these oldest old, there is also growth of the over 100 years old. This class, at the moment, is about 454.000 strong, but it will grow almost tenfold by 2050 to about 4.1 million (see Figure 2). It means that the older population is growing faster than the total population in practically all regions of the world, the oldest old population is growing even faster and the difference in growth rates between the older population and the total population is increasing (United Nations, 2009).

MAIN FOCUS OF THE CHAPTER

The Frail Elderly Concept

About 14% of elderly population lives alone. An ever growing part of this population is affected by multi-pathologies and various levels of invalidity. This brings to light the concept of "Frail Elderly People" which includes "the group of old or very old subjects affected by multi-pathologies, with an instable health situation, frequently disabled, in whom the effects of ageing and pathologies are often complicated by socio-economical problems. On the basis of this definition, frailty leads to a high risk of a rapid deterioration of health and performance, and therefore to an elevated resource consumption" (Ferrucci, 2001).

The concept of "frailty" as a geriatric syndrome has come to light in the last 20-25 years, as a requirement leading from social demographic changes. From an epidemiological point of view, there is no precise data on the prevalence of the phenomenon in the elderly population. In fact, this data depends strongly on the classification criteria used. For example, in the Cardiovascular Health Study, conducted in the United States in 1989 and re-elaborated in 2001 on 5317 subjects

Figure 2. Average annual growth rate of total population, aged 60 or over and aged 80 or over

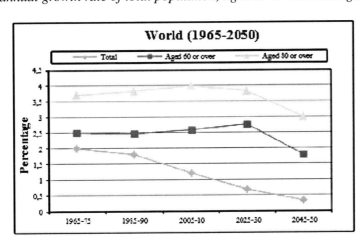

Figure 3. The five determinants of frailty

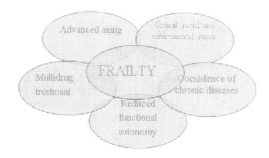

over 65, frailty was defined as a clinical syndrome in which three or more of the following criteria were present: unintentional weight loss (10 lbs in past year), self-reported exhaustion, weakness (grip strength), slow walking speed, and low physical activity (Fried, 1991 and 2001) (see Figure 3). The overall prevalence of frailty in this community-dwelling population was 6.9%; it increased with age (3% in subjects between 65 and 70, 26% between 85 and 89) and was greater in women than men (7% vs 5%). Four-year incidence was 7.2%.

Social-Sanitary Assistance Requirements

This part of the population needs an extremely complex socio-sanitary assistance. From this complexity, an assistance methodology, which is based on three key aspects, has been developed the Comprehensive Geriatric Assessment, to identify the frailest subjects and plan their assistance:

- Team work;
- Continuing care.

This assistance model requires the presence of a sanitary team specialized in the evaluation of the state of health and the needs of the elderly person. This team must also 'take global care' of the patient using a 'web' of structures and services, both Hospital and Territorial, founded on the strict collaboration between the General Practitioner,

the Geriatric Evaluation Unit, Integrated Home Care, Day Centres, Nursing Home, Hospital, Rehabilitation Centres.

There is a double objective: the first is to guarantee the continuing and punctual assistance of the chronic problems of the elderly person, keeping them in their own home and ensuring a psycho-physical stability. The second is reducing the need for Specialist Visits, Points of First Assistance and Hospital, to only really necessary cases.

At the present time, even if this assistance model is well defined and accepted as the solution to ensure old peoples' assistance, the realization of the project is not complete, and there is disparity between the various Nations, mainly due to a poor cultural interest in this part of the population. Therefore, in a lot of Countries, the basic assistance for the older patient is almost totally on the shoulders of the family. In the first instance the assistance is given by the partner, often old and needing care too, or, a growing phenomenon, by a carer, frequently foreign and without sanitary training, and by the General Practitioner who is often lacking in the specific preparation. This leads to frequent and unnecessary calls on ambulatory and hospital services. These services are often inadequate in terms of organization and function for this type of patient. This, along with the clinical and management complexity of these patients, often causes problems of correct destination and treatment in cases of hospitalization. Consequently, the elderly patient is often looked after by sanitary personnel without a specific competence and a functional decline occurs with the loss of autonomy and security; and with increase in frailty and re-hospitalizations.

Economic Aspects

Sanitary assistance for elderly patient has, of course, important repercussions also in the economic setting. The average world expenditure for health in 2008 was just less than 8,9% of the GNP (Gross National Product). The biggest spending was in United States (15,3% of the GNP), followed by France (11,1%), Germany (10,6%), Portugal (10,2%), Greece (9,19%), Italy (9%), Spain and Great Britain (8,4%), Japan (8,2%) and Turkey (5,7%).

Analysing the figures relative to one of the G8 countries like Italy, that is in the middle of the list of average expenditure, it can be seen that the total national health expenditure for 2008 was about 106,650 billion euros, divided as follows:

- **Personel:** 35,177 billion euros
- **Capital and other Services:** 30,865 billion euros
- **General Practice:** 6,084 billion euros
- **General Farmacies:** 11,208 billion euros
- **Specialistic Practice:** 3,923 billion euros
- **Rehabilitation:** 1,958 billion euros
- **Prosthesic Practice:** 1,764 billion euros
- **Other types of Assistance:** 5,642 billion euros
- **Hospital Practice:** 8,949 billion euros
- **Other:** 0,534 billion euros

In total, more than 1 milliard and 300 million sanitary activities were provided in 2008 with an average of 22 services for each one, most of which are microbiological and chemical-clinical laboratory analyses, in second place there are imaging diagnosis and in third place cardiologic activity. There were 12,100,696 hospitalisations, for a total of 75,371,789 days spent in hospital and an average time of ordinary acute hospitalisation of 6.8 days. The part of the population which is aged, even if it represents only 20% of the total population, determined about 40% of the hospitalisations and 50% of hospital days that are on average 20% more complex than the hospitalisation of the common population with consequent costs.

From the analysis of the Italian sanitary costs for the last 10 years, there emerges an exponential evolution of said costs of 100%.

Faced with such a marked increase in the sanitary costs, it is imperative to evaluate if the

Biological and Technological Research has been up to the population's necessities, and which may have been the possible determining factors for the shortfall.

From the above-mentioned figures, it clearly emerges that one of the fundamental factors of the sanitary costs is represented by the management of the elderly patients, particularly of their chronicle problems, and that Research needs to move also in this direction.

The E-Health Approach

An emerging approach to this problem is represented by the development of eHealth, the use of ICT (Information and Communication Technologies) for health (Ahern, 2006). Its objective is to increase the quality, access and efficacy of sanitary services for all the Users. The possible applications of ICT in Health Services are huge, involving numerous professional figures such as Medical Doctors and Nurses; the Managers and Technical staff who elaborate the social security date both administrators and patients. The E-Health concept is relatively young, in fact it was introduced in 1999 at the 7th International Congress on Telemedicine and Telecare in London by John Mitchell, the Managing Director of JMA (John Mitchell & Associates) an Australian consultancy company specialising in the areas of e-Health, e-education and videoconferencing. He defined E-Health "a new term needed to describe the combined use of electronic communication and information technology in the health sector... the use in the health sector of digital data, transmitted, stored and retrieved electronically, for clinical, educational and administrative purposes, both at the local site and at distance" (Mitchell, 2000). He described a national government study whose main result was the recognition that "cost-effectiveness of telemedicine and telehealth improves considerably when they are part of an integrated use of telecommunications and information technology in the health sector (Della Mea, 2001)." After this, national programs were created for the development of E-Health. In 2000, the University Health Network and the University of Toronto created the Program in health Innovation to develop the Centre for Global E-Health Innovation. The mission was to "imagine a world in which people, regardless of who they are or where they live, use state-of-the-art information and communications technologies with enthusiasm, proficiency and confidence, to achieve the highest possible levels of health and to help health systems make the most efficient use of available resources." In the United States the Robert Wood Johnson Foundation developed its Health e-Technologies Initiative in 2002 functioning as a National Program Office. The initiative is intended to promote E-Health for the health behavior change and chronic disease management sectors of the health care industry. An initiative to focus on E-Health was implemented in 2004 through an executive order by President George W. Bush. The result was that the Department of Health and Human Services created the Office of the National Coordinator for Health Information Technology to implement and use the most advanced health information technology and the electronic exchange of health information.

Also in the European Union, E-Health plays a key role in the plan of action for the innovation launched in 1999 and followed by a series of programs in 2002 and 2005, and by the Comunication "Preparing Europe's digital future i2010 Mid-Term Review" in April 2008.

The objective fixed by the EU State Members and Commission was the constitution, before 2009, of the foundations of the European e-Health service, for the administrative and clinical activities.

In October 2006, the results of the study "E-Health Impact: the economic benefits of implemented E-Health solutions at ten European sites," were published (Stroetmann, 2008). The information gathered from ten sites across Europe clearly shows the benefits of information and communication technology in routine healthcare settings, in fact all ten cases show a positive economic impact,

measured as a net benefit at present values. The benefits range from improvements in quality and better access of all citizens to care, to avoidance of unnecessary cost to the public purse. The ranges of the results are very wide, reflecting the material differences between each type of E-Health application analysed. The Authors considered the ten sites as part of an E-Health dynamic in the equivalent of a virtual health economy, and Figure 4 shows the potential of the economic impact of E-Health in this virtual system.

Over the period 1994 to 2008, the summarised annual present value of benefits grows continuously; conversely the associated costs stay broadly stable after the initial planning and implementation phases. Figure 5 shows the same surge in net benefits in the cumulative present values of costs and benefits.

The European View

None of the ten applications on its own show such an impressive performance, but these results may be taken as an indication of the potential overall benefits to be expected from a wide diffusion of successful E-Health applications across the European Union.

In May 2007, a meeting on the theme of e-Health was organised between the European Commission and the American Department of Health & Human Services in collaboration with the American-European Business Council: the first EU-USA Workshop on E-Health policy. The principal points of interest were the sanitary activities based on the information and communication technologies.

In November 2008, the Commission of the European Communities approved the document COM (2008)689 final: "Communication from the Commission to the European Parliament, the Council, the European economic and social Committee and the Committee of the Regions on telemedicine for the benefit of patients, healthcare systems and society." The Commission confirmed

Figure 4. Estimated present values of annual costs and benefits of e-health for a virtual health economy of 10 sites from 1994 to 2008, in € mill

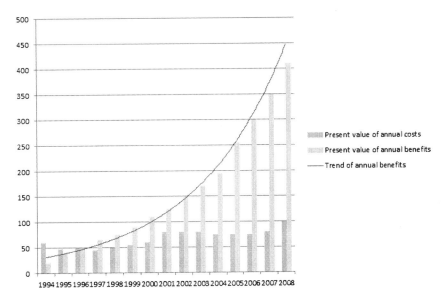

Figure 5. Estimated present values of cumulative costs and benefits of e-health for a virtual health economy of 10 sites from 1994 to 2008, in € mill

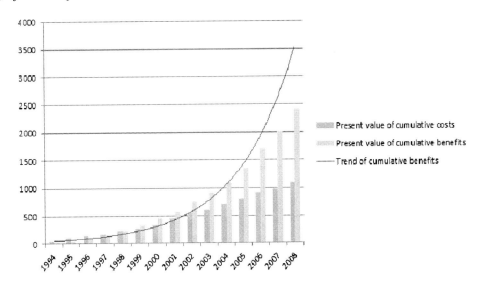

the importance of Telemedicine to improve access to specialised care in areas suffering from a shortage of expertise, or in areas where access to healthcare is difficult. The objectives were: improving quality of life, reducing hospital stays, optimise the use of resources and enable productivity gains. Telemedicine can also make a significant contribution to the EU economy. The Commission underlined that "despite the potential of telemedicine, its benefits and the technical maturity of the applications, the use of telemedicine services is still limited, and the market remains highly fragmented. Although Member States have expressed their commitment to wider deployment of telemedicine, most telemedicine initiatives are no more than one-off, small-scale projects that are not integrated into healthcare systems." To support Members States of UE in achieving large-scale use of telemedicine services, the Commission founded three strategic sets of action:

- **Building confidence in and the acceptance of telemedicine services:** The Commission will support the development of guidelines for consistent assessment of the impact of telemedicine services, including effectiveness and cost-effectiveness and it will also support a large-scale telemonitoring pilot project. Member States of EU have to collaborate in assessing their needs and priorities in telemedicine to define a national health strategy, to be presented and discussed at the 2010 E-Health Ministerial Conference.
- **Bringing legal clarity:** The Commission will establish a European platform to support Member States, in sharing information on current national legislative frameworks relevant to telemedicine, and proposals for new national regulations. Member States will have to assess and adapt their national regulations, enabling wider access to telemedicine services.
- **Solving technical issues and facilitating market development:** By the end of 2010, the Commission invites industry and international standardisation bodies to issue a proposal on the interoperability of telemonitoring systems, including both existing and new standards. By the end of 2011, the Commission, in cooperation with Member States, will issue a policy

strategy paper on how to ensure interoperability, quality and security of telemonitoring systems based on existing or emerging standards at European level.

At the present time, European E-Health research is controlled by the "Seventh Framework Program for research and technological development," the EU's principal financial instrument of European. The Seventh Framework Program will be operative from 2007 to 2013, with a 53.2 billion euro grant. The main part of the grant, about 32.413 billion euros, will be destined to the research program "Cooperation," which is the most important and the widest part of the project, structured to favour the collaboration between EU member states and the other partners in the research. Among the 10 themes of interest in the program, there are also information and communication technologies (ICT, for which there is a provision for a grant of 9.05 billion euros) therefore including Telemedicine. In this setting, three key points have been identified:

1. Personal Health Systems (PHS), that is to say the key technologies such as biosensors and secure communications.
2. Patient Safety (PS) represented by the software.
3. Virtual Physiological Human (VPH), the creation of multidisciplinary nets of researchers in bioinformatics, genomics and neuroinformatics, to help the creation of E-Health new generation systems for assistance; and prevention, diagnosis and treatment of diseases.

A lot of projects have been supported by the ongoing previous Sixth Framework Program, regarding both specific pathologies and general sanitary data control; for example:

- **BEPRO (Enabling Best Practices for Oncology):** The creation of a multinational net assistance in oncological valuation and assessment.

- **DIAFOOT (Remote Monitoring of Diabetic Foot):** This project is based on the use of remote home monitoring devices for measuring glycaemic levels. Following the transmitted data, the Remote Physician takes action.

- **E-SCOPE (Fully Digital Microscopy for routine diagnostics and integration into hospital information workflow):** The objective is to integrate standards in medical imaging, archiving and communication through the digitalisation of microscopy.

- **IHELP (Electronic Remote Assistance in the Operating Room):** The definition of the best practices for providing on-line assistance, on a 24h basis across the world, to surgeons using the latest neurosurgery systems in the Operating Room (O.R.) by the engineers who developed these systems.

- **PRIDEH (Privacy Enhancement in Data Management in E-Health).**

- **RESHEN (Regional Secure Healthcare Networks).**

- **SCREEN-TRIAL (The Screening Mammography Soft-Copy Reading Trial).**

- **SPIRIT (Priming the Virtuous Spiral for Healthcare:** Implementing an Open Source Approach to Accelerate the Uptake and Improvement of Best Practice, Regional Healthcare Network Solutions).

- **STEMNET (Information Technology for Stem Cell Transplantation).**

- **WOMAN II (European Network of Services for women health management).**

- **WRAPIN (World-wide online Reliable Advice to Patients and Individuals).**

It is clear that Telemedicine, and more generally E-Health, is an argument of interest in world sanitary circles. However, the economical investments in this sector are still limited; in fact, the E-Health market is currently just some 2% of total healthcare expenditure in Europe. There are also notable differences between the various EU state members in terms of investment, project advancement and application of the European Commission indications. In first place there is Great Britain, followed by Finland, Belgium, Ireland, France and Germany; Italy, Spain, Austria, Portugal and Greece result lower down.

Telemedicine in Italy

In Italy, investments in the ICT of the public and private sanitary structures, reach only about 1% (920 million euros) of the total sanitary expenditure. There is an evident difference between North and South Italy: the investments, in fact, are concentrated in 79% of the cases among the Northern structures, where the ICT expenditure is 21 euros per person, against just 9 euros a head in the South and Islands. The high budget ICT structures are localized, for 83%, in the Northern regions, only 11% in the Central regions and even less in the South and Islands (6%). Moreover, regions such as Piemonte, Lombardia, Veneto and Emilia Romagna are characterized by a low per person public health expenditure and by an elevated perceived quality of sanitary service, whereas regions like Lazio and Molise are characterized by the opposite situation. As a consequence, in the North there is the highest ICT investment level while in the South there is the lowest. Therefore, in Italy, in spite of the European Commission's indications from the document COM(2008)689 final: "Communication from the Commission to the European Parliament, the Council, the European economic and social Committee and the Committee of the Regions on telemedicine for the benefit of patients, healthcare systems and society," no large scale development of Telemedicine services were reported. There are, rather, fragmented and experimental projects limited to small areas, of uncertain duration and, sometimes without adequate financing and integration in the National Sanitary System.

There aren't either guidelines or standard tariffs in telemedicine services in the National Sanitary Program (School of Management Politecnico di Milano, 2011).

Mariano Corso, the Scientific Responsible of the Sanitary ICT Observatory, to explain the reasons for the Italy's backwardness, compared to the principal UE state members, declared that "there are a lot of reasons for this gap. Certainly there is the limitation in invested economical resources, but also the weakness of the chief information officer's role and the consequent absence of a single governance of the ICT development in the healthcare company. Furthermore there is the inadequate internal competence in the ICT Direction of each structure, and in the local vision by which the investments are planned and managed, and the incapacity to create a system by promoting the development and reuse of best practise." "The Research highlights the necessity of a unitary governance to promote and facilitate the involvement of both the lower and higher levels, together with the collaboration with the same level actors." Mariano Corso also said: "It is absolutely vital that no more time be lost in waiting for a providential intervention, a sort of 'deus ex machina', from on high to restore the correct balance. Everybody involved, the National and International Institutions, the Regions, the health structures right down to the single Health operatives, must commit themselves, at their own level, to playing their part in a system, that in order to survive, must renew itself. Without a concerted effort from all these figures for a shared governance, ICT innovation in Health runs the risk of being eternally 'in search of an author'."

CONCLUSION

In the last decades, demographic and cultural changes, have led to the development of a new population subgroup characterized by extreme frailty and subsequent necessity of appropriated and elevated standards of care. Telemedicine, and more generally e-Health, is proposed as a tool for ensuring this fundamental care assistance, trying, at the same time, to reduce related costs. A lot of projects and indications have grown, worldwide, to favour the insertion of the e-Health into the conventional healthcare practice. At the present time, however, there is an unequal and fragmentary development of these projects. The main limitation is not the lack of technology, that is in constant upgrade and that is reaching high standards, but is a lack of the proper mentality not only on the part of the patients but also, and above all, on the part of the medical and managerial classes. Therefore it is necessary, to transform isolated projects into a standardized and efficient service network, an evolution in the mentality and in the approach to e-Health that needs to start from the institutions and then educate and involve the entire Health Care System.

REFERENCES

Ahern, D. K., Kreslake, J. M., & Phalen, J. M. (2006). What is ehealth: Perspectives on the evolution of ehealth research. *Journal of Medicine on the Internet, 8*(1), 4. Retrieved from http://www.jmir.org/2006/1/e4/

Commission of the European Communities. (2008). *COM(2008) 689: Communication from the Commission to the European Parliament, the Council, the European economic and social Committee and the Committee of the Regions on telemedicine for the benefit of patients, healthcare systems and society.* Retrieved November 4, 2008, from http://www.epractice.eu/

Della Mea, V. (2001). What is e-Health: The death of telemedicine? *Journal of Medicine on the Internet, 3*(2), 22. Retrieved 2001 from http://www.jmir.org/2001/2/e22/

Federanziani, Centre for Economic and International Studies (Ceis) of University of Tor Vergata (Rome), Università Cattolica Sacro Cuore. (2009). *Compendio SIC – Sanità in cifre 2009*. Retrieved from http://www.sanitaincifre.it

Ferrucci, L., et al. (2001). Linee-Guida sull'Utilizzazione della Valutazione Multidimensionale per l'Anziano Fragile nella Rete dei Servizi. *Giornale di Gerontologia, 49*(Suppl. 11)

F.M. (2011). *Sanità, in Italia la spesa IT non decolla*. Retrieved May 3, 2011, from http://www.corrierecomunicazioni.it/

Fried, L. P., Borhani, N. O., Enright, P., Furberg, C. D., Gardin, J. M., & Kronmal, R. A. (1991). The Cardiovascular Health Study: design and rationale. *Annals of Epidemiology, 1*(3), 263–276. doi:10.1016/1047-2797(91)90005-W

Fried, L. P., Tangen, C. M., Walston, J., Newman, A. B., Hirsch, C., & Gottdiener, J. (2001). Frailty in older adults: Evidence for a phenotype. Cardiovascular Health Study Collaborative Research Group. *The Journals of Gerontology. Series A, Biological Sciences and Medical Sciences, 56*(3), 146–156. doi:10.1093/gerona/56.3.M146

Mitchell, J. (1999). *From telehealth to e-health: the unstoppable rise of e-health*. Canberra, Australia: National Office for the Information Technology.

Mitchell, J. (2000). Increasing the cost-effectiveness of telemedicine by embracing e-health. *Journal of Telemedicine and Telecare, 1*(6), 16–19. doi:10.1258/1357633001934500

School of Management del Politecnico delle Milano. (2011). *Quarto Rapporto dell'Osservatorio ICT in Sanità: L'innovazione in cerca d'autore*. Retrieved from http://www.osservatori.net/

Stroetmann, K. A., Jones, T., Dobrev, A., & Stroetmann, V. N. (2008). *eHealth is worth it: The economic benefits of implemented eHealth solutions at ten European sites*. European Commission. Retrieved from http://www.ehealth-impact.org

United Nations, Economic and Social Affairs, Population Division. (2010). *Population ageing and development 2009*. Retrieved from http://www.un.org/esa/population/publication/ageing/ageing2009.html

Williams, D. L., & Denz, M. D. (n.d.). *European Health Telematics Association EHTEL*.

KEY TERMS AND DEFINITIONS

E-Health: The use of information and communication tecnologies in clinical care; pratically all of the sector of clinical care can be managed by e-health such as diagnostic, therapeutic, gestional (i.e. medical record) and administrative practices.

Frail Elderly: A geriatric syndrome characterized by multi-pathologies, critical social and environmental status and reduced autonomy. It leads to an instable health situation and an increase in necessity of clinical care.

Information and Communications Technologies (ICT): Any communication device or application, such as cellular phones, computer and network hardware and software, as well as the various services and applications associated with them. The most important aspect of ICTs in the field of e-Health is the creation of a greater access to information and communication in underserved populations.

Seventh Framework Programme for Research and Technological Development: The European Union's main instrument for funding research in Europe; at the present time there is the seventh edition (FP7) and it will run from 2007-2013.

Telemedicine: A defined setting of e-Health to support remote clinical care. It implies a physical distance between the patient and the doctor or also between two physicians (i.e. the General Practitioner, who requires the consulting, and the "Remote Doctor" who performs it).

Chapter 4
The Role of Telemedicine in Paediatric Cardiology

Brian A. McCrossan
The Royal Belfast Hospital for Sick Children, Northern Ireland

Frank A. Casey
The Royal Belfast Hospital for Sick Children, Northern Ireland

ABSTRACT

Paediatric cardiology is a subspecialty ideally suited to telemedicine. A small number of experts cover large geographical areas and the diagnosis of congenital heart defects is largely dependent on the interpretation of medical imaging. Telemedicine has been applied to a number of areas within paediatric cardiology. However, its widespread uptake has been slow and fragmentary. In this chapter the authors examine the current evidence pertaining to telemedicine applied to paediatric cardiology, including their own experience, the importance of research and, in particular, economic evaluation in furthering telemedicine endeavours. Perhaps most importantly, they discuss the issues relating transitioning a pilot project into a sustainable clinical service.

INTRODUCTION

Telemedicine continues to expand its range and scope. Over the past 25 years telemedicine has matured and should have now moved beyond feasibility studies. However, there remains a wide gap between what telemedicine is technically capable of achieving and its utilisation/

DOI: 10.4018/978-1-4666-2979-0.ch004

incorporation into routine clinical services. A lack of communication and cooperation between the interested parties (people with technological knowledge and resources, clinicians, health service funders) is a significant, recurring obstacle. A failure to appreciate the different needs of various clinical subspecialties and geographical settings is an aspect of this problem.

This chapter aims to highlight limitations to the clinical practice of paediatric cardiology that are suitable for telemedicine intervention.

We shall describe our experience in addressing these problems and hown the solutions have been translated into sustained clinical services. We shall discuss the importance of economic evaluation of telemdicine research to its translation into routine care. This chapter will also suggest potential directions and themes for future research and development of telemedicine in paediatric cardiology. Finally, it is hoped that the reader will have a clearer understanding of the potential for telemedicine to meet the needs of patients with congenital heart disease and feel encouraged to utilise this exciting clinical tool!

BACKGROUND

In order to employ telemedicine technology in a congenital cardiac setting it is essential to understand what paediatric cardiology is, how clinical care is currently provided, what aspects of paediatric cardiology practice are suited to telemedicine and the evidence base.

What is Paediatric Cardiology?

Paediatric cardiology is the medical specialty concerned with diseases of the heart in the growing and developing individual.(Workforce Review Team, 2009) Paediatric cardiologists investigate and treat patients with congenital or acquired heart disease, diseases of cardiac rhythm and conduction, and disturbances of cardiac and circulatory function. The specialty provides a service for acute and chronic conditions from fetal life through childhood into adulthood (National Health Service).

Paediatric cardiology is a demanding and exciting specialty to work in. There have been great advances in paediatric cardiology over the last two decades. Improvements in diagnostic imaging, intensive care, introduction of prostaglandin therapy, catheter procedures and in particular surgical procedures have contributed to dramatically improved outcomes for patients with CHD.

In the UK, the national average 1 year survival rate for all operations and catheter intervention is 95%.(Congenital Cardiac Audit Database, 2009) In particular children with complex CHD, typified by single ventricle physiology, now have the possibility of life beyond the neonatal period. (Marino, 2002).

Current Service Provision for Paediatric Cardiology in the UK

Paediatric cardiologists are responsible for the care of patients ranging from fetus to adult with a wide range of defects, both congenital and acquired and even patients with no discernable cardiac disease. Paediatric cardiologists tend to monitor their patients' progress indefinitely so that the caseload appears ever increasing. There are approximately 80 consultant paediatric cardiologists in the UK which is 100 less than is currently recommended by the British Cardiovascular Society.(NHS - medical careers, 2009) Care is centralised in 14 paediatric cardiology centres throughout the UK, 12 of which provide a surgical service. At these tertiary centres, the workload of paediatric cardiologists includes the assessment of patients presenting as acute emergencies or routine outpatient referrals; performing specialised investigations and procedures such as MRI and cardiac catheterisation; and co-ordinating referrals to cardiac surgeons. Paediatric cardiologists are also closely associated with intensive care units, providing pre and post-operative care for their own patients but also supporting multi-disciplinary teams in the care of patients with severe and complex conditions.(Royal College of Physicians, 2009) There is close liaison with paediatrics and its sub-specialties, adult cardiology, obstetrics, radiology and pathology.

However, the care of patients with CHD is not confined to the tertiary centre. Paediatric cardiologists hold outreach clinics at a number of DGHs within their region, travelling on a half day or full day once a month or once every two or three months. Lower thresholds for referring asymptomatic children with clear cut innocent murmurs for "a second opinion" have swollen outreach clinics.(Dowie et al., 2009) Further pressures have been placed on service provision because of the need to comply with guidelines recommending screening of babies with various syndromes and family screening of certain inheritable conditions. Thus the paediatric cardiologist may be away from the tertiary unit on average at least once a week. Whilst an excellent service is provided at the outreach clinic, it does not seem to be efficient from the tertiary unit's perspective. (Qureshi, 2008) It is understood that most patient's first port of call will be their DGH. Therefore it is important to foster confidence and competence in managing children with CHD. On the other hand, patients with a clinical problem requiring a paediatric cardiology opinion that cannot wait for the next outreach clinic, need transferred to the tertiary centre for a specialist opinion.

A recent innovation has been the curriculum for paediatricians with special expertise in cardiology. Several posts have been appointed in DGHs throughout the UK.(Royal College of paediatrics and Child Health, 2009) The role of the paediatrician with special expertise in cardiology is to unload some of the outpatient work currently being done by the tertiary centres (e.g. evaluation of children with asymptomatic murmurs or chest pain), to be the link person for children with CHD followed up at that DGH and to be competent at performing 2-D echocardiography. These paediatricians will need to be supported by the relevant tertiary centre.

The British Congenital Cardiac Association has given consideration to paediatric cardiology outreach services.(Qureshi, 2008) Various models of care have been debated leading to the following recommendations:

- Provision of excellent clinical care.
- Location should be convenient to patients.

- One-stop out patient visit necessitating the availability of non-invasive investigations.
- Rationalise direct involvement by paediatric cardiology.
- Identification of paediatricians with special expertise in paediatric cardiology to jointly organise and run the outreach clinics.
- Telemedicine links with the tertiary unit in order to have echocardiograms interpreted by paediatric cardiologists at all hours, all the year round.

A proposed restructuring of paediatric cardiology services in the UK may reduce the number of paediatric cardiology surgical centres to seven, which would further centralise expertise and potentially isolate clinicians working in non-cardiac centres (Paediatric and Congenital Cardiac Services Review Group, 2003). In this setting paediatric cardiology centres are being encouraged to develop clinical networks of peripheral units and primary care providers. The supra-regional units at the centre of these networks will cover very large geographical areas (Figure 1).

Why is Paediatric Cardiology Suited to Telemedicine?

Paediatric cardiology is a highly centralised specialty which currently undergoing further concentration into larger centres. A small number of professionals are expected to cover large geographical areas and provide outreach clinics to DGHs. Telemedicine has the potential reconfigure this workload so that part of it may be delivered remotely (see Table 2).

Diagnosing, excluding and quantifying heart disease in children is largely dependent on data: heart sounds, ECGs, Chest radiographs, cardiac angiograms and more recently magnetic resonance images. In particular echocardiographic imaging is the mainstay of evaluating structural heart disease. All of these modalities are capable of being received, digitalised and then transmitted

Figure 1. The complex web of a managed clinical network

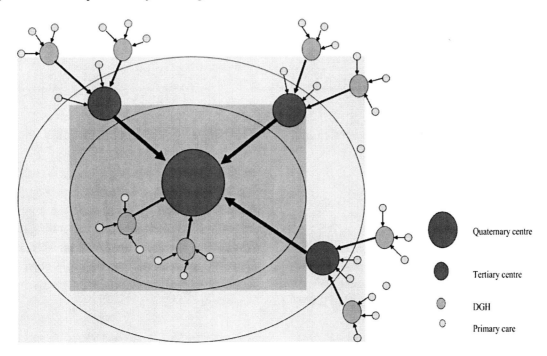

Quaternary centre

Tertiary centre

DGH

Primary care

via tele-links to remote locations for expert interpretation.

To summarise, paediatric cardiology is perfectly suited to telemedicine because it is a highly centralised specialty requiring interpretation of audiovisual data to diagnose potentially lethal conditions. Earlier diagnosis and institution of appropriate therapy, facilitated by telemedicine, may alter the outcome. This is what telemedicine hopes to achieve, is it not?

What Parts of Paediatric Cardiology Lend Themselves to Telemedicine?

Many aspects of paediatric cardiology may be facilitated by telemedicine (see Table 1). The key question to ask is: Is there a clinical problem in which distance separating the specialist from the patient is a significant factor? If yes, then telemedicine has the potential to help. As outlined above telemedicine may be utilised to collect and transmit various forms of clinical data that may

facilitate diagnosis and management of children with heart problems. The clinical scenario in which you employ telemedicine is dependent on what your needs are.

At our institution we have conducted research on four different clinical situations within paediatric cardiology: fetal cardiology, newborn presentation of severe congenital heart disease, tele-homecare of babies with severe congenital heart disease and the outpatient clinic.

Why Telemedicine Research is Important

The National Institute for Health and Clinical Excellence (NICE) is an influential institution that provides guidance to the NHS in the UK on the clinical and cost-effectiveness of new and established technologies. Consideration of a comprehensive evidence base is fundamental to the NICE appraisal process. NICE are particularly interested in technologies that have the potential

Table 1. Why is paediatric cardiology suited to telemedicine?

Small number of paediatric cardiologists in centres covering large geographical areas	Diagnosis of CHD depends on interpretation of data suitable for transmission -
Non-specialists increasingly less confident in excluding CHD.	- Still images: Chest X-Ray - moving images: Echo
Delay in diagnosis can negatively impact on outcome	- - Heart sounds

to (National Institute for Health and Clinical Excellence, 2008):

- Provide significant health benefits
- Promote health equality
- Impact on NHS resources

Telemedicine is a clinical tool with similar aims to those stated above. The dissemination of tele-health would be greatly facilitated by NICE guidance.

However, at present there is not enough good quality evidence to support a NICE guideline. Telemedicine has been frequently criticised for the lack of well conducted research trials. Much of the research concerns retrospective, uncontrolled studies involving small numbers of patients i.e. centres reporting their "experience" of telemedicine once they have gathered together enough numbers to put together a paper. This is a criticism that could also be leveled at paediatric cardiology!

In order to convince healthcare managers to invest in telemedicine services it is vital that there is evidence to support its application. Either the evidence is already available or you conduct a trial to acquire the evidence.

CURRENT EVIDENCE BASE

As this chapter is not only concerned with presenting the evidence for telemedicine applied to paediatric cardiology but also how it may be incorporated into routine practice, I shall separately discuss the literature available on both issues. However, as economic evaluation is such a vital aspect of service development I shall discuss this separately.

Telemedicine Applied to Neonatal Presentation of CHD

The main application of telemedicine in paediatric cardiology to date has been remote diagnosis of congenital heart disease by the transmission of echocardiograms from DGH to specialist. Several regional paediatric cardiology centres in the UK have instigated such a telemedicine service. The paediatric cardiology department at the RBHSC has been evaluating tele-echocardiography in paediatrics since 1995. Mulholland et al published the first study in the UK demonstrating accurate diagnosis and exclusion of CHD in neonates using an ISDN 2 link between the regional paediatric cardiology unit and a district general hospital (DGH). (Mulholland et al., 1999) There are many articles

Table 2. Telemedicine applications in paediatric cardiology

Researched	Not researched
Neonatal echocardiography	Counselling families/patients
Fetal echocardiography	Inter-professional teleconferencing
Telehomecare including remote monitoring	Ongoing education of non-specialists
Remote stethoscopy	

Table 3. Reasons for not getting involved in neonatal tele-echocardiography

Tertiary Unit perspective	DGH perspective
Do not perceive a problem with its current model for assessing sick neonates with potential CHD	Do not want to learn how to perform an echocardiogram
Do not have the time to set up a telemedicine service.	Do not have the time
Are put off by the technology	Are put off by the technology
Put-off by the start-up and running costs	Put-off by the start-up and running costs
The personnel at the tertiary unit are not paid for this additional service	Not being paid for this work
Do not want the hassle of guiding non-cardiologists through the acquisition of a complete echocardiogram	The personnel at the DGH just want to transfer the neonate out of their unit so that it is someone else' problem.

in the literature confirming the effectiveness of this telemedicine application (Alboliras et al., 1996; Cloutier, 2000; Cotton, Gallaher, & Henry, 2002; Finley et al., 1989; Finley et al., 1997; Fisher, Alboliras, Berdusis, & Webb, 1996; Justo et al., 2004; Lewin et al., 2006; Mulholland et al., 1999; Randolph et al., 1999; C. Sable et al., 1999; C. Sable, 2002; C. A. Sable et al., 2002; Tsilimigaki et al., 2001; Whitten, Mair, Haycox, May, Williams, & Hellmich, 2002b). The feasibility, reliability and clinical utility of neonatal tele-echocardiography are now well established. However, much of the literature reports short-term, start-up studies with or without poorly designed cost-analyses. We recently published an 8 year-review of a neonatal tele-echocardiography service for three DGHs in our region. This clearly demonstrated that real-time neonatal tele-echocardiography is accurate, affects patient management, does not excessively increase referral patterns and is cost-saving. Most importantly this telemedicine application is sustainable and has become an integral part of our regional service. On a clinical note, this study also cautions that if there is a clinical suspicion of major CHD that cannot be confidently diagnosed or excluded, following a tele-echocardiogram, then transfer to a tertiary unit for hands-on assessment should not be delayed. Its uptake by regional paediatric cardiology services depends on a number of factors relating to the tertiary units and the surrounding DGHs.

Solutions and Recommendations

These hurdles may be overcome by addressing real issues such as a lack of long-term funding/reimbursement for telemedicine activities and misconceptions such as the technical challenges: modern telemedicine systems are fairly idiot proof!

The value of telemedicine in education has been well documented if not fully researched (Casey, 1999; Justo et al., 2004; C. Sable, 2003; C. A. Sable et al., 2002; Tsilimigaki et al., 2001). Our experience of the educational benefit of real time transmission of echocardiograms has been very positive. Having performed echocardiograms under the guidance of a paediatric cardiologist, paediatricians report an improvement in their ability to interpret echocardiograms and have been observed to gain confidence in echocardiography.

Telemedicine Applied to Fetal Cardiology

The summary of fetal cardiology literature demonstrates that timely, antenatal diagnosis of CHD is important for improving outcomes for fetus and family by facilitating:

- Parental counselling
- Elective delivery at an appropriate centre
- Parental choice in terms of termination

- Fetal intervention – pharmacotherapy for dysrhythmias catheter intervention for severe complex lesions

In the UK, the most practicable method of promoting antenatal detection of CHD is by improving cardiac evaluation during the routine anomaly scan. Schemes that may support sonographers should therefore be encouraged.

There are a number of features of fetal cardiology that appear to make telemedicine an attractive proposition:

- Fetal cardiology is a highly centralized subspeciality. In Northern Ireland, there are 18 hospitals/clinics offering obstetric services and/or fetal anomaly scans. There is only one centre with fetal cardiology services provided by two paediatric cardiologists with a specialist interest in fetal cardiology. Unsurprisingly, the demand for appointments at one of the twice weekly fetal cardiology clinics is very high.
- Patients often travel large distances (up to 100 miles in Northern Ireland) to attend the fetal cardiology clinic. The distance between home and the specialist centre is even greater in larger countries. In Quebec, 34% of mothers referred to a fetal cardiology service travel more than 100km. (Cloutier & Finley, 2004)
- Fetal cardiology is predominantly a speciality of medical imaging as physical examination of the fetal cardiovascular system is obviously not possible and fetal catheter and surgical interventions are limited to a handful of centres worldwide. Telemedicine lends itself to areas where medical imaging is crucial to diagnosis. (Casey, 1999)

Telemedicine has the potential to facilitate earlier diagnosis of CHD by offering increased and quicker access to specialist opinion. Telemedicine may also support radiographers' education and training.

Experience of telemedicine in fetal cardiology is still in its infancy. The fetal cardiology telemedicine programs that are currently active appear to have developed from centres with a major interest in telemedicine and fetal cardiology.

Despite a potential role for telemedicine in fetal cardiology, there are very few studies investigating its potential. Apart from our own experience only one study is reported to date that investigates the feasibility and acceptability of performing remote, real-time 2-D fetal echocardiography (Sharma et al., 2003). Sharma et al performed a study in two phases. Phase one was a laboratory study, investigating the effect of bandwidth on image quality and overall adequacy of scan. Sixty-four fetal echocardiograms were performed and randomly assigned to transmission across 128, 384 and 768 kbps and recorded on Super VHS videotape for subsequent review. The researchers utilised a 31 item check list to ascertain the adequacy of the transmitted fetal echocardiogram and a five point Likert scale to assess the received image quality.

Six studies were excluded due to the presence of CHD. Of the 58 real-time studies interpreted, 15/58 were transmitted across 128 kbps, 21 across 384 kbps and 22 across 768 kbps. The image quality was felt to be significantly poorer at 128 kbps. At 128 kbps, the mean Likert score was 1.1/5 compared with 3.1/5 at 384 kbps ($p < 0.01$) and 3.4/5 at 768 kbps ($p < 0.01$). There was no significant difference in perceived image quality in transmission across 384 kbps compared with 768 kbps ($p = 0.08$). Similarly, there was no significant difference in the adequacy of studies transmitted across 384 kbps compared with 768 kbps. The mean number of items inadequately demonstrated were 2.1/31 and 2.5/31 at 384 and 768 kbps respectively ($p = 0.49$). Again transmission across 128 kbps was significantly less complete with a mean of 6.9/31 items inadequately demonstrated ($p < 0.01$). This study also found acceptable inter-observer variability. In this first phase, Sharma et al conclude that 384 kbps is an adequate bandwidth for the identification of normal heart structures.

In the second phase of the study, 40 patients were enrolled for live, real-time remotely guided fetal echocardiography. In two cases, appointments were not kept and in four cases (11%) technical problems prevented transmission. Therefore, 34 fetal echocardiograms were successfully transmitted and interpreted in this cohort. The fetal echocardiogram was performed by a fetal cardiac sonographer or a paediatric cardiology fellow with experience in fetal echocardiography. Again the adequacy of the transmitted fetal echocardiogram was assessed using the previous 31 item check list. This was compared with a video recording of the study made at the transmitting site. Mothers were followed up with a face-to-face fetal echocardiogram if a concern was identified on the transmitted fetal echocardiogram. In order to evaluate patient satisfaction, a questionnaire was completed by all 34 expectant mothers and a control group of 195 patients referred from peripheral hospitals to the regional fetal cardiology clinic. The most common referral reason was maternal insulin dependent diabetes mellitus (24/34). Other referral indications included extra-cardiac anomaly, possible arrhythmia, suspected CHD and a family history of CHD.

The mean number of items inadequately demonstrated on each transmitted fetal echocardiogram was 2.3/31 compared with 2.1/31 in the store-and-forward study in phase one (p = 0.2). CHD was identified correctly in two transmitted fetal echocardiograms with a third case of CHD being suspected but only confirmed on direct fetal echocardiography.

The satisfaction survey results were very positive. In all nine questions, the mean patient satisfaction score was $\geq$ 4.3/5, indicating high levels of satisfaction with the telemedicine consultation. In eight questions there was no significant difference in patient satisfaction between the telemedicine and control groups. In addition, only 6% of patients stated that they felt uncomfortable talking to the doctor across the tele-link and only 3% felt it was difficult to ask questions.

In this important study, the authors conclude that transmission of fetal echocardiograms across 384 kbps is feasible and adequate for the interpretation of screening fetal echocardiograms. Community acceptance of telemedicine screening and counselling is not adversely affected by a lack of direct personal contact with the specialist (Sharma et al., 2003).

However, the authors acknowledge a number of limitations to their study.

- The majority of transmitted fetal echocardiograms were not followed up with a face-to-face fetal echocardiogram which is the gold standard.
- The proportion of fetuses with CHD was small in this cohort. Therefore, the diagnostic accuracy of the telemedicine process was not adequately assessed.
- The fetal echocardiograms were performed by an operator already skilled in fetal echocardiography. This may falsely enhance the adequacy and quality of the fetal echocardiogram being transmitted. It is suggested that most difficulties in interpreting echocardiograms transmitted via a tele-link are related to image acquisition rather than transmission (Cloutier, 2000).
- Eleven per cent of studies were terminated due to technical difficulties. A routine clinical service would be significantly limited if 11% of consultations were aborted due to technical difficulties.

There are also reports of telemedicine facilitating 3-D fetal echocardiography by spatio-temporal image correlation (STIC) and datasets transmitted across an ADSL link. STIC is a relatively new approach for clinical assessment of the fetal heart. It is an easy technique for acquiring data from the fetal heart (a single, automatic volume sweep) and produces a 4D cine sequence.

Michailidis et al conducted a study whereby 3-D datasets were acquired, stored, compressed and then transmitted across an ADSL link to the regional centre. The datasets were then processed and interpreted by a specialist in fetal cardiology. In a cohort of 30 normal studies, an adequate four chamber view was obtained in every case and all other views were obtained in more than 80% of occasions. Complete studies were acquired in 77%. The mean acquisition time was 9.5 minutes and processing and interpretation time 17 minutes. The datasets did not include information on ventricular function or blood flow. The authors suggest that in this situation, a store-and-forward protocol has advantages over real-time transmission as both doctors are not simultaneously required (Michailidis, Simpson, Karidas, & Economides, 2001). However, a store-and-forward strategy demotes the referring sonography to the role of simply acquiring images of which they are ignorant. By implication all "high risk" pregnancies should have a dataset acquired and interpreted by an expert. However, this policy would not enhance the detection rate amongst "low-risk" pregnancies which account for greater than 90% of CHD. A group from Chile conducted a similar study STIC transmitted across an ADSL connection with bandwidths of 300 and 600 kbps. In total fifty scans were transmitted from two peripheral hospitals to the regional centre. On average complete fetal echocardiograms could be interpreted in 92%. (Vinals, Mandujano, Vargas, & Giuliano, 2005)

In or own study, an initial FE was performed by the sonographer as part of the routine fetal anomaly scan offered to all pregnancies. The sonographer recorded a diagnosis (D1). A second FE was performed by the sonographer. These images were transmitted in real-time via ISDN 6 tele-link to the regional unit and viewed by the fetal cardiologist. There was continuous, live audio-visual contact between patient, sonographer and fetal cardiologist. The fetal cardiologist provided guidance to the sonographer in terms of which structures were currently in view, necessary manoeuvres to view particular cardiac structures and highlighted any abnormalities as they appeared. At the completion of the fetal tele-echocardiogram, the fetal cardiologist explained the findings (D2) and the subsequent management plan. Parents had the opportunity to ask questions of the fetal cardiologist.

All patients were given an appointment for a "hands-on" FE at the regional unit. The "hands-on" FE was performed by the fetal cardiologist. D3 was documented at this point which is considered the reference standard for this study. Following the "hands-on" FE, the parents were informed of the diagnosis, what future management was required and had the opportunity to ask questions. The study protocol is summarised in Figure 2.

A structured six point questionnaire, using a 5-point Likert scale was completed by the obstetric sonographers involved in this study. Questions related to confidence in FE and attitudes towards telemedicine consultations. The questionnaire was completed at the start and end of the study period.

The results of this study were very positive. 69 fetal tele-echocardiograms were performed. All videoconferences connected successfully at the first attempt with no interruptions in transmission. The mean duration of the fetal tele-echocardiogram was 13.9 minutes (s.d. = 6.1 minutes, range = 6 – 35 minutes). The quality of the videoconference and transmitted fetal echocardiogram were rated highly by the paediatric cardiologist. Video quality (Median, IQR) = 7.5 /10, 7 –8, audio quality = 8 /10, 7 – 9, ease of use = 8 /10, 7 –8 and overall quality = 8 /10, 7 –8.

In 72% (50/69) cases all 12 aspects of the fetal echocardiogram were confidently assessed from the transmitted images. At least 11 /12 structures were confidently assessed in 94% cases. In 19/69 cases the quality of the transmitted image was adversely affected by a range of factors relating to the fetal lie, obstructing limbs, twin pregnancy and maternal obesity. Picture quality was rated as significantly lower in fetal tele-echocardiograms

Figure 2. Fetal telemedicine study protocol

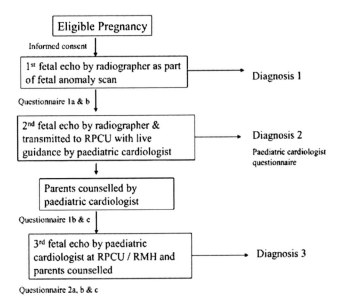

Diagnostic Accuracy

The initial FE (D1) agreed with the "hands-on" FE in 47/69 (68%) cases with disagreement in 22/69 (32%). On 19 occasions CHD was incorrectly suspected and in three cases CHD was missed. These results indicate a relatively poor level of agreement between the sonographer and fetal cardiologist (kappa score = 0.27, sensitivity = 0.75, specificity = 0.67). In 57/69 (82.6%) cases the fetal tele-echocardiogram (D2) indicated a normal fetal heart with 12/69 (17.4%) suggesting CHD. On 97% occasions D2 was confirmed by "hands-on" FE (D3). There was one false positive and one false negative diagnosis. These results indicate an excellent level of agreement between

affected by these problems (Median Likert score = 6/10 vs 8/ 10, p < 0.01 [Mann-Whitney U-test]). Using the "hands-on" FE as the reference standard, 57 of the 69 FEs demonstrated normal fetal hearts. In 12 (17%) cases the FE was not normal with 8 cases of major CHD, including three duct-dependent lesions which are life-threatening in the newborn period.

fetal tele-echocardiography and "hands-on" FE, Table 2.7 (kappa score = 0.90, 95% confidence interval = 0.66 – 1.0). Sensitivity = 0.92, specificity = 0.98, positive predictive value = 0.92, negative predictive value = 0.98.

Sonographers were highly satisfied with their involvement in the study. There was a consistent shift of responses towards increased confidence in fetal echocardiography technique and satisfaction with the telemedicine process. The mean total questionnaire score before the study was 16.8 /30 compared with 24.4 /30 after the study. This finding is confirmed on comparing individual radiographer's total questionnaire score (/30) at the start and end of the study. Using a Wilcoxon Signed Ranks test there was a significant increase in questionnaire score following participation in this study (p = 0.04).

Expectant mothers indicated a high degree of satisfaction with the telemedicine consultation. There was no significant difference in aggregate satisfaction scores for the telemedicine and face-to-face consultations. Indeed study participants stated that they preferred to have the fetal cardiology consultation conducted over the tele-link rather than travel to the tertiary unit for a hands-on fetal echocardiogram. Unsurprisingly, travel times and costs were much reduced for the telemedicine consultations.

This study demonstrates that fetal echocardiography, performed by radiographers with little experience of fetal cardiology, transmitted in real-time with live guidance by a paediatric cardiologist is technically feasible, reliable and not particularly time consuming. The images are sufficient to permit accurate diagnosis and exclusion of CHD. Expectant mothers are highly satisfied with the remote consultation and may even find it preferable to travelling to the regional centre for direct consultation with the paediatric cardiologist. The vast majority of fetuses with CHD are born from pregnancies without a recognisable antenatal risk factor. Obviously, formal evaluation by a fetal cardiologist cannot be offered to every single pregnancy. Therefore, in order to maximise antenatal detection of CHD, greater proficiency, from the non-specialist, is required at confirming normality and identifying pathology during the main formal evaluation of the fetus: the routine anomaly scan. A significant positive feature of real-time fetal tele-echocardioghraphy is the continued support provided to radiographers performing fetal anomaly scans in DGHs.

Solutions and Recommendations

The introduction of a remote fetal cardiology service would have attendant costs which are not offset by savings in inter-hospital transfers. However, the possible establishment of a "one-stop-shop" for "high-risk" pregnancies in which the routine fetal anomaly scan is followed by a remote fetal echocardiogram confidently identifying all relevant cardiac structures (55% in this cohort) could potentially be cost neutral, relieve pressure on the tertiary unit and present time and cost savings to the patient (McCrossan, Sands, Kileen, Cardwell, & Casey, 2011).

Tele-Homecare

Tele-home care has become established as a useful support mechanism for adults with particular chronic illnesses.(Clark, Inglis, McAlister, Cleland, & Stewart, 2007) There is good and increasing evidence that tele-home care can be an effective method of health care delivery. Indeed tele-homecare is *the* growth area in telemedicine. I shall describe an overview of the literature pertaining to paediatrics and cardiology with particular focus on paediatric cardiology.

In 2007 the BMJ published a separate meta-analysis of fourteen randomised control trials relating to home tele-monitoring and structured telephone support programs for patients with chronic heart failure. It reported a significant reduction in hospital admissions for chronic heart failure (21%), although not "all cause" admissions. A significant decrease in "all cause" mortality (20%) was also observed. These results were most marked in the tele-monitoring trials compared with structured telephone support. Tele-home care was also associated with improvements in quality of life measures.

There are many commercially available home monitoring systems varying in scope and sophistication. The devices operate without clinician input. The clinical data such as BP, oxygen saturations, heart rate, respiratory rate and weight are automatically recorded and sent to the health professional via an internet connection. There is also the facility for symptoms to be documented, either as yes/no answers to prompted questions or as free text. The observations may be daily or less frequently. Alternatively, regular phone calls may be scheduled with a clinician and the data communicated directly. These systems often employ an automated range of physiological parameters with specified protocols which if breached prompt a medical intervention usually in the form of a phone call from hospital/primary care staff. There are recent reports of ambulatory ECG monitoring leading to detection and early intervention of arrhythmias in patients with congestive heart failure (Hickey et al., 2010).

In a joint venture with pacemaker manufacturers, electrophysiologists have pursued remote monitoring of pacemakers and implantable cardiac devices. The electronic data stored by the the ICD/pacemaker may be transmitted to the hospital transtelephonically using equipment provided with the device. This has proven very successful. There is convincing evidence that remote monitoring of such devices is helpful in the early detection of arrhythmias like a trial fibrillation or ventricular tachyarrhythmias. Remote monitoring significantly reduces the number of follow-up visits, patients' and physicians' time spent per visit, and increases patients' adherence to follow-up visits (Gramegna et al., 2012; Mabo et al., 2011; Perings et al., 2011).

Whilst the scale of paediatric chronic illness is much smaller than in adult and elderly populations, it is certain the past twenty years has seen a significant increase in the number of children with chronic complex illness (Wise, 2007). Improvements in survival for a range of conditions across the paediatric spectrum e.g. congenital heart disease, cystic fibrosis, ex-premature infants and severe congenital gastro-intestinal defects have produced a cohort of patients requiring ongoing specialist care beyond discharge from hospital (Chiu & Hedrick, 2008; Farrell et al., 2005; Hintz et al., 2005; McElhinney & Wernovsky, 2001). Parental expectations have increased regarding the quality of life experienced by their child and the level of specialist input that should be provided. (little hearts matter, 2009; tiny life, 2009) This is especially pertinent to life-limiting illnesses such as neuro-degenerative disorders, severe epilepsy, home ventilated patients and children receiving palliative care. These expectations are unlikely to decline but rather to increase with time.

As detailed above, there is substantial good quality evidence supporting tele-home care in adult cardiology. However, there is a paucity of data in paediatric populations. In 2001, Hersh et

al conducted a systematic review of telemedicine home interventions on paediatric and obstetric populations for Medicare policy makers. The authors concluded that most of the studies were small and/or methodologically limited. However there appeared to be evidence that access to healthcare was improved when families had the opportunity to receive healthcare at home rather than face-to-face care at a hospital or clinic. Access was particularly enhanced when the tele-health system enabled timely communication between patient or family and care providers and facilitating adjustments that may prevent hospitalization (Hersh et al., 2001). One of the few tele-home care trials involving children to be published in mainstream, peer reviewed journal was reported from a Japanese centre. In 1997, Miyasaka et al published a case-control study involving children with home ventilation care. Study participants received a videophone connected to the specialist centre by an ISDN 1 (64Kbps) link. Although the sample size was very small (n=10), the authors observed large reductions in the number of home visits by physicians, unscheduled hospital attendances and hospital admission days. Whilst the number of phone calls between hospital and home increased during the study period, there was a net reduction in the number of hours of unscheduled medical care (Miyasaka, Suzuki, Sakai, & Kondo, 1997). This study is encouraging and appears to make sense. Therefore, it is disappointing that no follow-up or similar studies have subsequently been reported.

On reviewing the evidence base for tele-home care, several themes become apparent:

- Tele-home care is well established and continues to expand in the care of adults and elderly people with chronic illness.
- There is a wide spectrum of formats for tele-home care.
- Not all tele-home care programs confer significant benefit to the patient and/or family.

- The tele-home care program needs to be tailored to the needs of the patient and family.
- There are groups of children who would potentially benefit from tele-home care.
- There is a paucity of high quality data with respect to tele-home care in paediatric populations.

Tele-Home Care in Paediatric Cardiology

It is recommended that tele-home care be targeted at conditions that require close monitoring, clinical assessment and early intervention to avoid adverse events such as hospitalization or emergency visits (Dellifraine & Dansky, 2008). Paediatric cardiology is a highly specialized and centralized field of medicine. It seems logical that members of the paediatric cardiology team who have been involved in the daily management of these patients are ideally placed to monitor the patient's progress and deal with any problems as they arise. Paediatric cardiology is provided as a regional service and by its nature many families are distant from the tertiary care centre.

The group of congenital cardiac lesions that have attracted most interest over the past 15 years have been those which fall within the umbrella term - "hypoplastic left heart syndrome." In HLHS, there is severe under development of some or all left heart structures (Dhillon & Redington, 2002). Until relatively recently, surgical intervention was not widely available. However, it is now exceptional for babies with HLHS not to be offered surgical intervention. This usually takes the form of staged surgical palliation culminating in a total cavo-pulmonary anastomosis with a systemic right ventricle. The first stage is the Norwood procedure, performed during the early neonatal period, with the second stage occurring during mid-infancy (Bove, Ohye, & Devaney, 2004; Sano et al., 2004; Stasik et al., 2006). Although modifications to the Norwood procedure

have been associated with a reduction in early mortality, there remains a significant attrition rate between the first and second stages (Forbess, 2003). This group of patients could particularly benefit from additional monitoring and support following discharge from hospital.

A group from Wisconsin, USA, postulated that patients at risk of inter-stage mortality could be identified by a deterioration in their physiological status. A daily home programme of measuring arterial oxygen saturations and weight was combined with a protocol guiding the need for hospitalisation. There was significantly less mortality observed during the 15 month intervention period compared with the preceding 50 month control period (0% vs 16%, p = 0.039). The second stage operation occurred earlier during the intervention period (3.7 months vs 5.2 months, p = 0.028) (Ghanayem et al., 2003; Ghanayem, Cava, Jaquiss, & Tweddell, 2004; Ghanayem, Tweddell, Hoffman, Mussatto, & Jaquiss, 2006).

This study is valuable as it suggests that, even for one of the most severe forms of CHD, a home monitoring programme is safe, effects patient management and may reduce mortality. These are bold assertions that are not necessarily supported by the study design. There is a learning curve with any new congenital cardiac surgical programme. It is difficult to compare the results of a fledgling operative programme with one that has accumulated five year's experience (Bull, Yates, Sarkar, Deanfield, & de Leval, 2000).

Similar to the Wisconsin group, a group from Sweden have recently published their experience of using pulse oximetry to detect an impending critical deterioration in infants with severe CHD. Although the study is small, it does highlight the potential for home monitoring in well defined groups of patients (Ohman, Stromvall-Larsson, Nilsson, & Mellander, 2012).

We conducted an ambitious randomised controlled trial to evaluate the feasibility and efficacy of a videoconferencing home support programme for infants with major CHD compared with telephone support and a control group. Participants were randomly allocated to one of the three groups. If videoconferencing equipment was not available, the family was randomly allocated to either the telephone support group or control group (Figure 3). The intervention consisted of weekly or twice weekly videoconferences between the clinician and parent & patient which were scheduled over a ten week period. The assessments consisted of an oral history from the parents and visual examination of the patient including pulse oximetry (Figure 4).

We initially performed a pilot study to confirm the most suitable hardware and transmission modality. The videoconferencing hardware consisted of a Tandberg 880™ codec in the hospital and Tandberg 1000 ™ or Sony TL-30 codec in the home. At the inception of this study, home broadband was not of sufficient quality to support diagnostic quality videoconferencing. Therefore, ISDN6 lines (384Kbps) were installed in all families' homes. This was very reliable but also expensive and difficult to install in more emote areas. Over time we were assured that internet protocols and community internet connections had improved and should hopefully support reliable videoconsultations. Before installing any such connections in study subjects we undertook preliminary testing across the proposed ADSL connection at 256Kbps. Whilst this is one third less than the bandwidth available using ISDN 6 (384Kbps), it is generally agreed by videoconferencing companies that, using modern internet protocols (H.264), 256Kbps provides similar audio-visual quality to ISDN 6.(Questmark, 2008) The routers were specifically programmed so that their packages were given priority in traffic ("tagged"). Transmission above 256Kbps incurs a higher risk of transmission interruption.

We were impressed by the audio-visual quality and apparent reliability of the test videoconferences. We remained remained sceptical about embarking on internet transmission due to previous unimpressive experiences. However, internet transmission was attractive by our realisation that for this project to be scaled out to a full clinical service, then it needed to be less expensive and more geographically sustainable.

Over the 41 month study period, 370 video-consultations were conducted involving 35 patients and families. Family involvement in the home support program lasted on average 12.1 weeks (s.d. 5.7 weeks). A successful audio-visual connection was made at the first attempt in 342 consultations (92.4%).

Tele-consultations were scheduled on a weekly basis, or more often if requested, with the facility for "urgent" consultations. The consultations consisted of a videoconference which facilitated an interview with the patient and parent including an audiovisual assessment of the patient and a recording of the oxygen saturations, heart rate and respiratory rate.

Over the 41 month study period, 273 telephone consultations were conducted involving 24 families. Family involvement in the home support program lasted on average 11.3 weeks (s.d. 3.5 weeks). The mean consultation time was 8.0 minutes.

The clinical utility of the 370 video-consultations rated highly on a five-point Likert scale. The clinician strongly agreed that the child could be confidently assessed (Median = 4.5 /5, IQR = 4.3 – 4.8) and that the parents' concerns could be adequately addressed across the tele-link (4.6/5, IQR = 4.3 – 4.8). The clinician agreed that the video-consultations were beneficial (Median = 4.3, IQR = 4.1 – 4.5).

Whilst a similar proportion of video and telephone consultations included the parent expressing a specific concern (Median per patient = 63% vs 68%, χ^2 test p = 0.19), a very small percentage of video-consultations concluded with the parent being advised to seek further health care assessment compared with telephone consultations (Median per patient = 0 vs 25%, Mann-Whitney U test p < 0.01). In 97% of video-consultations the clinician felt he was able to address the parental concerns

Figure 3. Randomisation protocol

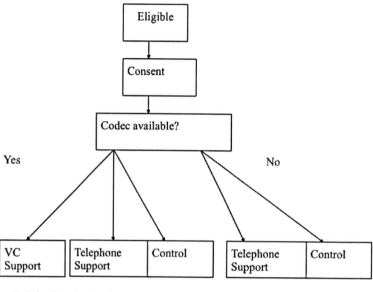

compared with 64% of telephone consultations. This finding is supported by the clinician's opinion as to the benefit of visually assessing the patient. At the conclusion of 30% of video-consultations, the clinician stated that the ability to visually assess the patient had influenced their management plan. Similarly, following more than one quarter of telephone consultations, the clinician stated that the inability to visually assess the patient had affected their management plan.

These results suggest that, whilst families in both videoconferencing and telephone groups were provided with similar levels of support (in terms of the personnel involved, duration of home support and number of consultations), expressed similar levels of concern and were equally anxious before each consultation video-consultations provided a more confident clinical assessment.

Parents were extremely positive about the video-consultations with a median four point Likert scale = 4 across all questionnaire domainss. In particular parents felt the telemedicine equipment was easy to use. This is especially gratifying as one of the main concerns at the inception of this study was parents having difficulties with the telemedicine equipment.

Parents in the telephone group were also very positive about telephone support. However, direct comparison of video to telephone consultations demonstrates that parents felt that video-consultations were superior in terms of facilitating communication and overall benefit.

Overall health service utilisation was significantly reduced in the video-conferencing group with approximately 40% fewer health service episodes than either telephone or control groups (Table 4). Linear regression of this data demonstrates that patients in the videoconferencing group had significantly fewer health service episodes per week than the telephone support or control group patients despite adjusting for all of the variables described in Table 1 (Adjusted difference in mean [95% confidence interval] 1.Video = -0.5 [-0.8, -0.3], 2. Telephone = +0.1 [-0.2, +0.4] and 3. Control = 0 [reference category]). Health service utilisation costs were accordingly lowest in the videoconference group.

Figure 4. Tele-homecare study protocol

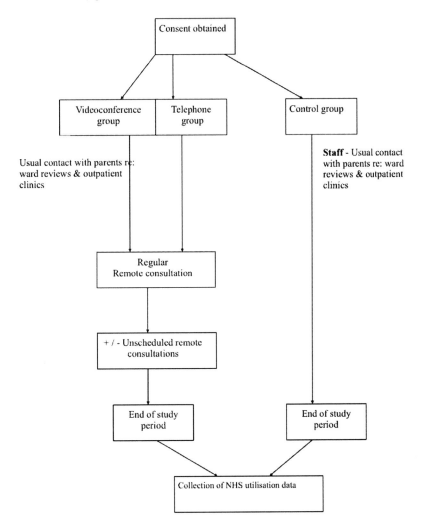

We performed a separate analysis comparing the quality and outcome of videoconsultations performed using ISDN vs IP transmission. We found that there were significantly more frequent technical problmes with internet transmission. The two most common problems were: 1. Loss of audio contact and 2. Requiring more than one attempt to successfully establish the video-link. These problems were almost always surmountable and led to the abandonment of the videoconsultation on only 5 occassions. The clinical utility of the two transmission methods was similar and there was no difference in the parents' perception of the videoconsultation neither was there any difference in frequency of health service utilisation (McCrossan, 2009).

Solutions and Recommendations

Overall our experience with a home support programme facilitated by videoconference consultations demonstrates:

- Real-time video-conferencing between hospital and home is technically feasible.
- The technical quality of videoconferences is sufficient to make clinical judgements.

Table 4. Tele-homecare applications researched in cardiology

Adult			Paediatric		
Home monitoring systems:	Height		Home monitoring systems:	Height	
	Weight			Weight	
	Blood pressure			Blood pressure	
	Pulse oximetry			Pulse oximetry	
	Heart rate			Heart rate	
	Resp rate			Resp rate	
	Spirometry				
ECG			INR (Monitoring warfarin levels)(Bhat, Upponi, Rakecha, & Thomson, 2010)		
Implantable cardiac defibrillators/ pacemakers					
Telestethoscopy					

- Clinicians felt more confident making clinical decisions on the basis of video-consultations compared with telephone consultations.
- Parents' experience of home support is very positive and reassuring.
- Parents expressed greater satisfaction with video-consultations compared with telephone consultations.
- Home support programmes significantly reduce parental anxiety. Home support delivered via video-conferencing results in a significantly greater reduction in anxiety compared with telephone support.
- Real-time videoconferencing may be supported by internet transmission available in most homes in developed countries.

Telemedicine Applied to Stethoscopy

In real-time telemedicine the patient, the clinician sending the data and the clinician receiving the data are working together simultaneously. The expert may guide the referring clinician and thus improve data acquisition and provide an educational experience. Therefore, the tele-link employed needs to be reliable and probably requiers a larger bandwidth to minimise the risk

of interruption. In store and forward studies the data is acquired, digitised and then sent via an internet connection (ie email) or even by post to the receiving clinician. The data may be reviewed at a later, more convenient time. However, there is no opportunity for the receiving clinician to review the quality of data acquired before it is sent. Table 5 summarises some of the key differences between real-time and store-and-forward formats. Certain telemedicine applications and individual clinicians may be better suited to one format over another. Tele-stethoscopy is the area of paediatric cardiology in which there has been the greatest division between real-time and store-and-forward telemedicine studies.

Real-Time, Live Studies

Although remote stethoscopy was reported as early as 1973, the first significant study, from Mattioli and Belmont et al, appeared in 1995(Belmont, Mattioli, Goertz, Ardinger, & Thomas, 1995; Mattioli et al., 1992; Murphy, Block, Bird, & Yurchak, 1973). Auscultation of the heart is a "test" to diagnose and exclude congenital heart disease. Tele-stethoscopy is a "test" comprising two main components: a) the individual examiner interpreting the heart sounds and b)

Table 5. Relative merits of real-time vs. store-and-forward telemedicine

	Advantage	**Disadvantage**
Real-Time	Specialist can guide consultation and data acquisition	More-time consuming for specialist
	Immediate diagnosis and management follows consultation	Requires simultaneous presence of staff at both ends of the tele-link
	Abundant educational opportunities for non-specialist	Requires large bandwidth
Store and Forward	More flexible: specialist and referrer do not need to be present at the same time	Incomplete and or inadequate information may be sent which would impede the specialist giving accurate advice
	Less time consuming for the specialist	Feedback more difficult to provide
	Do not need large bandwidths or videoconferencing equipment	Less educational opportunities
		May demote referrer to the role of "technician"

the telemedicine equipment and link facilitating tele-stethoscopy. Therefore, Mattioloi et al began their study by assessing the level of agreement in "hands-on" examination between the three clinicians using their day-to-day acoustic stethoscopes (AS) followed by hands-on examination using the electronic stethoscopes (ES) employed later in the study. Seventy-eight children were independently examined in this way.

In hands-on examination, there are three different comparisons that can be made between the two examiners: AS vs AS, ES vs ES and ES vs AS. The inter-observer agreement (κ) for the presence or absence of congenital heart disease was - AS vs AS = 0.80, ES vs ES = 0.67 and ES vs AS = 0.65. The study also examined other auscultatory variables including heart sounds and murmur characteristics. There was unsatisfactory agreement with respect to detection of S2 and S3. Having established that there is good to very good inter-examiner agreement in face-to-face auscultation using their own or electronic stethoscopes, the investigators progressed onto a comparison of "hands-on" with telemedicine consultation.

Thirty-eight children were auscultated by hands-on stethoscopy (ES and AS) and ES with transmission of the heart sounds to a remote clinician (TM). The telemedicine consultations occurred in real-time over leased telephone lines with simultaneous 2-way audio-visual contact. The bandwidth available was 384kbps, 32 kbps was allocated to the transmission of the ES output. Inter-observer agreement as to the presence or absence of congenital heart disease was $\kappa = 0.8$ for ES vs TM and $\kappa = 0.64$ for TM vs AS. This initial study suggested that tele-stethoscopy was viable and should be considered for further research.

The same group of investigators proceeded to a separate investigation concentrating on the validation of tele-stethoscopy (Belmont & Mattioli, 2003). Seventy-six patients were examined by face-to-face consultation using an acoustic stethoscope (reference standard) and by telemedicine consultation. A 2-D echocardiogram was also performed to confirm or refute the clinical findings. Tele-stethoscopy was considered clinically useful ($\kappa > 0.6$) for detecting murmurs, distinguishing specific murmurs (innocent, pathological, vibratory, diastolic aortic, diastolic pulmonary) and diagnosing congenital heart disease ($\kappa = 0.63$). However, agreement was poor for assessing heart sounds and presence of clicks ($\kappa < 0.5$). When tele-stethoscopy was compared with echocardiography, the results were less satisfactory for the diagnosis of innocent/pathological murmurs ($\kappa = 0.55$, Sensitivity $= 0.82$, Specificity $= 0.75$).

In particular, Belmont found that remote stethoscopy's accuracy suffered in younger children ($\kappa = 0.29$). Consequently, Belmont et al conclude that remote stethoscopy provided accurate, dependable detection of congenital heart disease but only in children five years old and above.

A smaller study was conducted by another group from the USA. McConnell et al evaluated 21 children, with murmurs, initially by face-face examination and then with a tele-stethoscopy system transmitted across a 768Kbps (ISDN 12) tele-link. Using the hands-on diagnosis as the reference standard, the telemedicine diagnosis was accurate in 19/21 cases. 2 small ventricular septal defects were missed by tele-stethoscopy. McConnell et al also examined the frequency of ancillary investigations and patient satisfaction for both consultation types. Request of additional investigations was similar following each consultation format. Patient satisfaction for the telemedicine consultation was reportedly high (McConnell, Steed, Tichenor, & Hannon, 1999).

A similar study to that of Mattioli was performed at this institution by Grant et al. Prior to the telestethoscopy test, the performance of two paediatric cardiologists' at acoustic auscultation was compared in a study with 39 children. There was excellent agreement between the two examiners as to the presence or absence of CHD (κ –score $= 0.87$). Having established the diagnostic equivalence of the two examiners, Grant proceeded to the telemedicine arm of the study. This was a real-time, live evaluation of a bespoke PC-based tele-stethoscope. The telemedicine equipment is described in more detail later in this chapter. Thirty-nine children all unknown to the examiners (33 new patients and six patients with established pathology) were examined initially face-to-face by one of the examiners and then remotely by the other examiner. Each paediatric cardiologist undertook a similar number of face-to-face and telemedicine consultations. The reference standard was based upon the clinical findings from the face-to-face examination. There was a high level of agreement observed with respect to the presence or absence of CHD (κ –score $= 0.82$). There was also a good level of agreement in the discernment of heart sound II (κ -score $=0.64$). (Grant, 2006)

Store and Forward Studies

In 2002, a Norwegian group published a remote stethoscopy study using a very different protocol. Heart sounds from 47 patients were sampled and recorded using an electronic stethoscope and sent as an e-mail attachment to a remote computer (7 with no murmur, 20 with innocent murmurs and 20 with pathological murmurs). Having retrieved the 47 recordings, 100 sound clips were compiled in a CD by repeating the initial recordings a variable number of times. The 100 sound clips were then assessed by four paediatric cardiologists at a later time. The mean analysis time per clip was 2.1 minutes. The investigators presented results for sensitivity, specificity and inter-observer agreement (κ -score). The mean inter-observer agreement in classifying the cases (presence or absence of congenital heart disease) was very good $\kappa = 0.81$. The mean sensitivity and specificity in classifying cases were 89.7% and 98.2%, respectively, which is excellent. Although Dahl et al do not present auxillary examination details e.g. detection of a murmur or normality of heart sounds, this study indicates that a "store and forward" protocol has the potential to be an accurate and efficient method of screening children with cardiac murmurs (Dahl, Hasvold, Arild, & Hasvold, 2002).

A further store and forward study was published by Finley et al in 2007. Fifty-five children known to have a murmur and considered significantly co-operative to take part in the study were enrolled. Heart sounds were acquired in a similar fashion as the Norwegian study but transmitted directly to a PC via an infra-red connection. The sound clips were blindly assessed by three paediatric cardiologists for clarity of heart sounds, nature of

2nd heart sound, murmur characteristics and final diagnosis. For the presence or absence of CHD, the mean sensitivity was 93%, specificity was 86%, positive predictive value was 94% and negative predictive value was 86%. The mean inter-observer agreement was $\kappa = 0.62$. Finley et al did not suffer any decrease in accuracy amongst younger children. In 14% of evaluations the recordings were considered unclear. However, this did not significantly impact on the diagnostic accuracy $(p = 0.18)$. Finley et al envisage this application as a useful method of triaging patients with murmurs. Despite employing a store and forward protocol, the researchers conclude by stating that auscultation education for referring physicians is crucial to allow appropriate selection of patients for specialist evaluation. How this education is to be delivered is not discussed in this paper. However, the issue of promoting auscultation skills in non-specialists is important (Finley, Warren, Sharratt, & Amit, 2006).

Although this chapter is mostly concerned with telemedicine applications to paediatric cardiology, there are two adult studies which merit discussion. Both studies are from Fragasso et al, an Italian group of adult cardiologists. Their first study, appearing in 2003, evaluated the feasibility and accuracy of a self-built, PC based tele-stethoscopy system using a live, real-time internet protocol (Fragasso et al., 2003). One-hundred and three cardiac patients were auscultated across an internet link with the physician blinded to the identity of the patient. The patients were then examined face-to-face by the same clinician in random order. The reference standard was 2-D echocardiography. Tele-auscultation was accurate in 92% of cases. In 8/103 patients the murmur described by tele-auscultation was incorrect. In no cases was a diagnosis of normal made when pathology present. The authors viewed this application as an adjunct to tele-homecare.

In a recent study, Fragasso et al, progressed to a purpose built tele-stethoscopy system, identical to that used in this study (Fragasso et al., 2007).

Fifty adult patients with heart failure (New York Heart Association grade II – IV) were assessed by hands-on auscultation followed by remote stethoscopy. There were two examiners, one face-to-face examiner and one telemedicine examiner, with no cross over. There was no pre-study validation between the two examiners. Both examiners had access to the patients' clinical notes containing details of previous cardio-pulmonary examinations.

It is not explicit in this study what the main outcome measures were. Presence of individual heart sounds (S1 - S4), qualitative specifics and magnitude of the murmur were considered. However, a diagnosis based on the auscultatory findings was not presented. Pulmonary auscultatory details were also documented.

Fragasso reports that tele-stethoscopy had 96% accuracy with the only mistakes being made in respiratory sounds. However, the physician's knowledge of the patient's diagnosis and previous clinical findings may well have biased the examination and positively skewed the reported accuracy. Indeed Fragasso believes that it would not be appropriate to utilise this system without knowledge of the patient's baseline cardiac and pulmonary examination. Fragasso also highlights that the remote physician's intervention was important for positioning the stethoscope and maintaining firm contact with the skin.

We conducted two studies at our own institution (ISDN6 and IP 128kbps) which support real-time tele-stethoscopy as a valuable tool in the outpatient setting. Both studies demonstrated high levels of inter-observer agreement. In the latter study conducted by myself, there was agreement in 95% (40/42) with respect to the presence or absence of a murmur, κ – statistic = 0.81, indicating very good agreement. There was also a good level of agreement as to whether the murmur was innocent or pathological, κ – statistic = 0.72. There was very good agreement between FF and TM in the specific diagnosis reached following each consultation, κ – statistic = 0.82. In 12% of cases (5/42), TM diagnosis was incorrect with respect to FF diagnosis. Two false positive and two false negative. There was also very good agreement in terms of the broad categorisation of diagnosis into presence or absence of CHD, κ – statistic = 0.80. Remote consultations were not associated with greater requests for echocardiography. Contrary to previous studies, age did not appear to adversely affect diagnostic accuracy.(McCrossan, 2009)

Problems

A major limitation of the real-time tele-stethoscopy studies discussed above is one that is constant throughout the evolution of telemedicine systems. The telemedicine systems employed to date, including this institutions' initial experience, have been self-built PC based systems. Self-built, stand alone telemedicine equipment is not supported technically by outside agencies and therefore requires on-site expertise to remedy any problems as they arise. Such a requirement would act as a deterrent to many institutions otherwise interested in telemedicine applications. Self-built systems tend to consist of components from different manufacturers which have variable compatibility. Upgrades in software in one particular company may not take account of the effect on compatibility with other systems. In fact some companies may actively seek to impede inter-product compatibility in order to protect their market share.(Questmark, 2008) It is difficult to replicate self-built systems and so scalability and standardisation of systems is limited.

We learnt this lesson the hard way! An elegant study by Grant et al conducted at our own department utilised a bespoke PC-based tele-stethoscopy system. We attempted to repeat this study as a prelude to performing actual remote clinics. However, despite many permutations of equipment the tele-stethoscopy system was not resucitatable. An alternative system from Aethra became available and we used this equipment in a further feasibility study. This system had the major advantage that

it could be supported by the manufacturer and by the seller. This system worked very well and facilitated high quality remote stethoscopy with similar results to published studies.

Solutions and Recommendations

Our experience in remote stethoscopy demonstrates very clearly the potential pitfalls in using bespoke, purpose built, telemedicine systems. Once a problem occurred with the system it was difficult to locate where the difficulty originated and if there was more than one problem. Even as a department experienced in telemedicine, and in this application, we were unable to proceed. This set of circumstances is not conducive to fostering wide spread adaption of a telemedicine application. In order to roll out this application of telemedicine into a routine service provided in rural hospitals, apart from being accurate, the equipment needs to be user friendly, reliable and must have technical support.

In our opinion such requirements are difficult to fulfil unless commercially built systems are validated and widely available. It is important to have acess to rapid expert technical assisstance should a fault occur. This is generally possible through support contracts with the seller or directly with the manufacturer.

The relative merits of store and forward vs real-time remote stethoscopy have been discussed. Although there may be an advantage to real-time tele-stehoscopy in acquiring quality data, busy clinical schedules may constrain uptake of this format. Greater adoption of remote stethoscopy using a store and forward format may be more likely especially if referrals to tertiary clinics come on-line. There is the possibility that clinical details, ECG, chest X-ray and heart sounds may be forwarded to the cardiologist for consideration resulting in more effective triaging of the outpatient service.

Economic Evaluation of Telemedicine Activities

In any health service, resources are limited. Choices always need to be made concerning resource deployment. Economic evaluation provides organised consideration of the factors involved and attempts to link costs with consequences to facilitate a decision to commit resources to one use instead of another (Drummond, Sculpher, Torrence, O'Brien, & Stoddart, 2005a). For telemedicine to become widely disseminated and incorporated into routine practice, decision makers in healthcare (those who deliver and fund health services) require assurance that telemedicine provides good value for money (Hailey, Ohinmaa, & Roine, 2004). However, to date there has not been enough conclusive proof to convince decision makers that telemedicine will generate rates of return on investments (D. L. Smith, 2005). This requires evidence of the attendant costs and potential savings and outcomes of telemedicine programs from well conducted studies.

Almost every published telemedicine study, reporting cost data, comments that there are few studies providing such economic evaluation. Most reported studies are small scale, methodologically flawed and are not based on control trials. In 2002, Whitten et al, performed a meta-analysis of cost-benefit studies relating to telemedicine. Of 612 potential articles, only 55 reported cost data and only 24 were suitable for meta-analysis. Although 56% of studies reported cost savings, the authors caution against making generalisable conclusions due to the variation in economic analysis, short duration of the studies and small sample size. A recommendation is made that future research is conducted in accordance with generally accepted, standards for health economic analysis (Whitten, Mair, Haycox, May, Williams, & Hellmich, 2002a). Knowledge of these agreed standards is important and not always evident in telemedicine literature.

Jacklin et al published an economic evaluation from a large randomised control trial of teleconsultations for patients referred by their GPs to a wide range of specialists in England. Over a six month period, 2,100 patients were randomised to either traditional face-to-face consultation or telemedicine consultations. The cost per patient was higher in the telemedicine group (mean difference per patient = £99). This study also captured the patients' personal costs and loss of productivity. Patients in the telemedicine group incurred lower personal costs (mean difference per patient= £8) and cost society less money from loss of productive time (mean difference per patient = £11). The authors comment that the scope of the study was perhaps too wide. Sub-analysis showed that certain specialties may be more appropriate for virtual outreach clinics than others and improved selection of patients may also improve the relative cost effectiveness (Jacklin et al., 2003).

An Australian group published a cost-minimisation study comparing the actual cost of providing a telemedicine consultation service for a paediatric population with a hypothetical alternative of no telemedicine service available. This study suggests, over a five year period, that the telemedicine service has produced a net saving of approximately AS\$ 600,000 to the healthcare provider (A. C. Smith, Scuffham, & Wootton, 2007).

The two studies quoted demonstrate that economic evaluations of telemedicine studies are not easily transferable due to:

- The clinical practices particular to an individual specialty.
- The location of the study – e.g. savings made from avoiding transport to a centre 1000km distant compared with 10km are likely to be very different.
- Health authorities in individual countries/ states have different models of purchasing and providing health care.

In short, for telemedicine to supplant or augment an existing service, it is important to recognise that a particular service may be highly clinically and cost effective in one context but highly ineffective when transferred to another context (Whitten, Mair, Haycox, May, Williams, & Hellmich, 2002a). It is not that generalisations can never be made but that caution is needed in transferring conclusions from one set of circumstances to another.

An important development has been in the shift away from cost-minimisation studies towards cost-effectiveness studies following the publication of Michael Drummond's textbook "Methods for the Economic Evaluation of HeralthCare Programmes"(Drummond, Sculpher, Torrence, O'Brien, & Stoddart, 2005a).

Economic Evaluation of Telemedicine in Paediatric Cardiology

There have been even fewer economic analyses of telemedicine application in paediatric cardiology. Most of the reports are from the paediatric cardiology department at the Royal Brompton Hospital, London, in conjunction with health economists from Brunel University. Subspecialty opinions are offered in fetal cardiology and paediatric cardiology for both neonates and older children. The Brompton hospital utilises a combination of real-time and store and forward telemedicine to deliver the service. In their published studies, the control group consists of patients conventionally referred for paediatric cardiology assessment from the four DGHs in the network. This group have published three articles whose main interest has been economic evaluation. Whilst the introduction and discussion sections of these papers lucidly describe the potential role of telemedicine in paediatric cardiology, the results in the economic analysis are less straight forward. Using Bootstrapping, NHS costs are calculated for the initial consultation and then at 14 days

and again at six months. Bootstrapping is an increasingly employed technique that estimates confidence intervals for cost analyses without making assumptions as to the distribution of the data (Drummond, Sculpher, Torrence, O'Brien, & Stoddart, 2005b). Costs are presented for: all four hospitals, the three hospitals with level 2 neonatal units and an individual analysis for one of the hospitals. The results suggest that, for all four hospitals, the mean cost of implementing and running the telemedicine service is higher at each time interval than conventional referral. However, owing to the large standard deviation, these differences are not statistically significant. For the three hospitals with level 2 neonatal units, telemedicine care was more expensive on the initial consultation day but became lower than conventional care at 14 days and six months. Again these differences are not statistically significant. The separate analysis of the Basildon DGH demonstrated that telemedicine care was significantly cheaper on the initial consultation day but then was not significantly different at 14 days and six months.

This analysis of the full range of paediatric tele-cardiology services is valuable. However, the amalgamation of the services evaluated, the different populations involved (fetuses, neonates and children) and the different telemedicine formats employed make it difficult to elicit generalisable conclusions. For any paediatric cardiology centre considering embarking on a telemedicine programme it is perhaps more helpful to individually assess the separate components of a tele-cardiology service.

To this end, the Brompton group describe an economic evaluation of their experience of a fetal tele-cardiology service. One of the four DGHs within the telemedicine network, also sends pre-recorded fetal echocardiograms from pregnancies meeting the criteria for referral to a fetal cardiology service. A before and after cohort design was employed. The authors conclude that the telemedicine assessment was more costly than a face-to-face examination in London (£206 vs £74 per patient, p < 0.001). However, using bootstrapped NHS costs, the telemedicine service became cost neutral at 14 days and six months. This study allows the reader to make more definite conclusions as to what the costs and savings of providing a similar fetal tele-cardiology service in their own region (Dowie, Mistry, Young, Franklin, & Gardiner, 2008).

Sicotte et al performed a cost-effectiveness analysis of a paediatric cardiology telemedicine program in Quebec. They found that whilst telemedicine care increased effectiveness and was cost saving for the patient, it represented a supplementary cost to the health service of approximately £750 per patient. In this study it was estimated that telemedicine consultations reduced patient journeys by 42% but only 12% of patients avoided an inter-hospital transfer. This much lower calculation of avoided transfers seems to mitigate against remote diagnosis of CHD. However, the study group was very different from the population under investigation in other studies. The mean age was 2.4 years and only 56% consultations related to CHD (Sicotte, Lehoux, Van Doesburg, Cardinal, & Leblanc, 2004).

Another criticism of cost analyses involving telemedicine projects is that they are based upon start up programs where the initial burst of interest and activity decreases the unit cost of a tele-consultation (Roine, Ohinmaa, & Hailey, 2001). Telemedicine cost analyses have been criticised for being small scale, short term pragmatic evaluations. In a systematic review of cost effectiveness studies in telemedicine, Whitten et al concluded that there is no good evidence that telemedicine is cost effective (Whitten & Cook, 1999).

At our institution we have recently conducted two cost-analyses of telemedicine projects. The first related to the neonatal tele-echocardiography study. Over an 8 year period, each DGH made a cost saving through the avoidance of ambulance transfers of patients to the tertiary unit despite

the relatively high start-up and running costs associated with ISDN6 lines. The tertiary unit did not bill for its services. The results presented in this study may not be representative of working practices across all paediatric cardiology units considering undertaking a telemedicine service. However, to increase generalisability and reduce regional variation, expert opinion (in conjunction with best practice guidelines) were used to estimate staff input at each stage of the process and PSSRU unit cost data were used. The aim of the analysis was to be transparent, such that individual units could substitute data from their situation to estimate if the cost savings achieved in Belfast could be transferred to their setting.

Ideally, a randomised controlled clinical trial would have been performed to determine cost and outcome differences between groups using patient specific data, however, this was not the original intent of the research. Similarly, it would have been useful to collect costs borne/saved by the family to ensure that no 'cost-shifting' occurred. This too was beyond the scope of this particular study. However, in light of the clinical utility of telemedicine in the remote diagnosis and exclusion of CHD, it is debatable whether a randomised control trial would be possible for a range of ethical and practical reasons (A. C. Smith, 2007).

The second cost-analysis has yet to be published but relates to the home support programme. There are obviously attendant costs to setting up and running a telehome care system for patients. The costs for any project are obviously specific to each setting but they may be generalised in start up and running costs. The start-up (Capital) costs consist of purchasing the telemedicine/ tele-homecare equipment. Therefore, they become more economical the greater number of patients enrolled into the project. The running costs consist of the fresh expense incurred each time a new patient is enrolled into tele-homecare The running costs may be sub-divided into the fixed costs associated with each installation and the running costs (Table

6). The start-up costs per patient were relatively cheap in both groups as the equipment was used repeatedly throughout the study. The running costs were significantly cheaper for internet transmission because the installation and especially rental of ISDN lines were very expensive. Therefore the overall cost per patient was significantly greater when using ISDN 6 transmission.

As described earlier, the patients in the video group had less health service episodes when compared with both the telephone support and control groups. The costs to the health service were consequently lowest in the video group. Therefore, we concluded that a telemedicine home support programme for infants with major CHD, facilitated by ADSL transmission, apart from its other benefits, may be cost saving to the health service.

Two other issues are pertinent to the future development of telemedicine services – the falling cost of telemedicine technology and learning effects. If as expected the cost of technology continues to fall, this will serve to increase the cost difference between care pathways, in essence strengthening the argument for use of this technology. However, the safety and efficacy of such next generation technology would need to be assured. Furthermore, in other telemedicine studies, learning effects have been attributed to the technology. Wootton et al estimated that the introduction of real time teledermatology (compared with conventional outpatient dermatological care) reduced the need for GP training by 6.3 days, at a cost of approximately £6,123.60 (Wootton et al., 2000). It is possible that remote diagnosis via telemedicine may confer upon staff in the DGHs some additional learning, expertise and confidence in their decision-making.

As a footnote to the importance of economic evaluation in the development and implementation of telemedicine applications we would add this: Economic evaluation is not the most important consideration. Patient outcomes are the key factor. Most cost-analyses should be treated with caution.

There have been very few innovations in healthcare that actually save the health service money. If a new tool improves patient care and professional working practices without costing a lot of money then it is worthwhile. However, demonstrating a clear cost-analysis is a vital component of a business case to convince health service managers to invest in a project.

Solutions and Recommendations

The economic solution depends on the economic problem. I shall briefly summarise our approach to two key issues.

1. **Economic considerations in starting a telemedicine application:** In the next section we shall discuss the importance of selecting an appropriate application. The economic implications of a telemedicine application very much depend on its success as a clinical tool. It is essential that a well designed trial is conducted in order to properly evaluate the clinical effect of the application but also to acquire data on which economic decisions may be made. To this end, employ a health economist to help design the study and analyse the economic data. One should use recognised methodology and attempt to make the study generalisable and therefore capable of replication. It is very important (the health economist will advice this) to link costs with a measurable outcome such as mortality or QALY (Quality Life Adjusted Year). It is advisable to concentrate the study on an individual application rather than a combination of servcies because there is a risk that the results become convoluted and diluted.

2. **Economic considerations in developing a service:** It is much easier to persuade health service funders and managers to invest resources into a telemedicine servcie if you have a track record of using telemedicine and

Table 6. Comparitive cost providing home support via ISDN compared with IP

		ISDN		IP	
		Hospital	Home	Hospital	Home
Fixed Costs	VC equipment installation	++	++	++	++
	Line installation	++	++	+	+
	Internet Router (re-programmed)	n/a	n/a	+	+
	Total per patient	Relatively expensive		Relatively cheap	
Capital Costs (Annual cost)	VC codec	++++	++++	++++	++++
	Technical support for codec	++	++	++	++
	Pulse oximeter	0	++	0	++
	Internet Routers (new)	n/a	n/a	++	0
	Total per patient	Realtively cheap		Relatively cheap	
Running Costs	Line rental	+++++	+++++	+	++
	Phone calls	0	++	0	0
	Running costs per patient	++	+++++	+	+
	Total per patient	Expensive		Very cheap	

have demonstrated its benefit for patients and the health servcie. The difference between developing the service and the research phase is working out the day-to-day management of a service. It impresses health service managers to be presented with a detailed description of what equipment and personnel are required and how they will be employed i.e. how the money will be spent. Health service managers are predominantly interested in what will save them money - not the patient!

It is highly advisable to continue auditing the service both from a clinical and economic perspective in order to justify future funding.

What Makes for Successful Telemedicine (and Telemedicine Research)

One of the leading figures in telemedicine, Richard Wootton, states that three components are essential for successful telemedicine (Harnett, 2006):

1. The personnel
2. The technology
3. A liberal measure of perseverance

To this I would add: Money!

Personnel

People with the necessary skills to undertake the clinical components are necessary. They must be comfortable with this mode of healthcare delivery. They must also understand its limitations as well as its potential.

There is a lot of background work required to ensure that a telemedicine research trial runs smoothly. Therefore, we advice that a research fellow is specifically funded to write grant applications, co-ordinate consultations, complete paperwork and write up the results. Depending on the clinical experience of the research fellow he/she may also be involved clinically in the project. In setting up a service, it is very useful to have an administrator dedicated to the telemedicine service.

Technology

The technical aspect is in many ways the most straightforward part of a telemedicine system. Once the telemedicine system has been set-up it usually requires little technical support.

There are numerous options, each with their own advantages and disadvantages. As with any medical device, reliability is the most important factor.

Perseverance

At least one committed individual is needed with the perseverance to overcome the inertia inherent in all established clinical routines.

In addition to these considerations, some specific points merit attention. Telemedicine applications tend to be more successful the greater the distance separating the expert and remote site (Finley et al., 1997). The expected cost is also a major factor in the development of telemedicine projects (D. L. Smith, 2005). Probably even more important is the expected "hassle" associated with telemedicine. The perceived or actual nuisance of using telemedicine can be overcome by improvements in user friendliness, employing dedicated technical support and the perceived benefits of using telemedicine. This leads on to what is, in my opinion, the vital component that must be present – the clinical need.

Telemedicine should only be applied to areas in which there is a recognised problem that could be helped by connecting people who are not normally in the same location. Telemedicine should not be applied merely because the technology is available and it is feasible to conduct a research trial. The fuel that drives telemedicine applications into routine practice is a continued clinical need which is identified by both the provider (expert) and the user (patient or generalist).

Outlining the clinical need for telemedicine within one's own practice will help define the research question. However, before purchasing any equipment or installing any transmission modalities it is important to consider which telemedicine format is most suited to the purpose of the proposed telemedicine application.

Project Funding

Research of any kind requires money! There are several sources for this and all should be explored.

University: The vast majority of paediatric cardiology units are situated in teaching hospitals affiliated to a university. University grants require a detailed and considered research proposal. They are more successful if led by a supervisor experienced in university research.

Healthcare organisation: This is a less reliable source of funding as most small scale research associated with healthcare will be channeled through the universities. However, if available it should be applied for. If your unit is not a "professorial unit" i.e. no direct links to a university, then this may be a more successful route.

Government Agencies: Telemedicine is recognised by governments across the globe as a potential means of improving patient access to care and reducing costs. There are substantial grants available for projects. However, government sources of funding are more likely to be granted to established researchers who are building a service. This point will be explained in more detail later.

Charitable Sources: Ranging from Welcome Trust grants to small scale charities associated with individual units, charities are a very important source of funding. Most hospitals have a charity associated with the entire hospital or separate charities with closer links to individual services. Our experience with charitable sources is very positive. Telemedicine research, is very acceptable to patient charities because it is patient centred and the families derive an immediate benefit from the application e.g. better access to the specialist.

Industry: Collaboration with industry can be very helpful in conducting any type of research and telemedicine is no different. There are two principal elements in the industrial sector of telemedicine: The manufacturers and the retail/technical support agencies. The manufacturers are making moves towards directly selling telemedicine equipment and providing day-to-day technical support vital to videoconferencing and telemedicine. However, most of the purchaser/seller interface still involves the independent videoconferencing retail/support companies.

It is obviously in the industry's interests that telemedicine research trials are conducted. They are therefore a potential source of funding or may lend equipment free of charge or at reduced rates. The independent retail/support companies can be an invaluable resource in terms of providing technical guidance, lending hardware, sourcing equipment at reduced fees and may even provide services free of charge.

Developing a Service

This is undoubtedly the pitfall of telemedicine. Far too few sustained clinical services have been built with respect to the number of research trials that have been published. Most of the reasons for this have been touched on before (Table 7).

Although funding is a major issue, this is not the most common problem (most people don't even apply for long term funding). The two main reasons that telemedicine research fails to translate into clinical services are:

- The initial idea did not address a real, pressing clinical problem.
- Cannot convince other clinical personnel outside of your institution that it is in their interests to turn this application into a clinical service.

The first reason feeds into the second. You might believe that there is a real problem with current service provision and think that telemedicine will help address it. However, health care professionals/managers at the referring end may not see it in this light and may be content with the current arrangement. Hopefully, the evidence from a well conducted research trial will support your claims and be convincing! However, personal relationships and building up a network of interested professionals is a key factor. Perseverance is crucial.

Funding a Service

Funding a telemedicine service requires more money and a longer outlook. If a telemedicine application is to become incorporated into a clinical service then it requires sufficient funding like other clinical services. This point is often underestimated! As outlined above, colleagues may be persuaded into "helping out" with a research project for a defined period of time but are unlikely to be sufficiently enthused to continue, unpaid, with the level of attention required to deliver a consistent clinical service.

The first step is to decide the aims of the service. Who is it aimed at? What are the benefits and how will you check that the service is delivering these benefits? These are key questions because a regular clinical service business case would also be expected to satisfactorily address these points. Do not make unrealistic claims regarding the potential of the service. Whilst it is not essential that the service is derived from your own research project it does lead to more reliable answers to these questions.

For example, a tele-homecare programme may aim:

1. To be acceptable to patients and health professionals.
2. To be time saving for health professionals and patients.
3. To reduce the number of face-to-face contacts with health professionals.
4. To reduce admissions to hospital.
5. To be cost saving to the health service and/or patient.

Table 7. Factors (real and perceived) which influence the success of a telemedicine enterprise

Helpful	Unhelpful
Clinical need	Application was not a good idea
Enthusiastic personnel	Apllication not practicable
Reliable technology	Telemedicine is a "hassle"
Perseverance	Researcher loses interest
Funding	Can't secure long-term funding
Good relationships with referring colleagues	Can't find suitable personnel to carry on service after research period

The benefits to the patient and health care system are contained within the aims. Although not research, clinical governance should prompt ongoing audit of the service and comparing outcomes with a previous era.

The second step to detail how the service is to be run, who is involved and what equipment is required. A telemedicine service should be run by health professionals competent to meet the needs of the clinical situation just as in hospital. Administrative staff may be an important part of a telemedicine team but only health professionals are suitably trained to deal with clinical situations and data. Preferably more experienced staff should be involved at the beginning to ensure the best possible start. A successful service will largely depend upon finding clinical staff who will identify with the need for and perceive an advantage from involvement in the telemedicine service. For example, an improvement in their patients' care or streamlining referral practices.

The equipment necessary is dictated by the nature of the telemedicine service. Close links with industrial representatives and networking with colleagues experienced in telemedicine will aid in this process.

The third step is to calculate the costs and potential savings. On this point, well conducted economic evaluation incorporated into a clinical trial of the application is vital. We strongly recommend enlisting the support of a qualified health economist in calculating the costs. It is not simply a matter of adding up the salaries of

everyone involved and the cost of purchasing/running the equipment. Your business case will taken much more seriously if you due attention is given to this point.

Calculating savings is more complex and may require evidence to support claims. Unless identical research has been performed elsewhere it will probably be necessary to perform one's own cost-analysis which in turn necessitates a research trial. As there are very few standardised telemedicine programmes, transferring cost-analyses from one clinical setting to another is hazardous and may be greeted with skepticism by healthcare managers.

It is also important to identify who will be making the potential saving. Most telemedicine applications will at the very least save the patient/family money. They may save society money through less days off work etc. However, these are not considerations that healthcare organisations are particularly concerned with. In fact current health economic studies avoid analysis of the patient/societal perspective. Therefore it is advantageous to demonstrate that hospitals - either the referring hospital or the tertiary centre will make savings due to a more efficient use of healthcare resources. Although this sounds daunting, it should be possible as this is one of the keys aims of telemedicine after all!

The fourth step is to identify possible sources of funding. The sources available are the same as for research but the suitability and likelihood of funding a service is different. Ideally, a telemedicine clinical service should be recognised by the bodies which fund healthcare organisations and become incorporated into the department's budget. This is the most stable source of funding but probably the most difficult to achieve. Health service organisations recognise that once a service has been recognised and permanently funded, it is difficult (but not impossible) to withdraw that funding. In the UK the most secure method is for telemedicine activities be incorporated into a consultant job plan. This is possible but only when the doctor has a proven track record of publishing research and a significant ongoing clinical commitment to telemedicine. In the US it is to have telemedicine activities reimbursed by Medicare and private health insurance companies. This is perhaps a better model for funding because it is more flexible and allows for expansion of a service without having to repeat the whole funding application process.

Government agencies often have separate agencies concerned with promoting translational research. These are generally defined but considerable sums of money. The money has to be used and will be granted to the most suitable applicant. In our experience, the application process, whilst thorough, is not as time consuming as research ethics proposals. These bodies are an ideal source of medium term funding but as stated the sum of money available is set and will run out! Again having a proven track record of researching and publishing in telemedicine will greatly enhance ones chance of successfully securing this type of funding because the agencies concerned have to justify how the money has been distributed.

The telemedicine industry may be willing to fill some of the gap in funding (although obviously not all) but it is not healthy for a clinical service to be financially dependent on a commercial enterprise. Complications in terms of the choice of hardware and which projects receive funding are bound to occur.

Research charities such as the Welcome Trust are unlikely to fund a clinical service but may provide longer term funding for an ambitious research project that could result in a clinical ser-

vice. Charities specific to your medical specialty are more likely to fund a telemedicine service if it is perceived as providing a superior service to patients. Charities may help fund a service by contributing to the salary of a nurse specialist who would be actively involved in the telemedicine service. Large charities such as the British Heart Foundation have a long history of a secure income and fund many specialist nurses. However, much of this funding remains on short-term contracts and cannot be completely relied upon.

Smaller local charities attached to individual hospitals and units may offer a reliable longterm source of funding depending on how much money they have and how much you need! Close collaboration between the interested parties can result in a clinical service tailored to meet the wishes of the patients represented by the charity and the needs of the health professionals. However, it should not be the role of charities to fund clinical services. Ideally telemedicine services should be funded as part of the overall clinical budget. All other sources should be seen as temporising.

TRANSLATING RESEARCH INTO CLINICAL SERVICE

Difference between Conducting Research and Running a Telemedicine Service

The litmus test for a telemedicine application is whether it is translated into a sustained clinical service. Conducting a research trial, whilst challenging, is easier because there is an initial burst of enthusiasm and activity. The novelty of the telemedicine hardware is alluring and it is possible to persuade colleagues to give up their professional time, free of charge, for a defined period. Often there is a backlog of patients ideally suited to the application waiting to be included in the trial. This can skew the usefulness of the application as short term studies often present results as indicative of normal working patterns. In reality there is usually a slow down in the use of the telemedicine equipment following a research trial.

Research trials are usually under the auspices of an academic body such as a university. There are stringent regulations to conducting research involving human subjects. The ethical approval process is time consuming. Often there are separate governance bodies for the university, health care organisation and the central government body. This can be off-putting but gets easier with practice!!

Starting up a clinical service (apart from the financial considerations) can be more straight forward but sometimes not. If your healthcare organisation deem that the application in question has not been sufficiently tested, then there will be a lengthy process of proving its safety and efficacy. However, our experience with telemedicine applications is that this is not usually a problem. This is may partly be due to the services in question emanating from research trials conducted within our department. As has been stressed earlier, the key driving factor is the presence of a clinical need for the application.

Differences between Inter/ Intra-Hospital and Community Telemedicine Services

Inter-Hospital Telemedicine

This usually occurs between a tertiary centre and a DGH involving two or more health care professionals discussing a patient's case. In paediatric cardiology the consultation will usually contain the transmission of data for expert evaluation e.g. neonatal and fetal echocardiograms, heart sounds but also ECGs and chest radiographs.

Intra-Hospital Telemedicine (or within a Healthcare Organisation)

In this scenario, videoconferencing is usually being employed to facilitate meetings of healthcare professionals, often inter-disciplinary, who are working at different campuses e.g. joint oncology meetings. This is especially well deployed in rural DGH networks. It is also an application that is more likely to acquire funding because these meetings often involve healthcare managers!

In both inter and intra hospital telemedicine, there is the benefit that the service may be shared by several users thereby diluting the start up and running costs.

Hospital to Community

In this setting there is a direct connection between patient and healthcare professional. The patient stays in their own home. The equipment is fixed for the tele-care duration in one patient's home. It may obviously be re-used but is a less efficient use of telemedicine hardware and more expensive per patient than the other two scenarios. However, these applications are perhaps closest to the ultimate aim of telemedicine: to improve public access to expert opinion and keeping patients out of hospital. Our experience of tele-homecare in the form of videoconferencing, but also telephone calls, is very positive. Patients/ parents are extremely grateful for the individual attention accorded. Home monitoring programmes probably induce less appreciation but current evidence also demonstrates patients not only accepting but being reassured by the presence of remote monitoring systems and the extra check that is being kept on their health.

POTENTIAL FOR TELEMEDICINE TO CHANGE CURRENT HEALTHCARE WORKING PRACTICES AND FLOW OF PATIENTS THROUGH A HEALTH SERVICE

Neonatal Tele-Echocardiography

As this is the best established telemedicine application in paediatric cardiology, the effect on healthcare processes and patients is best understood. Without the availability of telemedicine, all newborns suspected of having major CHD are transferred to the tertiary unit for hands-on assessment by a paediatric cardiologist including an echocardiogram (Figure 6). The transfer involves medical ambulance (or air) transportation. Subsequently, the patient is either admitted to the tertiary unit or transferred back to the DGH.

In the presence of a telemedicine programme, newborns suspected of having major CHD have a tele-consultation performed by a paediatrician/ cardiac sonographer with guidance by a paediatric cardiologist. The consultation also involves relaying details of the clinical history and examination and evaluation of the chest- x-ray and ECG. At the end of the tele-consultation a decision is made by the paediatric cardiologist as to any specific cardiac therapy required and the necessity of urgent or elective transfer to the tertiary unit or whether the patient is best managed at the DGH neonatal unit.

The effect of this telemedicine application on patients is very clear and beneficial. Those infants with major CHD are correctly identified and transferred to the paediatric cardiology unit for ongoing management. Sick babies without major CHD are also correctly identified and avoid the risk of medical transfer and their management may be focused more appropriately at the DGH neonatal unit.

The effect of this telemedicine applications on health professionals is more complex and difficult to predict. For the paediatrician at the referring site, a tele-echocardiography service means a responsibility to keep up echocardiography skills so that an effective tele-echocardiogram may be performed. However he/she is supported by the paediatric cardiologist in real-time telemedicine. The paediatricians will have less, stressful inter-hospital transfers to perform. This is also true for ambulance crews and accompanying nursing staff (see Figure 5).

The sick baby, in whom major CHD cannot be excluded, is a stressful situation for paediatricians in DGHs. The paediatrician does not want to transfer every baby with cyanosis to the tertiary unit as it is potentially hazardous for the patient and would not reflect well on them as most of these patients will not have significant CHD. The availability of telemedicine takes the stress out of this scenario. The issue may be resolved quickly and reliability with a tele-consultation.

There is the potential for this service to be overused and abused. However, this has not been our experience with four DGHs over 15 years.

For the paediatric cardiologist, this use of telemedicine changes working practices by necessitating a different skill set:

- (Patiently) guiding the sonographer/paediatrician through the echocardiogram.
- Counselling families over the tele-link.

An additional bonus of not transferring the patient to the tertiary unit is that ad hoc, complete assessment is a lengthy process and can take up to half a clinical session. As we have demonstrated, the majority of patients may be followed up at the outpatient clinic at a later date which is much more efficient. Neonatal tele-echocardiography is a bit of a "no-brainer" and its use should be more widely disseminated.

Fetal Tele-Echocardiography

In the absence of telemedicine, all pregnancies fulfilling referral criteria travel to the tertiary unit for a fetal cardiology consultation including a fetal echocardiogram. Therefore the patient attends at least two appointments (general anomaly scan and fetal echocardiogram).

This telemedicine application does not have the same clinical impact as neonatal tele-echocardiography but a fetal tele-echocardiography service may alter working practices to a greater extent.

Figure 5. Interactions between clinicians/patients and support agencies

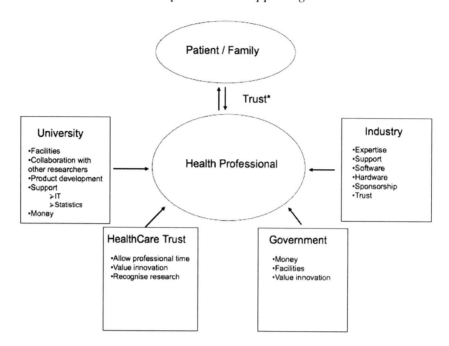

There is the potential for virtual clinics in which "high-risk" pregnancies are booked in for an anomaly scan at the DGH with time allowed for a fetal echocardiogram/consultation transmitted in real-time with guidance by a fetal cardiologist. A relatively large number of fetal echocardiograms could be performed in a single clinical session as long as the referring site are able to rotate patients through the telemedicine part of the consultation. This may be accomplished by having two sonographers scanning simultaneously at the DGH or linking in with more than DGH during the virtual clinic. The latter, although logistically more difficult, would improve the accessibility of the fetal cardiology service for urgent referrals. Eventually paediatric cardiac sonographers who run their own fetal cardiology clinics could lead the virtual clinics.

Such virtual clinics could obviate the need for many pregnant women to travel to the tertiary unit for hands-on assessment. It also promotes ongoing

interest in fetal echocardiography which can only facilitate improvements in antenatal detection rates of CHD. This telemedicine application would help reduce pressure on the regional fetal clinic which in our experience is considerable.

Tele-Stethoscopy

Tele-stethoscopy could significantly alter paediatric cardiology outpatient clinics depending on how it is utilised.

Real-Time

Virtual clinics with DGHs could be established which would decrease the need for paediatric cardiologists to travel to outlying hospitals and likely reduce families' travelling to the tertiary unit. At the referring site, the virtual clinic could be run by a doctor or by a trained nurse. To make this time-efficient form the paediatric cardiolo-

Figure 6. Patient pathways in presence and absence of a telemedicine service

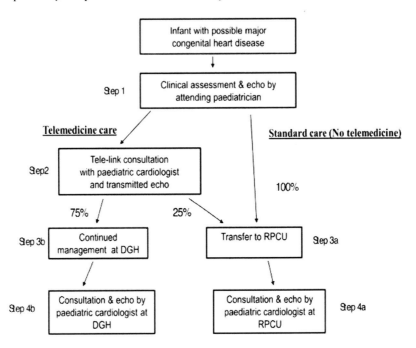

gist's perspective, it is important that a steady flow of patients is maintained throughout the clinic. Therefore, like fetal tele-cardiology, running virtual clinics with several DGHs simultaneously or having more than one doctor/ nurse preparing patients at the DGH would be important. However, as children are not always (or rarely) compliant when they most need to be, co-ordinating such clinics may be logistically challenging!

Store and Forward

The use of an electronic stethoscope to acquire and store auscultatory data which can then be forwarded to a paediatric cardiologist, along with other data e.g. clinical history/examination, chest x-ray and ECG, is more likely to be generally adopted than the real-time tele-stethoscopy model. It is flexible for both sending and receiving sites. A paediatric cardiologist may review each referral at his/her leisure and write back an opinion as to the necessity for formal cardiology evaluation. As described earlier, there is evidence that this could

streamline referrals to paediatric cardiology and potentially reduce outpatient clinics.

However, there is perhaps a danger that the seemingly limitless capacity of this referral system may lead family doctors and paediatricians to refer every patient with a murmur!

Tele-Homecare

The relationship between tele-homecare and traditional modes of out-patient follow-up is the most complex because it is a direct interface between specialist and patient. It is not a substitute but a complimentary service. In our experience, tele-homecare is effective at reducing the number of ad hoc attendances at the tertiary unit and unscheduled visits to the family doctor and DGH. It is also associated with reduced admissions to hospital. All of these features help keep the patient at home. The tele-consultations are much more efficient than face-to-face consultations. However, they are not a substitute for formal outpatient assessment.

How a tele-homecare service would affect one's practice is very much dependent on the set-up of your practice. In paediatric cardiology, the outpatient attendance will include an echocardiogram which obviously cannot be performed and transmitted from the home. Therefore, in paediatric cardiology, tele-homecare programmes are not going to reduce scheduled outpatient visits but they will help reduce the ad hoc attendances at various healthcare settings and possibly reduce the frequency of community nursing visits. It also ensures that the specialist has direct knowledge of the patient's clinical status on at least a weekly basis.

In our opinion, this telemedicine application (videoconferencing between hospital and home) is most suited to vulnerable patients in whom the attending clinician believes a substantial degree of outpatient support is needed.

FUTURE RESEARCH DIRECTIONS

The evidence to date demonstrates that telemedicine may be applied across multiple common paediatric cardiology scenarios: from fetus, to neonate, to infant to child; and from home, to outpatient clinic, to intensive care unit.

A wide range of clinical data, including visual examination, auscultatory sounds, physiological parameters and echocardiographic images, may be transmitted in real-time across low bandwidth telemedicine links facilitating accurate diagnosis, effective decision making and promoting access to specialist opinion.

- Telemedicine is an acceptable process to both health professionals and the public. It is associated with high levels of parental satisfaction.
- Telemedicine applications are shown to impact on patient managent and reduce health service utilisation with the net ef-

fect of keeping patients and their families closer to home.

- Established telemedicine programmes may continue to be cost saving beyond the initial start-up phase.
- Local Area Networks (LAN) and Wide Area Networks (WAN) that support internet/intranet systems within hospitals are large enough to facilitate inter-hospital real-time telemedicine activities reuiring high visual fidelity such as fetal echocardiograms and angiograms. Home broadband is still not consistent enough to achieve this goal. However, ADSL does permit videoconferencing of sufficient quality to permit audiovisual assessment of a patient.

Future research is dependent upon the perceived needs of the clinicians involved. Within paediatric cardiology, I believe there is further work needed in the following areas:

Home Monitoring

- Home monitoring applications could be expanded, beyond videoconferencing, to include ECG monitoring, for carefully selected patients, and INR monitoring to promote effective and safe anti-coagulation therapy.
- Videoconferencing home support programmes could be applied to other groups of vulnerable patients, for example: expreterm babies with chronic lung disease, home-ventilated patients and cystic fibrosis.
- The next large step for tele-health research could be an evaluation of the role of e-health in paediatric cardiology. For example, the use of internet applications to:
  - Improve patient/parent education.
  - Improve parental experiences during long inpatient stays e.g. patient diaries.

○ Streamline referrals as e-mails containing clinical information with attached files containing heart sounds, 12-lead ECG +/- chest x-ray.

Tele-Stethoscopy

Future research should concentrate on implementing telemedicine outpatient clinics. Parental and referrer satisfaction and acceptability of remote consultation will be key factors in the workability of this diagnostic tool. Comprehensive cost analyses will also be important in developing remote tele-stethoscopy clinics.

Fetal Cardiology

The next phase of research should concentrate on 2 themes.

- Evaluating the best modality and bandwidth across which to perform real-time fetal tele-echocardiography, taking into account cost.

- Performing a multi-site, randomised control-trial comparing telemedicine consultations with hands-on consultations including a detailed cost analysis. Remote consultations confidently excluding CHD would not receive a follow up outpatient appointment.

Ultimately the aim of future work should be aimed towards the establishment of a regional fetal tele-echocardiography service that supports DGHs, improves access to fetal cardiology, reduces pressure on the regional unit and reduces patient travelling and its attendant costs. In our opinion there is little need for further research into the clinical utility of neonatal tele-echocardiography. However, more rigorous cost analyses would be valuable.

CONCLUSION

Paediatric cardiology is a highly centralised medical specialty with a small number of clinicians covering large geographical areas. It is a speciality heavily reliant on the interpretation of clinical data such as echocardiography, ECG, MRI, chest-radiography and heart sounds all of which may be digitised and transmitted from one locality to another. Therefore paediatric cardioogy is ideally suited to telemedicine.

There is a substantial body of evidence supporting the feasibility, acceptablility and clinical utlity of telemedicine in paediatric cardiology. Neonatal tele-echocardiography become established as an important adjunct in many regions, supporting paediatricians and facilitating the work of cardiologists. We envisage a hub and spoke model for the provision of paediatric cardiology in our region. Telemedicine will be a valuable aid in supporting a paediatrician with a special expertise in cardiology. There is increasing evidence supporting the transferral of this technology to fetal echocardiography. Remote auscultation, whilst feasible and accurate, has yet to find its place in routine clinical practice. The likely advent of digital referral systems may bring this application to the fore. Tele-homecare and home monitoring are the main growth areas in telecardiology. There is good evidence that remote montoring systems and other telemedicine methods are associated with better patient care and may be cost saving.

Telemedicine aims to utilise health service resources more effectively and efficiently. Health departments are keen to pursue telemedicine because of this promise. However, a lack of well conducted studies investigating the economic impact of telemedicine applications is its retarding progress. Telemedicine is now at the stage where evaluation of large scale programmes is necessary to assess its real impact. In this setting research and service development are closely linked which we would recommend.

This chapter has described the current and potential role of telemedicine in paediatric cardiology. Telemedicine is capable of facilitating better quality care and a more efficient use of resources. Telemedicine is an important component in our regional service and its use will increase. We hope that the reader now has a clearer idea how to begin building a telemedicine programme specific to the needs of a paediatric cardiology service. The main recommendation from this chapter is for clinicians (for only clinicians can make telemedicine work) to consider whether areas of their clinical practice are negatively affected by distance separating themselves from either patients or colleagues. If so, then telemedicine is a useful tool in bridging this gap.

REFERENCES

Alboliras, E. T., Berdusis, K., Fisher, J., Harrison, R. A., Benson, D. W. Jr, & Webb, C. L. (1996). Transmission of full-length echocardiographic images over ISDN for diagnosing congenital heart disease. *Telemedicine Journal: The Official Journal of the American Telemedicine Association*, *2*(4), 251–258.

Belmont, J. M., & Mattioli, L. F. (2003). Accuracy of analog telephonic stethoscopy for pediatric telecardiology. *Pediatrics*, *112*(4), 780–786. doi:10.1542/peds.112.4.780

Belmont, J. M., Mattioli, L. F., Goertz, K. K., Ardinger, R. H. Jr, & Thomas, C. M. (1995). Evaluation of remote stethoscopy for pediatric telecardiology. *Telemedicine Journal: The Official Journal of the American Telemedicine Association*, *1*(2), 133–149.

Bhat, D., Upponi, A., Rakecha, A., & Thomson, J. (2010). Evaluating safety, effectiveness, and user satisfaction of home international normalized ratio monitoring service: Experience from a tertiary pediatric cardiology unit in the United Kingdom. *Pediatric Cardiology*, *31*(1), 18–21. doi:10.1007/s00246-009-9535-x

Bove, E. L., Ohye, R. G., & Devaney, E. J. (2004). Hypoplastic left heart syndrome: Conventional surgical management. *Seminars in Thoracic and Cardiovascular Surgery. Pediatric Cardiac Surgery Annual*, *7*, 3–10. doi:10.1053/j.pcsu.2004.02.003

Bull, C., Yates, R., Sarkar, D., Deanfield, J., & de Leval, M. (2000). Scientific, ethical, and logistical considerations in introducing a new operation: A retrospective cohort study from paediatric cardiac surgery. *British Medical Journal*, *320*(7243), 1168–1173. doi:10.1136/bmj.320.7243.1168

Casey, F. A. (1999). Telemedicine in paediatric cardiology. *Archives of Disease in Childhood*, *80*(6), 497–499. doi:10.1136/adc.80.6.497

Chiu, P., & Hedrick, H. L. (2008). Postnatal management and long-term outcome for survivors with congenital diaphragmatic hernia. *Prenatal Diagnosis*, *28*(7), 592–603. doi:10.1002/pd.2007

Clark, R. A., Inglis, S. C., McAlister, F. A., Cleland, J. G., & Stewart, S. (2007). Telemonitoring or structured telephone support programmes for patients with chronic heart failure: Systematic review and meta-analysis. *British Medical Journal*, *334*(7600), 942. doi:10.1136/bmj.39156.536968.55

Cloutier, A. (2000). Distance diagnosis in pediatric cardiology: A model for telemedecine implementation. *Telemedicine Today*, *8*(3), 20–21.

Cloutier, A., & Finley, J. (2004). Telepediatric cardiology practice in canada. Telemedicine Journal and e-Health *The Official Journal of the American Telemedicine Association, 10*(1), 33–37. doi:10.1089/153056204773644553

Congenital Cardiac Audit Database. (2009). Congenital heart disease website. Retrieved from http://www.ccad.org.uk/002/congenital.nsf/WMortality?Openview

Cotton, J. L., Gallaher, K. J., & Henry, G. W. (2002). Accuracy of interpretation of full-length pediatric echocardiograms transmitted over an integrated services digital network telemedicine link. *Southern Medical Journal, 95*(9), 1012–1016.

Dahl, L. B., Hasvold, P., Arild, E., & Hasvold, T. (2002). Heart murmurs recorded by a sensor based electronic stethoscope and e-mailed for remote assessment. *Archives of Disease in Childhood, 87*(4), 297–301. doi:10.1136/adc.87.4.297

Dellifraine, J. L., & Dansky, K. H. (2008). Home-based telehealth: A review and meta-analysis. *Journal of Telemedicine and Telecare, 14*(2), 62–66. doi:10.1258/jtt.2007.070709

Dhillon, D., & Redington, A. N. (2002). Hypoplastic left heart syndrome In Anderson, R. H., Baker, E. J., Macartney, F. J., Rigby, M. L., Shinebourne, E. A., & Tynan, M. (Eds.), *Paediatric cardiology* (2nd ed., pp. 1191–1211). Edinburgh, UK: Churchill Livingstone.

Dowie, R., Mistry, H., Rigby, M., Young, T. A., Weatherburn, G., & Rowlinson, G. (2009). A paediatric telecardiology service for district hospitals in South-East England: An observational study. *Archives of Disease in Childhood, 94*(4), 273–277. doi:10.1136/adc.2008.138495

Dowie, R., Mistry, H., Young, T. A., Franklin, R. C., & Gardiner, H. M. (2008). Cost implications of introducing a telecardiology service to support fetal ultrasound screening. *Journal of Telemedicine and Telecare, 14*(8), 421–426. doi:10.1258/jtt.2008.080401

Drummond, M., Sculpher, M., Torrence, G., O'Brien, B., & Stoddart, G. (Eds.). (2005a). *Methods for the economic evaluation of health care programmes* (3rd ed.). Oxford, UK: Oxford University Press.

Drummond, M., Sculpher, M., Torrence, G., O'Brien, B., & Stoddart, G. (Eds.). (2005b). Methods for the economic evaluation of health care programmes (3rd ed.). Oxford, UK: Oxford University Press.<[REMOVED IF= FIELD]></>

Farrell, P. M., Lai, H. J., Li, Z., Kosorok, M. R., Laxova, A., & Green, C. G. (2005). Evidence on improved outcomes with early diagnosis of cystic fibrosis through neonatal screening: Enough is enough! *The Journal of Pediatrics, 147*(3Suppl), S30–S36. doi:10.1016/j.jpeds.2005.08.012

Finley, J. P., Human, D. G., Nanton, M. A., Roy, D. L., Macdonald, R. G., & Marr, D. R. (1989). Echocardiography by telephone--Evaluation of pediatric heart disease at a distance. *The American Journal of Cardiology, 63*(20), 1475–1477. doi:10.1016/0002-9149(89)90011-8

Finley, J. P., Sharratt, G. P., Nanton, M. A., Chen, R. P., Bryan, P., & Wolstenholme, J. (1997). Paediatric echocardiography by telemedicine-Nine years' experience. *Journal of Telemedicine and Telecare, 3*(4), 200–204. doi:10.1258/1357633971931165

Finley, J. P., Warren, A. E., Sharratt, G. P., & Amit, M. (2006). Assessing children's heart sounds at a distance with digital recordings. *Pediatrics, 118*(6), 2322–2325. doi:10.1542/peds.2006-1557

Fisher, J. B., Alboliras, E. T., Berdusis, K., & Webb, C. L. (1996). Rapid identification of congenital heart disease by transmission of echocardiograms. *American Heart Journal, 131*(6), 1225–1227. doi:10.1016/S0002-8703(96)90103-9

Forbess, J. M. (2003). Pre-stage II mortality after the Norwood operation: Addressing the next challenge. *The Journal of Thoracic and Cardiovascular Surgery, 126*(5), 1257–1258. doi:10.1016/S0022-5223(03)01040-7

Fragasso, G., Cuko, A., Spoladore, R., Montano, C., Palloshi, A., & Silipigni, C. (2007). Validation of remote cardiopulmonary examination in patients with heart failure with a videophone-based system. *Journal of Cardiac Failure, 13*(4), 281–286. doi:10.1016/j.cardfail.2007.01.008

Fragasso, G., De Benedictis, M., Palloshi, A., Moltrasio, M., Cappelletti, A., & Carlino, M. (2003). Validation of heart and lung teleauscultation on an internet-based system. *The American Journal of Cardiology, 92*(9), 1138–1139. doi:10.1016/j.amjcard.2003.07.015

Ghanayem, N. S., Cava, J. R., Jaquiss, R. D., & Tweddell, J. S. (2004). Home monitoring of infants after stage one palliation for hypoplastic left heart syndrome. *Seminars in Thoracic and Cardiovascular Surgery. Pediatric Cardiac Surgery Annual, 7,* 32–38. doi:10.1053/j.pcsu.2004.02.017

Ghanayem, N. S., Hoffman, G. M., Mussatto, K. A., Cava, J. R., Frommelt, P. C., & Rudd, N. A. (2003). Home surveillance program prevents interstage mortality after the Norwood procedure. *The Journal of Thoracic and Cardiovascular Surgery, 126*(5), 1367–1377. doi:10.1016/S0022-5223(03)00071-0

Ghanayem, N. S., Tweddell, J. S., Hoffman, G. M., Mussatto, K., & Jaquiss, R. D. (2006). Optimal timing of the second stage of palliation for hypoplastic left heart syndrome facilitated through home monitoring, and the results of early cavopulmonary anastomosis. *Cardiology in the Young, 16*(1), 61–66. doi:10.1017/S1047951105002349

Gramegna, L., Tomasi, C., Gasparini, G., Scaboro, G., Zanon, F., & Boaretto, G. (2012). In-hospital follow-up of implantable cardioverter defibrillator and pacemaker carriers: Patients' inconvenience and points of view. A four-hospital Italian survey. *Journal of the Working Groups on Cardiac Pacing, Arrhythmias, and Cardiac Cellular Electrophysiology of the European Society of Cardiology, 14*(3), 345–350. doi:10.1093/europace/eur334

Grant, B. (2006). *The development of telemedicine systems applicable to the diagnosis and monitoring of children with congenital heart disease.* MD: Queen's University Belfast.

Hailey, D., Ohinmaa, A., & Roine, R. (2004). Published evidence on the success of telecardiology: A mixed record. *Journal of Telemedicine and Telecare, 10*(1), 36–38. doi:10.1258/1357633042614195

Harnett, B. (2006). Telemedicine systems and telecommunications. *Journal of Telemedicine and Telecare, 12*(1), 4–15. doi:10.1258/135763306775321416

Hersh, W. R., Wallace, J. A., Patterson, P. K., Shapiro, S. E., Kraemer, D. F., & Eilers, G. M. (2001). Telemedicine for the Medicare population: Pediatric, obstetric, and clinician-indirect home interventions. *Evidence Report/technology Assessment, 24,* 1–32.

Hickey, K. T., Reiffel, J., Sciacca, R. R., Whang, W., Biviano, A., & Baumeister, M. (2010). The utility of ambulatory electrocardiographic monitoring for detecting silent arrhythmias and clarifying symptom mechanism in an urban elderly population with heart failure and hypertension: Clinical implications. *Journal of Atrial Fibrillation, 1*(12), 663–674. doi:10.4022/jafib.v1i12.567

Hintz, S. R., Kendrick, D. E., Vohr, B. R., Poole, W. K., Higgins, R. D., & National Institute of Child Health and Human Development Neonatal Research Network. (2005). Changes in neurodevelopmental outcomes at 18 to 22 months' corrected age among infants of less than 25 weeks' gestational age born in 1993-1999. Pediatrics, 115(6), 1645-1651.

Jacklin, P. B., Roberts, J. A., Wallace, P., Haines, A., Harrison, R., & Barber, J. A. (2003). Virtual outreach: Economic evaluation of joint teleconsultations for patients referred by their general practitioner for a specialist opinion. *British Medical Journal, 327*(7406), 84. doi:10.1136/bmj.327.7406.84

Justo, R., Smith, A. C., Williams, M., Van der Westhuyzen, J., Murray, J., & Sciuto, G. (2004). Paediatric telecardiology services in queensland: A review of three years' experience. *Journal of Telemedicine and Telecare, 10*(1), 57–60. doi:10.1258/1357633042614258

Lewin, M., Xu, C., Jordan, M., Borchers, H., Ayton, C., & Wilbert, D. (2006). Accuracy of paediatric echocardiographic transmission via telemedicine. *Journal of Telemedicine and Telecare, 12*(8), 416–421. doi:10.1258/135763306779378636

Mabo, P., Victor, F., Bazin, P., Ahres, S., Babuty, D., & Da Costa, A. (2011). A randomized trial of long-term remote monitoring of pacemaker recipients (the COMPAS trial). *European Heart Journal, 33*(9), 1105–1111. doi:10.1093/eurheartj/ehr419

Marino, B. S. (2002). Outcomes after the Fontan procedure. *Current Opinion in Pediatrics, 14*(5), 620–626. doi:10.1097/00008480-200210000-00010

Mattioli, L., Goertz, K., Ardinger, R., Belmont, J., Cox, R., & Thomas, C. (1992). Pediatric cardiology: Auscultation from 280 miles away. Kansas Medicine *The Journal of the Kansas Medical Society, 93*(12), 326, 347–350.

McConnell, M. E., Steed, R. D., Tichenor, J. M., & Hannon, D. W. (1999). Interactive telecardiology for the evaluation of heart murmurs in children. *Telemedicine Journal: The Official Journal of the American Telemedicine Association, 5*(2), 157–161.

McCrossan, B. A. (2008). *Questmark*. Personal communication.

McCrossan, B. A. (2009). *Little hearts matter*. Personal communication.

McCrossan, B. A. (2009). *The role of telemedicine in paediatric cardiology. Unpublished Medical Doctorate*. Belfast, Belfast: Queen's University.

McCrossan, B. A. (2009). *Tiny life*. Personal communication.

McCrossan, B. A., Sands, A. J., Kileen, T., Cardwell, C. R., & Casey, F. A. (2011). Fetal diagnosis of congenital heart disease by telemedicine. *Archives of Disease in Childhood. Fetal and Neonatal Edition, 96*(6), F394–F397. doi:10.1136/adc.2010.197202

McElhinney, D. B., & Wernovsky, G. (2001). Outcomes of neonates with congenital heart disease. *Current Opinion in Pediatrics, 13*(2), 104–110. doi:10.1097/00008480-200104000-00003

Michailidis, G. D., Simpson, J. M., Karidas, C., & Economides, D. L. (2001). Detailed three-dimensional fetal echocardiography facilitated by an internet link. Ultrasound in Obstetrics & Gynecology *The Official Journal of the International Society of Ultrasound in Obstetrics and Gynecology*, *18*(4), 325–328. doi:10.1046/j.0960-7692.2001.00520.x

Miyasaka, K., Suzuki, Y., Sakai, H., & Kondo, Y. (1997). Interactive communication in high-technology home care: Videophones for pediatric ventilatory care. *Pediatrics*, *99*(1), E1. doi:10.1542/peds.99.1.e1

Mulholland, H. C., Casey, F., Brown, D., Corrigan, N., Quinn, M., & McCord, B. (1999). Application of a low cost telemedicine link to the diagnosis of neonatal congenital heart defects by remote consultation. *Heart (British Cardiac Society)*, *82*(2), 217–221.

Murphy, R. L., Block, P., Bird, K. T., & Yurchak, P. (1973). Accuracy of cardiac auscultation by microwave. *Chest*, *63*(4), 578–581. doi:10.1378/chest.63.4.578

National Health Service. (n.d.). Paediatric cardiology. Retrieved March 12, 2012, from http://www.nhscareers.nhs.uk/details/Default.aspx?Id=593

National Institute for Health and Clinical Excellence. (2008). *Guide to the methods of technology appraisal*. London, UK: National Institute for Health and Clinical Excellence.

NHS - Medical Careers. (2009). Paediatric cardiology. Retrieved from http://www.medicalcareers.nhs.uk/SpecialtyPages/Medicine/Paediatriccardiology/Pages/default.aspx

Ohman, A., Stromvall-Larsson, E., Nilsson, B., & Mellander, M. (2012). Pulse oximetry home monitoring in infants with single-ventricle physiology and a surgical shunt as the only source of pulmonary blood flow. Cardiology in the Young, online before print, 1-7.

Paediatric and Congenital Cardiac Services Review Group. (2003). *Report of the paediatric and congenital cardiac services review group*. London, UK: Department of Health.

Perings, C., Bauer, W. R., Bondke, H. J., Mewis, C., James, M., & Bocker, D. (2011). Remote monitoring of implantable-cardioverter defibrillators: Results from the reliability of IEGM online interpretation (RIONI) study. *Journal of the Working Groups on Cardiac Pacing, Arrhythmias, and Cardiac Cellular Electrophysiology of the European Society of Cardiology*, *13*(2), 221–229. doi:10.1093/europace/euq447

Qureshi, S. A. (2008). Requirements for provision of outreach paediatric cardiology service. London, UK: British Congenital cardiac Association.

Randolph, G. R., Hagler, D. J., Khandheria, B. K., Lunn, E. R., Cook, W. J., & Seward, J. B. (1999). Remote telemedical interpretation of neonatal echocardiograms: Impact on clinical management in a primary care setting. *Journal of the American College of Cardiology*, *34*(1), 241–245. doi:10.1016/S0735-1097(99)00182-5

Roine, R., Ohinmaa, A., & Hailey, D. (2001). Assessing telemedicine: A systematic review of the literature. Canadian Medical Association Journal = Journal De l'Association Medicale Canadienne, 165(6), 765-771.

Royal College of Paediatrics and Child Health. (2009). Cardiology training for paediatric SpRs. Retrieved from www.rcph.ac.uk/publications/education_and_training_documents/cardiology_for_paeds_march2005.pdf

Royal College of Physicians. (2009). Consultant physicians working with patients: The duties, responsibilities and practice of physicians in general medicine and the specialties - Paediatric cardiology. Retrieved from http://www.rcplondon.ac.uk/pubs/contents/39318d3e-4efb-49d6-994b-761892064f03.pdf

Sable, C. (2002). Digital echocardiography and telemedicine applications in pediatric cardiology. *Pediatric Cardiology, 23*(3), 358–369. doi:10.1007/s00246-001-0199-4

Sable, C. (2003). Telemedicine applications in pediatric cardiology. *Minerva Pediatrica, 55*(1), 1–13.

Sable, C., Roca, T., Gold, J., Gutierrez, A., Gulotta, E., & Culpepper, W. (1999). Live transmission of neonatal echocardiograms from underserved areas: Accuracy, patient care, and cost. *Telemedicine Journal: The Official Journal of the American Telemedicine Association, 5*(4), 339–347.

Sable, C. A., Cummings, S. D., Pearson, G. D., Schratz, L. M., Cross, R. C., & Quivers, E. S. (2002). Impact of telemedicine on the practice of pediatric cardiology in community hospitals. *Pediatrics, 109*(1), E3. doi:10.1542/peds.109.1.e3

Sano, S., Ishino, K., Kado, H., Shiokawa, Y., Sakamoto, K., & Yokota, M. (2004). Outcome of right ventricle-to-pulmonary artery shunt in first-stage palliation of hypoplastic left heart syndrome: A multi-institutional study. *The Annals of Thoracic Surgery, 78*(6), 1951–1958. doi:10.1016/j.athoracsur.2004.05.055

Sharma, S., Parness, I. A., Kamenir, S. A., Ko, H., Haddow, S., & Steinberg, L. G. (2003). Screening fetal echocardiography by telemedicine: Efficacy and community acceptance. *Journal of the American Society of Echocardiography: Official Publication of the American Society of Echocardiography, 16*(3), 202–208. doi:10.1067/mje.2003.46

Sicotte, C., Lehoux, P., Van Doesburg, N., Cardinal, G., & Leblanc, Y. (2004). A cost-effectiveness analysis of interactive paediatric telecardiology. *Journal of Telemedicine and Telecare, 10*(2), 78–83. doi:10.1258/135763304773391503

Smith, A. C. (2007). Telepaediatrics. *Journal of Telemedicine and Telecare, 13*(4), 163–166. doi:10.1258/135763307780908021

Smith, A. C., Scuffham, P., & Wootton, R. (2007). The costs and potential savings of a novel telepaediatric service in queensland. *BMC Health Services Research, 7*, 35. doi:10.1186/1472-6963-7-35

Smith, D. L. (2005). The influence of financial factors on the deployment of telemedicine. *Journal of Health Care Finance, 32*(1), 16–27.

Stasik, C. N., Gelehrter, S., Goldberg, C. S., Bove, E. L., Devaney, E. J., & Ohye, R. G. (2006). Current outcomes and risk factors for the norwood procedure. *The Journal of Thoracic and Cardiovascular Surgery, 131*(2), 412–417. doi:10.1016/j.jtcvs.2005.09.030

Tsilimigaki, A., Maraka, S., Tsekoura, T., Agelakou, V., Vekiou, A., & Paphitis, C. (2001). Eighteen months' experience with remote diagnosis, management and education in congenital heart disease. *Journal of Telemedicine and Telecare, 7*(4), 239–243. doi:10.1258/1357633011936462

Vinals, F., Mandujano, L., Vargas, G., & Giuliano, A. (2005). Prenatal diagnosis of congenital heart disease using four-dimensional spatio-temporal image correlation (STIC) telemedicine via an internet link: A pilot study. Ultrasound in Obstetrics & Gynecology *The Official Journal of the International Society of Ultrasound in Obstetrics and Gynecology, 25*(1), 25–31. doi:10.1002/uog.1796

Whitten, P. S., & Cook, D. J. (1999). School-based telemedicine: Using technology to bring health care to inner-city children. *Journal of Telemedicine and Telecare, 5*, S23–S25. doi:10.1258/1357633991932423

Whitten, P. S., Mair, F. S., Haycox, A., May, C. R., Williams, T. L., & Hellmich, S. (2002a). Systematic review of cost effectiveness studies of telemedicine interventions. *British Medical Journal, 324*(7351), 1434–1437. doi:10.1136/bmj.324.7351.1434

Whitten, P. S., Mair, F. S., Haycox, A., May, C. R., Williams, T. L., & Hellmich, S. (2002b). Systematic review of cost effectiveness studies of telemedicine interventions. *British Medical Journal, 324*(7351), 1434–1437. doi:10.1136/bmj.324.7351.1434

Wise, P. H. (2007). The future pediatrician: The challenge of chronic illness. *The Journal of Pediatrics, 151*(5Suppl), S6–S10. doi:10.1016/j.jpeds.2007.08.013

Wootton, R., Bloomer, S. E., Corbett, R., Eedy, D. J., Hicks, N., & Lotery, H. E. (2000). Multicentre randomised control trial comparing real time teledermatology with conventional outpatient dermatological care: Societal cost-benefit analysis. *British Medical Journal, 320*(7244), 1252–1256. doi:10.1136/bmj.320.7244.1252

Workforce Review Team. (2009). Workforce summary - Paediatric cardiology. Retrieved from http://www.wrt.nhs.uk/index

ADDITIONAL READING

Allan, L. (2007). Prenatal diagnosis of structural cardiac defects. *American Journal of Medical Genetics. Part C, Seminars in Medical Genetics, 145C*(1), 73–76. doi:10.1002/ajmg.c.30123

Augestad, K. M., Berntsen, G., Lassen, K., Bellika, J. G., Wootton, R., & Lindsetmo, R. O. (2012). Standards for reporting randomized controlled trials in medical informatics: A systematic review of CONSORT adherence in RCTs on clinical decision support. *Journal of the American Medical Informatics Association, 19*(1), 13–21. doi:10.1136/amiajnl-2011-000411

Bellavance, M., Beland, M. J., van Doesburg, N. H., Paquet, M., Ducharme, F. M., & Cloutier, A. (2004). Implanting telehealth network for paediatric cardiology: Learning from the Quebec experience. *Cardiology in the Young, 14*(6), 608–614. doi:10.1017/S1047951104006055

Casey, F. A. (1999). Telemedicine in paediatric cardiology. *Archives of Disease in Childhood, 80*(6), 497–499. doi:10.1136/adc.80.6.497

Casey, F. A., & McCrossan, B. A. (2011). Telemedicine in the diagnosis and management of congenital heart disease. In G. Graschew (Ed.), *Telemedicine techniques and applications* (1st ed., pp. 307-307-354). InTech.

Clark, R. A., Inglis, S. C., McAlister, F. A., Cleland, J. G., & Stewart, S. (2007). Telemonitoring or structured telephone support programmes for patients with chronic heart failure: Systematic review and meta-analysis. *British Medical Journal, 334*(7600), 942. doi:10.1136/bmj.39156.536968.55

Dowie, R., Mistry, H., Rigby, M., Young, T. A., Weatherburn, G., & Rowlinson, G. (2009). A paediatric telecardiology service for district hospitals in south-east england: An observational study. *Archives of Disease in Childhood, 94*(4), 273–277. doi:10.1136/adc.2008.138495

Dowie, R., Mistry, H., Young, T. A., Franklin, R. C., & Gardiner, H. M. (2008). Cost implications of introducing a telecardiology service to support fetal ultrasound screening. *Journal of Telemedicine and Telecare, 14*(8), 421–426. doi:10.1258/jtt.2008.080401

Finley, J. P., Sharratt, G. P., Nanton, M. A., Chen, R. P., Bryan, P., & Wolstenholme, J. (1997a). Paediatric echocardiography by telemedicine--nine years' experience. *Journal of Telemedicine and Telecare*, *3*(4), 200–204. doi:10.1258/1357633971931165

Finley, J. P., Sharratt, G. P., Nanton, M. A., Chen, R. P., Bryan, P., & Wolstenholme, J. (1997b). Paediatric echocardiography by telemedicine--Nine years' experience. *Journal of Telemedicine and Telecare*, *3*(4), 200–204. doi:10.1258/1357633971931165

Ghanayem, N. S., Hoffman, G. M., Mussatto, K. A., Cava, J. R., Frommelt, P. C., & Rudd, N. A. (2003). Home surveillance program prevents interstage mortality after the Norwood procedure. *The Journal of Thoracic and Cardiovascular Surgery*, *126*(5), 1367–1377. doi:10.1016/S0022-5223(03)00071-0

Inglis, S. C., Clark, R. A., & Cleland, J. G., & Cochrane Systematic Review Team. (2011). Telemonitoring in patients with heart failure. *The New England Journal of Medicine*, *364*(11), 1078–1080. doi:10.1056/NEJMc1100395

Morgan, G. J., Craig, B., Grant, B., Sands, A., Doherty, N., & Casey, F. (2008). Home videoconferencing for patients with severe congenital heart disease following discharge. *Congenital Heart Disease*, *3*(5), 317–324. doi:10.1111/j.1747-0803.2008.00205.x

Mulholland, H. C., Casey, F., Brown, D., Corrigan, N., Quinn, M., & McCord, B. (1999). Application of a low cost telemedicine link to the diagnosis of neonatal congenital heart defects by remote consultation. *Heart (British Cardiac Society)*, *82*(2), 217–221.

Sable, C. (2002a). Digital echocardiography and telemedicine applications in pediatric cardiology. *Pediatric Cardiology*, *23*(3), 358–369. doi:10.1007/s00246-001-0199-4

Sable, C. (2002b). Digital echocardiography and telemedicine applications in pediatric cardiology. *Pediatric Cardiology*, *23*(3), 358–369. doi:10.1007/s00246-001-0199-4

Weatherly, H., Drummond, M., Claxton, K., Cookson, R., Ferguson, B., & Godfrey, C. (2009). Methods for assessing the cost-effectiveness of public health interventions: Key challenges and recommendations. *Health Policy (Amsterdam)*, *93*(2-3), 85–92. doi:10.1016/j.healthpol.2009.07.012

Wootton, R. (2001). Recent advances: Telemedicine. *British Medical Journal*, *323*(7312), 557–560. doi:10.1136/bmj.323.7312.557

Zanaboni, P., & Wootton, R. (2012). Adoption of telemedicine: From pilot stage to routine delivery. *BMC Medical Informatics and Decision Making*, *12*(1). doi:10.1186/1472-6947-12-1

KEY TERMS AND DEFINITIONS

Asymmetric Digital Subscriber Loop: (ADSL): This is a method commonly used for delivering home broadband. It utilizes the telephone line entering homes. It is much less expensive than ISDN. However, the bandwidth is contended and variable although there are techniques to ameliorate this effect.

Echocardiogram: Also known as an echo or cardiac ultrasound. It uses standard ultrasound techniques to image two-dimensional slices of the heart.

Fetal Cardiology: The study of heart disease in fetuses. It is essentially an ultrasound application.

Health Economics: A branch of economics concerned with issues related to efficiency, effectiveness, value and behavior in the production and consumption of health and healthcare.

Integrated Services Digital Network (ISDN): This is a subset of the Public Switch Telephone Network and permits a fixed and reliable bandwidth over which telemedicine activities may be performed.

Paediatric Cardiology: The study of heart disease in childhood primarily concerned with congenital heart defects.

Tele-Homecare: This is one of several umbrella terms describing telemedicine applications that are concerned with providing care in a home setting with the primary focus of supporting the patient rather than the health professionals.

Chapter 5

Telemedicine, the European Space Agency, and the Support to the African Population for Infectious Disease Problems:
Potentiality and Perspectives for Asia Countries and China

Giorgio Parentela
European Space Agency, France

Franco Naccarella
Italian Society of Telemedicine, Italy

Pierluigi Mancini
European Space Agency, France

Zhang Feng
First People Hospital of Jiao Tong University, People's Republic of China

Giovanni Rinaldi
Italian Society of Telemedicine, Italy

ABSTRACT

Telemedicine and the broader field of eHealth as the application of Information and Communication Technology in the health sector offer opportunities for improving health world-wide. The European Space Agency (ESA) is, since 1996, active in this field and has initiated various projects which have demonstrated that satellite communications is a powerful technology for enlarging the reach of Telemedicine services toward geographically isolated regions, especially those with a high burden of diseases, such as many areas in Sub-Saharan Africa. In 2006 the Telemedicine Task Force (TTF) with the mandate to explore the potential of Telemedicine via Satellite for this region has been established on initiative of ESA and the European Commission, with representatives of African stakeholders and the World Health Organization (WHO). After a review of the current situation, the TTF has recommended short-term pilot projects to demonstrate the feasibility of an approach based on user demands, public private partnerships, African ownership, and building on existing successful initiatives. These projects shall begin in

DOI: 10.4018/978-1-4666-2979-0.ch005

2008, serving selected isolated areas in Sub-Saharan Africa by offering clinical services and eLearning via satellite for infectious diseases, in particular HIV, tuberculosis, and malaria. The projects should and will be presented in China for finding bilateral cooperation between Italian and Chinese Civilian and Military technologies and opportunities present already in the field.

INTRODUCTION

Information and Communication Technology (ICT) offers a large variety of opportunities for world-wide advancements in health and healthcare. eHealth (the use of ICT in the health sector, for clinical, educational and administrative purposes, both locally and at a distance) and its sub-domain Telemedicine (the provision of healthcare services from a healthcare provider to a patient) are key enablers for supporting health systems and delivery of healthcare.

The second phase of the World Summit on the Information Society (WSIS) held in Tunis in 2005, adopted a Plan of Action that urges different stakeholders to contribute actively in utilizing ICT for the achievement of the Millennium Development Goals (MDGs) and for bridging the so called digital divide. Also in 2005, the World Health Assembly (WHA) passed a resolution urging countries to take advantage of the potential offered by eHealth to strengthen their health systems. In 2006, the WHA also requested World Health Organization (WHO) Member States, in another resolution, to use ICT to help address the global shortage of health workers.

This health workforce crisis is particularly acute in Sub-Saharan Africa where thirty-six countries have a health worker density below a critical minimum necessary for effective provision of basic health services, and where in many countries the health service coverage (Table 1) and the readiness for information society (Figure 1) are critically low. With a broad range of possible applications in support of health service provision, communication, education, business, and governance, eHealth offers a significant number of opportunities to address this health crisis (Asamoah-Odei, E., et al. 2007).

Despite the potential benefit of ICT for health world-wide, its utilization is in many countries still difficult or impossible, due to a lack of connectivity and network coverage, and other reasons such as for example illiteracy, regulatory, or cultural barriers. The prospect of using satellite communications technologies and associated connectivity services to support the development and dissemination of Telemedicine and eHealth applications was the reason why ESA began to be active in this challenging field (Feliciani, F., 2003). In 2006, efforts toward the support of Africa have been initiated by ESA in collaboration with the European Commission (EC), the WHO, and African stakeholders.

ESA TELEMEDICINE PROJECTS

Several different projects have been undertaken within the Advanced Research in TElecommunication Systems (ARTES) programme to explore and promote the different facets of Telemedicine via satellite, taking a pragmatic approach, addressing broadband applications, medical simulation, emergency consultation, teleconsultation, clinical research, access to patient multimedia databases, and continuing medical education (Feliciani 2003). These projects have been targeted at developing the hardware, software and content elements required by the specific Telemedicine applications and then using the resulting system in a pilot utilisation phase with real users and under truly operational conditions.

An ESA Road Map for Telemedicine via Satellite was worked out in 2003 and 2004, identifying needs and opportunities for using ICT in specific areas of healthcare, and the role that satellite communications can play therein (Dario, C., et al.

Table 1. Health service coverage in sub-Saharan Africa (WHO 2006), (Asamoah-Odei, E,. et al. 2007)

Nr.	Country	Population	Immunization coverage among 1-year-olds			Antenatal care coverage			Births attended by skilled health personnel		Contraceptive prevalence rate	
			Measles	DTP3	HepB3	At least 1 visit	At least 4 visits					
		(millions) 2005	(%) 2004	(%) 2004	(%) 2004	(%)	(%)	Year	(%)	Year	(%)	Year
1	Angola	15.9	64	59	...	...	...		47	2000	6.2	2001
2	Benin	8.4	85	83	89	88	61	2001	66	2001	18.6	2001
3	Botswana	1.8	90	97	79	99	97	2001	94	2000	40.4	2000
4	Burkina Faso	13.2	78	88	...	72	18	2003	57	2003	13.8	2003
5	Burundi	7.5	75	74	83	93	79	2001	25	2000	15.7	2000
6	Cameroon	16.3	64	73	...	77	52	1998	62	2004	26.0	2004
7	Cape Verde	0.5	69	75	68	...	99	2001	89	1998	52.9	1998
8	Central African Rep.	4.0	35	40	...	...	...		44	2000	27.9	2000
9	Chad	9.7	56	50	...	51	13	1997	14	2004	7.9	2000
10	Comoros	0.8	73	76	77	...	...		62	2000	25.7	2000
11	Congo	4.0	65	67	...	...	...		...		...	
12	Dem. Rep. of Congo	57.5	64	64	...	...	...		61	2001	31.4	2001
13	Côte d'Ivoire	18.2	49	50	50	84	35	1998-99	63	2000	15.0	1998-99
14	Equatorial Guinea	0.5	51	33	...	...	37	2001	65	2000	...	
15	Eritrea	4.4	84	83	83	...	49	2001	28	2002	8.0	2002
16	Ethiopia	77.4	71	80	...	27	10	2000	6	2000	8.1	2000
17	Gabon	1.4	55	38	...	94	63	2000	86	2000	32.7	2000
18	Gambia	1.5	90	92	90	92	...	2000	55	2000	9.6	2000
19	Ghana	22.1	83	80	80	90	69	2003	47	2003	25.2	2003
20	Guinea	9.4	73	69	...	74	48	1999	35	1999	6.2	1999
21	Guibea-Bissau	1.6	80	80	...	89	62	2001	35	2000	7.6	2000
22	Kenya	34.3	73	73	73	88	52	2003	42	2003	39.3	2003
23	Lesotho	1.8	70	78	67	91	88	2001	55	2004	30.4	2000
24	Liberia	3.3	42	31	...	...	84	2001	51	2000	...	
25	Madagascar	18.6	59	61	61	91	38	1997	51	2003-04	27.1	2003-04
26	Malawi	12.9	80	89	89	94	55	2000	61	2002	30.6	2000
27	Mali	13.5	75	76	73	53	30	2001	41	2001	8.1	2001
28	Mauritania	3.1	64	70	...	63	16	2000-01	57	2001	8.0	2000-01
29	Mauritius	1.2	98	98	98	...	...		99	1998	...	
30	Mozambique	19.8	77	72	72	71	41	1997	48	2003	16.5	2003
31	Namibia	2.0	70	81	...	85	69	2000	76	2000	43.9	2000
32	Niger	14.0	74	62	...	39	11	1998	16	2000	14.0	2000
33	Nigeria	131.5	35	25	...	61	47	2003	35	2003	12.6	2003
34	Rwanda	9.0	84	89	89	93	10	2001	31	2000	13.2	2000
35	Sao Tome and Principe	0.2	91	99	99	91	...	2000	79	2000	29.3	2000
36	Senagal	11.7	57	87	54	82	64	1999	58	2000	10.5	1999
37	Seychelles	0.1	99	99	99	...	...		...		...	
38	Sierra Leone	5.5	64	61	...	82	68	2001	42	2000	4.3	2000
39	Somalia	8.2	40	30	...	...	32	2001	34	1999	...	
40	South Africa	47.4	81	93	92	89	72	1998	84	1998	56.3	1998
41	Sudan	36.2	59	55	...	...	75	2001	...		...	
42	Swaziland	1.0	70	83	78	...	...		70	2000	27.7	2000
43	Tanzania	38.3	94	95	95	96	69	1999	46	2004-05	25.4	1999
44	Togo	6.1	70	71	...	78	46	1998	49	2000	25.7	2000
45	Uganda	28.8	91	87	87	92	40	2000-01	39	2000	22.8	2000-01
46	Zambia	11.7	84	80	...	94	71	2001-02	43	2001-02	34.2	2001-02
47	Zimbabwe	13.0	80	85	85	82	64	1999	73	1999	53.5	1999
48	Mayotte	0.2	...	...	...	...	...		...		...	
	Total	749.86										
	Minimum		35	25	50	27	10		6		4.3	
	Maximum		99	99	99	99	99		99		56.3	
	Average		66	66								
	# Countries with ≥ 80%		16	21	14	22	4		5			
	# Countries with < 50%		5	6	0	2	17		21			

91

Figure 1. Digital opportunity indices for Africa (WISR 2006)

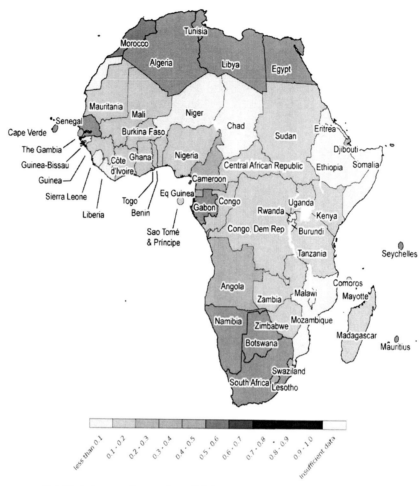

Note: The Index ranges between "0" and "1", where 1 would be complete digital opportunity.

2005). The Telemedicine areas studied included: interconnectivity for healthcare services, management of trauma, emergencies, and disasters, health early warning for environmental risks, eHealth education, healthcare at home, services for the citizens, and mobility. Strong involvement of health professionals in the process of defining this road map reflect ESA's strategy to complement initiatives mainly driven by industry and service operators with initiatives driven by demand.

More Telemedicine projects followed, in line with this new strategy. In 2005, the SIMONA project established the connection of a teach-ing hospital in Baghdad, Iraq, with the Hospital Umberto I of La Sapienza University in Rome, Italy, which helped by tele-consultations via video-conference e.g. in reducing childhood mortality. In the beginning of 2005, the project I-DISCARE has been initiated to support medical treatment of the victims along the coastal areas ravaged by the December 2004 tsunami in Asia, by connecting mobile teams of rescue workers with hospitals via satellite.

The Satellite for Health Early Warning and for Epidemiology (SAFE) Telemedicine project has recently successfully completed a pilot run and demonstrated the feasibility of providing assistance via satellite, from remote locations, in the event of natural disasters and for post-crisis management.

SUPPORT TO THE AFRICAN POPULATION FOR INFECTIOUS DISEASE PROBLEMS

A workshop held in Brussels in January 2006, sponsored by EC and ESA, focused on the potential of satellite telecommunication technology to strengthen health systems in Africa, recognising that given the current limitations of land based and mobile telecommunication, satellite technology could significantly extend the reach of communication to remote and isolated areas of the continent.

A Telemedicine Task Force (TTF) was therefore set up with a mandate to develop a comprehensive picture of Telemedicine opportunities in Africa, focussing in particular on the Sub-Saharan region, and to formulate recommendations for future action. The TTF was composed of representatives from: the African Union Commission (AUC), the New Partnership for Africa's Development (NE-PAD), the African Development Bank (AfDB), the Communauté Economique et Monétaire de l'Afrique Centrale (CEMAC), the Organisation de Coordination pour la lutte contre les Endémies en Afrique Centrale (OCEAC), the East African Community (EAC), the Economic Community of West African States (ECOWAS), the Secretariat of the African, Caribbean and Pacific Group of States (ACP Sec), WHO, EC, and ESA.

In its report the TTF stresses that among the world's regions, Sub-Saharan Africa, with its 47 countries and 750 million inhabitants (2005 figures), is the one with the highest burden of communicable diseases such as HIV/AIDS, tuberculosis, and malaria. The average life expectancy at birth in Sub-Saharan Africa was 46 in 2004. Health service coverage is low, as for example figures

for immunisation coverage and the numbers of births attended by skilled personnel show. The region faces a serious health workforce crisis, due to the migration of doctors and nurses to more developed countries, and also due to the death of skilled personnel from disease (Asamoah-Odei, E., et al. 2007).

The TTF has reviewed health policies and strategies for African development of NEPAD, WHO and the European Union (EU). The review revealed that overall ICT penetration in most African countries is low, the availability of computers and, in particular, the internet access is extremely low. The TTF is convinced that by complementing terrestrial infrastructure with satellite communications, complete coverage of the African region can be achieved. In its report (Asamoah-Odei, E., et al. 2007) the TTF emphasizes the important role of private public partnerships in the implementation of e Health programs and projects in Africa, mentioning NEPAD e Africa Commission's e-Schools project as an excellent example. In this project five major consortia of private companies work in African countries with national industry and government partners to provide interconnectivity and ICT infrastructure to schools.

The TTF has aligned itself with the health policies and strategies for African development of NE-PAD, WHO and EU. These strategies all address the UN Millennium Development Goals (MDGs) and recognise ICT as an important enabler for progress towards these goals in the African region. Consequently, the TTF recommends a user and demand driven approach to support better access to information and knowledge for African health workers and citizens, based on well-delineated local needs and health priorities, laying emphasis on support to existing initiatives which address the needs of the stakeholders, by observing and harmonising related activities, promoting open markets, facilitating open systems, implementing demonstrators and proposing governance models and financial options.

THE WAY FORWARD

In the short-term the TTF proposes concrete action to demonstrate the feasibility of satellite technology to extend the reach of eHealth and to contribute to regional efforts to overcome health workforce shortages. Short-term actions include piloting the extension of existing programmes on eHealth. It is envisaged that this piloting process will permit an immediate start for using ICT in management and use of information and knowledge for improved health in Sub-Saharan Africa in order to demonstrate the potential benefits and to allow an estimation of the costs of effective use of the available technology.

Piloting activities shall begin in 2008. General requirements include: address highly relevant strategic goals; demonstrate a clear benefit in satisfying an urgent demand of African inhabitants; achieve strong African ownership; commitment of the stakeholders; innovative services, yet be based on existing and easy-to-use components; take advantage of successful service implementations, including infrastructure, governance models, and regulatory aspects; create a clear business plan ensuring a good chance for sustainability of the created services after initial funding.

In order to reduce the risk of failure, special attention will be put on: the geographical choice of target areas, which shall build upon already existing mechanisms, e.g. used those used by NEPAD in their e-Schools project; the training of users and technicians in the isolated area, since it is crucial for a reliable operation of the communication facilities; the language issue; in order to keep it manageable, the piloting activities should not need the involvement of too many stakeholders; to ensure feasibility, they should not depend on complicated and/or failure-prone technical configurations; to address connectivity, not only one single country shall be served; no considerable amount of new content shall be creates, since this is a time-consuming and costly

task; the creation of a business case for migrating the project scenario into a sustainable service.

Both eLearning services and clinical services, targeted towards carefully chosen remote areas in Sub-Saharan Africa, can meet the criteria set up by the TTF. Therefore, two objectives shall be addressed:

1. Offer continuing professional education via satellite to health workers in selected remote areas. The target areas shall be chosen within different countries. They shall be isolated and suffer from a significant burden of disease. Though, there must be health workers on site who are able and willing to utilize ICTs for continuing education purposes.

Existing medical content for doctors and nurses shall be chosen, preferably from African sources, paying special attention to its maintenance. Satellite-based access to the eContent shall be facilitated through different end-user devices, especially mobile devices. Low-cost, easy to use components with low electricity consumption shall be combined to serve a broad range of application scenarios and to achieve good acceptance.

2. Establish electronic communications between healthcare facilities in a few isolated areas with high burden of diseases and medical centres of excellence in Africa, for HIV/AIDS, tuberculosis, and malaria. Implement a satellite-based clinical service to support health workers in diagnosing and treating these diseases.

Medication follow-up, logistical and other types of support shall be given via communication services for speech, images, and sensor data. In addition to communication with centres of excellence, communication between inhabitants of the isolated areas shall be facilitated.

The potential of using the service for providing telepharmacy functionality, which is highly relevant for the treatment of infectious diseases, shall be explored.

These piloting activities will be of particular interest to the EC in considering the potential expansion of eHealth as part of the EU Strategy for Africa objective of increasing interconnectivity, which will be taken forward under the 10th European Development Fund.

All envisaged activities are, directly or indirectly, addressing the support for infectious disease problems, especially HIV/AIDS, tuberculosis, and malaria. The medical content and expertise shall preferably be provided by African centres of excellence.

CONCLUSION

There is still a long way to go in order to gain substantial contribution from Telemedicine and eHealth to the achievement of the MDGs. Therefore, based on earlier experiences and the lessons that will be learned from the piloting activities described, a programmatic framework shall be developed, outlining actions on a medium and long term scale, toward a sustainable eHealth infrastructure for the African continent.

We are looking, in collaboration with ESA, and other Italian institutions, including Rome Celio Military Hospital Satellite Telemedicine for Italy Europe China collaboration in the field, due to Our long lasting knowledge of the China health care reform approached problems and friendships with many hospitals and health Bureaus Municipality. The projects should and will be presented in China for finding bilateral cooperations between Italian and Chinese Civilian and Military technologies and opportunities present already in the field. (Naccarella F., et al. 2012).

A very relevant international experience using military telemedicine for health problems in both civilian and military contexts has been settled in the last ten years at Celio Hospital in Rome. (Anaclerio M., et al.2007-2012).

ACKNOWLEDGMENT

We thank Prof Franco Naccarella MD FESC, FACC, FAHA MESPE for the kind permission to publish the paper from MESPE JOURNAL 2009 We thank for collaborating reviewing and preparing the final draft of the present paper.

REFERENCES

Asamoah-Odei, E., de Backer, H., Dologuele, N., Embola, I., Groth, S., & Horsch, A. (2007). eHealth for Africa – Opportunities for enhancing the contribution of ICT to improve health services. *European Journal of Medical Research*, *12*(Suppl. 1), 1–38.

Dario, C., Dunbar, A., Feliciani, F., Garcia-Barbero, M., Giovannetti, S., & Graschew, G. (2005). Opportunities and challenges of ehealth and telemedicine via satellite. *European Journal of Medical Research*, *10*(Suppl. 1), 1–52.

Feliciani, F. (2003). Medical care from space: Telemedicine. *ESA Bulletin*, 114.

Naccarella, F., Sun, L., Zhou, S., et al. (2012). *2012 Beijing Workshop in collaboration with Embassy of Italy*. Euro China Society for Health Research and Dao Health Care Management Company.

WHO. (2006). *WHS: World health statistics 2006*. Retrieved July 20, 2012, from www.who.int/entity/whosis/whostat2006.pdf

WISR. (2006). *World information society report 2006*. International Telecommunications Union. Retrieved July 20, 2012, from http://www.itu.int/osg/spu/publications/worldinformationsociety/2006/wisr-web.pdf

KEY TERMS AND DEFINITIONS

EHealth: The term eHealth came into use in the year 2000, but has since become widely prevalent. The scope of the topic was not immediately discernible from that of the wider health informatics field for which a lot of definition are presented in literature. e-health is an emerging field of medical informatics, referring to the organization and delivery of health services and information using the Internet and related technologies. In a wider sense, the term characterizes not only a technical development, but also a new way of working, an attitude, and a commitment for networked, global thinking, to improve health care locally, regionally, and worldwide by using information and communication technology.

ESA: European Space Agency.

Telemedicine Task Force (TTF): It has been established on initiative of ESA and the European Commission with the mandate to explore the potential of Telemedicine via Satellite for African regions, with representatives of African stakeholders and the World Health Organization.

Chapter 6
DREAM Programme:
Use of Telemedicine as a Model to Cooperation with Africa

Michelangelo Bartolo
S. Giovanni Addolorata Hospital, Italy

Andrea Nucita
University of Messina, Italy

ABSTRACT

This chapter is the description of the authors' experience in providing healthcare consultation and support in African countries. The project, named DREAM, was developed to provide support to in fighting pandemic diseases such as HIV using telematics for data gathering and remote consultations.

INTRODUCTION

DREAM (Drug Resource Enhancement against AIDS and Malnutrition) is a programme made from the Community of S.Egidio started in 2002 in Mozambique and now spread in 10 countries of sub-Saharan Africa (Mozambique, Malawi, Tanzania; Kenia, Rep. Guinea; Guinea Bissau, Nigeria, Angola; Cameroon, Congo). It is a holistic programme to fight HIV and Malnutrition. Up today DREAM has 33 centres already operational and 13 molecular biology laboratories that guarantee constant monitoring to DREAM patients. More than 95.000 patients are under assistance and 55.000 of them are in HAART treatment.

DOI: 10.4018/978-1-4666-2979-0.ch006

BACKGROUND

This pandemic has characteristics that make it unique in its kind and which can be summed up as follows.

The HIV/AIDS infection is mainly concentrated in countries with limited resources, and in particular, in sub-Saharan Africa. It has become the first cause of death here and the new infections per year still outnumber the deaths. In fact, according to the WHO statistics, there are 33 million infected people in the world, around 60% of whom live in sub-Saharan Africa. Every year it is estimated that around 2 million people die from HIV/AIDS, and over 70% of them in sub-Saharan Africa.

No vaccines are available yet, neither preventive nor therapeutic. Nonetheless great progress has been made in the field of antiretroviral drugs, which have been administered in a triple combination since 1996 and have reduced the death rate in the West by 90%.

However, the antiretroviral drugs are not able to eradicate the virus: therefore the patients' health depends on them taking the drugs for their whole life. One can thus understand that the richness and complexity of the clinical records generated and of the history of the patients is unequalled by any other pathology.

Moreover, both the infection and the therapy need to be carefully monitored with a sophisticated diagnostic system organised on four levels: progression of the disease and the patient's clinical condition; his immune status (mainly expressed in terms of his CD4 cell count); the "quality" of the viral infection (viral load and resistance mutations); surveillance for any adverse events and toxicity related to the pharmacological treatment.

Another critical point is that the whole system has to be integrated into the health systems of countries with limited resources and has to take into consideration other widespread conditions in these countries, like for example, malnutrition, the low level of access to health services and the poor level of health education.

One more point is that the poor knowledge about the disease and above all the need to consolidate solutions for several aspects of the public health system (like for example, the prevention of mother-to-child transmission, the knowledge of the best time to start therapy, the control and prevention of co-infections and of opportunistic diseases) mean that the African programmes have to be able to carry out research, in particular operational research. This then means that the data collected have to be available for drawing up reports, but also for data mining, cost/benefit evaluations, and epidemiological analyses in general (Palombi et al., 2012).

Finally DREAM had to deal with another key problem in sub-Saharan Africa, which is the dramatic shortage of qualified health staff, as reported recently by the WHO. In other terms both the clinical centres and the laboratories had to combine adequate apprenticeships with the theoretical training of new biologists, doctors, laboratory technicians and obviously computer experts.

The DREAM Project

Considering the above, the DREAM Project aims to introduce the essential components of an integrated strategy for the prevention and treatment of HIV/AIDS within the framework of national health systems. The project is intended to serve as a model for the wide-ranging scale-up of the response to the epidemic. Its main objective is achieved through the establishment of services providing diagnosis and comprehensive treatment.

The prevention of HIV transmission in the general population and of mother-to-child transmission through Community Care and Home Care services (CCHC) and Mother and Child Prevention and Care (MCPC), respectively, are additional key components of the programme. The Community Care and Home Care services look after the rest of the family, that is the male partners in the first place, and also the children. Mother and Child Prevention and Care is DREAM's approach for achieving results in caring for the mothers and preventing mother-to-child transmission. This link is crucial to ensure the survival of women and good adherence to the treatment programme.

Since adherence to ARVs and treatment follow-up are essential for the effective use of HAART in large-scale public health settings, DREAM provides the treatment package free of charge to all patients. This is a crucial element; for many patients, even the cost of transport may prevent them from adhering to treatment. By eliminating the cost of treatment, high adherence rates have been achieved.

DREAM Software and Telemedicine Services

In order to follow one by one all these patients we realized a specific software that every DREAM centre must use: DREAM® Software (Nucita et al., 2009). The software is multilanguage and supports Italian, French, English and Portuguese languages.

DREAM® Software is a crucial tool in order to check, by remote control and by mirror databases in different servers, all the clinical data of patients and the daily work of all health professional workers.

The software has different sections: Reception for the personal data, family and social data of each patients; the clinic situation with symptoms and diagnosis, according to the ICD10; treatments, blood examinations, a lot of vital parameters and a Dashboard that shows the values of Cd4, Viral Load, Hgb and BMI by means of graphs.

The software has a dedicated section in order to manage the drugstore and the food store.

Moreover, there is a section for the pregnancies and several tools to evaluate the adherence at the treatment. All sensitive data of patients are anonymous.

In some rural zones the Internet connection is provided by a satellite connection.

DREAM Software was born of the need to computerise the management of the clinical files of DREAM patients.

This need envelops three main objectives:

- Optimising access of the patients to the clinic so as to guarantee the highest possible number of daily visits;
- Having at one's disposal a database with information on the clinical history of individual patients and on the overall running of the DREAM centre, which is useful for refining therapies and for the sound running of the centres;
- Providing researchers with a useful database, by making use of the experience accumulated over the years.

The first objective of DREAM, and consequently for DREAMS (DREAM Software), is to guarantee a standard of quality comparable with that of developed countries. In this sense, the genesis of the software is strictly related to that of DREAM.

In the main form of the software is shown in Figure 1.

Teleconsultation

The Teleconsultation service is implemented by a particular section of the software: it is sufficient to type the patient ID and the Clinical issue. All the data of medical records will be checked subsequently by accessing the local server. About 10 doctors from Italy can access and verify clinical data and give therapeutic indications and suggestions.

Figure 1. DREAM terminal GUI

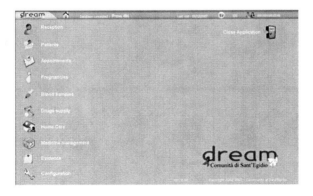

Up to now more than 12.000 Teleconsultation have been performed.

A large part of the work on DREAM Software has been dedicated to the design of a relational database for the management of data contained in clinical files. This is an important resource both for the management of the clinical data of patients, as well as for the possibility it gives to analyse information found therein, from clinical and organisational perspectives.

As has already been acknowledged, creating a dictionary of terms used is of crucial importance for the management of the database. In particular, there was a felt need for encoding with regard to the more important information – pathologies and drugs although not exclusively – as this has the capacity of making such information usable in an epidemiological context while maintaining a friendly approach towards clinical users. ICD X and ATC codifications in particular were used. The transcoding dictionaries compile 2,700 items for pathologies in the following languages: English, French, Portuguese and Italian. This feature is all the more useful in the case of DREAM, where the presence of many centres spread across different countries makes the homogenisation of terminology necessary. In the DREAM Software, pre-codified data is consequently used for the specification of symptoms, of diagnosis and of drugs, to avoid the possibility of inserting free text, which would lead to non-homogeneity of data.

This feature is crucial in the context of tele-medicine, in the sense that different medical doctors, from different countries and with different mother languages can access clinical data avoiding ambiguities.

Architectural Organization of a DREAM Centre

This section briefly presents the typical architecture of a DREAM centre.

The DREAM database and Software are on the computer server in every DREAM centre. For security reasons, access to the database can take place only indirectly through the DREAM Software: the users (the coordinator, doctors, nurses and operators) do not have the privilege of direct access to the database. This precaution is to prevent a malicious (or inexpert) user from damaging the database or from deliberately spreading sensitive information. Moreover, sharing the same software on the server simplifies the configuration of the computers used. The architecture of a DREAM centre is illustrated in (Figure 2).

Figure 2. DREAM network configuration

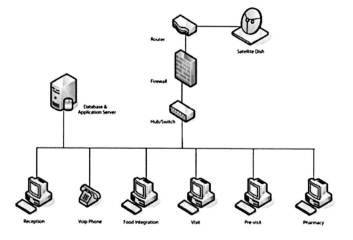

As may be seen, every service within the DREAM centres (the examination room, the pharmacy and so on) has a computer, which is linked to the server and to the rest of the computers through a LAN, giving individual operators the possibility of following the patient for his/her entire course of treatment in the centre, with the most updated data always at hand, without having to refer to files on paper.

Communication between the various centres is guaranteed by an Internet connection, and through satellite in those places where it has proved impossible to get connected through an already existing cable network. Communication has turned out to be of considerable importance for two fundamental reasons, namely the centralised compilation of data and communication/consultation with specialised personnel. Through Internet communication (instant messaging or VoIP), every user can communicate with the personnel of other African or European centres. This has made the extensive use of teleconsultation possible (with no additional cost save that of the Internet connection), and this is very useful when the doctor feels the need to interact with colleagues about more complex clinical cases.

CONCLUSION

The DREAM programme, together with Telemedicine Service, represents a real proposal for a model of international cooperation that makes it possible, nowadays, to remotely support developing countries.

The experience of DREAM overall, and in particular of the software and the telemedicine services, has shown how the catastrophe of HIV and AIDS in Africa also holds an opportunity: that of equipping the continent, in response to this emergency, with the necessary and appropriate technologies to overcome old and new problems: the digital divide, the poor possibilities of communications, the sprawling distances and poor

logistics. The repercussions of the implementation of such technologies actually go well beyond the specific context of the epidemic. There are strong possibilities for the development of formation too, since it would be possible, for example, to have long-distance formation with centres.

REFERENCES

Nucita, A., Bernava, G. M., Bartolo, M., Di Pane Masi, F., Peroni, M., Pizzimenti, G., & Palombi, L. (2009). A global approach to the management of EMR (Electronic Medical Records) of patients with HIV/AIDS in Sub-Saharan Africa: The experience of DREAM Software. *BMC Journal of Medical Informatics and Decision Making, 9*(42).

Palombi, L., Bernava, G. M., Nucita, A., Giglio, P., Liotta, G., & Nielsen-Saines, K. (2012). Predicting trends in HIV-1 sexual transmission in sub-Saharan Africa through the drug resource enhancement against AIDS and malnutrition model: Antiretrovirals for reduction of population infectivity, incidence and prevalence at the district level. *Clinical Infectious Diseases, 55*(2), 268–275. doi:10.1093/cid/cis380

KEY TERMS AND DEFINITIONS

Drug Resource Enhancement Against AIDS and Malnutrition in Africa (DREAM): DREAM is a programme based on a holistic approach of treating AIDS in Africa, launched in February 2002 by the Community of St Egidio.

DREAM® Software: A software used in the DREAM Programme to manage EMR and telemedicine services.

Elecronic Medical Records (EMR): Computerised medical records that are the core of a database for medical information systems.

HAART: Highly Active Antiretroviral Therapy.

HIV: Human Immunodeficiency Virus.

Teleconsultation: Remote clinical consultation, by the use of information and communication technologies.

Telemedicine: Telemedicine uses information and communication technologies in order to provide health care at a distance.

Chapter 7
The Effects of Telehealth on Patients with Long-Term Conditions in Routine Healthcare Use and Lessons from Practical Application

Victor Vuni Joseph
Leeds Institute of Health Sciences (LIHS), University of Leeds, UK & Doncaster Primary Care Trust (PCT), UK

ABSTRACT

There is increasing uptake of telehealth for long-term conditions (LTCs). However, evidence of their effectiveness remains largely inconclusive. Similarly, success factors for implementation of telehealth into routine healthcare practice are not fully understood. The objectives of this chapter are to determine the effectiveness of telehealth; and to update existing checklist on key success factors for implementation of telehealth. Both randomized controlled trial (RCT) and observational study methods were used as case-studies. Analysis was carried out using logistic regression model and summary statistics. There was a statistically significant reduction in hospital admissions in favour of the intervention groups in the RCT, with an odds ratio (OR) of 0.08 (95% CI: 0.01, 0.81); p-value = 0.03, while in the observational study, the mean hospital admission per person reduced from 2.19 (95% CI: 1.67, 2.69) to 1.20 (95% CI: 0.88, 1.52); p-value 0.0004. Key success factors identified were used to update the second version of telehealth checklist tool. Telehealth was effective in reducing hospital admission in patients with COPD, heart failure, and diabetes. Key success factors were updated to support telehealth practitioners in embedding telehealth in routine practice.

DOI: 10.4018/978-1-4666-2979-0.ch007

INTRODUCTION

The past decade has seen an increase in telehealth activities, especially in the United Kingdom. Much of these increased activities was driven by the claim that telehealth is effective in reducing hospital activities and thereby reducing associated healthcare costs to health organisations (Audit Commission, 2004). However, it was unknown whether the above claim could translate in local settings in routine healthcare practice. In the United Kingdom, the Government supported a programme to promote piloting telehealth (as part of assistive technology) and many local authorities and healthcare organisations in England started to undertake telehealth activities from around 2006 onwards (Department of Health, 2005). Doncaster, one of the English districts, was one of the areas that managed to get initial Government grant to pilot the implementation of telehealth in 2007 and funding was subsequently met from the resource of Doncaster Primary Health Care Trust. The initial pilot was designed as a randomized controlled trial (RCT) to test the effectiveness of telehealth. After one year of the RCT, the telehealth project was transformed into a service development to all patients with long-term conditions (mainly patients with chronic obstructive pulmonary disease (COPD), heart failure and diabetes), with embedded service evaluation. The project was run by community nurses for patients living in their own homes. While this work was based in the community, it raised the need for interface between hospital and community services working together to coordinate and achieve optimum benefit for patients. This chapter reports on the findings of a local delivery of telehealth and the lessons learned in embedding telehealth in routine healthcare use, across community and hospital interface. The objectives were (1) to determine the effectiveness of telehealth; and (2) to report on updated key success factors that enable telehealth to embed in routine healthcare use.

BACKGROUND

Definition of Telehealth

The World Health Organisation (WHO) defined telehealth as:

The delivery of healthcare service, where distance is a critical factor, by all healthcare professionals using information and communication technologies for the exchange of valid information for diagnosis, treatment and prevention of disease and injuries, research and evaluation, and for the continuing education of healthcare providers, all in the interest of advancing the health of individuals and their communities (Scalvini, Vitacca, & Paletta, 2004; World Health Organisation, 2003).

While the above definition offers a broad base, and inclusivity, it also poses a problem in translating what is meant for the purpose of international comparison of evidence of effectiveness of telehealth. Telehealth has been used in the published literature to encompass a range of devices including: computer, videophone, still image video phones, mobile phone, fax radio, and the use of internet, among others (Grigsby, Brega, & Devore, 2005; Wootton, Dimmick, & Kvedar, 2006). It has been used for the management of a range of conditions such as mental health, heart failures, diabetes, lung diseases, as well as for public health interventions e.g. smoking cessation, and weight management programmes (Sheikh, McLean, Cresswell, Pagliari, Pappas, Car et al., 2011; Wootton, Craig, & Patterson, 2006).

Another issue that causes confusion among practitioners of telehealth is the lack of consensus on array of terminologies that are in common usage. Experts in the field of telehealth view telehealth as having different subsets, which overlaps with each other, and these include terminologies such as: telemedicine, mobile health (m-health), remote patient monitoring, mobile patient monitoring (Pawar, Jones, Van Beijnum, & Hermaens, 2012). On the other hand, telehealth itself is considered to be a subset of electronic health (e-health) (Pawar et al., 2012).

In view of the uncertainty in definitions in the published literature, it was felt necessary to define telehealth as used in this chapter:

Telehealth is defined as telecommunication device where patients can remotely monitor their vital signs (oxygen saturation level in their blood (SpO2), pulse, breathing, or blood pressure), and answer some questions on their conditions which are transmitted online to a healthcare professional to respond to them.

Evidence of Effectiveness: What is Known?

Systematic Reviews

The evidence of effectiveness of telehealth is generally not fully established yet. According to latest evidence, based on systematic reviews, there were mixed findings reported. For example, a systematic review of 80 review articles published between 2005 and 2009 found that 20 of the 80 articles (32.7%) concluded that telehealth was effective, while 19 (31.1%) concluded the evidence was promising, and 22 (36.1%) concluded that the evidence was limited and inconclusive (Ekeland, Bowes, & Flottorp, 2010). The limitations of the review included the issues related to definition of telehealth or telemedicine used in the articles included, as they encompassed various types of telehealth interventions as a result comparison could not be made easily between studies; different diseases were targeted; and poor quality of studies reported.

Another larger systematic review, which involved 162 systematic review articles published between 1997 and 2010, also concluded that the evidence of effectiveness of telehealth was limited in improving patients' outcomes, except in specific

areas such as chronic obstructive pulmonary disease (COPD), asthma, and heart failure (Sheikh et al., 2011). This was a more positive conclusion than an earlier review by the same group of authors who initially concluded that there was no evidence of effectiveness (Black, Car, Pagliari, Anandan, Cresswell, Bokun et al., 2011). The change in conclusion was due to publication of recent studies that changed the authors' perspective on the subject. The review by Sheikh and colleagues was quite broad, encompassing e-health, which of course included telehealth, but this meant that the studies reviewed were heterogeneous; making comparison between studies difficult (Sheikh et al., 2011). Their review did not pose a clearly focused question about the effectiveness of telehealth; outcomes were varied; and low quality of the studies reviewed. However, the authors found that patients were satisfied and they accepted telehealth if offered as an addition to face-face consultations.

It had been shown that telehealth industries appeared to be more positive about the effectiveness of telehealth than what the prevailing evidence suggested in the published literature (Sheikh et al., 2011). Similarly, the evidence threshold at which Governments appear to accept telehealth is lower than that held by the academic community, for example, in the UK, based on the findings of the Whole System Demonstrator (a cluster randomized controlled trial in England involving 6000 patients in three geographical areas), the Government decided to roll out telehealth to 3 million people in England (Department of Health, 2012a). Despite the publication of their study findings (Steventon, Bardsley, Billings, Dixon, Doll, Hirani et al., 2012), there remain a lot of questions regarding the study's main findings and the extent to which it would warrant such a wide-scale roll out of telehealth to three million users in England.

Systematic review which focused on specific disease areas (e.g. COPD, asthma and heart failure) appeared to offer more positive conclusions. For example, a review on asthma found that a significant reduction in hospital admissions over a 12 months' period, with an odds ratio (OR) of 0.21; 95% CI: 0.07, 0.61) (S McLean, Chandler, Nurmatov, Liu, Pagliari, Car et al., 2010). This study appeared to be well conducted; as it asked a clearly focused question, clear inclusion and exclusion criteria and a meta-analysis was conducted. However, the study's findings could not be generalized to other settings due to varying contexts and lack of guarantee in replicating the findings. Among heart failure patients, a meta-analysis involving 2710 participants (11 RCTs) found a reduction in mortality (risk ratio (RR) of 0.66; 95% CI: 0.5, 0.81); as well as a reduction in hospital admission (RR of 0.79; 95% CI: 0.76, 0.94) (Anker, Koehler, & Abraham, 2011). Similar findings were reported by other authors on heart failure (Inglis, Clark, McAlister, Ball, Lewinter, Cullington et al., 2010). On COPD, a systematic review found significant reduction in emergency department attendance over 12 months' period with an odds ratio of 0.27 (95% CI: 0.11, 0.66); while those with more than one hospital admission within 12 months had an odds ratio of 0.46 (95% CI: 0.33, 0.65) (S. McLean, Nurmatov, Liu, Pagliari, Car, Sheikh et al., 2011).

Randomised Controlled Trial (RCTs)

A number of randomized controlled trials (RCTs) on telehealth can be found in the published literature. However, it is worth identifying some few and major notable RCTs in the field of telehealth. For patients with heart failure, a multicenter RCT involving 1653 patients followed up over a six months period found no significant difference in health outcomes in terms of hospital readmission and mortality (Chaudhry, Mattera, Curtis, Sperlus, Herrin, & Lin, 2010). On the other hand, another RCT carried out over a 5-year period in New York State (USA) among patients with diabetes

found evidence of effectiveness in improving HgbA1c, LDL-cholesterol and blood pressure (Shea, Weinstock, Teresi, Palmas, Starren, Cimino et al., 2009). As telehealth technology changed over the 5-years of follow, this was likely to have influenced the study outcome as comparison could not be made easily over time for patients who received telehealth. In addition, there was a high drop-out rate over the 5-year time period, especially in the intervention group (60.9%) as compared to 43.6% in the control group. However, this study contrasts with one in the same location in New York which indicated that telehealth did not reduce cost among patients with diabetes, as the average cost per patient was found to be over US$8000 in the intervention (71-116%) compared to control; (Moreno, Dale, Chen, & Magee, 2009). The findings from Whole System Demonstrator RCT in England, based on 3230 patients with COPD, heart failure and diabetes found a reduction in hospital admission; odds ratio of 0.82 (95% CI: 0.70, 0.97) in favour of intervention group; as well as reduction in mortality (odds ratio of 0.54, 95% CI: 0.39, 0.75) (Steventon et al., 2012).

Cost Effectiveness

Various studies appear to show some evidence of cost-effectiveness, but they suffer from poor methodological designs; as many of them were not derived from well-designed RCT, but observational studies. Among diabetes patients, a study designed for delivering diabetic retinopathy screening indicated that there was potential for cost-effectiveness (Jones & Edwards, 2010). For patients with long-term condition, a systematic review of 4871 patients involving 22 published articles between 1998 and 2008 also concluded that telehealth had potential for cost saving (Polisena, Coyle, Coyle, McGill, Polisena, Coyle et al., 2009). Similar findings of potential cost-saving were also found in teledermatology (Whited, 2001). However, earlier systematic reviews on telehealth around the year 2000 found no evidence of cost-effectiveness of telehealth (Whitten, Mair, Haycox, May, Williams, & Hellmich, 2002), which could be partly due to limited studies undertaken at that time.

In the United States, one of the largest observational study undertaken by Veteran Health Administration (VHA) referred to as Care Coordination/ Home Telehealth (CCHT) programme examined not only the effectiveness but cost-effectiveness of telehealth (Darkins, Ryan, Kobb, Foster, Edmonson, Wakefield et al., 2008). Based on 31,570 patients who took part in the programme, they found that the average cost per person per year was US dollars 1600, compared to US$ 13,121 among patients in home-based primary care service, and US$ 77,745 for those in market nursing home care. They reported a reduction in bed-days in hospital by 25%, hospital admissions by 19%, and satisfaction rating of 86%. The limitation of the study included the fact that it was observational study and comparison between those on the programme could not be validly compared with those elsewhere; no baseline characteristics were available to indicate similarity or dissimilarity in population profile. However, the study showed that large scale telehealth deployment was feasible.

In cardiology, a 19-year old programme which was administered twenty-four hours a day and 7-days per week in Israel and Germany reported cost saving of 677,000 Euro per 10,000 population (Roth, Korb, Gadot, Kalter, Roth, Korb et al., 2006). The authors examined 1870 patients over the above period and found patients were generally reassured of their complaints related to coronary artery disease.

Patient Satisfaction

In general, various studies reported high level of satisfaction with telehealth. One systematic review, which covered the period 1998-2008 found that patients were generally satisfied with telehealth; and patients preferred it as an addition to face-to-face consultation by healthcare staff

rather than replacing them (Sheikh et al., 2011). The level of satisfaction was found to be between 80 and 100% in another systematic review (Williams, May, & Esmail, 2001). The high levels of satisfaction were reported in studies related to other long-term conditions such as dermatology (wound care) (Whited, 2001), COPD, and heart failure (Finkelstein, Speedie, Demiris, Veen, & Lundgren, 2004).

Gaps in Knowledge

From the foregoing literature review, uncertainty still remains in determining the effectiveness of telehealth for various long-term condition, and the conditions under which successful implementation can be expected. Definitions of telehealth vary and this pose problem for comparison of assessing health outcomes and effectiveness of telehealth in various settings. A successful outcome of telehealth in one area does not mean that similar findings can be replicated either in the same or different area where the context maybe different. Other authors have also acknowledged the gaps in research around economic evaluation, and the need to capture the views of patients about telehealth interventions (Ekeland et al., 2010).

MAIN FOCUS OF THE CHAPTER

Methodological Issues

The premise of telehealth is based on the fact that it will pick up problems early, while recognizing that it may potentially results in an increase in traffic of communication between patients and the healthcare staff concerned, usually a community nurse as in this study setting (Figure 1). This increase in initial contacts between patients and their community nurse is expected to pay off in the long-term by reducing emergency hospital admissions compared to patients who receive usual care.

Figure 1. A depiction of telehealth service in comparison with usual care

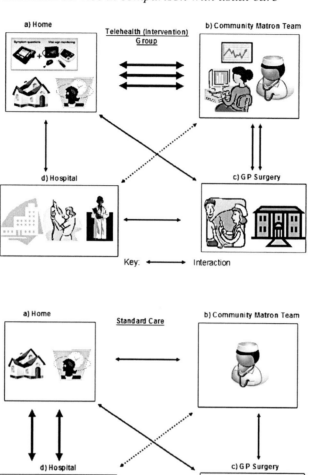

There were two main study methods used to recruit patients into the study; initially by means of randomized controlled trial (RCTs); and subsequently at a later stage (after 12-months) an observational study using service evaluation method was employed. The home telehealth was undertaken initially as an (RCT) with a focus on patients with COPD who had previous hospital admission in the previous 12 months. Patients were identified from hospital admissions records, based on discharge records and their diagnostic status were confirmed with general practitioners (GPs – doctor), where they were registered. Patients were included into the study if they had at least one previous hospital admissions from COPD in the preceding year; were on disease register for COPD; were both living in, and registered with a GP, in the local area. Exclusion of cases was based on those who did not have the physical and mental ability to use the equipment nor a carer to help them; who did not have COPD according to the disease register; not living in the local area; and if they had no landline telephone.

While the RCT design demanded such a rigorous process, it was found that the strict inclusion and exclusion criteria set made it difficult to recruit participants into the study. The first obstacle was encountered in identifying potential patients from hospital admissions record, which proved less reliable as they were based on patients who were admitted in the previous 12 months. By the time of identification of potential cases, some of the patients had died, others could not be contacted. A prospective identification of patients at the point of discharge would have been much easier. However, the choice of design was based on identifying patients with the disease who were living in the community, which had the majority of pool of patients.

After 12 months period, the RCT design was stopped and the eligibility to have patients on telehealth was delegated to community nurses (community matron or heart failure specialist nurses) who had patients on their caseload. They determined who, in their professional opinion, was suitable to be put on home telehealth monitoring. There were unstructured interviews with patients and staff, as well as focus group discussion, based on normalization process model (CR

May, Harrison, & Finch, 2003). The change of study design from RCT to observational study (service evaluation of the observational study) was well received with community nurses, as they disliked RCT which gave them no control of who they would like to put on telehealth machine. An inherent part of RCT was based on identification of similar group of patients some of whom would then be randomized to receive the intervention care, while others would receive usual care. This loss of RCT design was considered to be a price worth paying if local health practitioners were to be engaged in the local telehealth delivery.

The Results

Recruitment

From the RCT, there was a total of 36 participants included in the study, of which 20 were in the intervention group while 16 were in control arm of the study, with analysis undertaken based on intention to treat (ITT). The numbers of participants that were considered and finally selected for inclusion into the study through and those analyzed are shown in Figure 2.

Figure 2. Recruitment process into the RCT

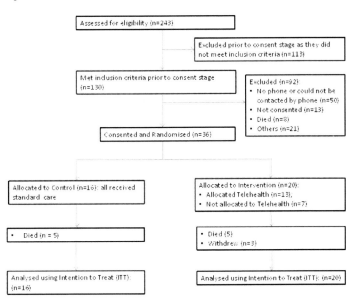

This contrasted with the number of participants recruited into the observational study after stopping RCT design, which saw a progressive increase of participants between April 2010 and October 2011, when the analysis was carried out. A total of 204 patients were referred to telehealth service, and 176 (86.3%) actually used telehealth. As of October 2011, the number of active users of telehealth was 119 participants and monthly figures of update showed a steady increase (Figure 3). They included patients with heart failure (49%), COPD (41%), multiple comorbidity (9%) and diabetes (1%). In reality, even patients who were assigned as having COPD and heart failure only might have also other long-term conditions.

Impacts on Hospital Admissions

Findings from the RCT indicated that there was a statistically non-significant reduction of hospital admission rate per person per year by 45.4% in the intervention group compared to that in the controlled group. The intervention group had 0.77 hospital admissions per person per year during telehealth period, and the equivalent rate for control group was 1.41 (Figure 4).

Further analysis using logistic regression model showed statistically significant reduction in hospital admission in favour of intervention arm of the study, adjusted odds ratio (OR) of 0.08; 95% CI: 0.01, 0.81; p-value 0.03. The OR for hospital admissions in males was 12.36 (95% CI: 1.25, 122.57); p-value 0.03 compared to females. Patients with more previous hospital admissions had higher odds ratio of being admitted, with OR of 4.85 (95% CI: 1.34, 17.52); and p-value of 0.02 (Table 1).

The analysis of the observational studies, which involved 119 participants revealed that the mean number of hospital admissions per person 12-months before telehealth period was 2.19 (95% CI: 1.67, 2.69), while during telehealth period, the rate of hospital admission reduced to 1.20 (95% CI: 0.88, 1.52); a reduction of 45%; p-value of 0.0004. While the average cost of hospital admissions per person 12 months prior to telehealth was £ (Great British Pound or GBP) 4951.05 (95% CI: 3680.03, 6222.05); and during telehealth period the equivalent cost was £2968.76 (95% CI: 2092.74; 3844.78); p-value of 0.005 (Table 2).

Both the RCT and observational study of telehealth showed that telehealth was effective in reducing hospital admissions. In addition, the observational study also showed that telehealth was cost effective for patients with long-term

Figure 3. Participants actively using telehealth between April 2010 and October 2011

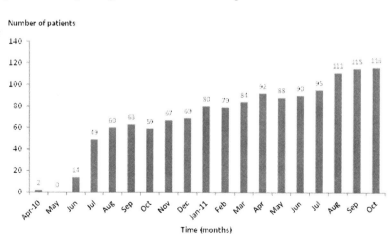

Figure 4. Hospital admission rates per person per year by intervention and control groups

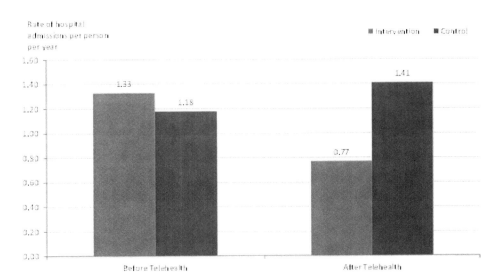

Table 1. Logistic regression modelling (adjusted odds ratio) to predict the likelihood of hospital admission

Predictive Variables	Adjusted Odds Ratio (OR)	P-value	95% CI
Sex (male)	12.36	0.03	1.25, 122.57*
Study design (Intervention)	0.08	0.03	0.01, 0.81*
Previous hospital admission rate	4.85	0.02	1.34, 17.52*

*Significant results

conditions such as COPD, heart failure and diabetes.

Key Success Factors

Here, the findings related to whether telehealth was embedding locally is presented; along with success factors that enable telehealth to embed in routine practice. To address the former, an electronic health implementation tool (eHIT) was used as a qualitative tool, based on assessment of a committee overseeing the implementation of telehealth. The committee comprised of about a dozen members, which included clinicians, commissioning managers, public health practitioners, and coordinator of telehealth service. A formal assessment were made at 6-months' intervals three times within a time frame of 15 months of the implementation of the observational study. A graphical illustration of the assessment on the dimensions of the tool indicated that over time the score by the group increased (the higher the score, the likelier was for telehealth to embed in routine use), suggesting that telehealth was embedding locally (Figure 5 and 6). Detail methodology of the eHIT tool can be found elsewhere (Murray, May, Mair, & Rocket Science UK Ltd, 2010), which is underpin by normalization process model (NPM) (C May, Finch, Mair, Ballini, Dowrick, Eccles et al., 2007; CR May et al., 2003).

The first version of key challenges for developing and implementing telehealth was produced

Table 2. Impact of telehealth on hospital admissions in Doncaster: March 2010 to August 2011

Variables	Pre-telehealth period	Post-telehealth period	Difference: n (%)	P-value (s=significant; ns=not significant)
A) PROFILE:				
(i) Number of patients	119	119	0	n/a
(ii) Total duration of follow up:				
Years	119.0	95.2	23.8 (20.0)	
Months	1428	1156.3	271.7 (19.0)	
(iii) Mean duration of follow up per person:				
Years	1.0	0.8	0.2 (20.0)	p=0.0000 (s)
Months	12.0	9.7	2.3 (19.2)	p=0.0000 (s)
B) ADMISSIONS:				
(i) Total number of hospital admissions	259	143	116 (44.8)	
(ii) Admission rate per year of follow up:	2.18	1.50	0.68 (31.2)	
(iii) Admission rate per month of follow up: rate (95% CI)	0.18 (0.16, 0.20)	0.12 (0.11, 0.14)	0.06 (33.3)	
(iv) Mean number of hospital admission per person: mean (95% CI)	2.18 (1.67, 2.69)	1.20 (0.88, 1.52)	0.98 (45.0)	p=0.0004 (s)
(v) Number of admissions during 1156.3 months (95.2 years) of follow up (telehealth period)	210	143	67 (31.9)	

Table 2 (cont.): Impact of telehealth on hospital admissions in Doncaster: March 2010 to August 2011 (n=119)

Variables	Pre-telehealth period	Post-telehealth period	Difference: n (%)	P-value (s=significant; ns=not significant)
C) LENGTH OF STAY (LOS)				
(i) Total LOS in days	1992	1381	611 (30.7)	
(ii) Mean LOS in days (95% CI)	16.7 (12.3, 21.2)	11.6 (7.5, 15.7)	5.1 (30.5)	p=0.06 (ns)
(iii) LOS per year of follow up	16.7	14.5	2.2 (13.2)	
(iv) LOS during 1156. months (95.2 years) of follow up (Telehealth period)	1594	1381	213 (13.4)	
D) COST (£) OF ADMISSIONS:				
(i) Mean cost of admissions (95% CI)	4951.05 (3,680.03, 6,222.05)	2968.76 (2,092.74, 3,844.78)	1982.29 (40.0)	p=0.005 (s)
(ii) Cost per admission per year of follow up	4951.04	3709.62	1241.42 (25.1)	
(iii) Total cost of admission during 95.2 years of follow up (Telehealth period)	471,507.75	353,282.00	118,225.00 (25.1)	
(iv) Total cost of admission during 119 years of follow up (12 months period).	589,174.00	441,444.64	147,729.36 (25.1)	

and published in the Journal of Telemedicine and Telecare (Joseph, West, Shickle, Keen, & Clamp, 2011). Here, an update of the key challenges is presented, which was informed by stakeholders' event that brought together around 30 participants with interest in telehealth and telecare. At the event, participants were asked for their views on key barriers and success factors in order to embed telehealth (and telecare) in the local area. The outcomes of this exercise was used to revise the original version of key challenges in developing and implementing telehealth, to form the second version of the tool for developing and implementing telehealth (Table 3). The key elements of tool focused on identifying needs and partners; developing a strategy; securing funding; project imple-

Figure 5. Summary scores on implementation of telehealth in Doncaster

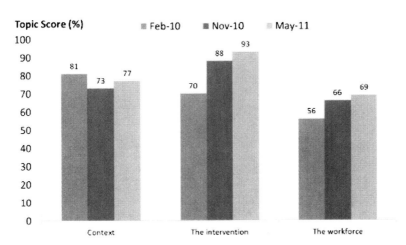

Figure 6. Scores on intervention dimension of implementation of telehealth

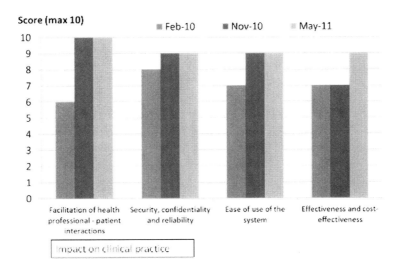

mentation, and monitoring & evaluation. The tool should be used as a qualitative assessment guide for practitioners and policy makers. Addressing all elements may not automatically mean that a particular project will succeed, however, the more elements of the tools addressed satisfactorily, the likelier it is for it to succeed.

Patients and Staff Perspective

The following perspective from patients summarized their views in relation to telehealth experience. They felt that home Telehealth monitoring offered them reassurance and helped build their self-confidence in managing their conditions, including taking decisions related to taking their medication. One patient with heart failure commented that:

Table 3. An essential telehealth checklist for practitioners (version 2)

Items of challenges	Remarks (Y,N,NA)

(A) NEEDS AND PARTENRS:
1. A clear statement of healthcare service delivery problem / issue; needs assessment has been undertaken.
2. Relevant evidence of effectiveness has been considered in relation to the condition (problem) in question and telehealth.
3. Telehealth is seen as a solution to a political and/or medical issue.
4. Joint assessment of needs has been undertaken to ensure balance between supply and demands of telehealth equipment.
5. Buy in from senior management and clinicians; overcoming professional resistance.
6. Telehealth is formally agreed as a priority.
7. Is run by a knowledgeable team working closely together.
8. Robust structures and integration is in place.
9. Increase engagement with voluntary sector and befriending community to improve social context for people using telehealth service.
10. Early input to clinical commissioning organisation to ensure they are aware of benefit of telesupport.
11. Established functional steering group (committee or board) for telehealth.
12. Having telehealth support groups to share information and provide peer reassurance.
13. A lead staff and agency has been identified.
14. All relevant partners are engaged.

(B) STRATEGY
1. There is a telehealth strategy in place for the organisation that contains a clear vision, objectives, action plan, targets and business models.
2. The organisation's management board is engaged with the strategy on telehealth.
3. Key priorities for change have been identified.
4. Telehealth system is a virtual one (not a single large database).
5. A central hub working with and for clinicians at satellite sites; there is a balance between horizontal (too many sites) vs. vertical implementation (few highly specialised sites).
6. The design of the service delivery has been considered (e.g. service evaluation vs. Randomised Controlled Trial (RCT); community vs. hospital base; short-term vs. long-term monitoring; selecting the right patients; considering how long people are going to have the equipment).
7. Communicates well with specialist groups.
8. Client-centred solution.

1. A seamless and coordinated service between health and social care. Coordinated approach to assessment and monitoring of users through a single assessment process and team that are co-located.
2. Sharing of information across health and social care.
3. Arrangement in place to address potential increase in staff workload, include cover for leaves.
4. Integrated IT (Information Technology) system and access to computers connected to internet for staff.
5. There is a plan to market telehealth in the area.
6. Training of staff has been considered; and measures on how to overcome potential barriers from staff have been formulated into action plan.
7. Approval has been granted from Information Governance point of view (confidentiality and access, data sharing).
8. Ethical approval has been considered.
9. There is legislation and regulation covering telehealth service.
10. The impact of telehealth service on health inequalities has been considered (e.g. people without landline telephone, vulnerable groups, minority groups, etc.).

(C) FUNDING
1. Is completely mainstreamed into health and social care systems.
2. Equipment is free to service users.
3. There is secured joint local authority and health service recurrent funding.
4. There is a service level agreement (SLA) with the service provider in place. The contract reflects actual machine used or rented.

(D) IMPLEMENTATION
1. A suitable supplier of telehealth has been chosen.
2. There are dedicated staff to co-ordinate and manage the service.
3. There is adequate support (e.g. education) to patients on the equipment.
4. Appropriate alert parameters are set for individual patients.
5. There are adequate arrangements for installation of the equipment.
6. Telehealth telecare is mainstreamed and integrated into standard care pathway of health and social care service provision. It is considered by all health and social care professionals as a matter of good practice (the "norm").
7. The equipment envisaged to be used is compatible with landline telephone providers in the area.
8. Consideration is given to any potential software problems to ensure access to patients record.
9. There is provision for decontamination of the equipment, where appropriate.
10. There is a written code of practice (manual) for telehealth, which defines how the whole system works, who is responsible, and key performance indicators.
11. Planned implementation of telehealth has been considered (starting with a small number, making sure it works, before increasing the number).

1. 24-hour availability for technical support.
2. Extended service including weekend and out-of-hours service (24/7)
3. A clear pathway that is fully integrated and mainstreamed.
4. Telehealth has service champions in different areas.
5. Mandatory training for certain groups of staff exists.
6. Joint awareness-raising of telehealth, creative advertising using various means.
7. Having provision for storage of equipment.
8. Change in culture for telehealth among clinicians, organisation, and general population.
9. Identified specific points on service user pathway where benefit may be gained for telehealth e.g. hospital discharge, intermediate care, GP appointments, Continuing Health Care, etc.

(E) MONITORING AND EVALUATION
1. Demonstrate benefits / outcomes; reduction in hospital activities.
2. Measures actual cost savings.
3. Has a review process in place to monitor improvement or deterioration.
4. Has positive service user and carer feedback.
5. Clear understanding of who is monitoring and responding to alert.
6. Flexibility to adapt how the service works following outcomes of review.
7. Accuracy and reliability of telehealth machine that captures patients true vital signs status (e.g. BP, spO2, temperature, etc.).
8. Reliability and sensitivity of selected questions used in telehealth machine.
9. Fewer red alerts, which are meaningful and sensitive to changes in patients condition. Setting appropriate alert parameters for individual patients.
10. Time out for staff to review progress with relevant stakeholders.
11. There is a plan to publish / disseminate the results of telehealth project.

Keynote: Remarks (Y = Yes fulfilled; N = Not fulfilled; N/A = Not applicable)

When I have been doubtful about my fluids it has been good to have the equipment as I have noticed that I have put on weight and started to take my medication without having to call the nurse or the GP [doctor]. I feel I am keeping an eye on myself (Heart failure patient).

The sense of self-confidence was generated by the fact that patients felt they were being monitored by healthcare professionals at the other end of remote home telemonitoring.

The positive impact of telehealth home-monitoring was also supported by the views of healthcare staff who felt that telehealth had helped in enhancing patient-staff relationship, as illustrated below:

The ones that I have used it with have been really positive and they really like it actually and give a lot of good feedback. They feel that they are being monitored and supported. So, I suppose from our point of view we can go in initially and give an awful lot of information and be making lots of changes to their treatment and plus we talk to them about 'do your weight, do this, let me know', but actually some of that burden is taken away a little bit I think. So they seem quite on board with it and I get a lot of positive feedback really (Heart Failure Nurse).

Solutions and Recommendations

One of the issues encountered in telehealth implementation was to address its evidence of effectiveness in routine use. Based on hierarchy of evidence, a randomized controlled trial or well conducted systematic review should address the issue of effectiveness. However, it has been found that available systematic review faced the challenge of poor quality studies, which renders their conclusions less valid, coupled with the varying definitions of telehealth that is critical in determining which studies to include. Although an RCT ranked as one of the high quality study in the hierarchy of evidence, there is difficulty in undertaking it in routine healthcare use. This chapter reports on the challenge of undertaking an RCT in local context and the associated difficulties that were faced in recruiting participants, including resistance of staff to RCT design. It was appropriate that the RCT was considered as a pilot with a small number of participants that was aimed to be recruited; as it later proved difficult to recruit into the study if a large sample size was aimed for. This work shows that it was more difficult to recruit into RCT when patients are in the community settings, using hospital admission records as these records became quickly outdated over time. Targeting eligible patients for recruitment into RCT study involving telehealth, including observational study, would appear to be much easier if patients are approached while they are in hospital prior to their discharge home, as they are captive audience. Another practical approached used in the observational study in this study was to use patients who were already part of the caseload of community nurses, another captive audience, which improved the uptake rate of telehealth.

Practitioners of telehealth may like to strengthen service evaluation of telehealth implementation as part of service development in routine healthcare service, with mix methods encompassing both qualitative and quantitative approaches as advocated by a number of authors (Campbell, Fitzpatrick, Haines, Kinmonth, Sandercock, Spiegelhalter et al., 2000; Ekeland, Bowes, & Flottorp, 2012). This is in light of the difficulties in implementing RCT in routine healthcare settings. The other alternative is a cluster randomized controlled trial, similar to that undertaken as part of the Whole System Demonstrator in England (Steventon et al., 2012). Implementations of RCTs are resource intensive, and if successful they still do not offer guarantee that any roll out in routine healthcare would be expected to be replicated with similar results. In the real world, resources are limited for delivering healthcare service, and any additional demands placed by undertaking RCTs will be resisted by health service providers.

Despite the small sample size, the RCT on Telehealth presented here managed to show statistical significant results, based on adjusted odds ratio (OR) of 0.08 (95% CI: 0.01, 0.81; p-value of 0.03) in relation to reduction of hospital admissions. The observational study also showed consistent finding in mean admission per person; 45% reduction in hospital admission in favour of telehealth, which was statistically significant (p-value 0.0004) when the period before and after telehealth was compared. These findings are consistent with those reported in a number of systematic reviews e.g. on COPD where they found the odds ratio OR of 0.46 (95% CI: 0.33, 0.65) for patients with more than one hospital admission within 12 months (S. McLean et al., 2011); major RCTs like the WSD (Steventon et al., 2012), and big observational studies such as the VHA Care Coordination Home Telehealth project in the United States (Darkins et al., 2008).

Although it has been shown that there was significant cost saving during the period before and after telehealth implementation, this analysis did not include costs of the machines and time of staff who were involved in running telehealth service. If all the costs were added up, it was likely that there would have been no significant difference in costs among patients with, and without, telehealth. It is reassuring to note the telehealth offers confidence to patients and it is seen also to embed into how healthcare staff begins to deliver healthcare differently.

Focusing telehealth either as a community-based or hospital-based programme in isolation run the risk of poor coordination, and partnership working that is required to ensure telehealth users are known to the whole health system. While the telehealth in Doncaster, started as an initiative based in the community, however, its subsequent roll out engaged hospital service providers, especially on the agenda of early hospital discharge scheme where patients who were deemed to be fit enough to be discharged home could be safely sent home with the support of telehealth. Such coordinated partnership approach of implementing telehealth across community-hospital interface needs to be promoted by practitioners of telehealth, while recognizing that the drivers may vary for the different parties involved.

FUTURE RESEARCH DIRECTIONS

1. Research is needed to understand benefits of telehealth by severity levels of various diseases. Such study has been carried out in a systematic review of patients with asthma and their use of telehealth, but it needs to be expanded to other disease areas e.g. COPD where there are patients with mild, moderate, severe, and very severe disease. It is unknown which of these groups are best suitable for, or most benefit from, telehealth.

2. There is still some gap in our understanding of which long-term conditions are best for telehealth, despite some work in demonstrating the use of telehealth in a range of disease areas.

3. A partnership approach is needed where staff from academic institutions and service providers work together in order to undertake real world research that reflects local contexts and has real prospect of embedding telehealth in routine practice. This may entail designing robust service evaluation (mix methods) in routine service development rather than undertaking RCTs. Such partnership also needs to involved the whole health system spanning from community (primary care) level to secondary (hospital) care.

4. The challenge of demonstrating evidence of cost-effectiveness of telehealth require a concerted efforts, as various elements required to measure cost are often difficult to quantify and collect in routine health setting, without expert support. As telehealth technologies develop and varies, it is important to determine which telehealth devices are more cost-effective; comparing low to high cost devices. For a wider population level adoption of telehealth, an ideal technology needs to be that which is commonly available, relatively cheap, and can be adopted for health monitoring.

5. Is it telehealth that is responsible for the outcomes seen in some studies or is it the increased contacts of patients by healthcare staff that is the cause? This is a research question that needs exploring, perhaps by increasing contacts of those in usual care by low-cost telehealth e.g. telephone versus more expensive form of telehealth. Some have referred to telehealth (as defined in this work) as the "black box", suggesting the uncertainty of its effectiveness. In clinical context of medical drug trial, this would have merited consideration of "drug-placebo" trial, but such thought is difficult to entertain from ethical perspective.

CONCLUSION

Telehealth is effective in reducing hospital admission among patients with long-term conditions: COPD, heart failure and diabetes. It provides reassurance and confidence to patients in managing their own conditions, and it plays an important role in enhancing patient-staff relationship. An updated checklist of key success factors are produced to support such a process of embedding telehealth in routine healthcare use.

REFERENCES

Anker, S., Koehler, F., & Abraham, W. (2011). Telemedicine and remote management of patients with heart failure (Heart Failure 4). *Lancet, 378*, 731–739. doi:10.1016/S0140-6736(11)61229-4

Audit Commission. (2004). *Assistive technology: Independence and well-being*. National Report No. 4.

Black, A. D., Car, J., Pagliari, C., Anandan, C., Cresswell, K., & Bokun, T. (2011). The impact of ehealth on the quality and safety of health care: A systematic overview. *PLoS Medicine, 8*(1). doi:10.1371/journal.pmed.1000387

Campbell, M., Fitzpatrick, R., Haines, A., Kinmonth, A., Sandercock, P., & Spiegelhalter, D. (2000). Framework for design and evaluation of complex interventions to improve health. *British Medical Journal, 321*, 694–696. doi:10.1136/bmj.321.7262.694

Chaudhry, S., Mattera, J., Curtis, J., Sperlus, J., Herrin, J., & Lin, Z. (2010). Telemonitoring in patients with heart failure. *The New England Journal of Medicine, 363*(24), 2301–2309. doi:10.1056/NEJMoa1010029

Darkins, A., Ryan, P., Kobb, R., Foster, L., Edmonson, E., Wakefield, B., et al. (2008). Care coordination/home telehealth: The systematic implementation of health informatics, telehealth, and disease management to support the care of veteran patients with chronic conditions. *Telemedicine and e-Health, 14*(10), 1118-26.

Department of Health. (2005). *Building telecare in England*. London, UK: Author.

Department of Health. (2012a). *A concordat between the Department of Health and the telehealth and telecare industry*. London, UK: Author.

Department of Health. (2012b). *COPD commissioning toolkit: A resource for commissioners*. London, UK: Author.

Ekeland, A. G., Bowes, A., & Flottorp, S. (2010). *Effectiveness of telemedicine: A systematic review of reviews* (pp. 736-771).

Ekeland, A. G., Bowes, A., & Flottorp, S. (2012). Methodologies for assessing telemedicine: A systematic review of reviews. *International Journal of Medical Informatics, 81*, 1–11. doi:10.1016/j.ijmedinf.2011.10.009

Ellis, T. (2008). *Evaluation of the whole system demonstrators - An overview of the key features*. Department of Health.

Eysenbach, G. (2001). What is e-health? *Journal of Medical Internet Research, 3*(2). doi:10.2196/jmir.3.2.e20

Finkelstein, S., Speedie, S., Demiris, G., Veen, M., & Lundgren, J. (2004). Telehomecare: Quality, perception, satisfaction. *Telemedicine Journal and e-Health, 10*(2), 122–128. doi:10.1089/tmj.2004.10.122

Grigsby, J., Brega, A., & Devore, P. (2005). The evaluation of telemedicine and health services research. *Telemedicine Journal and e-Health, 11*(3), 317–328. doi:10.1089/tmj.2005.11.317

Inglis, S., Clark, R., McAlister, F., Ball, J., Lewinter, C., & Cullington, D. (2010). Structured telephone support or telemonitoring programmes for patients with chronic heart failure. *Cochrane Database of Systematic Reviews, 8*.

Jones, S., & Edwards, R. T. (2010). Diabetic retinopathy screening: A systematic review of the economic evidence. *Diabetic Medicine, 27*(3), 249–256. doi:10.1111/j.1464-5491.2009.02870.x

Joseph, V., West, R., Shickle, D., Keen, J., & Clamp, S. (2011). Key challenges in the development and implementation of Telehealth projects. *Journal of Telemedicine and Telecare, 17*(2), 71–77. doi:10.1258/jtt.2010.100315

May, C., Finch, T., Mair, F., Ballini, L., Dowrick, C., & Eccles, M. (2007). Understanding the implementation of complex interventions in health care: the normalization process model. *BMC Health Services Research, 7*(148).

May, C., Harrison, R., & Finch, T. (2003). Understanding the normalisation of telemedicine services through qualitative evaluation. *Journal of the American Medical Informatics Association, 10*, 596–604. doi:10.1197/jamia.M1145

McLean, S., Chandler, D., Nurmatov, U., Liu, J., Pagliari, C., & Car, J. (2010). *Telehealthcare for asthma (review). The Cochrane Collaboration.* John Wiley & Sons, Ltd.

McLean, S., Nurmatov, U., Liu, J. L., Pagliari, C., Car, J., & Sheikh, A. (2011). Telehealthcare for chronic obstructive pulmonary disease. *Cochrane Database of Systematic Reviews, 7*, CD007718.

Moreno, L., Dale, S., Chen, A., & Magee, C. (2009). Costs to Medicare of the informatics for diabetes education and telemedicine (IDEATel) home telemedicine demonstration: Findings from an independent evaluation. *Diabetes Care, 32*(7), 1202–1204. doi:10.2337/dc09-0094

Murray, E., May, C., Mair, F., & Rocket Science, U. K. Ltd. (2010). *E-health implementation toolkit (e-HIT): A guide for senior managers to implement e-health initiatives in the NHS.* UCL, SDO, University of Glasgow, Newcastle University.

Pawar, P., Jones, V., Van Beijnum, B., & Hermaens, H. (2012). A framework for the comparison of mobile patient monitoring system. *Journal of Biomedical Informatics, 45*, 544–556. doi:10.1016/j.jbi.2012.02.007

Polisena, J., Coyle, D., Coyle, K., McGill, S., Polisena, J., & Coyle, D. (2009). Home telehealth for chronic disease management: A systematic review and an analysis of economic evaluations. *International Journal of Technology Assessment in Health Care, 25*(3), 339–349. doi:10.1017/S0266462309990201

Roth, A., Korb, H., Gadot, R., Kalter, E., Roth, A., & Korb, H. (2006). Telecardiology for patients with acute or chronic cardiac complaints: The 'SHL' experience in Israel and Germany. *International Journal of Medical Informatics, 75*(9), 643–645. doi:10.1016/j.ijmedinf.2006.04.004

Scalvini, S., Vitacca, M., & Paletta, L. (2004). Telemedicine: A new frontier for effective healthcare services. *Monaldi Archives for Chest Disease - Pulmonary Series, 61*(4), 226-233.

Shea, S., Weinstock, R., Teresi, J., Palmas, W., Starren, J., & Cimino, J. (2009). A randomised trial comparing telemedicine case management with usual care in older, ethnically diverse, medically underserved patients with diabetes mellitus: 5 year results of the IDEATel study. *Journal of the American Medical Informatics Association, 16*(4), 446–456. doi:10.1197/jamia.M3157

Sheikh, A., McLean, S., Cresswell, K., Pagliari, C., Pappas, Y., Car, J., et al. (2011). *The impact of ehealth on the quality and safety of healthcare: An updated systematic overview and synthesis of the literature: Final report for NHS Connecting for Health Evaluation programme* (p. 772). London, UK: The University of Edinburgh; and Imperial College.

Steventon, A., Bardsley, M., Billings, J., Dixon, J., Doll, H., & Hirani, S. (2012). Effect of telehealth on use of secondary care and mortality: findings from the Whole System Demonstrator cluster randomised trial. *British Medical Journal, 344*(e3874). doi:10.1136/bmj.e3874

Whited, J. D. (2001). Teledermatology: Current status and future directions. *American Journal of Clinical Dermatology, 2*(2), 59–64. doi:10.2165/00128071-200102020-00001

Whitten, P., Mair, F., Haycox, A., May, C., Williams, T., & Hellmich, S. (2002). Systematic review of cost effectiveness studies of telemedicine interventions. *British Medical Journal, 324*, 1434–1437. doi:10.1136/bmj.324.7351.1434

Williams, T., May, C., & Esmail, A. (2001). Limitations of patient satisfaction studies in telehealthcare: A systematic review of the literature. *Telemedicine Journal and e-Health, 7*(4), 293–316. doi:10.1089/15305620152814700

Wootton, R., Craig, J., & Patterson, V. (Eds.). (2006). *Introduction to telemedicine*. London, UK: Royal Society of Medicine Press Ltd.

Wootton, R., Dimmick, S., & Kvedar, J. (Eds.). (2006). *Home telehealth: Connecting care within the community*. London, UK: Royal Society of Medicine Press Ltd.

World Health Organisation. (2003). *Information technology in support of health care.*

World Health Organisation. (2011). *Health topics: Chronic diseases.*

ADDITIONAL READING

Campbell, M., Fitzpatrick, R., Haines, A., Kinmonth, A., Sandercock, P., & Spiegelhalter, D. (2000). Framework for design and evaluation of complex interventions to improve health. *British Medical Journal, 321*, 694–696. doi:10.1136/bmj.321.7262.694

Darkins, A. W., & Cary, M. A. (2000). *Telemedicine and telehealth*. London, UK: Free Association Books.

Heeks, R. (2008). *Causes of ehealth success and failure: Design-reality gap model egovernment for development.* Public Sector Health Information Systems.

Heeks, R., Mundy, D., & Salazar, A. (1999). Why health care information systems succeed or fail. *Information Systems for Public Sector Management: Working Paper Series* (p. 25). Manchester, UK: University of Manchester.

Kidholm, K., Bowes, A., Dyrehauge, S., Ekeland, A., Flottorp, S., Jensen, L., et al. (2010). *The MAST manual: Model for assesment of telemedicine.*

KPMG International. (2012). *Accelerating innovation: The power of the crowd.* University of Manchester.

May, C., Finch, T., Mair, F., Ballini, L., Dowrick, C., & Eccles, M. (2007a). Understanding the implementation of complex interventions in health care: the normalization process model. *BMC Health Services Research, 7*(148).

May, C., Mair, F., Dowrick, C., & Finch, T. (2007b). Process evaluation for complex interventions in primary care: Understanding trials using the normalization process model. *BMC Family Practice, 8*(42).

Murray, E., May, C., Mair, F., & Rocket Science, U. K. Ltd. (2010). *e-Health implementation toolkit (e-HIT): A guide for senior managers to implement e-Health initiatives in the NHS.* UCL, SDO, University of Glasgow, Newcastle University.

Scottish Centre for Telehealth. (2009). *Online resources.* Retrieved from http://www.sct.scot.nhs.uk/online-resources.html

Swinfen Charitable Trust. (2012). *Telemedicine.* Retrieved March 14, 2012, from http://www.swinfencharitabletrust.org/what-we-do

Telemedicine. (2012). *Online support for HIV/ AIDS care*. Retrieved from http://telemedicine. itg.be/telemedicine/Site/Default.aspx?Menu=M enuMain&MIID=119&WPID=1&L=E

The Norwegian Centre for Integrated Care and Telemedicine. (2009). *Developing best practice in telemedicine research.*

Wootton, R., Craig, J., & Patterson, V. (Eds.). (2006). *Introduction to telemedicine*. London, UK: Royal Society of Medicine Press Ltd.

Wootton, R., Patil, N. G., Scott, R. E., & Ho, K. (Eds.). (2009). *Telehealth in the developing world*. London, UK: Royal Society of Medicine Press Ltd.

Yellowlees, P. M. (1999). Successfully developing a telemedicine system. In Wootton, R., & Craig, J. (Eds.), *Introduction to telemedicine* (p. 100). London, UK: Royal Society of Medicine Press Ltd.

KEY TERMS AND DEFINITIONS

Chronic Obstructive Pulmonary Disease (COPD): "COPD describes lung damage that is gradual in onset and that results in progressive airflow limitation. This lung damage, when fully established, is irreversible and, if it is not identified and treated early, leads to disability and eventually death. The principle cause of COPD is smoking. Other factors include Workplace exposure, genetic mak-up and general environmental pollution." (Department of Health, 2012b)

Electronic Health (E-Health): "E-health is an emerging field in the intersection of medical informatics, public health and business, referring to health services and information delivered or enhanced through the Internet and related technologies. In a broader sense, the term characterizes not only a technical development, but also a state-of-mind, a way of thinking, an attitude, and a commitment for networked, global thinking, to improve health care locally, regionally, and worldwide by using information and communication technology." (Eysenbach, 2001; Pawar et al., 2012)

Long-Term Condition (Chronic Conditions): "Diseases of long duration and generally slow progression." (WHO, 2011)

Mobile Health (M-Health): "… The application of mobile computing, wireless communications and network technologies to deliver or enhance diverse healthcare services and functions in which the patient has a freedom to be mobile, perhaps within a limited area." (Pawar et al., 2012)

Telecare: "Telecare is the continuous, automatic and remote monitoring of real-time emergencies and lifestyle changes over time in order to manage the risks associated with independent living." (Ellis, 2008)

Telehealth and Telemedicine: These are used in the published literature for the same thing. Others authors attempts to make distinction between these terminologies; attributing telemedicine as device that supports communication between patients and a doctors, or doctor-to-doctor communication; while telehealth being that which supports communication between patient and a healthcare professional. This attempts can be misleading and confusion. Telehealth is a more encompassing terminology, as defined at the beginning of this chapter.

Chapter 8
Telemedicine Utilization, Availability of Physicians, Distance, and Urbanity:
An Exploratory Study

Ricky C. Leung
University of Missouri School of Medicine, USA

ABSTRACT

This study examines the relationship between telemedicine utilization, the availability of physicians, the level of urbanity of a locality, and the physical distance between a locality and an urban health facility at the county level within a rural state in the United States. As an exploratory study, the author conducts correlation analysis and analysis of variance to test if the chosen exploratory variables may account for variations in telemedicine utilization. The author obtained statistically significant results, but recognizes that there are other potential variables to be included in further studies. The results are useful for practitioners and may motivate further studies. The chapter discusses the implications of the study in its conclusion.

INTRODUCTION

Shortage of physicians in underserved areas creates unmet demands for health services. These unmet demands are aggravated by an aging population (Glasgow 2000; Ziembroski 2006). To identify these underserved areas, researchers have utilized large-scale data in various ways. For example, using data from the National Center for Health Statistics, the Kaiser Family Foundation has shown that physicians in patient care per 10,000 ranged from 17.0 to 65.9 across the fifty states in the U.S. in 2008 (The Kaiser Family Foundation 2008).

BACKGROUND

While demands for health services may not be reduced easily, it is possible to increase the availability of health services by utilizing new medical

DOI: 10.4018/978-1-4666-2979-0.ch008

technology. One plausible solution is the utilization of telemedicine. Telemedicine may be defined as the provision of medical services that involves the exchange of medical information from one site to another via electronic communications for purposes of improving patients' health status (American Telemedicine Association 2012). Using telemedicine, a physician located in virtually anywhere can consult patients in underserved areas, prescribe treatment and even perform remotely directed minor surgeries (Bashshur & Shannon 2009; Courtney 2008; Paul 2004).

More specifically, telemedicine enables diagnosis and consultation by health providers to patients who reside in remote areas (Morrison et al. 2010; Pronovost et al. 2009). The term telehealth is sometimes used to indicate that telemedicine can be provided to patients at home or in medical facilities. In the former case, patients do not need to travel outside of home to receive services. This is desirable for older patients and for those who are physically disabled (Magnusson & Hanson 2005). Alternatively, patients can go to local clinics or medical centers to receive consultation from physicians in a telemedicine session, with the aid of nurses or medical assistants in the local medical facility (Kalternina et al. 2011). This study focuses on this latter case.

Intuitively, availability of physicians (McCarthy 1995), urbanity of a locality (Higgs 1999), and distance to an urban medical facility (Hassol et al. 1997) are decisive factors regarding the level of telemedicine utilization as an alternative form of medical consultation or treatment. For example, patients who reside in an underserved area, such as a rural town, need to travel for a long distance to an urban medical center to receive medical services. To avoid these travels, patients in underserved areas may be more likely to seek telemedicine in lieu of traditional, face-to-face health services. Yet, few studies in the literature examined how the supply of physicians, distance to an urban medical facility and the level of urbanity of a locality are associated with the utilization of telemedicine services with statistical precision. Figure 1 displays a model that may be developed systematically to account for the variations in the utilization of telemedicine.

This study aims to gather preliminary statistical evidence for the above model. The next section will explain the method of this study, including the data sources and statistical techniques. Then, the results section will summarize the main findings of this study. The discussion session will present the implications of the findings, particularly the economic value of telemedicine for patients in rural and underserved areas.

Figure 1. A model of telemedicine utilization

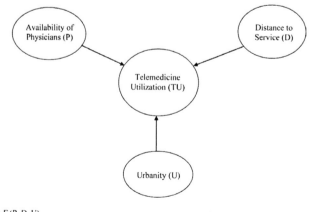

TU = F (P, D, U)

MAIN FOCUS OF THE CHAPTER

Issues, Controversies, Problems

While access to medical care represents a major factor regarding the utilization of telemedicine, three indicators seem particularly relevant: First, the availability of physicians in a locality may be a strong factor in explaining how willing patients would use telemedicine to substitute and/or supplement traditional, face-to-face health services. In relation to this first factor, the level of urbanity of a locality is likely to matter. In particular, in rural communities, there may not be sufficient health professionals and well-equipped facilities. Finally, the actual physical distance between the locality and an urban facility may explain how much patients tend to use telemedicine. This research aims to add evidence to the existing literature.

Solutions and Recommendations

For this purpose, the research evaluates the relationship between telemedicine utilization, the availability of physicians, the level of urbanity of a locality, and the physical distance between a locality and an urban health facility with descriptive statistical techniques. The level of analysis is counties in the United States. In countries with substantive health disparities such as the United States, county-level study is able to reveal variations among localities, and such findings could shed light to the provision of health services practically (Thomas et al. 2009). The current study draws on two datasets: First, the Bureau of Health Professions, under the United States Department of Health and Human Services, has created the Area Resource File (ARF). ARF is a publicly available for a fee, which includes rich data at the county-level of fifty states in the U.S. This study extracts data from the 2009-2010 release of ARF, and focuses on counties within a state in the Midwest region of the United States

(US). This state has a relatively large proportion of rural residents.

Second, this study draws on the support of a university-based telemedicine network provider. This telemedicine network technical and educational support to various sites that receive remote consultation, diagnosis and treatment within the state, and is one of the oldest networks of its type in the US. Data were managed by an information system called the IBM Cognos Powerplay, which stores data using cubic structure. Simply put, the researcher has to pre-select which data cubes are of interest in extracting data and leave unwanted (or confidential) information intact (e.g. patients' personal information was ignored in this study).

With these two datasets, the following variables are used (or created):

1. **Population Estimate (POP EST):** This variable is about how many people reside in a specific county within the selected state;
2. **Telemedicine Utilization (TEL UTIL):** This variable is about how many times a telemedicine session has been scheduled in a specific within the selected state;
3. **Active Physicians per 1000s Population (MD):** This variable is about how many active physicians are available for providing services in a specific county within the selected state;
4. **Rural/Urban Continuum (R/U):** This variable is about the level of urbanity of a specific county. The value of this variable ranges between 1 and 9, with "1" being the most urban and "9" being the most rural;
5. **Distance to urban facility (DISTANCE):** This variable is about the physician distance in miles between the local host of a telemedicine session where the telemedicine session was received and the remote urban facility where the telemedicine session was provided.

Table 1. Variables of interest

County ID	Population Estimate	Total Tel Utilization	MDs per 1000s Pop	Distance to UMHS	Rural/Urban Continuum
1	24943	34	0.48	95.7	7
2	16923	8	0.12	195	3
3	26049	12	1.27	43.7	4
4	36301	15	0.80	231	5
5	12531	8	0.32	208	6
6	18349	9	0.33	94	9
7	11990	3	0.08	237	9
8	89408	2	1.90	172	3
9	41383	41	2.63	241	7
10	43464	87	0.74	27.7	3
11	40664	15	1.45	87.3	7
12	73243	30	3.56	218	5
13	9756	8	0.31	105	6
14	5890	10	0.00	206	9
15	13652	5	0.22	168	6
16	7740	11	0.13	72	9
17	75479	51	0.97	182	2
18	7180	13	0.00	151	9
19	215707	10	1.57	140	1
20	74313	4	1.96	37.9	3
21	17535	1	0.57	33.5	6
22	23970	1	0.25	117	6
23	7418	5	0.13	195	8
24	16844	1	0.06	126	2
25	15199	7	0.26	132	7
26	13438	15	0.07	183	6
27	31454	29	1.18	319	7
28	15261	10	0.52	79.7	6
29	6185	1	0.65	193	8
30	22179	7	0.90	115	6
31	39000	35	1.44	181	7
32	116813	57	2.27	225	3
33	52016	8	0.81	108	4
34	4020	5	0.00	113	9
35	35524	46	0.73	114	6
36	37757	32	0.74	200	6
37	9951	3	0.00	115	9
38	12580	113	0.40	106	7
39	14213	44	0.35	124	6
40	15621	43	0.38	73.6	7
41	12276	3	0.41	201	7

continued on following page

Table 1. Continued

County ID	Population Estimate	Total Tel Utilization	MDs per 1000s Pop	Distance to UMHS	Rural/Urban Continuum
42	9046	2	0.22	69.1	8
43	28225	5	1.98	99.4	5
44	3523	1	0.28	178	9
45	24949	3	0.28	68.8	6
46	13504	24	0.30	269	7
47	15121	2	0.13	48.1	3
48	9127	1	0.00	62.6	9
49	11804	3	0.42	50.3	8
50	20861	4	0.19	71.9	8
51	17589	52	0.17	288	7
52	56120	17	0.25	233	3
53	22054	6	1.22	225	6
54	10264	6	0.29	206	9
55	13465	1	0.07	53.2	3
56	9227	2	0.11	209	9
57	41006	94	1.00	74.6	4
58	42205	21	1.66	99.6	5
59	18476	4	0.32	83.4	6
60	30404	23	1.15	139	2
61	44546	90	0.58	97.8	5
62	4862	18	0.00	139	9
63	9832	1	0.10	88.2	9
64	25723	5	0.43	44.8	6
65	6388	4	0.47	169	9
66	13485	2	0.52	234	9
67	22505	54	0.84	62.1	6
68	4110	8	0.00	123	9
69	4798	7	0.42	135	9
70	40673	96	1.18	243	5
71	8423	14	0.24	160	9
72	6411	1	0.31	89.1	9
73	9270	4	0.97	142	8
74	63214	4	0.95	183	4
75	29537	29	0.54	265	7
76	31551	4	0.48	208	8
77	6629	14	0.00	134	9
78	47023	36	1.47	215	6
79	24598	18	0.49	137	9
80	20009	32	0.85	184	7
81	36473	50	0.49	145	2
82	18443	35	0.38	147	6

In the analysis, TEL UTIL is a continuous variable, and is treated as the dependent variable. POP EST is presented to show the size of different counties, and is also used to compute available physicians per 1000 populations. To facilitate the analysis, the explanatory variables (C-E) are converted into categorical variables with several groups. For example, MD is categorized into grouped as 0.1 or less per 1000 populations, 0.11 to 0.2 per 1000 populations, and the like.

This study presents descriptive statistics of all the above-mentioned variables of interest. Table 1 provides the data for the analysis. Table 2 groups counties by the utilization of telemedicine per 1000 populations. In addition, the correlations between the dependent and explanatory variables are analyzed (Table 3). Finally, several sets of one-way analysis of variance (ANOVAs) are performed to show if telemedicine utilization (TEL UTIL) differs significantly across counties grouped by MD, R/U and DISTANCE (Tables 4-6). In the analysis below, only counties with at least 1 scheduled session of telemedicine service in 2010 are included. Some counties are dropped due to missing data or outliers.

Results

As Table 1 shows, the populations of the chosen counties range between 4020 and 215707. In 2010, a total of 1,938 telemedicine sessions were schedules. Of all counties in the data set, the highest number of telemedicine utilization was 113. Several counties had only 1 scheduled telemedicine utilization in the entire year.

Table 2 shows how many counties have utilized telemedicine in different levels. Thus, 25 counties (their names are included in the third column of the table) had at least one telemedicine session per 1000 populations; 16 counties had between 0.500 and 0.999 sessions per 1000 populations; and 41 counties had 0.499 sessions or less per 1000 populations.

Between the dependent variable and the three explanatory variables, the analysis shows only moderate correlations. As Table 3 shows, the strongest correlation is between MD and R/U, with a value of -0.424. The weakest correlation is between TEL UTIL and DISTANCE, with a value of 0.008.

Next, the analysis examines whether between-groups variations are stronger than within-groups variations, treating TEL UTIL as the dependent variable and MD, R/U and DISTANCE as explanatory variables. For these analyses, MD is divided into 10 groups; R/U is divided into 8 groups; and DISTANCE is divided into 8 groups. See Tables 4-6 for the actual groupings.

Table 2. Telemedicine utilization in the selected counties

Telemedicine Sessions per 1000 Populations	Number of Counties
2.500 or more	5
2.000 to 2.499	6
1.500 to 1.999	7
1.000 to 1.499	7
0.500 to 0.999	16
0.499 or less	41

Table 3. Correlations between variables

	Tel Util by 1000 Pops	Distance to UMHS (miles)	MD by 1000 Pops	Rural/ Urban Continuum
Tel Util by 1000 Pops	1.000			
Distance to UMHS (miles)	0.008	1.000		
MD by 1000 Pops	-0.141	0.158	1.000	
Rural/ Urban Continuum	0.126	0.093	-0.424	1.000

Table 4. One-way ANOVA: differences in telemedicine utilization between groups of physician availability

Groups	Count	Sum	Average	Variance		
MDs per 1000s Pop = 0.10 or less	13	93	7.154	38.308		
MDs per 1000s Pop = 0.11 to 0.2	7	84	12.000	321.667		
MDs per 1000s Pop = 0.21 to 0.30	10	80	8.000	60.667		
MDs per 1000s Pop = 0.31 to 0.40	9	265	29.444	1275.278		
MDs per 1000s Pop = 0.41 to 0.50	9	128	14.222	285.444		
MDs per 1000s Pop = 0.51 to 0.80	10	313	31.300	1131.567		
MDs per 1000s Pop = 0.81 to 1.00	8	254	31.750	1065.357		
MDs per 1000s Pop = 1.01 to 1.50	8	252	31.500	796.286		
MDs per 1000s Pop = 1.51 to 2.00	5	42	8.400	58.300		
MDs per 1000s Pop = 2.01 or more	3	128	42.667	184.333		
ANOVA						
Source of Variation	SS	df	MS	F	P-value	F crit
Between Groups	10790.05	9	1198.895	2.200	0.032	2.013
Within Groups	39238.94	72	544.985			
Total	50028.99	81				

Table 5. One-way ANOVA: differences in telemedicine utilization between groups of urbanity

Groups	Count	Sum	Average	Variance		
Rural/Urban Continuum = 1 or 2	5	135	27.000	521.500		
Rural/Urban Continuum = 3	8	178	22.250	1033.643		
Rural/Urban Continuum = 4	4	118	29.500	1859.667		
Rural/Urban Continuum = 5	6	257	42.833	1579.767		
Rural/Urban Continuum = 6	18	320	17.778	319.948		
Rural/Urban Continuum = 7	13	457	35.154	740.308		
Rural/Urban Continuum = 8	7	23	3.286	1.905		
Rural/Urban Continuum = 9	21	151	7.190	32.262		
ANOVA						
Source of Variation	SS	df	MS	F	P-value	F crit
Between Groups	12250.184	7	1750.026	3.428	0.003	2.136
Within Groups	37778.803	74	510.524			
Total	50028.988	81				

Tables 4-6 reveal the average and variance of telemedicine utilization in each group of the explanatory variables. For MD, the highest average utilization is found in the "MDs = 0.81 to 1.00 per 1000 populations" group, with 31.75 sessions. The largest variance is found in the "MDs = 0.31 to 0.40 per 1000 populations" group, with 1275.28. Grouping MD in the specific way as Table 4 shows, between-groups variations in TEL UTIL are significantly larger than within-groups variations. Thus, the Mean Squares (MS) for between groups are 1198.895, and within group variations are 544.985, producing a F statistics of 2.200 (i.e. 1198.895/544.985). This statistic is significant at a P value of less than 0.05.

For R/U, the highest average utilization is found in the "Rural/Urban Continuum = 5" group, with 42.833 sessions. The largest variance is found in the "Rural/Urban Continuum = 4" group, with 1859.667. Grouping R/U in the specific way as Table 5 shows, between-groups variations in TEL UTIL are significantly larger than within-groups variations. Thus, the Mean Squares (MS) for between groups are 1750.026, and within group variations are 510.524, producing a F statistics of 3.428 (i.e. 1750.026/510.524). This statistic is significant at a P value of less than 0.05.

Finally, for DISTANCE, he highest average utilization is found in the "Distance to Urban Facility = 241-300 miles" group, with 48.400 sessions. The largest variance is found in the "Distance to Urban Facility = 91-120 miles" group, with 1289.744. Grouping DISTANCE in the specific way as Table 6 shows, between-groups variations in TEL UTIL are significantly larger than within-groups variations. Thus, the Mean Squares (MS) for between groups are 1142.617,

and within group variations are 519.258, producing a F statistics of 2.200 (i.e. 1142.617/519.258). This statistic is significant at a P value of less than 0.05.

FUTURE RESEARCH DIRECTIONS

As an exploratory study, the results shown above are useful in several ways: First, they provide useful descriptive statistics about telemedicine session in a relatively rural state of many underserved areas. This statistics is quite intriguing on its own. More importantly, the analysis identifies three explanatory factors to account for variations of telemedicine utilization at the county-level (Kindig & Movassaghi 1989). These factors may be explored in further studies for predictive purposes.

In this respect, a simple linear model may not be appropriate (Shea et al. 2009). For example, even though the ANOVA results are statistically significant, they do not indicate linearity. That is, it is not the case that the farther away a county is, the more telemedicine utilization one will find necessarily. Thus, while there were 26.923

Table 6. One-way ANOVA: differences in telemedicine utilization between groups of distance to urban health facility

Groups	Count	Sum	Average	Variance		
Distance to Urban Facility = 30 - 60 miles	7	28	4.000	14.667		
Distance to Urban Facility = 61 - 90 miles	13	243	18.692	796.064		
Distance to Urban Facility = 91 -120 miles	13	350	26.923	1289.744		
Distance to Urban Facility = 121 - 150 miles	13	239	18.385	243.256		
Distance to Urban Facility = 151 -180 miles	6	39	6.500	31.500		
Distance to Urban Facility = 181 - 210 miles	15	216	14.400	237.400		
Distance to Urban Facility = 211 - 240 miles	8	166	20.750	366.214		
Distance to Urban Facility = 241 - 300 miles	5	242	48.400	826.300		
ANOVA						
Source of Variation	**SS**	**df**	**MS**	**F**	**P-value**	**F crit**
Between Groups	7998.318	7.000	1142.617	2.200	0.044	2.140
Within Groups	37386.569	72.000	519.258			
Total	45384.888	79.000				

telemedicine sessions for counties with a distance of 91-120 miles away from an urban facility, there were only 6.500 sessions for counties with a distance of 151-180 miles away from an urban facility. Results from other ANOVA tables do not indicate simple linearity between the explanatory and dependent variables, neither. Simply put, further studies aiming at prediction need to adopt more complex or sophisticated models.

Still, this study shows that telemedicine can be a very useful alternative form of health services, especially for patients resided in rural or other underserved areas. In a separate analysis with the same data sets used in this research, it is found that the average distance saved for the patient was approximately 117.3 miles. That is, since patients only needed to go to a local clinic or medical center to receive telemedicine, they could avoid the travel to an urban facility that they would have gone otherwise. These 117.3 miles can be translated into a saving of $131.90 per trip in gas money. In 2010, these savings would be multiplied by almost 2000 of scheduled telemedicine sessions.

CONCLUSION

While this study focuses on potential determinants of telemedicine utilization, it is also important to examine the clinical effectiveness of telemedicine (Loane et al. 2000), including patients' satisfaction (Allen & Hayes 1994). On the one hand, patients can reduce travel and wait times by utilizing telemedicine. On the other hand, they may experience a lower level of perceived personal attention and affection by receiving "virtual care". It is useful to examine how patients evaluate these two outcomes jointly in further studies.

Finally, this study has not paid attention to the variables of medical specialty and shortage of physicians in specific specialties (Paul et al. 1999). The author has examined the data and found that the majority of patient visits was serviced by five

specialties, namely autism, behavioral change, burn unit, dermatology and pediatric endocrinology. It is useful to find out whether physicians of these specialties are lacking in supply and how they affect the utilization of telemedicine.

REFERENCES

Allen, A., & Hayes, J. (1994). Patient satisfaction with telemedicine in a rural clinic. *American Journal of Public Health*, *84*(10), 1693. doi:10.2105/AJPH.84.10.1693

American Telemedicine Association. (2012). *Telemedicine defined*. Retrieved from http://www.americantelemed.org/i4a/pages/index.cfm?pageid=3333

Ashby, S., Nyenwe, E., Tidewell, J., Nouer, S., & Kitabchi, A. (2011). Improving diabetes care via telemedicine: Lessons from the Addressing Diabetes in Tennessee (ADT) project. *Diabetes Care, March*.

Baker, E., Ford, R., Newell, M., & Schmitz, D. (2007). *Idaho family physician rural work force assessment pilot study*. Idaho Department of Health and Welfare, June 2007.

Bashshur, R., & Shannon, G. (2009). *National telemedicine initiatives: Essential to healthcare reform*. Telemedicine and e-Health, July/August. doi:10.1089/tmj.2009.9960

Bischoff, R., Robinson, W., & Swinton, J. (2009). Telehealth and rural depression: Physician and patient perspectives. *Families, Systems & Health*, *27*(2), 172–182. doi:10.1037/a0016014

Bowers, B., Nolet, K., Roberts, T., & Esmond, S. (2009). Implementing change in long term care. In Nolet, K., Roberts, T., & Esmond, S. (Eds.), *Implementing change in long-term care* (pp. 1–129).

Boxer, R. (2009). *Telehealth can enable convenient, high-quality and affordable care for children and their families.*

Courtney, K. L. (2008). Needing smart home technologies: the perspectives of older adults in continuing care retirement communities. *Informatics in Primary Care, 16,* 195–201.

Davalos, M. E., French, M. T., Budrick, A. E., & Simmons, S. C. (2009). Economic evaluation of telemedicine: Review of the literature and research guidelines for benefit-cost analysis. *Telemedicine and eHealth, 15*(10), 933-948.

Higgs, G. (1999). Investigating trends in rural health outcomes: A research agenda. *Geoforum, 30*(3), 203–221. doi:10.1016/S0016-7185(99)00021-4

Kleiboer, A. G. (2010). Monitoring symptoms at home: what methods would cancer patients be comforable using? *Quality of Life Research, 19,* 965–968. doi:10.1007/s11136-010-9662-0

Loane, M. A., Bloomer, S. E., Corbett, R., Eedy, D. J., Hicks, N., & Lotery, H. E. (2000). A randomized controlled trial to assess the clinical effectiveness of both realtime and store-and-forward teledermatology compared with conventional care. *Journal of Telemedicine and Telecare, 6*(Suppl 1), S1–S3. doi:10.1258/1357633001933952

McLean, T. R., & McLean, P. B. (2007). Is a black market in telemedicine on the horizon? *International Journal of Medical Robotics and Computer Assisted Surgery, 3*(4), 291–296. doi:10.1002/rcs.167

Paul, D. L. (2004). A field study of the effect of interpersonal trust on virtual collaborative relationship performance. *Management Information Systems Quarterly, 28*(2), 183–227.

Paul, J. H., Patrick, Y. K. C., Olivia, R. L. S., & Kar Yan, T. (1999). Examining the technology acceptance model using physician acceptance of telemedicine technology. *Journal of Management Information Systems, 16*(2), 91.

PHI. (2003). Long term care financing and the long-term care workforce crisis: Causes and solutions. *Citizens for Long-Term Care,* 1-42.

Rojas, S. V., & Gagnon, M. P. (2008). A systematic review of the key indicators for assessing telehomecare cost-effectiveness. *Telemedicine and e-Health, 14*(9).

Shea, S., Weinstock, R. S., Teresi, J. A., Palmas, W., Starren, J., & Cimino, J. J. (2009). A randomized trial comparing telemedicine case management with usual care in older, ethnically diverse, medically underserved patients with diabetes mellitus: 5 year results of the IDEATel study. *Journal of the American Medical Informatics Association, 16*(4), 446–456. doi:10.1197/jamia.M3157

Singh, M., & Das, R. (2010). Utility of telemedicine for children in India. *Indian Journal of Pediatrics, 77*(1), 73–75. doi:10.1007/s12098-009-0292-x

Stone, J. (2010). Long-term care (LTC): Financing overview and issues for congress. *Congressional Research Service,* 1-22.

Swinton, J. J. (2009). Telehealth and rural depression: Physician and patient perspectives. *American Psychological Association, 27*(2), 172-182.

Thomas, K. C., Ellis, A. R., Konrad, T. R., Holzer, C. E., & Morrissey, J. P. (2009). County-level estimates of mental health professional shortage in the United States. *Psychiatric Services (Washington, D.C.), 60*(10), 1323–1328. doi:10.1176/appi.ps.60.10.1323

Torre, A., Rodriguez, C. H., & Garcia, L. (2004). Cost analysis in telemedicine: Empirical evidence from sites in Arizona. *Health Services: Telemedicine, 20*(3), 253–257.

World Health Organization. (2009). Preventing hospital visits through telemedicine. *World Health Organization Bulletin, 87*(10), 739–740. doi:10.2471/BLT.09.021009

ADDITIONAL READING

Brown, G., & Leung, R. (in press). Strategic valuation of enterprise information architecture. In Brown, G., Pasupathy, K., & Patrick, T. (Eds.), *Strategic management of information systems in healthcare*. Health Administration Press.

Brown-Connolly, N. (2002). Patient satisfaction with telemedical access to specialty services in rural California. *Journal of Telemedicine and Telecare, 8*, 7–10. doi:10.1258/135763302320301812

Bungard, T. J., Smigorowsky, M. J., Lalonde, L. D., Hogan, T., Doliszny, K. M., & Gebreyesus, G. (2009). Cardiac EASE (ensuring access and speedy evaluation) - The impact of a single-point-of-entry multidisciplinary outpatient cardiology consultation program on wait times in Canada. *The Canadian Journal of Cardiology, 25*(12), 697–702. doi:10.1016/S0828-282X(09)70530-6

Clawson, B., Seldon, M., Lacks, M., Deaton, A. V., Hall, B., & Bach, R. (2008). Complex pediatric feeding disorders using teleconferencing technology to improve access to a treatment program. *Pediatric Nursing, 34*(3), 213–216.

Cummings, J., Kresk, C., Vermoch, K., & Matuszewski, K. (2007). Intensive care unit telemedicine: Review and consensus recommendations. *American Journal of Medical Quality, 22*(4), 239–250. doi:10.1177/1062860607302777

DeVany, M., Alverson, D., D'Iorio, J., & Simmons, S. (2008, November). Employing telehealth to enhance overall quality of life and health for families. *Telemedicine and e-Health, 14*(9), 1003-1007.

Foster, C., Scott, I., & Addington-Hall, J. (2010). Who visits mobile UK services providing cancer information and support in the community. *European Journal of Cancer Care, 19*, 221–226. doi:10.1111/j.1365-2354.2008.01007.x

Garrelts, J. C., Gagnon, M., Eisenberg, C., Moerer, J., & Carrithers, J. (2010, September 1). Impact of telepharmacy in a multihospital. *American Journal of Health-System Pharmacy, 67*, 1456–1462. doi:10.2146/ajhp090670

Grisby, W. J. (2002). Telehealth: An assessment of growth and distribution. *The Journal of Rural Health, 18*(2), 348–358. doi:10.1111/j.1748-0361.2002.tb00896.x

Kobb, R., Chumbler, N., Brennan, D. M., & Rabinowitz, T. (2008, November). Home telehealth: Mainstreaming what we do well. *Telemedicine and e-Health, 14*(9), 977-981.

Lee, S., Mun, S. K., Jha, P., Levine, B. A., & Ro, D. (2000). Telemedicine: Challenges and opportunities. *Journal of High Speed Networks, 9*, 15–30.

Leung, R. (2012). Health information technology and dynamic capabilities. *Health Care Management Review, 37*(1), 43–53. doi:10.1097/HMR.0b013e31823c9b55

Magnusson, L., & Hanson, E. (2005). Supporting frail older people and their family carers at home using information and communication technology: Cost analysis. *Journal of Advanced Nursing, 51*(6), 645–657. doi:10.1111/j.1365-2648.2005.03541.x

Morrison, L., Cai, M. S., & Davis, N. (2010). Clinical and economic outcomes of the electronic intensive care unit: Results from two community hospitals. *Critical Care Medicine, 38*(1), 2–8. doi:10.1097/CCM.0b013e3181b78fa8

Noel, C., Vogel, C., & Erdos, J. (2004). Home telehealth reduces healthcare costs. *Telemedicine Journal and e-Health, 10*(2), 170–183. doi:10.1089/tmj.2004.10.170

Palmas, W., Shea, S., & Starren, J. (2010). Medicare payments, healthcare service use, and telemedicine implementation costs in a randomized trial comparing telemedicine casemanagement with usual care in medically underserved participants with diabetes mellitus IDEATel). *Journal of the American Medical Informatics Association, 17*(2), 196–202. doi:10.1136/jamia.2009.002592

Pronovost, A., Peng, P., & Kern, R. (2009). Telemedicine in the management of chronic pain: a cost analysis study. *Canadian Journal of Anaesthesia, 56*(8), 590–596. doi:10.1007/s12630-009-9123-9

Ramos, V. (2010). *Contributions to the history of telemedicine of the TICs*. Paper presented at the 2nd Region 8 IEEE Conference on the History of Telecommunications: A Century of Broadcasting, HISTELCON 2010. Retrieved from www.scopus.com

Rangaswamy, T., Sujit, J., & Kotteswara, R. (2008). Telepsychiatry in Chennai, India: The SCARF experience. *Behavioral Sciences & the Law, 26*, 315–322. doi:10.1002/bsl.816

Shivji, S., Metcalfe, P., & Khan, A. (2011). Pediatric surgery telehealth: Patient and clinician satisfaction. *Rediatric Surgery International, 27*, 523–526. doi:10.1007/s00383-010-2823-y

Speedie, S. M., Ferguson, A. S., Sanders, J., & Doarn, C. (2008, November). Telehealth: The promise of new care. *Telemedicine and e-Health, 14*(9), 964-967.

Sutherland, J. E., Sutphin, D. H., Rawlins, F., Burton, J., & Redican, K. (2009). A comparison of telesonography with standard ultrasound care in a rural Dominican clinic. *Journal of Telemedicine and Telecare, 15*(4), 191–195. doi:10.1258/jtt.2009.080909

Tracy, J., Rheuban, K., Waters, R. J., DeVany, M., & Whitten, P. (2008, November). Critical steps to scaling telehealth for national reform. *Telemedicine and e-Health, 14*(9), 990-994.

van Baar, J. D., Joosten, H., Car, J., Freeman, G. K., Partridge, M. R., & van Weel, C. (2006). Understanding reasons for asthma outpatient (non)-attendance and exploring the role of telephone and e-consulting in facilitating access to care: Exploratory qualitative study. *Quality & Safety in Health Care, 15*, 191–195. doi:10.1136/qshc.2004.013342

Young, T. L., & Ireson, C. (2003). Effectiveness of school-based telehealth care in urban and rural elementary schools. *Pediatrics, 112*, 1088–1094. doi:10.1542/peds.112.5.1088

KEY TERMS AND DEFINITIONS

Alternative Health Services: Health services other than traditional face-to-face interactions between a health provider and a patient.

Area Resource File: A publicly available data source with county-level data in the United States.

Availability of Physicians: The number of active physicians (or "MDs") in a certain geographical area.

Determinants of Utilization: Decisive social, physical and biological factors that account for the level of usage of health services.

Health Disparities: The discrepancies between health status and other health-related variables across geographical areas.

Telemedicine: The provision of medical services via electronic communications.

Urbanity: An indicator of population and resources defined by public agencies such as the U.S. Census Bureau.

Utilization of a Health Service: The level of usage of a specific type of health service within a well-defined time span.

Section 2

Chapter 9
Leading the Technological Innovation in Healthcare Systems:
The Telematic Medicine Approach

Vincenzo Gullà
Aditech SRL, Italy

ABSTRACT

The adoption of Telematics medicine or Telemedicine marks an important structural change in the mode in which deployment of medical care is being routinely provided. It is not a matter of using more or less developed technologies but mainly a deep change to the way in which countries and governments decide to provide and manage their national health care system. There is definitely a new paradigm taking place. Thus, the telemedicine approach implies deeply changing the way healthcare is provided. The authors are aware that this will take time, as does any cultural revolution, but for the time being, we need to start adapting our mentality and our networks to integrate and allow the two methods to cohabit together. Technology is one of the leading tools to allow this to happen, and it is necessary to understand what requirements are needed to get the maximum success. Years of experience have dictated the main rules and guidelines exploited in detail in this chapter.

INTRODUCTION

The telemedicine approach implies a much more modern and long range vision of health care, being prepared to take advantage of modern and cutting age technology solution, implement powerful tools and understand accordingly the enormous advantage that may derive in terms of resource optimization and services performance increase for social and healthcare assistance. With no doubt it is a political decision when to face or not this new challenge, that in the long term can only provide to governments many economic advantages and patients a much better care service and quality of life. In the short term such decision requires a deep change to the existing healthcare organizations and adjustments to the new service provisioning models. One could compare it to a

DOI: 10.4018/978-1-4666-2979-0.ch009

cultural revolution, a political or industrial epochal change but must keep in mind that historically any important transformation is caused by a critical combination of human and economic needs and indeed the world is slowly facing such change (Cleland, 2006; Gulla 2007). The background to all this picture is drawn by the aging statistics, the growing trend of lonely living people, the economic globalization scenarios, the need of more appropriate cost effective and ergonomic cares, which lead to an incredible increasing request of more and better distributed healthcare resources, consequently to higher cost requirements. In such constraining environment it is necessary to move towards new and better ways to deliver healthcare services and the only feasible and reliable tool today ready, worldwide tested and industrialized is the telematics medicine approach. Now we need to take a new more brave step forward for making all needed efforts to merge these solutions into the existing healthcare systems (COCIR, 2010) (see Figure 1).

THE TECHNOLOGY

Telemedicine, recently included under a wider concept and named Telematics Medicine approach, technology speaking, has reached a very high maturity stage. Most of the critical items have been removed, industry has invested heavily to improve and achieve cost-effective solutions. The market is offering tens of solutions addressing any disease management, relatively expensive, roughly simple and easy to use, covering most of daily needs and requirements for provisioning of efficient remote healthcare. Thanks to the technology progress, services such as telemonitoring and teleconsulting or Ambient Assisted Living models and any other medical information systems has now become a feasible and reliable tool. Ready to provide new efficient platforms, being offered by the industry as sustainable turnkey telemedicine solutions (Gulla, 2007, 2008, 2009).

Telematic Medicine Platform Model

A flexible telemedicine system is designed to provide efficient and low cost medical remote assistance, aiming to decrease the request for hospital recovery, allow patients and doctors to be connected when need raises or offer daily monitoring and patients healthcare information, simply using telematics means and networks. This in brief is the description of what a telemedicine system is required to do. The questions are "how is this performed? and " Are there guidelines to follow?" The best way to try to give an answer is to make use of empiric models, in reality there are a number of "main components" that collaborate together in a sort of dynamic mechanism that makes the engine run in the appropriate manner and become a real useful tool. Comparing the telematics medicine model with a simple system engineering approach it has the configuration shown in Figure 2.

Figure 1. Telematic medicine model: merging telemedicine, e-health, teleconsulting, and AAL

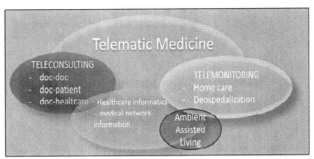

It may appear at first sight as an isolated and standalone system, but this is not the real scenario in which a telematics medicine system designer will ever work. The environment is usually diversified with geographical and cultural barriers, one will need to use tools to allow an easy integration of the system in the local organization service provisioning procedures. From a technical prospective there is the need to interface with a number of existing features and adapt the proposed solution to the real scenario, as for instance with local legacy regional data handling information systems, solving well-known data communication and telecommunication issues, granting secure access storage data, etc. In Figure 2's block diagram each element is an essential part of the system. Its role must be deeply exploited and developed in order to reach the most appropriate solution to provide a service suitable to the patient and to his daily living environment. The following paragraphs will better analyze each part and highlight the most significant elements to allow the reader to create its own set of guidelines and rules (TAO, 2005; Pech, 2004).

The Patient

The patient is always the central and main subject of the scene, wherever he resides or whatever he does, everything runs around him. His psychophysical data, disease, received medical care and quality of life improvements are the real mater upon which

and for which the telemedicine system is built. The patient, his health conditions, habitudes, life style and living environments are the variables one needs to carefully considered in solving this "equation." Every monitoring solution must fit in the patient's life style without generating any sort of alteration or additional concern, taking in due account that other than wellness monitoring cases, most of the events in which remote tele-monitoring is required, address elderly, chronicle or weak patients, characterized often by no technical informatics skills, debilitating diseases and sometimes being psychologically unstable. In such environments it is very important to provide simple and efficient tools, understandable and easy to use, focusing equipment already in use or for which the patient has gained sufficient confidence.

Data Collection

Vital data measurements is part of the mission for which a telemedicine system is meant for. Experience in the past have shown that it's not likely to provide sets of complicated medical equipment, filling rooms space just to make some simple vital measurements. Patient's data gathering must be implemented adopting a set of combined sensors. The most efficient system will address advanced noninvasive self-use medical devices, for multi parameter detection, allowing the patient a certain degree of freedom, not affecting his daily life habits. The body network concept is at the state

Figure 2. System engineering block diagram

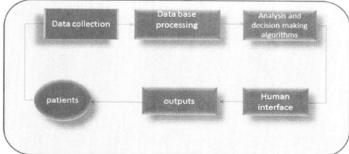

of the art the most advanced idea on how vital data should be collected even interacting with additional environmental data detection sensors, in order to permit efficient monitoring system to perceive any critical event which could compromise safety and healthy life style. Today's advanced models integrate vital data with ambient data and domotic remote controlled sensors, allowing an external decision making agent to decide whether or not an alarm occurs and communicate with a remote monitoring center. This solution is very appreciated to face heavy debilitating disease or monitor lonely living elderly, permitting patients to feel protected and to be less anxious in their daily life. With the aim to provide an efficient and economic support it is necessary to reduce human intervention as much as possible (avoiding false alarms) that is to say reaction from remote operators should be limited to real and essential cases. This milestone could be achieved developing a number of "scenarios" identified by the combination of a set of vital parameters and ambient sensors, managed by the local "decision making "device which will activate an alarm procedure based on the comparison and matching together health and environmental parameters. Each scenario will be built around the user's main weaknesses points, in order to secure prevention, appropriate wellness and medical care provisioning. In addition patient's data gathering must be grant with a multichannel approach, that is to say allow doctors and patients to connect with the database, update health status and keep vital parameters under control, by means of a set of multimedia terminals, chosen on the basis of the patients profile, life style and comfort, granting mobility with noninvasive methods. As mentioned above medical data are preferable gathered using, where possible, wearable wireless noninvasive devices. The market today offers plenty cost-efficient systems having such requirements, most using wireless Bluetooth, but even Zigbee technology is taking up the stage.

Database Processing and Handling System

Main body of any monitoring system is the database which links together information such as: patients' personal data, histories, disease information, vital parameter trend, medical reports, high resolution images (X-Ray, Imaging, MRI, MRT, etc.), data collected from different sources but all linked to one patient's account. As stated above access to data must be allowed from any media mean, therefore implies the use of high reliable security and safety protocols on one side and on the other it implies a much more heavy correlation with other local medical or administrative information systems. In other words the implementation of an efficient database must take in due account the interactive protocols and standards (HL7, Dicom, XML) to efficiently interface any other information system. As for instance many hospitals or healthcare services provider own legacy information system to keep trace of patients' data and diseases history. It will not be very appropriate and useful to develop a system for gathering remote patient's vital data that cannot interact with the patient's records stored in a local healthcare information system. It is strongly recommended that such systems be nationally wide spread, therefore designing a telemedicine network one must bear in mind multi interface approach simply adopting the database communication standards.

Privacy and data safety is one other very critical aspect for medical data management. Efficiency and safe data transfer includes: data storage within privacy respect, guaranteeing immediate access to health care stakeholders and data owners. It is not sufficient to protect data in their storage house but one must also protect data during the data transfer using encryption methods together with a number of "anti-intrusion" anti-malware tools for data servers or web portals, which could be very attractive for hacker attacks. The data base structure will need to take into account all the components that take place during a telemonitoring session and record all the data transferred between patient and doctor and place them in the correct location (see Figure 3).

Data Interaction HL7

Hospitals and other healthcare organizations typically make use of different informatics solutions and systems necessary to manage billing records, patient tracking, reports, data bases, etc. An efficient information system requires all systems to exchange data between each other when they receive new information. Many communication and interoperability tools have been developed and some standardize as for instance the HL7. The HL7 specifies a number of flexible standards, guidelines, and methodologies by which various healthcare systems can communicate with each other. Such guidelines or data standards are a set

Figure 3. Example of data base organization chart

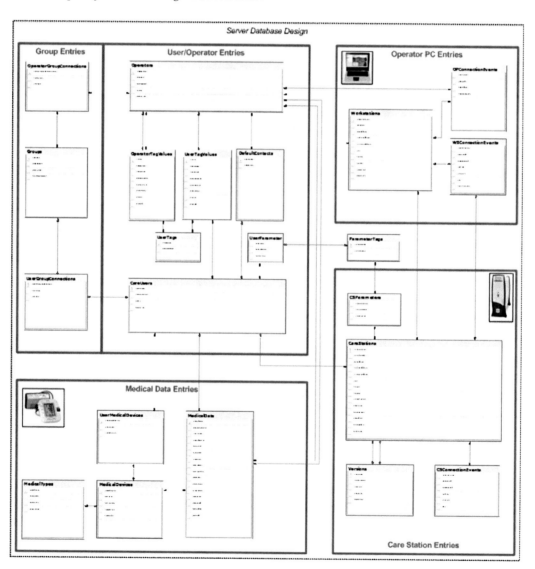

of rules that allow information to be shared and processed in a uniform and consistent manner. These data standards are meant to allow healthcare organizations to easily share clinical information. Theoretically, this ability to exchange information should help to minimize the tendency for medical care to be geographically isolated and highly variable.

Health Level Seven (HL7), is an all-volunteer, non-profit organization involved in development of international healthcare informatics interoperability standards, "HL7" is also used to refer to some of the specific standards created by the organization.

HL7 and its members provide a framework (and related standards) for the exchange, integration, sharing, and retrieval of electronic health information. v2.x of the standards, which support clinical practice and the management, delivery, and evaluation of health services, are the most commonly used in the world.

ANALYSIS AND DECISION MAKING

The model can appear a doctor-centric design, but once again the real prime actor is the patient, being his health, disease, pains and life style the real subject of the sheen, which a good art director cannot forget. Bearing this in mind one will develop algorithms integrated with robust and heavy handling data systems to create the decision making process route, designed to manage multiple patients, fit multi dimension and multilevel hierarchies models, manage incoming request, record, store and retrieve patients medical data health trend. That is to say manage multiple user data and multiple disease parameter control. Clinical "intelligence" routing integrated into management programs developed to combine vital data, must provide instant analysis and alarm detection to doctors and caregivers, allow to handle any complex needs of elderly and frail patients, in order to provide them a better quality of life and a cost efficient monitoring system.

Human Interface

Interacting with any new technology may create anxiety and this is exactly what a health aid tool should absolutely avoid. This aspect plays a very important role being the entering door, the dashboard by which one may receive or provide remote tele- healthcare assistance and is crucial for the efficient use of the system itself. The aim of the project designer is to provide an efficient and EASY TO USE tool that allows specialist, doctors, care givers to supervise remote patients vital parameters behavior and provide remote assistance and psychological support without the need to be informatics specialist. (Klapan, I, 2005, Gulla, V 2007).

In a centralized configuration approach a control center is the key element allowing care givers to:

- Access the system,
- Manage the database,
- Collect vital data,
- Control medical devices or any instrumental measurements from remote,
- Access patient data and history,
- Communicate with patients or other care givers making use of telecommunication aids to provide live communication, bidirectional or multidirectional video, together with synchronized or a-synchronized vital data.

One other important and even more critical aspect is the patient's terminal. It must be designed in a manner that allows easy use of its features to any user, not influenced by age culture and location. Plenty solutions are available today, based on the most appropriate multimedia means (phones, TV, PC, Tablets, smartphones, ad hoc touch screen device, etc.) which, connected to a telecommunication media (preferably broadband if available), link the patient to the healthcare system, no matter where he is and what he is doing (staying in home, walking in a street, shopping, jogging, laying on a bed, etc.).

Therefore both Control Center and User Terminal (see Figure 5) must interface with easy and comprehensive procedures and command medical operators and patients. The human interface must be very simple to use and easy to understand (see Figure 4 for its evolution), keeping in mind the target user which in many cases is not completely autonomous or technological oriented. As for instance a 80 years old elderly will have much more confidence with a TV remote control and a 60 years old person will be more confident with a smartphone or lab top. (Benny P.L. Lo, Surapa Thiemjarus, Rachel King and Guang-Zhong Yang, 2005)

Reference System Architecture

We have shown that implementation of a telemonitoring home care assistance network requires a number of components to be fit together. Following our rational and what has been stated above one can imagine a simple network configuration built around a central operation station or control center where al data is gathered, alarms are controlled, operators and caregivers cooperate together to provide service to remote patients. The other part of the network is merely composed by the user terminals, shaped with technology strictly depending on the use and type of telemonitoring model addressed. Simplifying the provisioning of

tele-monitoring facilities imply exploitation of a network built upon three main blocks:

- User Sensors
- Operation center
- Data management and storage

Figure 6 shows how this concept can be implemented and puts the components in the right position to give a better idea of how a telemonitoring network should look like.

Some further details about the components:

Sensors

Data gathering modules or sensors can be grouped in two key sets:

- **Body sensors:** Necessary to measure vital parameters such as: blood pressure, SpO2, heart rate, breath rate, activity, ECG, weight, etc. Body sensors are usually wearable and wireless (Bluetooth and Zigbee are the most used techniques). Some solutions have integrated together different sensors to give a more appropriate and complete health picture in other experimental projects, sensors have been combined in a sort of Body Network, able to provide the overall health conditions of patients.
- **Ambient living sensors:** Mainly used to manage and monitor the patients living environment, grant safety and comfort monitoring temperature, gas, water, movements, food consumption etc. Environmental sen-

Figure 4. Human interface evolution

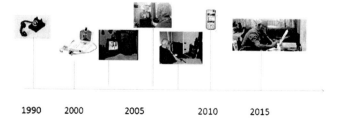

Figure 5. Home care terminals and electromedical equipment

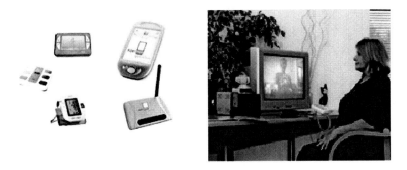

Figure 6. Reference homecare assistance network configuration

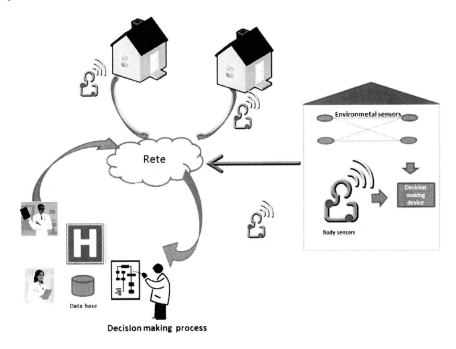

sors are very useful to gather additional information about the patients main living activities: sleeping, moving or eating to determine individuals healthy status and prevent support.

- The combination of body sensors and environmental sensors outputs could be integrated into a number of living "scenarios" which could give raise to alarms when impropriate living conditions occur (see Figure 7).

Operating Center

Health care provisioning is a centralized social service. Patients in a classic healthcare model receive cares from doctors, nurses or specialist directly or remotely using communication means. The same model is applied to telemedicine services provisioning. It's important to replicate a familiarly model which does not create critical issues or additional stress to patients or operators. For instance in a hospital the patient normally interacts with the nurse at first level, the second level is the doctor

Figure 7. Home care users

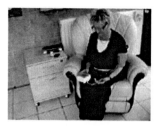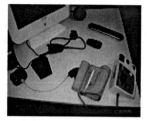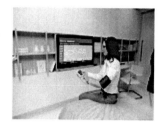

and the third level is the specialist. To provide efficient health care the model must replicate the role of each actor of the distribution chain.

INNOVATION FOR HEALTHCARE PROFESSIONAL NETWORK: THE WEB 2.0

There is no doubt at all when stating that IN-TRENET has speeded up the information, communication and is among the main players of the world's latest progress. The new web, or as it was named in 2004 by Tim O'Reilly Web 2.0, can offer even better facilities and opportunities. The higher degree of interaction is the driver for applications such as e-Health or healthcare assistance systems and the WEB 2.0 is an excellent interactive tool, showing how the communication world has moved forward from a static WEB1.0 to a more dynamic, easy and interactive WEB2.0.

As for instance WEB2.0 allows blog, forum, chat, wiki, Flickr, YouTube, Facebook, MySpace, twitter, Google+, LinkedIn, Wordpress, and lot more interactive entertainment means. To have a better understanding of the benefits and tools made available with the new web instruments, just think about how implementing a personal web site required knowledge of programming tools or HTML, now using simple blog tools one can easy share content, create interactive sites, chat with other internet users.

In telemedicine applications, such approach in the short term is responsible for a higher access to information, content made available by professionals, specialist, helping patients to get a better understand of their own disease or more simply a new connection channel for caregivers. Furthermore such technology allowed to develop a number of applications and products for remote monitoring services, first addressing wellness and sports providing GPS tracking maps speed and so on, latter being integrated with live vital parameter measurements to address more appropriate healthcare and prevention services. One example is shown in Figure 8, where data provided from a wearable multi-parameter sensor are show in real time, including an ECG graph, while the user is walking or jogging somewhere.

Organizational Impact of Telemedicine on Healthcare Services and Provisioning Models

The introduction of a new way to deliver healthcare using telemedicine solutions could create uncertainties and doubts about its applications affecting the most important aspects of today methodology of healthcare provisioning. If we analyze for instance the service models today generally adopted, we may find a common line in the relationship between the doctor providing the service and the patients receiving the cares. In between lay the healthcare organization, the service structures, all the legal bureaucracy, and finally, on top of all, lay the business models that allow the service to run. The most critical effect for adopting telemedicine may fall upon this "middle frame", shown in Figure 9. Notwithstanding that telemedicine improves the link between doctor

Figure 8. Example of website application showing vital parameters (www.zephyranywhere.com)

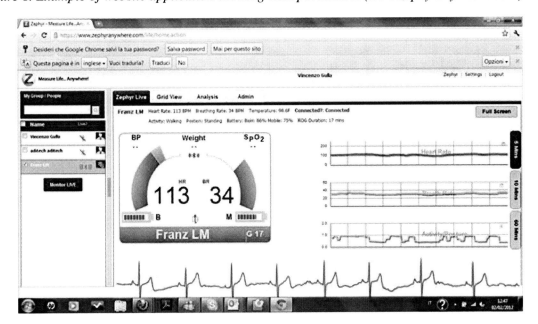

and patient, thanks to a higher degree of availability, trust and faster reaction, the middle frame must model itself to take advantage of the new technology's benefits, fitting into a new "dress" otherwise it will become just a disconnected wheel slowing down any modernization process, but this in anyhow is a general rule applicable to any innovation scenario.

As a matter of fact, *simplicius simpliciter,* if we take into consideration the basic model between patient and doctor, telemedicine could become for the doctor just a new communication channel to provide cares. Simplifying this concept a doctor connected with a patient via multimedia means. In a routine model the doctor will receive periodical or on demand measurements of a patient and will deliver response, diagnosis, reports and care prescriptions. The patient will have a better understanding of its disease, a better acknowledge of its vital parameters and a more efficient healthcare relationship. To grant such advantages the telemedicine basic model must fit into the "middle frame" connecting together the main actors,

aiming to limit the impact reactions and improve the service (Cleland, 2006).

Getting into a closer analysis of hospital organization we can define the main hospital stakeholders as:

- Department
- Personnel
- Information system
- Finance and administration

The Relationships, Roles, and Links

The personnel is composed by the head of the department, the specialist doctors, the nurses. The direct relationship with the patient is held by nurses and specialist. A patient in such environment will be subject to a number of visits and analysis depending on his disease and after a number of hospital stay days, where appropriate cares or surgery intervention have been undertaken, he will be released to reach his home where to continue the prescribed medicals cares.

Figure 9. Telemedicine fitting into the middle frame

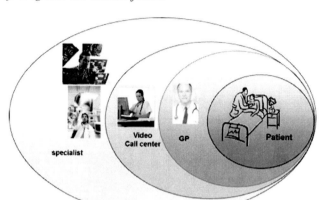

In some cases such as chronicle disease patients, they will be asked to follow periodical visits, necessary to monitor his evolution healthy conditions.

In such environment a telemedicine monitoring system could provide its major advantages allowing the patient to be released after a shorter hospital stay and receive appropriate cares in his own home, being remotely monitored. Thus technology can make the difference about how, when and where medical healthcare may be provided over a wide territory, not being limited by any geographical boundary. In other words a patient can live in his own home thousands of miles away from the doctors and continuously receive adequate cares using telemonitoring tools. In a hospital care delivery model the operating system is detected by the hospital itself, the patients are continuously connected and the GP's are the territorial operational and local controllers of the patient's disease.

A successful hospital telemedicine service needs an efficient management hierarchy model where roles are established in light of the profiles required to remote manage the patient. As for instance the experience shows that a patient and his relatives when receiving home cares feel more comfortable but in the initial phase may require a higher degree of attention to become confident with the new situation. In this case a physiological personnel profile would be needed to managed it in the most appropriate way. The management of such "new variable" into the hospital care delivery model may require to define a sort of filter or new "patient's tutor" profile. No special requirements are needed as long as this is a friendly approach support to follow the patient and his relatives in the initial home accommodation, becoming a point of reference for the service, notwithstanding that medical cares will be provided by doctors and care givers. Thus the profile could be a Call Center operator with appropriate skills, always available to provide information to the patient, manage doctors and patients visit agenda and prescriptions, contact the doctor or care giver and provide the necessary support.

TELEMEDICINE SERVICE DELIVERY MODELS

Delivering a service, whatever it may be, requires always to define a reference model, a procedure and the roles of each actor. In addition the model is a functionality of the service and can be different depending on the provisioning foreseen to be implemented. In the following we have developed 4 different models addressing medical assistance but each with different mix of players and services. All configurations are based on the most updated technology solutions today available on the marked including:

- Videocommunication
- Wireless and broadband IP connection (ADSL,Wifi, 3G)
- Noninvasive wearable medical devices
- Web-based networks

The models are developed keeping a centralized configuration with the integration of different entities depending on the user and service objectives. The center of the networking being a hospital, an NHS structure or a private service provider.

Model 1: Timeliness and Appropriateness in Emergency

This model is designed to support and manage emergency scenarios aiming to:

- Reduce timing for appropriate hospital recovery of a patient in emergency,
- Create immediate access on online specialist tele-consultation networks,
- Manage low risk triage codes to restrict hospital access to patients having real needs, intended as a filtering tool to reduce hospital time consuming for low –risk triage codes and reduce first aid ques.

This model can be further expanded over the same infrastructure management network to include locations other than hospitals such as: pharmacies, shopping malls, railway stations, airports, etc. for the provisioning of medical aids and consultation, addressing users anywhere at any time.

Such network must be designed concentrating most of the functionalities and activities in the Coordination and Management Operation Center, acting as the head quarter of the network.

Functions and Interactions

Upon an incoming emergency request the Coordination and Management Operation Center will start the triage procedure, identifying the most suitable available health care structure and the fastest mode to transfer the patient, if required, the operator will alert the specialist for an immediate consultation. The operation flow for this architectural configuration is as follows:

- Operation Center interacts only with ambulances, emergency crews and first aid posts
- Has access to territorial healthcare database to verify the availability of hospital beds
- Finds the appropriate specialists available on line
- Provides online advice for multi-channel triage

The use of video-communication and web based networks foreseen in the network, provide 3 main advantages to improve the service delivery:

1. The call center operator can see the sheen and allow doctors to interact with the crew.
2. The online specialist can be involved in the call and take real-time decisions.
3. If hospital recovery is needed the database will immediately detect the nearest available hospital, retrieve the patients data from central database and open an electronic admission sheet, available to doctors at the patients selected recovery site.
4. The on line doctor can provide guidance to crew or care giver to locally support the patient.

Territorial Location: Centralized territorial coverage, information links with territorial structures, fixed and mobile stations located in health facilities, hospitals and public areas.

Configuration: The telemedicine network required to provide the services mentioned above must have the following configuration. Also see Figure 10 for the delivery model.

- Operations Center managing incoming calls from fixed posts or mobile stations
- Fixed and mobile user terminals
- Access to geographic information systems for hospitalizations, availability beds and specialized recovery healthcare structures
- Regional information systems and interface
- Patient medical records
- Multivideo call center
- Specialist medical stations
- User terminal for fixed and mobile units with medical remote controlled equipment (ECG, SpO2, pressure, blood sugar, etc.)
- Public station healthcare "Totem"

Model 2: Optimizing the Use of Hospital Resources

One of the most critical items in many geographic areas is the expenditure to maintain and provide efficient hospital services (see Figure 11). This

model has the aim to optimize such cost addressing two main aspects of a hospital recovery:

1. In hospital days - stay
2. Post dismissal cares and support, and in particular:
   a. Early dismissal with follow-up in intermediate or local structures
   b. Early dismissal with home care follow-up
   c. Post hospital discharge rehabilitation activities

The three activities are grouped together because:

- Express different aspects of the same problem: post hospitalization remote assistance.
- Involve the same actors (Central Hospital, local healthcare facilities, remote patient domicile).
- The difference lays into the service provisioning mode and delivery locations.

Functions and Interactions

To allow a correct and efficient recovery of the patients healthcare conditions, upon the patients

Figure 10. Emergency telemedicine delivery model

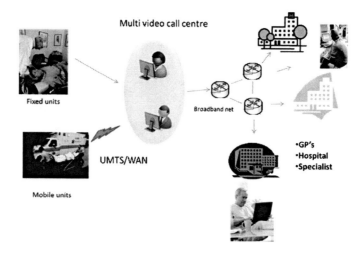

146

Figure 11. Hospital optimization model

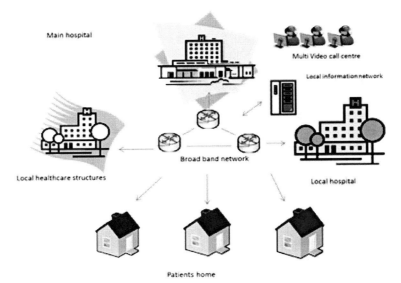

early discharge an appropriate healthcare procedure must be provided. Thus may require the involvement of hospital personnel resources, GP's, specialist and caregivers. The main interactions being limited to patient and medical staff can be listed here after:

- Discussions with the hospital medical staff in a remote healthcare structure for tele-consultation and receive daily -cares.
- The hospital doctor can perform a remote examination of the patient from home or the nearest healthcare structure in order to check the progress of convalescence, emerging complications and patient's resignation.
- The hospital personnel may interact with the patient and his family in his home.
- The doctor carries out a remote visit.
- The specialist or rehabilitation care givers may follow the patient evolution and activity recovery from a remote hospital or in his place of residence.
- Update the hospital patient's clinical record.

Territorial Location: Centralized over the hospital area of competence.

Configuration: The network model must take into account that service can be provided in a public structure or a private home therefore allow easy reach of the patients by caregivers or nurses where ever they are, when a need arises. The following configuration ideally fits the above requirements:

- Operations Center managing incoming calls from remote healthcare structures or home patient
- Regional information systems and patient medical records interface
- Multivideo call center to manage simultaneous calls
- Portable medical video terminals with medical operator software
- Patient's workstation for remote healthcare facilities
- Portable user terminals for temporary homecare use
- Medical equipment and rehabilitation monitoring (diabetes, heart failure, COPD, Alzheimer's)

Model 3: Continuous Care Provisioning for Chronicle Patients

Probably is the most critical item for any national healthcare system. As a matter of fact the number of chronicle patients requiring frequent hospitals resources is directly linked to the population aging, on the other hand an appropriate homecare service can provide a better output and significantly reduce the requirements for further cares and costs raise. The service applications foreseen in this framework are:

1. Integrated management of chronically ills
2. Systematic interaction between a health professional and chronic or fragile patients

The two objectives can be grouped together as they represent two different stages of the same problem:

*   Handling dependent patients with chronic diseases,
*   Request for assistance to a doctor or healthcare provider.

The normal procedure requires some interaction with GP's and between the local NHS. Being a service provided on the basis of a pre-existing schedule or on-demand request, it may need centralized coordination tools to manage appointments, visit schedules, doctors agenda and keep patients history updated. The actors involved are: GPs the local NHS and Social services. See Figure 12 for the delivery model.

Functions and Interactions

The main body of the telemedicine network may be managed by the local Social and or Healthcare organization depending on the national model. It is not strictly necessary to be included or driven by a hospital structure as the patients most of the times requires a psychological and moral support other than specific medications. The activity flow could be as follows:

*   The call center Operator interacts with the patients, the GP and home care caregivers.
*   The call center handles calls, visits and the agendas for doctors.

Figure 12. Chronicle of patients' continuous care delivery model

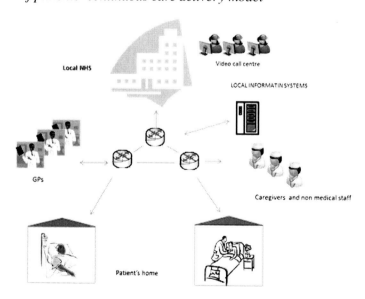

- The doctor may perform a remote visit to the patient's home from his studio, to check the progress of the disease, giving personal support.
- Non-medical staff in the call center may interact with the patient and his relatives.
- Medical staff update the patient's clinical record.

Territorial Location: Local NHS or centralized zone health structure
Configuration:

- Operations Center managing incoming calls from GP's, patients and medical staff
- Regional information systems and interface to patient medical records
- Multivideo call center to manage simultaneous calls
- Medical terminal stations at GP's location
- User terminal stations for long-term usage
- Medical equipment and rehabilitation monitoring (diabetes, heart failure, COPD, Alzheimer 's)

Model 4: Integrated Health and Social Services

Other important aspects that must be taken into account when planning a remote medical assistance network are those relative to psychological status of a patient, elderly or weak person. As a matter of fact many times the person is not inn real medical condition need but rather in a psychological sufferance sometimes generated by living alone, age, post trauma, panic attach etc. In general such situation could be handled providing adequate support with psychological experts.

I terms of objectives we may highlight following:

- Social services for elderly frail and weak subjects,
- Health and social integration, elderly patients and/or fragile.

The two goals are a continuous interaction between different care settings according to shared care plans, because the patient does not always need to interact with physicians or healthcare providers being more oriented towards the provision of a service to persons needing psychological medical support.

The actors involved may belong to social welfare structures and facilities sometimes provided by local health organizations or by public and private structures (cooperatives, utility companies and personal care, etc.) present on the territory.

In the hypothesis here examined the local NHS social service is involved as the Coordinator and owner of the monitoring network, which can provide directly or entrust the service outsourcing it to private companies. See Figure 13 for the delivery model.

Functions

Are mainly concentrated into the call center:

- Interacts with patients, GPs and home care caregivers l
- Handles emergency assistance calls and alerts the medical/psychologist staff
- Handles any alarms from home automation sensors for non -self-sufficiency people
- Handled the agendas of support personnel for the patients
- Offers psychological supportive medical personnel that activates when needed
- Connect to the GPs to perform a remote visit to the patients

Territorial Location: Local centralized area or structure with remote assist facilities
Configuring:

- Operations Center managing incoming calls, alarms from remote home sensors
- Multivideo call center to manage simultaneous calls

Figure 13. Integrating healthcare and social network

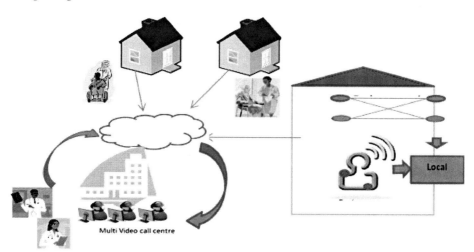

- Medical stations at GPs ambulatory for remote patients visit
- User stations for long-term usage
- Home sensors network
- Regional information systems and interface to patient medical records

Benefits of a Telematic Medical System

After years and hundreds of experimentation and local applications (see Table 1 for a summary of their requirements) there is no doubt that telematic medicine provides immediate and tangible benefits to patient, clinical staff, society and governments economies.

A brief but very significant list of benefits follows here after:

- **Reduced Mortality:** Patients using telemedicine live longer, compared to people receiving usual care (15-55% compared to people receiving usual care).
- **Reduced Hospital stay:** The use of telemedicine and telemonotoring results in a more healthy population requiring less acute healthcare resources: hospital recov-

ery can be reduced (30-50%), as well as hospital recovery stay (24-48%).

- **Increased quality of life of patients:** Patients enrolled in telematics medicine programs have enjoyed a better quality of life. Thanks to a better healthcare perception, more active connection with care givers team, involvement in the healthcare process ending in a significant decrease of anxious status.
- **Decrease chronicle diseases:** More appropriate cares addressing single patients' needs culminate in a much more efficient care, provided in a regular monitoring of vital parameters service, allowing doctors to prevent risk of health worsening conditions and reduce chronicle diseases, in other words reduce unwanted hospitalizations and improve healthcare conditions.
- **Education:** A better and ease access to patients medical information increases personal knowledge of healthy behaviors and allows patients to be educated about their diseases. This educating patient to become more sensible to understand their own medical conditions and adopt a more appropriate life style.

Table 1. Summary of models application requirements

Models common implementation requirements	
Item	**Description**
Central Operation Station	
HW	Redundant management servers -network - protected environment
	Video call center Operator stations
SW application	network management and database
	video call center for remote management of users
	GPs medical & communication sw
	home automation sensors management sw
	integration with existing information systems
User Terminal	
HW	Video Set top box. communication gateway
	medical devices environmental sensors
SW	User terminal communication software
	Device interface software
Telecommunication	
Infrastructure	Broadband availability in remote homes, peripherals and central structures

- **Time saving:** Telemedicine allows doctors to optimize time, performing visits and measurements from remote, thus saving travels to reach patient's homes, schedule visits and patients to save time for reach doctor's office.

Barriers Hindering the Development of Telehealth

Why is telematics medicine still in a beginning stage? Even thou the potential benefits of telematics medicine are enormous there are a number of barriers which continue to delay the introduction of such technology or preclude achievements of optimal demonstrated benefits.

- Among all the most important lays in the lack of reimbursement for telematics medicine services and visits. Governments have not yet made a clear decision if this is part of the national health service and how access is allowed.

- Second is the identification of an efficient business model: probably more linked to the above mentioned item, services providers do not seek a short term return of investments.

- Third but very important point is the lack of a common standardization of IT items and interfaces allowing telehealth technology to interact between different networks, infrastructures and medical devices. Most of the projects and solutions developed worldwide have ended in isolated experiences, providing excellence of results but never connected to each other, with a significant lack of interoperability. This expects are not much related to technology issues but mainly to political and economic aspects. Emerging standardization bodies such as IHE3 or Continua4 are slowly driving to overcome this barriers, pushed ahead by industry and political interest.

- Fourth position is the insufficient communication and acknowledge: many medical experts are still not persuaded about the benefits of telehealth. Acceptance from physicians and patients probably needs a more deep support from medical guidelines and a better evolution of solution usability for both patient and doctors.

- Fifth is the integration of telehealth services into care delivery structure: One of the primary challenges challenging telehealth today is the lack of effective workflow integration into existing care delivery structures. In other terms hospitals and local medical structures should adopt telematics medicine solutions and systems to provide efficient home cares, deliver de-hospitalization services allowing a major number of patients to receive efficient cares in their own home, in order to enable payers, providers and patients to fully benefit from telehealth.

- Last but not least stand the legal responsibilities: There is a certain lack of legal clearance in the area of telehealth that local governments have in some degree considered. Some countries are in an advanced stage but still rules and procedures are not mature to allow a wide deployment. This is a major challenge in particular with re-

gards to liability, jurisdiction and licensing, registration of telehealth services and professionals.

SUMMARY

In the above paragraphs we have considered the main aspects that influence the choice and implementation of a telemedicine system, analyzing the components, the requirements and the critical items that need to be dimensioned and correctly applied.

This chapter collects a number of articles provided by experts and researchers covering some of the most worldwide exciting experiences in the field of telemedicine network for hospital applications. The reader will have the opportunity to learn about the technical solutions approached and the achieved results in a complete field of pathologies including cardiology, pulmonary diseases, Alzheimer, cytology image processing and emergency. The aim of this chapter is to show how technology maturity has improved the way in which healthcare can be provided and allow the reader to understand from these examples what is required and how to design, implement and run a telemedicine network.

REFERENCES

Cleland, J. C. F. (2006). *The Trans-European Network –Home care management system study: An investigation of the effect of telemedicine on outcomes in Europe*. DIS Manage Health Outcomes 2006.

Gulla, V. (2004). *Broadband in Europe: Markets and trends*. Paper presented at the WCIT 2004, Information Technology Conference - Athens 19-21 May 2004.

Gulla, V. (2005). *The telemedicine market: A fast growing technology.* Paper presented at the E-Merging/E-Learning Conference, Dubai 19-21 Nov. 2005.

Gulla, V. (2007). *Tele-medicine is a driver for quality of life improving broadband application.* Paper presented at the 3rd Croatian & International Congress on Telemedicine and e-Health, June 2007

Gulla, V. (2008). Telemedicine potential business models. In Pillai, M. V. (Ed.), *Telemedicine concepts and applications.*

Gulla, V. (2009). How can tele-medicine benefit from broadband technologies? In Khoumbati, K., Dwivedi, Y. K., & Srivastava, A. (Eds.), *Handbook of research on advances in health informatics and electronic healthcare applications: Global adoption and impact of information communication technologies.* Hershey, PA: IGI Global. doi:10.4018/978-1-60566-030-1.ch006

Klapan, I. (2005). *Telemedicine.* Zagreb, Croatia: Telemedicine Association Zagreb.

Lo, B., Thiemjarus, S., King, R., & Yang, G.-Z. (2005). Body sensor network – A wireless sensor platform for pervasive healthcare monitoring. *Proceedings of the International Conference on Pervasive Computing.*

Pech, E. (2004). *Making innovation happen.* Technical paper produced by Detecon, Inc.

Tao, W. (2005). *IP broadband access network construction.* Network Marketing Department Technical paper produced by Huawei Technologies Co., Ltd.

ENDNOTES

[1] HL7 was founded in 1987 to produce a standard for hospital information systems. HL7, Inc. is a standards organization that was accredited in 1994 by the American National Standards Institute (ANSI).[5] HL7 is one of several American National Standards Institute accredited Standards Developing Organizations (SDOs) operating in the healthcare arena. Most SDOs produce standards (sometimes called specifications or protocols) for a particular healthcare domain such as pharmacy, medical devices, imaging or insurance (claims processing) transactions. Health Level Seven's domain is clinical and administrative data. Today, HL7 has been adopted by several national SDOs outside the United States. Those SDOs are consequently not accredited by ANSI. However, HL7 is now adopted by ISO in international standardization and accredited as a partnering organization for mutual issuing of standards. The first mutually published standard is ISO/HL7 21731:2006 Health informatics—HL7 version 3—Reference information model—Release 1. HL7 has allowed for the interoperability between electronic Patient Administration Systems (PAS), Electronic Practice Management (EPM) systems, Laboratory Information Systems (LIS), Dietary, Pharmacy and Billing systems as well as Electronic Medical Record (EMR) or Electronic Health Record (EHR) systems. Currently, HL7's v2.x messaging standard is supported by every major medical information systems vendor in the United States.(source Wikipedia)

Chapter 10

Telemedicine Service of San Giovanni–Addolorata Hospital in Rome:
Analysis of About Two Years of Activity (2008– Early 2011)

Michelangelo Bartolo
S.Giovanni Addolorata Hospital, Italy

Gianpiero Guerrieri
S.Giovanni Addolorata Hospital, Italy

Andrea Nucita
University of Messina, Italy

ABSTRACT

Telemedicine service has dramatically increased in San Giovanni-Addolorata hospital in Rome in the last two years. Stated as an experimental service in 2005, telemedicine has gained the status of usual service in 2008 and now has reached a good functional level since the creation of a dedicated department within the hospital in late 2009. The authors intend to present the results obtained since the beginning of the usual service and a brief description of the operational workflow.

INTRODUCTION

Telemedicine is the branch of the health care, which lets health operators control and cure patients remotely, freeing people from the constraint of a direct and tight connection to the hospital.

Patients can experience normal life as if they were not affected by pathologies while physicians have a constant ad updated view of their clinical situation. This way of acting in health care dramatically increases patients' life style level while, in the meantime, saves huge amount of money

DOI: 10.4018/978-1-4666-2979-0.ch010

for the hospitals sparing hospitalization beds, cures, sickbay accesses and lowers waiting lists. What we are going to describe is our experience in telemedicine in the San Giovanni-Addolorata hospital in Rome (Italy), as far as the adopted methodologies and the recorded results.

DESCRIPTION

The telemedicine service held in the San Giovanni-Addolorata hospital in Rome is one of the most significant and innovative services in Italy. It has grown from experimental to full operational status in 2008 after a 2 years training period and has become an independent clinical department in late 2009. Its key points and peculiarities are that is one of the few telemedicine wards created in Italy, with dedicated structure and personnel and that all the hardware and software architecture was designed by ward's and technological partners' personnel, avoiding to use already implemented stuff, but customizing the solution to the department needs and trying to continuously refine and improve it. Up to the end of 2010 the technological partner was Hewlett Packard Italy, which demanded software implementation to some of its partners. Since February 2008 software was developed by Format Systems & Networks.

In the following, the analysis of the collected data during the observation period is described in details.

Started as a prototypal service for selected patients in 2005, the telemedicine service is based on some portable clinical devices which create a "virtual hospitalization bed" (see Figure 1), a Service Centre for communication between patients and doctors, and a certain amount of specialist physicians who daily check the remote patients' life parameters remotely interacting with them as if they were making the normal department daily visit checkout.

This way of checking patient's health is called TeleMonitoring. It is greatly useful in some non-

Figure 1. Virtual bed devices

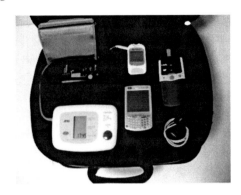

critical, long-term pathologies, such as hypertension, or many forms of cardiac diseases or for a territorial assistance and screening. We have adopted two different ways of using the Tele-Monitoring.

The first option has been named "Standard TeleMonitoring Service". It consists in a "virtual bed" composed of various and specific clinical devices that are supposed to be used by the patient or by his/her care giver to take and automatically send life parameters to the Service Centre in San Giovanni hospital.

The other option is called "MultiPatient Tele-Monitoring System". Its operational way is similar to the one described above, but, in this solution, many people might be monitored with the same apparel at the same time. In this case a more professional operator is required because clinical devices are more advanced than the single patients ones and a non-professional person might not be able to operate alone. The MultiPatient solution has been developed to be installed in nurseries, sickbays, or wherever many people may be treated at the same time.

A third option, the TeleConsultation Service, is also available: a spot request may be sent to a specialist physician via MultiPatient or custom software, with the option of sending the needed patient's life measurements in the meantime.

Only a certain amount of diseases may be treated by the telemedicine service (no emergencies, i.e.), so only selected patients can enter in the monitoring program. Typical patients come out of cardiological diseases (such as atrial fibrillation, heart failure, arrhythmias), diabetes, hypertension, bronchopneumonia, skin ulcers or angiology, but also terminally ill patients have been treated with such service.

Very often patients are sent to the service directly after First Aid treatment, avoiding hospitalization time and costs for public health, as it has been already noticed in other contexts (Stensland et al., 1999; Agha et al., 2002). The advantage is clear: they can be monitored in the same way of the normal hospitalization, maintaining the same level of diagnostic accuracy, but in a more familiar and retrieving environment: their homes (see Figures 2 and 3). Their care givers (typically relatives or professional nurses) are tasked to take measurements at given due dates and to automatically send them to the hospital.

An automatic alerting system and Service Centre phone calls supply the contacts with patients and care givers when needed.

Patient's Route in the Service

After being selected as adequate for the telemedicine, the patient comes to the telemedicine department where a virtual clinic paper is opened by the Service Centre. This virtual clinic paper is part of a custom web software that allows physicians and clinical operator to monitor and interact with patients almost in every place on the planet.

Fundamental information for patient's diagnosis must be inserted by the Centre's operator, as well as his/her anamnestic history and his/her present therapy. After that "bureaucratic" portion of the acceptance protocol, the patient and/or the care giver is instructed on how to use the instruments that will be given to monitor the required

Figure 2. Dashboard for blood pressure and glycaemia in chronological order and by time slots

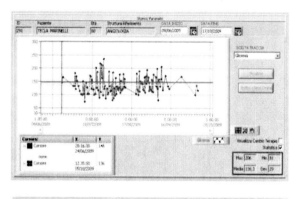
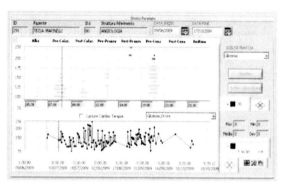
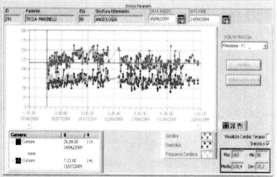
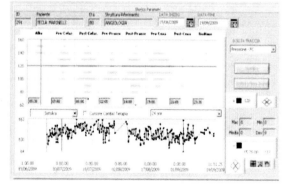

Figure 3. Ulcer monitoring: calibration and determination of the actual size

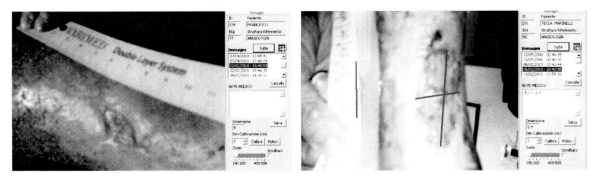

life parameters. The telemedicine operator checks that the persons are able to repeat all the needed operations alone, and then lets the patient return home. At due time he/she takes the requested measurements, that are automatically sent to the telemedicine receivers, and are instantly available for the health personnel to be watched (see Figure 4). If a therapy refinement is required, the doctor adjusts it in the virtual clinical paper only. Automatic alerts by sms, e-mail and internal notification system informs patient, care giver and Service Centre of the change. Service Centre operators ring the patient to ensure that he/she has acknowledged the information and to remotely assist him/her in case help is needed.

When the responsible physician decides that no further monitoring is required, the patient comes back to the department to give instrumentation back. If he/she agrees, he/she can compile a brief interview to feedback operators about his/her level of satisfaction on the service.

It is his/her second and only time of coming to the hospital even if he/she has taken tens of different clinical measurements. He/she has been called several times by Service Centre nurses and has been continually checked by hospital doctors instead. A very great advantage for his/her life style level, as many of them have declared in the interview.

Apparel Description

What is given to the patient (the so called "virtual bed") is a modular kit composed by some clinical devices (a portable electrocardiograph, a digital sphygmomanometer, a glucometer, an oxymeter, a camera or just some of them depending on the patient's pathology), and a PDA that acts as data concentrator and automatic sender. All these devices were selected by specialists among those on market. The only fundamental requirement was the possibility to interact to a PC or PDA via one

Figure 4. Multipatient station and technical laboratory of the telemedicine ward

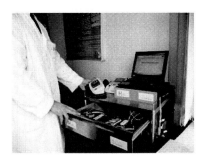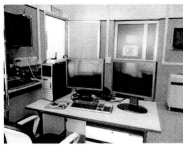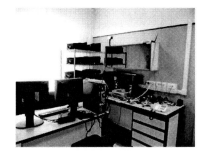

of the available communication ways (serial port, Bluetooth, infrared connection). The software has been implemented with an open code approach, which lets the software developers to add any new possible device as soon as it is compliant to system's requirements. Very few telemedicine solutions can grant this level of modularity.

An easy-to-use custom software on the PDA reminds the patient the operations that must be fulfilled to correctly take and send measurements. In case of problems or forgetfulness a technician is ready to solve the problem online. The PDA software is continually refined to simplify and reduce patient's operations at home, considering that very often users are old, non-technologised people living alone. Of course, only one person may take measurements from one single kit.

Even the kind of instrument is selected accordingly to the patient's skill. We have serial or Bluetooth based electrocardiographs as well as sphygmomanometers that we can choose to give on patient's supposed ability to handle technological devices. Often older people prefer a cable connected device instead of a wireless transmitting one (like Bluetooth technology), because they are more confident and reassured by the physical connection by wire. So we can prepare a differently organized kit on the base of patient's supposed reactions in front of the devices. Everything is absolutely modular in our service.

The multipatient device maintains the same philosophy but uses more advanced clinical devices, able to treat different patients at the same time. The data concentrator is different as well: a small portable PC with a custom software that interacts with the station personnel. No limits of contemporary patients have been created for this kind of service and devices. As in the situation described before, even for the multipatient device the control software was developed and customized by department's technological partners and is open to new instrumentation integration.

The virtual clinical paper is a web-based software that, together with custom server receiving software and appropriate database, lets operators read and interact with patients' data. The choice of a web-based software comes from the need to let physicians monitor patients' health not only during normal hospital job time, but even at home or abroad. Wherever an accounted doctor is, he/she can watch patients' data and be reached by alert notification via sms or e-mail (the use of SMS/MMS/E-mail has already been adopted with success, as reported in previous telemedicine studies (Figueredo et al., 2004; Setyono et al.,2010)). Ward's consultants doctors were able to report ECGs even during conferences in China or during their holidays!

A capillary system of notifications and alerts has been built as well. Every time a physician alters the patient's therapy or measurement protocol an automatic sms where all the required information are explained is sent to patients, care giver and GP is sent. Service Centre nurses receive a notification of the change adopted and ring the patient to check if he/she has correctly understood the message. When some medical data sent by the patient is out of customizable bounds selected during the monitoring period, an automatic sms is sent to the responsible ward physician to let him/her know that he/she must check patient's clinical paper. This method of alerting was selected by the overall diffusion of cellular phones in the world as the simplest and more efficient way to send information to people (especially over 60 year old patients) who are not very familiar with technology. During these years we have confirmed that this method of alerting is highly efficient and easily understood by patients and physicians.

A huge amount of physical and virtual servers acts in background as the basis for the entire system. Redundancies, load balancing, multiple scheduled backups, giant amounts of data storage space and a huge security level let us the confidence to have a stable hardware system that can operate constantly for years without significant unexpected stops or malfunctions.

RESULTS

At the end of March 2011 the service reached an amount of more than 500 treated patients, which is a very significant number, considering that the service has only 30 "virtual beds" and 2 multipatient installations available. We want to analyse these data.

Up to March 31st 2011, 502 patients were enrolled by the Telemedicine service. The mean age was 66 ± 14 years old; 46% were women, 54% men.

In Table 1, the patients were divided by the source and the treated pathology.

Table 2 shows the number of clinical parameters recorded by the patients in the same time period.

The growing of the service's amount of patients is shown in Figure 5.

The increasing of the amount of patients enrolled is clearly visible. Collaboration with other departments will allow further increase in the next future.

More than 18000 contacts with patients via sms, telephone and e-mail have been achieved. The mean is about 35 contact per patient.

Table 1. Patients grouped by pathologies

Patient Source	Treated pathology	No. of patients
Cardiological First Aid; Cardiological department	Atrial Fibrillation, Heart failure	347
Medicine departent; sickbays	Parkinson, Diabetes, cancer	57
Hypertension department	Systemic hypertension	62
Angiology	Leg ulcers	22
Wards	Terminally ill patients	10
Bronchopneumology	Chronic Obstructive Pulmonary Disease	4
TOTAL		502

Table 2. Clinical parameters recorded by the patients

Features of measures	No.
Blood Pressure/ Heart rate	25,840
ECGs	4,687
Glycemia	1,820
Sat O$_2$	3,222
Weight	325
Pictures	1,132
TOTAL	38,081

Figure 5. Growth of the service over time

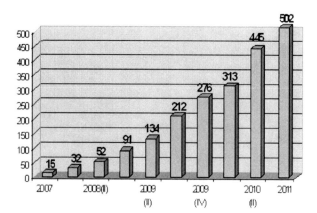

Table 3. Patients' responses to interviews

Question	Excellent	Good	Acceptable	Bad	Very bad
Did you find this service useful?	71.00%	24.00%	4.00%	0.00%	1.00%
Were explanaitions by operators clear enough?	74.00%	22.00%	2.00%	1.00%	1.00%
Did you find the kit easy to use?	59.00%	33.00%	6.00%	2.00%	0.00%
How did you find the staff?	83.00%	16.00%	1.00%	0.00%	0.00%
Do you find the service useful to better life conditions?	77.00%	20.00%	2.00%	0.00%	1.00%

Table 4. Cost savings due to telemedicine program

Amount	Decreased performance	Saving (estimation in €)
-347	Hospitalization (*)	874,000.00
-76	Days in hospital for early discharge	68,000.00
-84	ED admission	58,000.00
-430	Outpatient admission	19,000.00
	TOTAL	1,019,000.00

Different therapies, variation of drug's type or dose, was prescribed 681 times, 1.3 for each patient.

The time absorbed for single patient for enrolling, web and phone controlling, follow up was:

- 4 physician hours,
- 5 nurse hours,
- 1.5 help desk hours (engineering, web technicians).

The outcoming satisfaction interview compiled by 312 patients gave the result shown in Table 3 as far as the satisfaction degree is concerned.

The estimated saving for Regional finance, due to decrease of hospitalization, days in hospital, ED or outpatient admission can be shown in Table 4.

- Average hospitalization of 2.8 days calculated at a cost of 900 € per day.

CONCLUSION

Telemedicine shifts some patients from the hospital to an integrated home assistance, poly-specialistic, on-line, taking doctors and nurses virtually at home. The quality and the level of care are guaranteed, the patient's satisfaction too. No distance, no time, no waiting are conflicting with a good practice and attention to the health as the data presented in this article clearly show.

The telemedicine department of the San Giovanni-Addolorata hospital in Rome is a clear of good health innovation that can and must be, however, continually refined and bettered, that is and always will be our main goal. We are proud of the results obtained up to today but we know this is just a little step in the way of a new generation of health cares that can shift people's quality of life to layers we can only imagine at present. The spread of solutions like the one we are experiencing and we have just presented may be a first step to this scenario, but we know that too many bureaucratic, financial, operational and political problems should be faced and overcome before we might be able to say that telemedicine is a new health care reality also in Italy.

REFERENCES

Agha, Z., Schapira, R. M., & Maker, A. H. (2002). Cost effectiveness of telemedicine for the delivery of outpatient pulmonary care to a rural population. *Telemedicine and E-Health, 8*(3), 281–291. doi:10.1089/15305620260353171

Figueredo, M. V. M., & Dias, J. S. (2004). Mobile telemedicine system for home care and patient monitoring. In *Annual International Conference of the IEEE Engineering in Medicine and Biology Society* (pp. 3387-3390). Piscataway, NJ: IEEE Service Center.

Setyono, A., Alam, M. J., & Al-Saqour, R. A. (2010). Design of multimedia messaging service for mobile telemedicine system. *International Journal of Network and Mobile Technologies, 1*(1), 15–21.

Stensland, J., Speedie, S. M., Ideker, M., House, J., & Thompson, T. (1999). The relative cost of outpatient telemedicine services. *Telemedicine Journal: The Official Journal of the American Telemedicine Association, 5*(3), 245–256.

KEY TERMS AND DEFINITIONS

ICT: Information and Communications Technology.

Teleconsultation: Remote clinical consultation, by the use of information and communication technologies.

Telemedicine: Telemedicine uses information and communication technologies in order to provide health care at a distance.

Telemonitoring: Remote clinic control for several days.

Chapter 11
Remote Follow-Up of Implantable Cardioverter Defibrillators:
Technology, Patient Management, Integration with Electronic Records, and ICD Product Surveillance

David L. Scher
Pinnacle Health System, USA

Franco Naccarella
Euro China Society for Health Research, Italy

Zhang Feng
First People Hospital of Jiao Tong University, People's Republic of China

Giovanni Rinaldi
Italian Society of Telemedicine, Italy

ABSTRACT

In this chapter, the authors introduce some concepts about the remote follow-up of Implantable Cardioverter Defibrillators (ICD). Even if this type of remote monitoring system is relatively new, literature has demonstrated the utilization in clinical practice and during the last few years, the medical industry has provided different devices. Starting from the background, some models of utilizations are presented, focusing on the description of the main functions provided by some devices offered on the market. Next the motivations for which remote follow-up is needed are explored; a better management of the patient is described in several studies, and the integration of clinical information from monitoring devices in Electronic Medical Records is presented as the important step in order to provide comprehensive clinical information about the patient. Also, economic issues are shown. Then, some experiences realized in U.S. are explored, and at last, a number of questions are proposed to the discussion as contribution to the next research. Some Italian recent experiences in the field of remote monitoring and home care of patients with heart failure with and without implantable devices are reported.

DOI: 10.4018/978-1-4666-2979-0.ch011

INTRODUCTION

The remote monitoring systems (hereafter referred to as RMS) for follow-up of ICDs is a relatively new technology (Schoenfeld & Reynolds, 2005). It has been utilized in clinical practice for approximately three years.

The first large feasibility study, using Medtronic's Carelink System, was published in 2004 (Schoenfeld et al., 2004). This study demonstrated clinical usefulness as well as physician and patient satisfaction.

Recent large scale ICD generator and lead advisories and recalls have significantly increased the requirement to monitor devices more closely.

The Heart Rhythm Society has recommended the use of wireless and remote monitoring technologies for improved detection of device or system malfunctions (Carlson et al., 2006). Financial and ethical constraints by device manufacturers will likely soon result in significant decrease in industry participation in surveillance of devices in clinics and offices.

Wider use of electronic medical records begs the integration of device follow-up data with them in a seamless manor. All of these factors have accelerated the need and use of Internet-based monitoring systems. These systems are now offered without charge to the physicians and patients. Reimbursement policies for remote monitoring have been established by Medicare and most other insurance carriers. Remote monitoring is therefore needed and feasible as routine follow-up of ICDs.

It is logical to think that this type of follow-up will eventually be extended to pacemakers as well. The focus thus far has been on ICDs for a variety of reasons, but the advantages and rational for the extension of this technology to pacemaker follow-up are the same.

This article will address the technology of RMS, its potential impact on patient and device management, the integration of RMS with EMR, and the potential need to exploit RMS as a means of post market surveillance from a quality control standpoint, of ICDs. There remain unanswered questions about this technology which will be discussed as well.

It is clear that remote follow-up of cardiac rhythm devices in the USA is both accepted, welcomed, and growing, as it should be the home care and remote monitoring and data base assisted follow up of patients with heart failure without implantable devices.

REMOTE MONITORING SYSTEMS (RMS): BACKGROUND

Internet-based follow-up of ICDs was first commercially available in 2002. The appeal of the technology is to decrease time per follow-up, improve patient convenience by decreasing routine office visits, and to improve patient care by utilizing it to rapidly transmit data from patients with symptoms or arrhythmic events. It has significantly increased in usage over the past two years.

Clinics or physician practices were initially charged on a subscription basis by the first device company to market the technology (Medtronic) for utilizing the service.

Physicians and clinics operating within an environment of decreasing reimbursement were against this unprecedented model of having the physician subscribe for a service like this. Once comparable competition appeared with the LATITUDE system, which did not involve a subscription fee, adoption increased significantly, eventually becoming the economic model of the technology.

The advent of wireless devices which makes transmission logistically easier for patients also contributed significantly to increased acceptance. The utilization of the Carelink system in identifying trends of failure of the Sprint Fidelis leads has brought to the forefront the potentially most important role of remote follow-up: a source of early detection of failure of devices and leads (Groves & Medtronic, 2007).

RMS: FUNCTION

All the major cardiac rhythm device manufacturers currently have remote monitoring capabilities for ICDs. This involves a transmitter within a short distance from the patient, and a land line telephone connection. Some ICDs have antennae on the header of the device which communicates with the transmitter wirelessly. Others require a communication wand placed in close proximity of the ICD which allows communication with the transmitter.

The transmitted information, depending upon the company, may have the information sent to a proprietary Internet server with the practitioner able to download the information to a PC. Integration with some electronic medical record systems is a fertile area of active work among the companies, driven by the desire by clinicians to consolidate clinical information as well as eliminate paper-based records (see section Future of the Technology below).

Information obtained from the device is identical to that which would be generated by a printed report at the time of a device interrogation in the office. This includes functionality of the ICD generator and leads (battery status, lead impedances, last thresholds clinically obtained), arrhythmia logbook information with stored electrograms, and device settings. These systems are not designed at this time and are restricted by the FDA to allow changes in the device programming or test thresholds.

The Medtronic Carelink and Boston Scientific LATITUDE remote follow-up systems are Internet-based, where data is sent via the patient's transmitter (via land line phone modem) to a central proprietary repository Internet server. This information is able to be viewed and then downloaded to computers by the physician following the patient.

Both of these systems have the ability to detect 'alerts' issued by the device itself. Some alerts are automatically active and some are programmable on or off by the clinician (must be done via the ICD with Medtronic, but can be done via the Internet with LATITUDE). Wireless technology allows for automatic transmission of alerts to the company servers, which trigger a communication (via Internet, email, or telephone) to the clinician. Medtronic nominal alerts include electrical reset, asynchronous pacing modes programmed on, and charge circuit timeout. Programmable alerts include device and lead integrity alerts, and clinical management alerts (AF burden or with rapid ventricular rates, multiple shocks for an episode, or exhaustion of therapies for an episode).

Medtronic alerts are transmitted in non-wireless devices when the patient hears audible tones and then initiates a transmission. Wireless devices will automatically transmit alerts, and the physician determines which alerts to be personally notified for. Examples of nominal alerts of the LATITUDE system are: pacing and high voltage impedances out of programmed acceptable range, generator end of life (EOL), high or low shock lead impedance detected when attempting to deliver a shock, high voltage detected on shock lead during charge, tachy mode change due to magnet, tachy mode set to value other than Monitor + Therapy, possible device malfunction, or device parameter error.

Programmable alerts include low sensing amplitudes or impedances, arrhythmias prompting shock therapy, arrhythmia acceleration as a result of therapy delivery, atrial tachyarrhythmias, and device reaching the elective replacement time. With non-wireless devices, the transmitter will once weekly flash an indicator to the patient to download device info, looking only for alerts. With wireless devices, the information pertaining to alerts is automatically downloaded every 24 hours. The physician or clinic is notified on a schedule according to predetermined agreement with the company.

St. Jude's Housecall Plus system is not Internet-based, and has its basis in transtelephonic monitoring, consists of transmission to the follow-up clinic or to a commercial device monitoring company. This nature of the transmission allows for real-time electrograms. St. Jude has developed for use in the near future an Internet-based system, Merlin.net. It is comparable to Carelink and LATITUDE in design. St. Jude is about to launch the Merlin.net system which is not only Internet-based, but utilizes IHE (Integrating the Healthcare Enterprise) technology which is superior to the HL7 technology used by Boston Scientific and Medtronic with reference to integration with EMRs (see below).

Carelink and LATITUDE systems have functions of monitoring patients with heart failure who have CRT-D devices. Carelink will display data derived from their devices that have the capability to monitor transthoracic impedance over time (Optivol)®. Studies are under way to determine how intervening using this data may affect patient outcome. The LATITUDE system is called INSIGHT™. Information namely weight, blood pressure, % activity (via accelerometer), heart rate, and heart rate variability are available to view. Arrhythmias, counters and histograms are also available on the INSIGHT ™ report.

In addition, clinical questions the patient answers are posed by the communicator (dyspnea, edema, and others). Currently, the CHF part of remote monitoring is not approved for reimbursement. Outcome studies are needed to determine clinical utility and, if so, the optimal frequency of transmission, and appropriate medical interventions based on the data.

Biotronik's remote monitoring system, in widespread use predominantly in Europe, and notably, is cellular phone technology-based (versus land line modem-based systems of Medtronic, Boston Scientific, and St. Jude Medical). The information is sent to a central center, and reports are then sent to the follow-up physician. This data is also accessible via Biotronik's website by the physician.

Because of the utilization of special bandwiths, patient-specific transmitters are currently utilized by the Carelink, LATITUDE, and Biotronik systems. The new St. Jude Merlin.net system will use these as well.

WHY IS REMOTE FOLLOW-UP NEEDED?

1. Patient and Device Management

Though studies looking at remote follow-up versus in-clinic follow-up are lacking, the usefulness of information derived from remote follow-up of ICDs affecting patient management has been described (Schoenfeld et al., 2004; Lazarus, 2007; Brugada, 2006). Newly discovered atrial tachyarrhythmias and/or those with rapid ventricular rates many be detected.

Antiarrhythmic drug therapy can then be instituted and further transmissions used to assess the patient's rhythm thereafter. Appropriate institution of antithrombotic therapy for atrial tachyarrhythmias may also be prompted by events transmitted. Patients may initiate a transmission due to symptoms which may be arrhythmia related: VT treated with ATP, AF, bradyarrhythmias, pacemaker syndrome, pacing output failure, pacemaker-mediated tachycardia, or rhythm disturbances caused by device under or oversensing.

A large retrospective study using the Biotronic Home Monitoring system (6,548 ICD pts.) and 445 pts. with CRT-D was recently published (Lazarus, 2007). There were 66 alerts from 40 devices for abnormal function detection. 38 devices were in an inactive mode, and two devices exhibited a random malfunction. Interestingly, 4.1% of devices transmitted alerts of ineffective maximum output shocks.

One retrospective study of 271 patients followed for 12 months using the Biotronik Home Monitoring system by Brugada et al examined the utility of remote monitoring in forecasting the necessity of a previously scheduled routine in-clinic visit (Brugada, 2006). There was a 67% true negative rate, 16% true positive rate, 3% false positive rate, and 14% false negative rate. Interestingly, lead problems were all detected either with the first follow-up or with subsequent follow-ups when a problem was initially detected in the first follow-up. Based on their findings, a decision tree was formulated in which the following events since the previous remote follow-up would lead to an in-office follow-up instead of the subsequent routine remote follow-up: previous lead problem, hospitalization, arrhythmias requiring therapy, or significant clinical symptoms.

A short prospective data from the Carelink feasibility study (53 pts with two transmissions seven days apart) revealed more device-related observations than patient related ones.[2] Device-related issues were: atrial undersensing (2 pts), T wave oversensing (2 pts), and far-field R wave sensing (4 pts).

Patient-related observations consisted of: atrial fibrillation (5 pts with egrams), and VT episodes (2 pts).

Detection of incessant VT has also been reported (Siaplaaouras et al., 2006). Inappropriate shocks can be detected with remote monitoring possibly eliminating emergency room visits as well as prompting an office visit for reprogramming the ICD or prompt referral for lead revision. In one study of 230 pts. being followed with remote monitoring, 18/72 pts. receiving either ATP or shock therapy had experienced atrial tachyarrhythmias as the cause (Res, Theuns, & Jordaens, 2006).

2. Integration with Electronic Medical Records

Practices and clinics with electronic medical records realize the power of technology to improve management of patients. All physician practices and hospitals will have electronic medical records (EMRs) in the near future as mandated by the federal government. Currently there are at least two bills on the floor of Congress dealing with EMRs. The marriage of remote monitoring systems with EMRs is a natural one.

A sophisticated cardiology practice with an EMR system is currently paperless-except for its cardiac rhythm device follow-up clinic. It is ironic that a technology-heavy subspecialty such as EP is hindered by the current IT constraints on integrating RMSs with EMRs. There are only a couple of EMRs that have been integrated with remote monitoring. Medtronic's Carelink currently only has the Medtronic Paceart® system is as a portal to an EMR system.

Paceart is one of the most widely used cardiac rhythm device data storage programs. The remote monitoring data is transferred via Carelink into the physician's Paceart system. The data from Paceart then needs to be transferred to an office EMR. As of now, Paceart serves as a portal for only for Medtronic Carelink data to be transferred into it. Medtronic is now working with other companies to have their remote data enter Paceart. Currently one modality of getting around this is to download data from LATITUDE for example, into a PC.

It is saved as a pdf file and then can be transferred into the Paceart program on the computer.

Paceart as a repository of downloaded remote monitoring data and will eventually be replaced by the integration of RMSs directly with EMRs. An easy integration with seamless flow of data is certainly a natural progression and expectation of clinicians already using EMR systems.

There are other technical issues to resolve with integration. The way in which the data is formulated in the computer program is of paramount importance. Boston Scientific and Medtronic utilize HL7 and this is cumbersome and difficult to use from an IT perspective for transfer of data. St. Jude's system is the only one to have written to the IHE (Integrating the Healthcare Enterprise) Device standard. This is actually an international endeavor aimed at having healthcare data transfer seamlessly regardless of the application or IT system. All companies will eventually need to conform to IHE standards. Ideally there needs to be bidirectional communication between the RMS and EMR for easy transfer of data. This means that the two systems can communicate back and forth to recognize and transfer data easily.

Currently, only Medtronic's Carelink has bidirectional capability and it is rudimentary. Patient identifiers may be different in the RMS and EMR. The patient's identifier at the time of implant may be that used by the hospital, which is what is generally entered at implant by the device company rep when enrolling the patient for remote follow-up. One way to resolve this is to enroll the patient in the office. If necessary, the identifier in the RMS can be changed when the patient is seen later in the office. Integration of RMSs and EMRs will eventually be realized. At this time it seems that there is not much clamoring for this from either clinicians or the device companies.

Most physicians still do not have EMRs, and of those that do, most are not utilizing RMSs to a major extent yet. The device companies aren't running to do it because not many customers are demanding it, and it is something that is not going to result in direct profit. The force behind the integration of the RMS and EMR will be the rapid expansion of both RMS and EMR in the next few years.

3. RMS as an ICD System Registry

The issue of utilizing remote monitoring for post-market surveillance of leads and devices is a burning one in view of recent device and lead advisories and recalls. Since most devices are implanted for primary prevention, bad outcomes psychological as well as physical due to system malfunction or other complications, need to be avoided at all costs.

Problems with ICD system failure are not new (Hauser & Kallinen, 2004; Hauser et al., 2006).

The Carelink system was utilized by Medtronic to survey the most recent leads which were eventually recalled. This system was instrumental in helping to identify the problem. Most interestingly, a set screw issue was identified in up to 20% of the confirmed lead integrity issues (Groves & Medtronic, 2007). This represents the first time that a device or system failure was successfully identified using a remote monitoring system database. There are many issues involved with the use of these systems for ICD post-market release surveillance. Not all patients are or will be using the system, by choice. Most patients like the sys-

tem. It decreases visits to the office which is time and cost-saving to the patient. Patient acceptance and satisfaction are high (Schoenfeld et al., 2004; Lazarus, 2007).

However, some patients are technology-averse or just desire an in-office check. In my personal experience these are in the minority (approximately 10%). For remote monitoring systems to become a de facto registry, all patients must be in the system. Perhaps one way to do it is to mandate that all patients be followed remotely in a system. If the patient doesn't wish to transmit from home, this can be done from the physician's office during the visit.

Remote monitoring systems are proprietary. For example, patient alerts are similar, though not the same among the companies.

Presently companies use proprietary algorithms in looking at the data to determine if there is a problem. Some uniformity would be beneficial from an oversight perspective. HRS has recommended remote monitoring of ICDs as a tool of surveillance (Carlson et al., 2006). HRS cannot mandate or enforce this and industry has no incentive to give up stewardship of the remote monitoring data (there are still legal questions as to who owns the data and who can use it for reasons for research, for example), nor of the surveillance itself. In light of perception (and/or perpetuation of it via the press) that companies have acted too slowly in contacting the FDA, and that the FDA itself has been slow in acting, perhaps a different mode of surveillance is warranted.

The use of data derived from remote monitoring may be the answer. HRS, industry, and the FDA all must work together to resolve these issues. The focus of patient safety must not be lost. The devil would certainly be in the details of the who and how of the process. A certain amount of standardization of alerts, and data collection would be in order. One may propose a model whereby an independent panel of expert physicians not affiliated with industry in any way, would review data on a regular basis and determine if an early trend was occurring which would then trigger closer scrutiny, earlier than company quality control departments would, perhaps. These physicians would not have any apparent conflict of interest in the process. This is certainly not to say the companies are acting with a conflict, but it would remove a public perception of one.

The importance of the issue of device surveillance and the potential role of remote monitoring in the process cannot be overstated.

The failure of devices is devastating to patients, industry, and health care professionals alike. But the big elephant in the room is the number of high risk patients (primary or secondary prevention) who will choose not to receive an ICD because of these failures, publicity surrounding them, and eager trial lawyers. It is time for industry to use remote follow-up technology for its highest purpose and provide the support for all of us to monitor ICDs with transparency.

MEDTRONIC CARELINK®: THE USA EXPERIENCE

Carelink was approved for use by the US Food and Drug Administration in 2002.

It was launched with the GEM family of ICDs.

In 2003, The Marquis platform of ICDs and CRT-D devices were added. In addition, the Veterans Administration signed a national contract with Medtronic for the VA clinics.

In 2004, The Maximo and Marquis InSync II were added to devices covered.

All newer models of ICDs and pacemakers are now covered.

Older devices required a patient-activated transmitter, but newer devices are coupled with the transmitter via RF (wireless).

There are currently over 1000 clinics and 100,000 patients enrolled in the Carelink network for Medtronic CRM device follow-up.

Currently there are 940 physician-based clinics enrolled, seven of which are university physician practices. There are 881 non-university hospital-based clinics and 68 university hospital-based clinics enrolled.

Carelink was the first Internet-based remote CRM device monitoring system utilized in the USA and the reimbursement approval was given first in Pennsylvania. The reimbursement code is different than an office code but is financially equivalent to an office-based interrogation without reprogramming.

OUTSTANDING AND RECENT RESULTS OF OTHER COMPANIES

Biotronik developed a worldwide monitoring system with wireless technology very appreciated in Italy and in China from our direct experience with courses so called of "training of trainers" to further develop telemedicine and remote monitoring of implanted devices patients in Italy, Europe and China (Santini & Ricci, 2011; Zhang S. Beijing Fuwai Hospital, 2011; Zhang Feng Shanghai First People Hospital, 2012).

St Jude is developing the same technology in US, Europe and China associated with courses so called of "training of trainers" to further develop telemedicine and remote monitoring of implanted devices patients in China (Zhang S. Beijing Fuwai Hospital, 2011).

NECESSITY OF HOME CARE AND REMOTE MONITORING OF PATIENT ALSO WITHOUT IMPLANTABLE DEVICES

We must consider the increased and further increasing number of patients with Chronic Heart Failure in different countries including US, China, Europe and Italy. The patient population is also showing an increasing mean age and most of the time associated chronic heart diseases. Not all of them could or should be implanted with implantable devices.

For a many of them the traditional and low technology Home Care and the remote telemedicine or telecardiology monitoring should be more simply applicable (Naccarella, 2009, 2010, 2012).

A recent advanced software application for Home Care and Telecardiology has been developed by Fragomeni & Naccarella, to be applied to the magnitude of chronic heart failure patients whom are to be taken care more frequently and more appropriately in out of hospital facilities and in the home care regimen (Naccarella et al., 2012).

Telemedicine and remote monitoring using satellite technology instead of internet is another very valuable perspective, at present time used only by military physicians also for educational purposes, possibly to be used in the future for dual application both in military and civilians contexts, and in international cooperation activities between developed and developing countries (Anaclerio & Cucuzza, 2006-2012]

A study conducted by Human Factors International showed that device checks with the Medtronic CareLink® Network can be done in under 8 minutes—one-third the time of a typical in-office device check.

The ability to communicate wirelessly between newer CRM devices and Carelink makes it easier for remote follow-up, and will expand usage of this technology with Medtronic devices in the USA.

Boston Scientific Latitude System: The American Experience

The Latitude system is just beginning to be utilized in the USA.

Hard Marketing data is not available at this time, however it is projected that there will be 70,000 patients enrolled by the end of 2007. Thus far there are approximately 12,500 patients enrolled utilizing the wireless (radiofrequency) technology.

The technology retrofitted for non-wireless implanted devices (wand technology, which began enrolling patients March 1, 2007) has approximately 2000 patients enrolled (as of March 15). There are already approximately 800 follow-up clinics utilizing the Latitude system. There are slight differences between Carelink and Latitude

Figure 1. November 2003: US Medtronic CareLink Network ICD/CRT-D reimbursement status

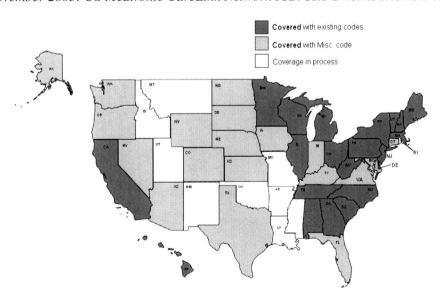

regarding the physician alerts. The Latitude system has some basic alerts which signify device or system malfunction. These are called "red alerts." In addition, there are other non-critical alerts that the individual physician or clinic can choose to be notified about. Neither red nor yellow alerts are programmable via the device itself.

In contrast, Carelink notifies physicians or clinics only about alerts that are activated on, via device programming by the physician. Both systems, however, are proven, excellent ways to alert physicians of system malfunctions and significant arrhythmia developments in their patients.

Economic Considerations: The American Experience

A very significant issue is economics. When Carelink was introduced in the USA, it was looked at as a time and cost saver for the customer (physician or clinic), and marketed as such. It was offered on a contractual basis, with the physician or clinic paying a fee to Carelink to enroll patients. The fee was based on the number of patients (cost going down for more patients).

This was met very negatively by physicians for a number of reasons. The reimbursement

Figure 2. July 10, 2006: Medtronic CareLink Network ICD/CRT-D reimbursement status

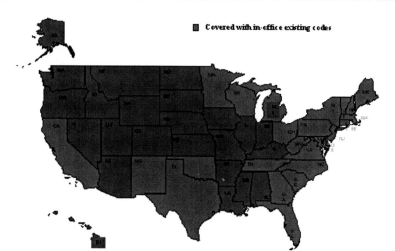

Figure 3. Falk D, Straub K. Practice efficiency improvements resulting from the use of Medtronic CareLink Network remote monitoring service. Fairfield, Iowa: Human Factors International, July 2004.

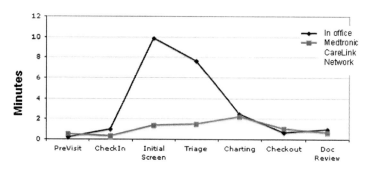

model that Carelink proposed was not realistic (see Figures 1 and 2), thereby throwing off the theoretic cost savings in time and efficiency that the system would generate (see Figure 3). In addition, as government reimbursement in the USA historically declines over time, the fixed costs of Carelink enrollment would relatively increase. The concept of paying to follow a patient was a strange and upsetting one to physicians.

Due to markedly disappointing enrollment statistics over time, Medtronic drastically reduced their enrollment fees and just weeks ago eliminated them totally. This was driven by Boston Scientific not having any enrollment fees for the Latitude system.

It is clear that remote follow-up of cardiac rhythm devices in the USA is both accepted, welcomed, and growing. It will become standard of care for more convenient patient follow-up (well-suited to patients receiving ICDs for primary prevention indications), as well as meeting HRS recommendations for better quality control of post-market released systems. There is much marketing and medical data first being gathered from surveillance of these devices remotely. It will be a significant while before any of this is released. Factors for this delay include the freshness of the technology as well as the debate over property rights of the data (companies versus physicians/clinics).

UNANSWERED QUESTIONS

There remain other questions about RMS unanswered since the advent of this technology. Who owns the data? Can physicians access it for the purpose of conducting research (without patient identifiers, of course)? Some electronic medical record companies claim *they* own all data in their repositories. If RMS integrates with an EMR, who then owns the data?

This new technology will eventually be integrated in follow-up clinics in all academic centers.

New training requirements as per COCATS will need to be put into place for cardiology fellows for minimum device follow-ups with RMS, to familiarize them with the follow-up process, in different European and Asia Countries.

All allied professionals involved in device follow-up should become familiar with RMS.

Requirements of physician qualifications for RMS follow-up should conform to HRS guidelines.

There are medico legal questions regarding this technology. Patients should download data only with an appointment.

Downloading information without an appointment may result in data not being reviewed or lost. Patients should sign an agreement when enrolling, stipulating they will transmit only by appointment.

RMS is here to stay and its potential for improving patient and device management is unquestioned. The more intriguing and perhaps just as important role of this technology lies in its potential for post market quality control of ICD generators and leads. The future is now!

REFERENCES

Brugada, P. (2006). What evidence do we have to replace in-hospital implantable cardioverter defibrillator follow-up? *Clinical Research in Cardiology; Official Journal of the German Cardiac Society, 95*(Suppl 3), 3–9. doi:10.1007/s00392-006-1302-x

Carlson, M. (2006). Recommendations from the Heart Rhythm Society Task Force on Device Performance Policies and Guidelines. *Heart Rhythm, 3*(10), 1250–1273. doi:10.1016/j.hrthm.2006.08.029

Groves, R., & Medtronic. (2007). *Sprint Fidelis® lead patient management recommendations.* Letter Appendix A Oct.

Hauser, R. G., Hayes, D. L., & Epstein, A. E. (2006). Multicenter experience with failed and recalled implantable cardioverter-defibrillator pulse generators. *Heart Rhythm, 3*(6), 640–644. doi:10.1016/j.hrthm.2006.02.011

Hauser, R. G., & Kallinen, L. (2004). Deaths associated with implantable cardioverter defibrillator failure and deactivation reported in the United States Food and Drug Administration manufacturer and user facility device experience database. *Heart Rhythm, 1*(4), 399–405. doi:10.1016/j.hrthm.2004.05.006

Lazarus, A. (2007). Remote, wireless, ambulatory monitoring of implantable pacemakers, cardioverter defibrillators, and cardiac resynchronization systems: Analysis of a worldwide database. *Pacing and Clinical Electrophysiology, 30,* S2–S12. doi:10.1111/j.1540-8159.2007.00595.x

Res, J. C. J., Theuns, D., & Jordaens, L. (2006). The role of remote monitoring in the reduction of inappropriate implantable cardioverter defibrillator therapies. *Clinical Research in Cardiology; Official Journal of the German Cardiac Society, 95*(Suppl 3), 17–21. doi:10.1007/s00392-006-1304-8

Schoenfeld, M. H., Compton, S. J., & Hardwin Mead, R. (2004). Remote monitoring of implantable cardioverter defibrillators: A prospective analysis. *Pacing and Clinical Electrophysiology, 27,* 757–763. doi:10.1111/j.1540-8159.2004.00524.x

Schoenfeld, M. H., & Reynolds, D. W. (2005). Sophisticated remote implantable cardioverter-defibrillator follow-up: A status report. *Pacing and Clinical Electrophysiology, 28,* 235–240. doi:10.1111/j.1540-8159.2005.09554.x

Siaplaaouras, S., Buob, A., & Neuberger, H. R. (2006). Femote detection of incessant slow VT with an ICD capable of home monitoring. *Europace, 6*(8), 512–514. doi:10.1093/europace/eul050

KEY TERMS AND DEFINITIONS

Electronic Medical Record (EMR): It is an electronic collection of clinical information about the patient regarding his/her lifelong health situation. Clinical information are gathered by doctors, nurses or health stakeholders during clinical encounters or medical events; can be collected automatically by monitoring devices or in some cases by patients also. EMR is used to make health decisions. It is maintained in a secure and private environment, with the individual determining the rights of access.

ICD: Implantble Cardioverter Defribillators.

Remote Monitoring System (RMS): It is a technological system in which clinical information about patient pathology are detected by devices and sent electronically to a central system. The central system provides facilities for analyzing information and for presenting clinical scenarios to doctors. Wireless or mobile devices are also used in order to improve the life style of the patient.

Chapter 12
Remote Electronic Monitoring in Chronic Pulmonary Diseases

S. Bella
Bambino Gesù Paediatric Hospital, Research and Care Institute, Italy

F. Murgia
Bambino Gesù Paediatric Hospital, Research and Care Institute, Italy

ABSTRACT

In this chapter the main aspects of telemonitoring are described and discussed in the field of chronic respiratory diseases. The authors describe the various challenges they faced, in the order in which they did. First, they face the problem of effectiveness of the method, then, the problems related to the economic viability, and finally, the problems related to the operating method. The authors conclude that remote monitoring is a promising method in terms of effectiveness of follow-up that must be performed under well controlled conditions. They still require further validation studies to improve the effectiveness and reduce the effects of new issues that arise.

1. CLINICAL ASPECTS

Background

Innovative technologies and informatics applied to medicine offer both health operators and patients a wide range of services that have changed the traditional concept of health care. In the last few years, the availability of handy equipment, easy to transport and use, and suitable to collect and transmit various clinical data, have resulted in a fast development of Homecare. The earliest application of Telemonitoring has involved the follow-up of acute patients affected by arrhythmia or heart failure, diabetes, acute respiratory insufficiency as bronchial asthma, the control of breast-feeding mothers during lactation and the assessment of post surgery patients (Scalvini, 2004).

Only recently Telehomecare (THC) became an opportunity for the follow-up of chronic diseases such as cardiopulmonary, bronchial asthma and heart failure (Meystre, 2005), although the impact of Telemonitoring on patients' conditions still remains uncertain (Paré, 2007).

The natural course of Cystic Fibrosis (CF) is characterized by a progressive lung destruc-

DOI: 10.4018/978-1-4666-2979-0.ch012

tion, caused by obstruction of the airways due to dehydrated thickened secretions, resultant endobronchial infection and an exaggerated inflammatory response leading to development of bronchiectasis and progressive obstructive airways disease (Flume, 2006).

Prevention and control of lung infections is one of the main objectives of therapy in CF patients with the aim to slow down the progressive decline of the pulmonary function (Que, 2006).

Many researchers demonstrated that, in case of infectious relapse, pulmonary function modifications often precede the clinical symptoms and that monitoring variations in pulmonary function can be useful in children and in adults (Davis, 2001) (Mohon, 1993).

Early recognition of infectious relapse allows to promptly administer an antibiotic therapy, to prevent serious complications, and to use less aggressive therapies (Rajan, 2002).

Since 2001 distance monitoring of lung parameters has been used in the follow-up of patients with CF in the Cystic Fibrosis Centre of the Bambino Gesù Children's Hospital - IRCCS - in Rome.

In 2009 we have published data from the first years of this activity (Bella, 2009).

Purpose of this study was to assess the effect of THC in the follow-up of CF patients, by systematically monitoring respiratory parameters (O2 saturation during the night and spirometry), to early detect pulmonary infectious relapses, and to measure the impact on respiratory function over time.

Materials and Methods

Study Design

We performed an open label trial in a population of CF patients followed in our reference centre for CF from 2001 to 2005.

Patients were considered eligible to enter the study if they presented multiple infectious lung relapses (more than 3-4 episodes in a year) and/

or significant decrease of mean FEV1 (more than 10% in a year).

The intervention consisted in administering THC in addition to standard therapy. THC was assigned to the first patient seen in the week, who satisfied the eligibility criteria. A group of controls was chosen among patients visited on the same week, matching for respiratory function, bacterial colonization, sex, age and complications. The main outcome parameter measured considered in the study was the FEV1 values over time. To standardize for individual characteristics, FEV1 Zscores were calculated considering average FEV1 and standard deviation measured in the 12 months before entering the study. FEV1 was then measured during follow up, and Zscores calculated and compared in the two groups. To all patients, regardless of intervention assignment, were provided antibiotic treatment and therapies according to current treatment guidelines (Cystic Fibrosis Foundation, 1997).

Intervention

Telemonitoring was performed using Vivisol OXITEL M32 (www.vivisol.com), a digital multiparametric recorder with integrated saturimeter. Oxitel M32 is a multi-channel recorder, which is able to receive data from external devices, such as spirometers. Spirometries were obtained using a Vivisol One Flow Spirometer linked to Oxitel by cable. Both patients and parents were trained by the physicians centre, being part of the multidisciplinary CF care team, using the equipment. OXITEL can record and store overnight SaO2 and pulse rate. Home recording of SaO2 was carried out through the night. Spirometer measurements were performed in the morning, after chest physiotherapy for mucous drainage. The collected data were automatically sent by a modem via the public telephone line to a dedicated Personal Computer located in the CF Unit, and decrypted by a dedicated software. Data were collected and interpreted by the CF Unit medical team during work shifts. Patients were reached by a physician by telephone and the clinical situation was evaluated. Depending on the patient's conditions, further data transmissions could be requested or oral antibiotic therapy straight prescribed. Otherwise patients could be invited to the hospital for more detailed surveys and therapies. Data collection of respiratory parameters through Telemonitoring was performed generally twice a week. Patients could autonomously decide to transmit depending on the individual clinical condition. We used data from OXITEL instrumentation only for monitoring variations in pulmonary function at home, with the aim to early recognize the relapses of pulmonary infections. Acute FEV1 variations less than 10% from the individual baseline were considered as an indication for antibiotic treatment for the intervention and control groups (Ramsey, 1992).

Statistical Analysis

Beside FEV1 we calculated also outpatient visit rate and hospitalization rate during the follow up together with rates of intravenous antibiotic therapy and we expressed them as number of events per 100 person per month. Difference in rates have been studied comparing rate ratios and their 95% confidence intervals with the mid-p exact test. Continuous variables, including age at enrolment, FEV1 at enrolment, and follow up duration were compared by the Student t test, once verified the normality of the distribution. To analyze FEV1 variations we considered monthly average Zscores by the use of THC. Observations were interpolated through simple linear regression to look for trends. To adjust for multiple measures in the same patient, we compared the two groups by robust regression.

Results

Out of 60 CF patients enrolled in the study 30 were assigned to THC and 30 to the routine care program only. Thirteen out of the 30 patients assigned to THC have been subsequently excluded: 11 because of a short period of enrolment (< 6 months) or because they provided incomplete data registration, whereas 2 patients had unpredictable complications and have died during the study, with a resulting dropout of 43,3%. Two control group patients withdraw participation in the study within six months. We analyzed thus the data of 17 CF subjects who received THC for a minimal period of 7,04 months and of 28 control patients.

The general characteristics of patients participating in the study are illustrated in Table 1.

Although assignment to THC was not randomized, the baseline characteristics of the two groups were similar and none of the comparisons were statistically significant.

Table 2 shows a comparison of mean hospitalization rates, mean outpatient rates, and number of therapy cycles in the 12 months before enrolment in the trial and during the follow up.

THC patients had a higher outpatient visit rate (p=0,024) and a higher number of therapy cycles (p=0,01) compared to controls during the follow-up.

Table 1. General characteristics of subjects exposed and not exposed to THC

	Telehomecare	Controls	p
Number of patients analysed	17	28	
Males/Females	6/11	13/15	0.463
Age at enrolment, years (mean ± SD)	15,74 ± 5,8	14,77 ± 5,22	0,338
FEV1 at enrolment % of expected value (mean ± SD)	67,48 ± 21,28	76,47 ± 24,56	0,218
Follow-up duration, months (mean ± SD)	29,30 ± 13,32	30,13 ± 20,49	0,882

Table 2. Hospital access and therapy cycle rates before and after the intervention

	Baseline			During intervention		
	THC	Controls	Rate ratio; 95% CI; P	THC	Controls	Rate ratio; 95% CI; P
Mean hospitalization rate (Admissions per 100 person months)	13,73	15,2	0.90; 054-1.51; 0,699	26,5	24,09	1.1; 0.86-1.41; 0,451
Mean outpatient visit rate (Visits per 100 person months)	55,39	44,61	1.24; 0.94-1.64; 0,124	46,38	37,14	1.25; 1.03-1.52; 0,024
Mean therapy cycles (Cycles per 100 person month)	21,08	15,2	1.41; 0.87-2.21; 0,165	22,29	15,26	1.46; 1.09-1.96; 0,01

Figure 1 shows comparison of the FEV1 monthly mean in THC patients and controls during the follow- up, expressed as Zscore. The trend over time is showed both in THC subjects and in controls by a regression line. Both groups showed a progressive decrease of FEV1 over time and no statistically significant difference was detected when comparing the two groups over time. However, the linear trend calculated on Zscore FEV1 values of controls tended to lower values with follow-up time. Moreover, several mean FEV1 values in patients without THC were lower than –2 standard deviations with respect to the 12 months before enrolment, whereas the minimum mean Zscore FEV1 value recorded in THC patients was -1.46.

Discussion

Our study suggests that THC may be helpful in reducing the decline of respiratory function in patients who are compliant with THC. Our data are coherent with previous studies (Finkelstein, 1992) showing the non-interference of home monitoring and daily diary recording with physical or psychological status of FC patients, and (Magrabi 2005) showing the feasibility of THC for monitoring CF.

Subjects monitored through THC had a higher number of therapy cycles compared to controls.

On the other hand, no statistical difference was detected in mean FEV1 values over time when the two groups were compared, although a tendency toward lower FEV1 values was detected in controls.

The decrease in the number of outpatient accesses (p=0,02) and the increase in the number of therapy cycles (p=0,01) between treated subjects and controls are statistically significant in both cases. We observed an increase in the number of hospitalizations from the pre-intervention period to the follow-up period in all patients.

Therefore, statistical tests resulted significant only in the intervention period, because the period of observation was longer than baseline period and confidence limits of rate were narrowed. Despite these rates seemed significant only during intervention, they were similar in the two periods. This means that was no effect of THC treatment on the measures considered.

Our results should be interpreted with caution due to the lack of randomization and a limited number of CF subjects participating in the study.

However, in the THC-treated group we noted a higher stability of FEV1 values according to lower SD values of FEV1. This trend, if confirmed, might suggest a situation of higher stability of the FEV1 and, therefore, of the respiratory function, in THC treated subjects.

Figure 1. FEV1 monthly averages and trend lines

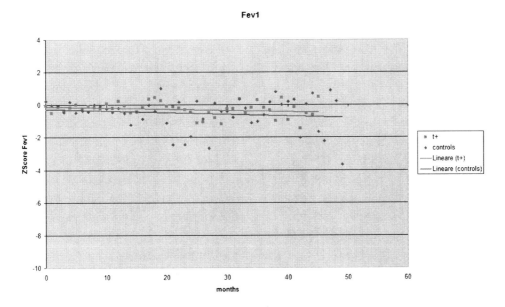

In conclusion our study suggests that THC programs seems to increase in general the rate of access to health care. A positive effect of THC use in CF, therefore, has to be conclusively demonstrated.

Further larger randomized studies on the effect of THC on pulmonary function are necessary to clarify if it represent a real benefit for CF patients.

2. ECONOMIC ASPECTS AND BENEFITS

We attempted to quantify the real economic significance of the use of respiratory function remote monitoring on the scale of NHS economics, in order to strike a balance between health spending and health needs (Murgia, 2010).

Materials and Methods

The calculation of the budget statement was made by examining the costs of: medical equipment, medications used, the cost of a day hospital and of an outpatient visit. We do not have deliberately

calculated indirect costs because variable and difficult to assess and in any case with low incidence.

We considered as revenue the fees relating to admissions avoided through early detection of acute events and therefore to remaining free beds that the hospital could use for other patients. Simultaneously we administered to patients a questionnaire with multiple answers partly open to confirm the level of satisfaction with this method and related matters. As regards the mode of administration of the questionnaire, the use of direct interview appeared generally preferable. In fact, compared to telephone and/or mail, the interviews allow you to add information and explanations and to limit the number of no answer (Mattoscio, 2003).

The main risk of bias lies in a strong interaction between interviewer and interviewee: the interviewer may influence the responses(answers), especially if the interviewee is not familiar with the matter. It is obvious, however, that the possibility of distortion is relatively high if the respondent is an ordinary citizen, which normally has a limited knowledge of the object of evaluation. In contrast, the risk is reduced in the case that the questionnaire is administered to a patient, as a rule, conscious of the intervention being analyzed (Nuti, 1998).

In the preparation of the questionnaire, the patient should be given only the necessary information, relating to that aspect that we intend to evaluate, to avoid the so-called "information bias". In our study, to keep as low as possible all the above concerns, we used a single person as editor of the questionnaire and as an interviewer. The economic aspects about payment and service cost appears rather more complex, through which and how would the respondent contribute to the costs required to implement the health technology (Torrence, 1996).

The magnitude of the cost proposal must be realistic in the sense that the respondent should not think of a charitable donation, but only a real contribution to the costs. A further possibility of bias is given by the method of payment, it is different if you are referring to a ticket or a one-off payment.

In 2004 in Italy a multicenter study has already been proposed, involving 2380 doctors registered as AIPO (Italian Association of Hospital Pulmonologists) on the question whether or not to begin systematically use of telemedicine in patients with CODP (Chronic Obstructive Pulmonary Disease). The responses received were 261, i.e. just over 10%. This shows that even among the experts on that date, telemedicine had not yet taken a leading role considered important (De Tullio, 2004).

In our case, the questionnaire, formulated ad hoc, was sent via e-mail. We used three categories of persons, homogeneous for age and all with chronic diseases:

1. CF patients currently using the Telemonitoring,
2. CF patients who do not use the remote home monitoring,
3. Non CF chronic patients who do not use the remote home monitoring.

In the questionnaire we also attempted to evaluate some parameters which do not correspond to a market value such as anxiety, pain and the hoped-being using the method of "willingness to pay of the individual (WTP). Mishan points out that the principle of willingness to pay is the only one consistent with the general basics of market economy and, therefore, of monetary valuation (Torrence, 1996) (Mishan, 1971).

Is important to note that the meaning of willingness to pay does not end necessarily in the life of the individual, but may also include family members, friends and all who are interested in its welfare. Obviously, the assessment of these benefits is in addition to strictly economic components, as compared to lower risk of declines in productivity due to illness. The exchange ratio between the amount of money you are willing to pay and changes of duration and/or quality of life is fixed from time to time by the individual concerned, to avoid change. According to a widespread point of view in economics and psychology, an individual should always be able to exchange a change in its survival probability or likelihood of improving the quality of his life, with a sum of money.

The amount of money that an individual will be willing to pay will depend on such variables as the level of individual wealth and the current location of each individual in its life cycle (Rosen, 1994) it is clear that young people are less willing to pay because their probability of dying is lower.

The approach based on willingness to pay is based on the assumption, known as the principle of Pareto improvement, that a public decision is acceptable if they are net benefits for at least one member of the community, and not result in net costs for any other member. This condition is particularly restrictive, born from the impossibility of measuring utility, and then to make trade-offs between individuals who are receiving benefits and those who suffer costs as a result of the decision.

Consequence of the above is that the individual is the best judge of his actions and related consequences. It also assumes that he is still able to make at least the operations that are strictly necessary to make choices consistent with their preferences and consistent with each other. Ultimately it is deemed to be able to evaluate and take the final decision, in total respect of hierarchy of interests.

In reality, the meaning of what is said is not always applicable to the market of consumer goods, much less to markets where situations involve decisions that lead to an exchange between health and money. It is difficult to argue that it is known in advance in its entirety, and then accepted, the risk to which port the decision. Severe criticisms have been made on the use of WTP by Broome (Broome, 1978), who said that identifying the interests of an individual with his or her preferences and, more importantly, with his choices, is particularly suspect especially when it comes to decisions affecting the life or health of the individual itself. Broome insists on the fact that the adoption of the principle of WTP can give rise to a conflict between a democratic principle, that decisions would reflect individual preferences, and the principle of rationality, which is based instead on be consistent with a value-judgment. Often who governs will evaluate then situations related to health problems in apparent conflict with the benefits of the individual. It may be remarked that this criticism is not a contradiction to the principle of WTP, but a conflict between

different ways of taking decisions of collective importance. Bearing in mind that in recent years the availability of State funding is declining, it is necessary to understand what each citizen, sick or not, it would be willing to pay for this service. To this end we have included in the questionnaire questions that concern both the WTP both knowledge of telemedicine, its usefulness and increase expected in the quality of life.

Is also required, finally, if the telemedicine changes doctor-patient relationship.

For completeness, appendix 1 includes the questionnaire proposed.

Cost Analysis Results

The cost analysis showed an annual saving of €. 5241 per patient/ in telehomecare, compared to the average cost of patients followed in the conventional way. The results of the questionnaire are reported in graphical form in Figures 2 to7 (our elaboration).

Discussion

The annual savings achieved through the use of home telemedicine in the management of patients with CF is not very relevant, especially in view of the national average expenditure per patient.

Figure 2. Knowledge of the methodology by patients

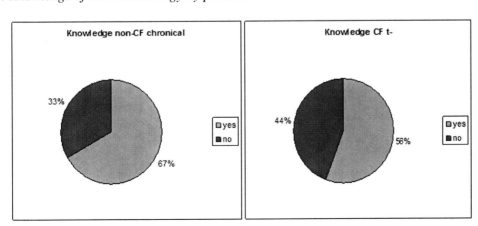

It should however be noted that this saving is achieved in conformity to an improvement in the levels of care and to an higher satisfaction of the patient subject

The considerations we can make on the results of the questionnaire are many.

Figure 2 shows the level of knowledge of the methodology among the patients. As one can see, in spite of telemedicine in Italy has not yet been adequately spread, a large number of patients, however, are aware of the existence of it. What is even more remarkable is that even not CF patients, namely the majority of patients with chronic gastrointestinal diseases, say they have learned about it (over 66% of respondents). The telemedicine group patients are not considered in this table because their knowledge is obviously equal to 100% of the respondents. Not CF patients know about telemedicine because they have read in magazines, while 38.9% of patients with CF who are not included in the telemedicine group know the subject because they heard about our Care Centre.

Figure 3 shows for how long our CF patients have been using home care telemedicine. This

finding seems important because reinforces the significance of their responses, direct expression of their knowledge of technology.

Another figure in our reference questionnaire is the utility of telemedicine in terms of efficiency, convenience and economy, results are reported in Figure 4. It is evident that all three groups of patients (CF in THC, CF without THC, other chronic patients) have no doubts about the efficacy and practicality of telemedicine. As for the economic data, especially the group of CF patients not in telemedicine expresses many doubts on the economy of the method. This is in apparent contradiction with the fact that patients with CF, recognized by the NHS as 100% invalids and recipients of welfare health services free of charge, should have no more than a general understanding of the burden for the community of their pathology.

The answer regarding the question if telemedicine may change the doctor-patient relationship shows a concept that seems very important: according to our CF patients: telemedicine can not replace the doctor, and can help patients to better follow the course of the disease. The CF

Figure 3. Percentage distribution of CF patients based on time of use of home care telemedicine

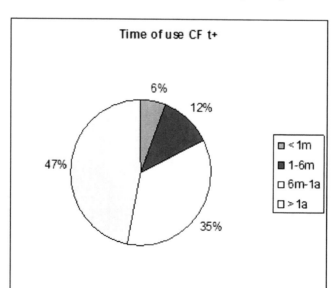

Figure 4. Opinion of patients on the utility of telemedicine: percentage of positive responses about its usefulness

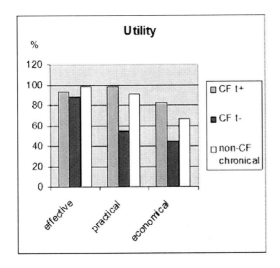

patients using telemedicine are those among the three groups showing the higher percentage confirming this finding (Figure 5). We then asked whether telemedicine saves time in the daily management of the therapy, of course, not by changing the effectiveness of the same, and how long, approximately, we can quantify the savings (Figure 6). As seen above, the responses of the group of patients with CF in telemedicine appear more homogeneous than the group not in telemedicine.

Regarding the question on whether or not to increase this practice, there was a positive unanimity response

The latter figure, and perhaps the most important issue concerns the WTP. The result indicated, in Figure 7, follows a clear rationale. One must consider separately each group of patients. Those using telemedicine are the most realistic, in fact their WTP does not reach 300 Euro/month. It is worth to remind in this context that the rent paid for local use of healthcare devices to the company providing the service is around 210 Euro/month, so patients with CF in Telemonitoring have provided a report very close to reality. The CF patients,

not in telemedicine, have an expectation that this method would be requiring to pay from their own pockets around 750 €/month, more than twice in the first group of patients. Patients in the third group, belonging to gastroenterological chronically ill, not in telemedicine, are positioned in a central location, showing 550 €/month. That's because they probably do not have a direct interest in the technique, but as chronic patients, however, have similar expectations on innovative technologies compared to patients in the second group.

It should be emphasized, that one of the main limitations of the WTP is that the "quantum" that the user would be willing to pay depends directly on the knowledge of the subject in question. The patient without a deep knowledge of the argument is likely to conceive of a notion of risk more complex and broader than that provided by technicians and therefore the readings of the WTP can not but reflect this different way of defining the risk. The risk assessments provided by those who for professional reasons, can be considered experts in a given subject are thus more precise than those provided by non-experts.

Figure 5. Opinion of patients on the change of doctor-patient relationship from the use of tele-homecare: percentage of positive responses

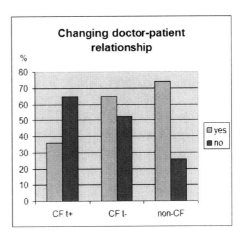

Figure 6. Opinion of patients on the time savings from the use of telehomecare: percentage of positive responses

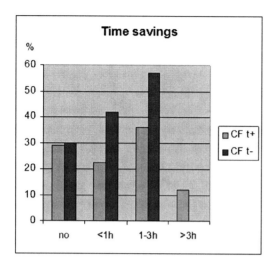

Figure 7. Patients' willingness to pay for a home telemedicine service, expressed in Euro per month.

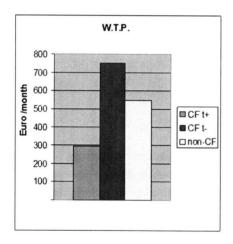

3. ORGANIZATIONAL ASPECTS

In this section we describe and discuss the way we daily act in remote telematic tracking of CF outpatients, a procedure which has been improved through our daily experience in telehomecare.

Materials and Methods

To date 30 patients are included in our telehomecare program. We use currently the Spirotel instrumentation (www.spirometry.com), provided as part of a domiciliary service called "Vivitel Control Service" (www.vivisol.it), able to collect the following parameters: spirometry with determination and recording of FVC, FEV1, FEV1%, PEF, FEF 25-75, FET, flow-volume and volume-time curves; pulse oximetry with registration of oxygen saturation (SaO2) and heart rate also in 24 hours recordings with regard to desaturation events. Data gathering and transmission is performed by home telephone just with a normal telephone call. The data transmission is performed by acoustic coupling, putting the instrument near to the phone and pushing the right button. Data are recorded automatically through a dedicated web server. Physician can easily download data in a protected way on their own computer. Data interpretation is performed using a dedicated application software and are displayed in graphical mode. Spirotel is a transportable device of small dimensions (70x80x30 mm), light (100 g) battery powered (lithium 3 V) projected to be used by patients.

Procedure

Patients and parents were trained on the use of the device and for data transmission by physicians, from the reference centre. The telemonitoring activity cycle has the following sequence:

1. The trained patient, at home on their own make the registration of oxygen saturation and heart rate all night long.
2. The next morning the patient performs chest physiotherapy and drainage of mucus and, soon after, performs spirometry, after answering a simple questionnaire on respiratory symptoms.

3. Data are transmitted with the home telephone by a modem to a dedicated server.

4. Healthcare trained professionals in the hospital download the data, using the dedicated software, which runs on a computer connected by the hospital intranet to the Net. Additional transmission may be received on patient's demand. Data from each patient are manually downloaded and stored in a local database.

Data Measurements and Transmission

The data are recorded on scheduled intervals agreed with the CF centre physicians, which may vary from patient to patient, depending of the patient's clinical situation, usually twice a week. Patient may autonomously decide to transmit data even without informing or asking the doctors.

Patients included in telehomecare program are treated from the physicians of the CF centre according to the same guidelines used for patients not using it (Cystic Fibrosis Foundation, 1997).

The application software can display the spirometric curves and main parameters (FEV1, FVC, PEF, FEF25-75). The trend of FEV1 in time is showed on the graph and it's always possible to compare previous parameters with the new ones. Variations are expressed as percentage difference.

About nocturnal pulse oximetry the software shows the graph of the SaO2 and hearth rate trend for the entire duration of the registration (usually all night). Data showed include mean, minimum and maximum SaO2 and T89 and T90 (percentage of total time spent with SaO2 below 89% and 90%, respectively).

We consider pathological acute reduction of FEV1 (>10% compared to previous value recorded in stable clinical conditions (Ramsey, 1992).

Reduction below 80% of the maximum value of oxygen hemoglobin saturation, reduction of mean SaO2 and increase over 5% of T90 are considered significant.

Every transmission for each patient is printed and stored also in a paper archive.

Every patient who send a transmission is called back on his phone to recall anamnestic data and to share the results.

Anamnestic data and graphs obtained are discussed in a briefing meeting between CF Centre healthcare professionals for an overall evaluation and to decide on any therapeutic action.

Patients who show significant decrease of SaO2 and/or FEV1 are invited to rapidly transmit further tests. In some cases, if suggested by anamnestic history or by data collected antibiotic home therapy is prescribed on the basis of the last sputum culture collected in hospital. In other cases patients are invited to attend to the CF Centre for a clinical evaluation, to perform further testing, or to be admitted. In any case the next data transmission is scheduled.

Since February 2010 we started keeping and electronic database of transmissions in spreadsheet format.

For each transmission the following data are collected:

- Date,
- Time,
- Patient's name,
- Number and type of tests sent,
- Test's results,
- Evaluation of the test,
- Telephone number used to call back the patient,
- Person who answer the operator's call,
- Clinical information reported,
- Any therapeutic measure decided by physicians,
- Name of the doctor who prescribed the therapy,
- Eventual need for hospital admission.

Every calibration procedure or technical assistance needed on the devices is also recorded on the database. Monthly summary of the test transmitted and patient's adherence to telemonitoring program is calculated.

Database is compiled by professional healthcare dedicated to telehomecare and is securely available for doctors of the CF Centre involved in clinical care of patients through hospital intranet.

Data collected on transmissions are available on demand of the single patient with a secure system that protects privacy according to current law disposals. That was very useful in case of patients followed also by other CF Centre (for example patients waiting for lung transplant).

Maintenance

The patients are asked to take back their device on every hospital scheduled admission for a check-up and calibration. In case of problems, when it is not possible to fix the instrument in the hospital, Assistance Service is asked to perform maintenance of the device. In some cases is possible to repair the device at patient's home.

For all the duration of telehomecare program CF Centre healthcare professionals overtake a training program with patients and family members on the correct use of the device and on the different possibilities and evolution of this technology.

To facilitate contacts between healthcare professional and family members an electronic email account was activated. Questionnaires about any issue on the device and on the psychological impact of the procedure are sometimes administered through email.

Continuous contact with Vivisol Assistance are maintained to report any noticed issue with the purpose of improve service's quality.

Healthcare professional dedicated to telehomecare periodically revise data collected for writing report and scientific works.

Gathered Results

Since 15th February 2010 to 15th June 2011 we received 882 transmissions including 1317 spirometries and 291 nocturnal pulse oximetry.

To understand and give a dimension of the adherence of our patients to the telehomecare system we considered the number of days in which our patients performed a transmission. Medium adherence (transmissions/total days) in the indicated period was 8,91%.

We established a contact 722 times after transmissions (80,9% of total). Remaining patients were called back mainly on the mobile phone. On 494 calls in 68% patients answered on the first try. All remaining patients were called back later.

Since June 2010 we admitted patients in hospital 19 times after a transmission.

Discussion

During the follow-up, we recorded an average compliance (transmissions/total days) of about 10%.

Considering our recommendation to patients for transmitting data twice a week, the optimal expected compliance should be 40%. We couldn't find any previous data about THC compliance in CF literature. We may hazard that chronic patients who receive several different therapies may be overwhelmed by additional interventions. Certainly compliance must be considered when planning such an intervention and possible related clinical trials.

After receiving a transmission, in most cases (80,9%) a contact was soon established, direct if the patients were in the hospital or by phone. On 494 calls performed only 68% had a good outcome in the first try. In our opinion this is a critical point that could be improved working on organizational aspects of the project.

In CF there is a lack of a unique definition of a pulmonary exacerbation. In many clinical studies a definition was adapted from US CF Consensus Conference (Ramsay, 1994) (Cystic Fibrosis Foundation, 1994).

According to this definition a relapse consists in the presence of clinical symptoms such as cough, dyspnea, increase or change in sputum quality, asthenia with or without decrease of FEV1.

Isolated FEV1 decrease, on the other side, should not be considered as a symptom of relapse (Sarfaraz, 2010).

Those statements suggest that pulmonary relapse may be individuated even from just symptoms analysis. To this end it's indispensable that each transmission should be integrated with direct contact with patient's or parents to recall anamnesis data necessary to a correct interpretation of obtained data even if they result into the normal range used for the telehomecare procedure. The device we used allows the transmission, along with functional respiratory parameters, of a brief questionnaire regarding clinical symptoms. The efficacy of this questionnaire and it's practice outcome is still to be validated.

Legal and Privacy Aspects

Regarding law issues telehomecare services should be considered as any other medical procedure performed for the patient in its clinical and legal aspects (Gensini, 2010).

About data it is fundamental to consider that every transmitted data may be crucial in the management of the patient so it should be used with the maximum care, security and privacy during transmission.

In Europe standards about medical informatics are regulated by CEN/TC251 committee (http://www.cen.eu), a working group belonging to European Union caring about standardization of data and procedures in Health Information and Communications Technology (ICT).

This group establish minimum requirements about data transmission in medicine in order to support clinical and administrative procedures.

It should be noted that while for some arguments defined standards are available, for others they are still under evaluation so it is fundamental to keep caution in manipulation of data and use of instrumentation.

Telemedicine enhance possibility that patient's data could be manipulated or simply used by not authorized third persons. As worldwide are enacted increasingly precise laws about privacy it is fundamental to consider this issues also in telemedicine.

In particular, in Italy, those issues are regulated by Decreto del Presidente della Repubblica 10 novembre 1997, n. 513, defining the meaning of electronic document, digital signature and giving legal validity to electronic documents.

This law also lays down rules for the certification and characteristics of the certification authority so that the overall approach to the problem of secure communications in telemedicine should be studied according to it.

Readability of the Services

In light of the foregoing, it is clearly necessary to provide the utmost reliability to the entire diagnostic and therapeutic procedure performed at a distance and in the designing of the system, to study well the ability to control and rebuild at any time in a precise manner the flow of work. In order to timely identify episodes of exacerbation, it seems appropriate in the light of our experience limited at this stage only in CF, to download transmissions at least once a day in order to ensure the essential timeliness to clinical interventions.

For this purpose will be preferable and appropriate, depending on the operating environment, to provide dedicated staff for the management of telemedicine activities which may be entrusted with operations and simple control system maintenance and equipment. This professionals should cooperate with the physicians of the CF centre, whose workloads are generally cumbersome and often in day difficult to predict.

Another important aspect is the registration of critical or sentinel events that may occur during the execution of the procedure. Only through a systematic analysis of these episodes will be possible to improve the reliability and safety of the overall system, by submitting the entire program to periodic reviews aimed at controlling and minimizing the possible clinical risk (Ministero della salute, 2011).

CONCLUSION

The use of telemedicine highlights several advantages that will surely become even more evident when its use will spread more.

Being able to monitor patients at home is certainly a turning point for the "quality of life of people with chronic conditions that, with the progress of medical knowledge, will become more and more numerous.

The reduction of hospital accesses is a goal of considerable magnitude in the long-term management of chronic diseases. The use of telemedicine in the follow-up provides a further guarantee of better monitoring of exacerbations often cause of the gradual decay of the general conditions of these patients.

From the economic point of view, we pass through a historical phase in which health is increasingly considered a right for all. In the phase of increasingly limited economic resources, it still shows a steady increase in health expenditure, which is now a substantial part of the National Gross Domestic Product. At this stage, economic telemedicine can be a rare source of savings.

The hope is that new studies confirm our initial data to begin with the conviction the "development phase" of telemedicine in health care.

Finally, Telemedicine represents a promising new tool for patients and healthcare professionals, that under certain conditions can improve the quality of assistance and possibly also to reduce costs. It is necessary, however, that its adoption is supported by careful study of validation and a general focus on some new issues arising from them.

REFERENCES

Bella, S., Murgia, F., Tozzi, A. E., Cotognini, C., & Lucidi, V. (2009). Five years of telemedicine in cystic fibrosis disease. *La Clinica Terapeutica, 160*(6), 457–460.

Broome, J. (1978). Trying to value a life. *Journal of Public Economics, 9*, 91. doi:10.1016/0047-2727(78)90029-4

Cystic Fibrosis Foundation. (1994). *Microbiology and infectious disease in Cystic Fibrosis: V.* Bethesda, MD: Author.

Cystic Fibrosis Foundation. (1997). *Clinical practice guidelines for cystic fibrosis.* Bethesda, MD: Author.

Davis, S., Jones, M., & Kisling, J. (2001). Comparison of normal infants and infants with cystic fibrosis using forced expiratory flows breathing air and heliox. *Pediatric Pulmonology, 31*, 17–23. doi:10.1002/1099-0496(200101)31:1<17::AID-PPUL1002>3.0.CO;2-8

De Tullio, R., Dottorini, M., et al. (2004). La telemedicina in Pneumologia: I risultati di un questionario in Italia. *Rassegna di Patologia dell'Apparato Respiratorio, 19*, 11–17.

Decreto del Presidente della Repubblica. (10 novembre 1997). *Regolamento contenente i criteri e le modalità per la formazione, l'archiviazione e la trasmissione di documenti con strumenti informatici e telematici.* A norma dell'articolo 15, comma 2, della legge 15 marzo 1997, n. 59.

Finkelstein, S. M., Wielinski, C. L., & Kujawa, S. J. (1992). The impact of home monitoring and daily diary recording on patient status in cystic fybrosis. *Pediatric Pulmonology, 12*, 3–10. doi:10.1002/ppul.1950120104

Flume, P. A., O'Sullivan, B. P., & Robinson, K. A. (2007). Cystic fibrosis pulmonary guidelines: Chronic medication for maintenance of lung health. *American Journal of Respiratory and Critical Care Medicine, 176*, 957–969. doi:10.1164/rccm.200705-664OC

Gensini, G. (2010) Manifesto Italiano della medicina telematica. *Giornate nazionali di studio in medicina telematica.*

Magrabi, F., Lovell, N. H., & Henry, R. L. (2005). Designing home telecare: A case study in monitoring cystic fibrosis. *Telemedicine Journal and e-Health, 11*, 707–719. doi:10.1089/tmj.2005.11.707

Mattoscio, N., & Colantonio, E. (2003). La valutazione contingente quale strumento per la determinazione di un ticket prestazionale. *Il Risparmio, 3*.

Meystre, S. (2005). The current state of telemonitoring: A comment on the literature. *Telemedicine Journal and e-Health, 11*, 63–69. doi:10.1089/tmj.2005.11.63

Ministero della salute, Dipartimento della qualità. (2011). *Sicurezza dei pazienti e gestione del rischio clinico: Manuale per la formazione degli operatori sanitari.* Retrieved from http://www.salute.gov.it/imgs/C_17_pubblicazioni_640_allegato.pdf

Mishan, E. J. (1971). Evaluation of life and limb: A theoretical approach. *The Journal of Political Economy, 79*, 687. doi:10.1086/259784

Mohon, R. T., Wagener, J. S., & Abman, S. H. (1993). Relationship of genotype to early pulmonary function in infants with cystic fibrosis identified through neonatal screening. *The Journal of Pediatrics, 122*, 550–555. doi:10.1016/S0022-3476(05)83534-6

Murgia, F., Cilli, M., Renzetti, E., Popa, N., Romano, T., Alghisi, F., & Bella, S. (2010). Valutazione economica del telemonitoraggio domiciliare in malattie polmonari croniche. *La Clinica Terapeutica, 162*(2), e43–e48.

Nuti, F. (1998). *Introduzione all'economia sanitaria e alla valutazione economica delle decisioni sanitarie* (Giappichelli, G., Ed.). Torino.

Paré, G., Jaana, M., & Sicotte, C. (2007). Systematic review of home telemonitoring for chronic diseases: The evidence base. *Journal of the American Medical Informatics Association, 14*(3), 269–277. doi:10.1197/jamia.M2270

Que, C., Cullinan, P., & Geddes, D. (2006). Improving rate of decline of FEV1 in young adults with cystic fibrosis. *Thorax, 61*, 155–157. doi:10.1136/thx.2005.043372

Rajan, S., & Saiman, L. (2002). Pulmonary infections in patients with cystic fibrosis. *Seminars in Respiratory Infections, 17*, 47–56. doi:10.1053/srin.2002.31690

Ramsey, B. W., & Boat, T. F. (1994). Outcome measures for clinical trials in cystic fibrosis: Summary of a cystic fibrosis consensus conference. *The Journal of Pediatrics, 124*, 177–192. doi:10.1016/S0022-3476(94)70301-9

Ramsey, B. W., Farrell, P. M., & Pencharz, P. (1992). Nutritional assessment and management in cystic fibrosis: A consensus report. The Consensus Committee. *The American Journal of Clinical Nutrition, 55*(1), 108–116.

Rosen, S. (1994). The quantity and quality of life: A conceptual framework. In Kenkel, D., Tolley, G., & Fabian, R. (Eds.), *Valuing health for policy: An economic approach* (p. 221). Chicago, IL: University of Chicago Press.

Sarfaraz, S., Sund, Z., & Jarad, N. (2010). Real-time, once-daily monitoring of symptoms and FEV1 in cystic fibrosis patients – A feasibility study using a novel device. *Clinical Respiration Journal, 4*(2), 74–82. doi:10.1111/j.1752-699X.2009.00147.x

Scalvini, S., Vitacca, M., & Paletta, L. (2004). Telemedicine: A new frontier for effective healthcare services. *Monaldi Archives for Chest Disease, 61*, 226–233.

Torrence, G. (1996). Measurement of health state utilities for economic appraisal – A review. *Journal of Health Policy, 5*, 1–3.

ADDITIONAL READING

Cox, N. S., & Alison, J. A. (2011). Telehealth in cystic fibrosis: A systematic review. *Journal of Telemedicine and Telecare, 18*(2), 72–78. doi:10.1258/jtt.2011.110705

APPENDIX

Questionnaire

1.   Are you familiar with telemedicine?...y/no

    If so...
    Because have you spoken?..y/no
    Because are you using?...y/no
    If you use it...

2.   How long you use it?

    One month
    Six months
    One year
    More than one year

3.   Do you think that telemedicine give you:

    A more efficient service ...
    More efficient ....y/no
    More pratical ....y/no
    Cheaper ....y/no

4.   Telemedicine, in your opinion,

    Change the relationship with the doctor?..y/no
    If so, why? ....
    ....
    If not, why?...
    ....

5.   Believe this type of assistance you can save time with the same efficiency?............................ y/no

    As if in hours per week?
    1 h
    3 h
    more than 3 h

6.   Do you think that you should increase this kind of service? …………....................................y/no

If so, why?………………………...
…………………………………….
If not, why?………………………
…………………………………….

7.   If you were the manager of a company, allocate funds to sponsor this type of assistance?……y/no
8.   If yes, what do you think you could quantify € in a speech like that? ……………(put different data)
9.   If health care were private, how would you willing to pay, as a patient, per month, the possibility of such assistance?... (insert data)

Thanks for your cooperation.

Chapter 13
Telemedicine and Alzheimer Disease:
ICT–Based Services for People with Alzheimer Disease and their Caregivers

Letteria Spadaro
*IRCCS Centro Neurolesi "Bonino-Pulejo",
Italy*

Silvia Marino
*IRCCS Centro Neurolesi "Bonino-Pulejo",
Italy*

Francesca Timpano
*IRCCS Centro Neurolesi "Bonino-Pulejo",
Italy*

Placido Bramanti
*IRCCS Centro Neurolesi "Bonino-Pulejo",
Italy*

ABSTRACT

The focus of this chapter is to asses a new model of care in dementia, particularly Alzheimer's Disease (AD). According with sociotechnical approaches, the authors describe a proof of concept, Information and Communication Technologies (ICT) intervention, as a technical and organizational model of robust, reliable, and efficient clinical practice to meet the medical, psychological, and social needs of AD people and their family. The authors also propose the "Identification-Recognition-Evaluation-Application Model" as process methodology in a telemedicine project. In this perspective, the technology has to be analyzed as technology-in-use, a process coming out from an ecology of specific actions and actors. Finally, the authors describe their experience of a longitudinal study in which ICT networking technologies are used to implement coping strategies, in order to improve the quality of life of AD families.

DOI: 10.4018/978-1-4666-2979-0.ch013

1 INTRODUCTION

1.1 Aging Population, Alzheimer Disease: Cost and Health Needs

A long life is a desirable goal, a significant indicator of quality of life in a Country, an expression of the advances in medicine, nutrition and technology. By 2050, almost 2 billion people in the world will be aged 60 years or over, with an average life expectancy of 75.4 years (Department of Economic and Social Affairs of the United Nations [DESA], 2007). The aging population is an important conquest of modern society, but few data about long-term trends in incidence or prevalence of chronic disease are available. At the present time the elderly usually have more healthy lifestyles, that are important protection factors against some chronic diseases. The deterministic combination of old age and disease seems to overcome but it is true that, in the coming decades, there will be a different society and we will need new models of lifestyle and new tools to cope with treatable but not curable diseases for those, who have more years to live.

The focus of this chapter is about new model of care in dementia, particularly Alzheimer's disease (AD). Dementia is a frequent chronic disease in the elderly population: the age is a risk factor. It is a neurodegenerative disease defined as progressive cognitive decline with important interferences in activities of daily living accompanied by any behavioural problems. On 2010 about 35.6 million people with dementia in the world are estimated with an important increase in countries with limited resources (Alzheimer's Disease International [ADI], 2010). The total estimated worldwide costs of dementia, including family care as well as direct medical and social care, are US$604 billion in 2010 (ADI, 2010). AD is the primary cause of dementia among older people, representing 60-80% of diagnosed dementias. The cognitive impairment of AD patients and the loss of the ability in daily life make the disease course difficult to cope for the patient and her/his family with direct and indirect costs for States and patient's family (Wimo, Winblad, & Jo¨nsson, 2010; Brookmeyer, Johnson, Ziegler-Graham, & Arrighi, 2007). AD people need specific supports and services: drug therapy for cognitive and behavioural disorders, neuropsychological and psychosocial rehabilitation, environmental adaptations to reduce the impact of cognitive and behavioural symptoms, education and support for caregivers. The growing financial pressure and funding cuts have a negative effect on the possibility of an increase in usually health care services. Also, Alzheimer's disease is increasingly present in high as in low resource countries, where care systems are further less ready to provide specialized services. We need new affordable and specialized care delivery model to meet healthy needs of AD patients and their families.

2 BACKGROUND

2.1 Alzheimer Care: The Families' Perspective

The insidious onset and the slow and gradual progression characterize the beginning of AD. Every disease stage has specific behavioural and cognitive characteristics, that deplete a person of her/his ability to complete dependence on the other. In high and low resource countries, usually, the families care for AD person (ADI, 2010): an especial family member becomes the primary caregiver. The most studies on family caregiver are focused on problematic caregiving aspects (Rosa et al., 2010; Ravio et al., 2007; Schneider et al., 1999). AD patient's care may be a chronic distress with physical, emotional, social and economic burden for the caregiver (Wai-Chi Chan, 2010; Censis, 2007; Pearlin, Mullan, Semple, & Skaff, 1990). In particular, the cognitive impairment and disability in daily living activities increase caregiver's physical work (Amirkhanyan,

& Wolf, 2003; 2006). The behavioural problems rather affect psychological stress: the caregiver may feel tiredness, depression and anxiety (Karttunen et al., 2011; Neri et al., 2007; Yueh-Feng Lu & Guerriero Austrom, 2005; Gaugler, Davey, Pearling, & Zarit, 2000; Levesque, Cossette, & Lachance, 1998; Schulz, O'Brien, Bookwala & Fleissner, 1995). Then, the caregiving appear as a dynamic process that involves the patient and the caregiver in a special relationship, characterized by the constant adjustments of the caregiver to the situation (Gaugler et al., 2000). The involvement between the patient and her/his primary caregiver becomes central for both. During the disease course, the patient's needs are different such as caregiver's needs. Healthcare services may support as people with dementia as their primary caregiver (Figure 1).

In clinical and research practice, patient and caregiver well-being are deeply linked and numerous studies show that medical, neuropsychological and social intervention for the patient as psychosocial intervention for the caregiver improve the well being of both (Van Mierlo, Meiland, Van der Roest, & Dro¨es, 2011; Hort et al., 2010; Ryan et al.,2010; Yamaguchi, Maki, & Yamagami, 2010; Callahan et al., 2006; Nobili et al., 2004). Against these evidences, in Italy, for example, health care systems arrange AD services focused on the supply of drug therapy by the

physician, reducing these experiences in pilot projects not integrated in the care system. The problems of implementing these projects in clinical practice are:

- Need of a specialist multidisciplinary team (neurologist, neuropsychologist, rehabilitation therapist, social assistant, and other specialists),
- Appropriate times and places,
- New organization of clinical practice,
- Need for training in the use of telehealth delivery systems and the necessary technology infrastructure.

We believe however that the major problem is the planning of health care systems in which the care is often identified only by medication and not by global management of the sick person and the family, at the same time in medical, psychological and social perspective. For AD, as other diseases, this point of view is outdated.

In this perspective telemedicine can supply in terms of available specialized personnel and customized service, linking patients to specialized service without difficulties in time and distances, reducing direct and indirect cost. Indeed the new technologies are increasingly being used in rehabilitation and support of AD people and families.

Figure 1. Needs of AD patients and their caregiver

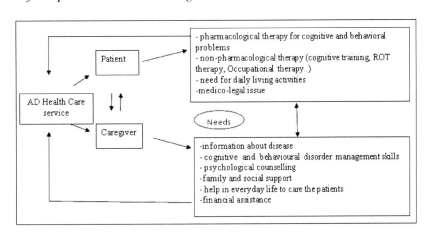

3 MAIN FOCUS OF THE CHAPTER

3.1 Issues, Controversies, Problems

3.1.1 ICT Solution for People with Alzheimer Disease and their Family

The terms telemedicine is a neologism relating to a whole of use of Information and Communication and Technologies (ICT). This view extends the concept of telemedicine including, beyond health and diagnostic practices, also management applications, such as computerized medical records or the coordination above health staff and administrative matters (Craig, Russell, Patterson, & Wootton, 1999; Rajani & Perry, 1999). This acronym is to be intended as a disposition and a global effort to improve local and world public health, through the use of ICT (Eysennbach, 2001).

On the base of the different definitions of telemedicine the sense and the ground of its application is established. The most literature on this topic considers technology as a datum beyond argument: it is an independent variable whom effects are analyzed, studying its usability, but not its planning. These studies often concentrate on the interaction between type of technology used and on the consultation method, producing "strong programmes", in which telemedicine is seen as an intrinsic development of medicine; and "weak programmes", in which it is only a means to provide a service (Finch, Mort, May, & Mair, 2005). Some authors (Grisby, Kaehney, Sandberg, Schlenker, & Shaughnessy, 1995; Robinson et al., 2003; Roine, Ohinmaa, & Hailey, 2001) define telemedicine as the use of communication technology, in order to provide health services to persons living far away from the provider. May et al. (2003) argue that this limited view comes from the medicalization of the ICT solutions, that can be understood only if they are englobed in a specific scientific field.

In this chapter we consider technology in its dynamic side, that is socially established within the social relationship and action system. Contrary to

Technicist, that consider technology as a transferable product to different places, regardless of the users and the environment, we consider technology as indivisible from its users, and so from its context of use. It's seen as a circular process, in which society establishes technologies, inscribing them within social relationship (Trist & Murray, 1993). In other words, society shapes technology on its needs and technology, in its turn, obstructs or makes some form of social relationships possible.

A sociotechnical system (Gherardi & Strati, 2004) is a relational system in which machine, users and context of use are not separated, but in mutual interaction (Figure 2).

In this view, technology doesn't be considered as a decontextualized object, but as a dynamic process used by a community in relationship with other tools. Thus the context of use become a very important testing ground to assess the usability and the effectiveness of the technology. The shift from technology to "technology-in-use", allows, methodologically and conceptually, to highlight all the procedures, sometimes hidden, that users have to do in order to make the technology "usable" within a context of use and in relationship to users needs and other technologies. It's just this

Figure 2. Graphic exemplification of the sociotechnical system, in which the three actors (context of use, machine and users) are interconnected within society

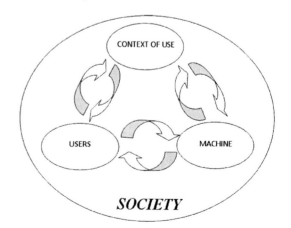

approach to telemedicine that led us in the planning of the below described telecare project.

The studies on the interaction between human and non-human demonstrate that remote interaction represent both the major awaited benefit, and the biggest difficulty (Suchman, 1987). Only if all the actors form a context of use, working together in a "new way", we can study telemedicine and ICT as a social practice, adopting an interpretative model in which the technology-in-use is analyzed as a process coming out from an ecology of actions and actors (Cicourel, 1999). Telemedicine necessary conditions are work in remote and shape a virtual ground between different actors; make the hidden practice explicit, in order to improve the usability of the system; insert different expertise and knowledge and affect the daily management of public health.

In order to better comprehend how ICT are useful in the field of health care it is necessary to think in term of users needs and technology usefulness to satisfy these needs. For this reason, holding a systemic perspective, we introduce a classification of the different ICT solutions that are adaptable to the different needs of AD patients and their families. This new way of thinking ICT solutions comprehend the identification of needs and features of several actors involved, such as clinicians, technical experts, financial and project managers, politicians and users, to a better implementation of telemedicine design.

Although, when we treat with AD it is very difficult to draw clear-cut among the different kind of services, for explicative reasons, it is important to make a classification. The most common way to classify interventions and fields of application is to refer to the specialist expertise of medicine (Roine et al., 2001; Burt & Taylor, 1998). Others authors follow different criteria. We use Taylor (1998) classification of telemedicine services, as a framework, to describe ICT application in health projects for AD people and their families:

Treatment services: In different studies (Galante, 2009) are presented programs of non-pharmacological treatment of cognitive and behavioural diseases devoted to patients and caregivers, followed by telemonitoring intervention, aimed to verify compliance to treatments, to offer constant support to caregivers and ensure patients and caregivers with a prompt access to operators of the Alzheimer Unit in case of sudden onset of health or assistance needs. It is expected that combined cognitive-behavioural intervention devoted to patients and caregivers could produce many positive effects. In particular, slowing down of cognitive decline, a better control of behavioural disturbances and a delay in patients institutionalization. Moreover, the accomplishment of improved information on disease and assistance options, and the reduction of caregivers feelings of loneliness and hopelessness might engender the reduction of their anxiety and depression symptoms.

Diagnostic services: Within this services area, we can identify four sub-categories:

- Teleconsultation, useful to obtain a medical advice or a second opinion from a health worker. It can involve not only the patient and the specialist, but also a further contact with a specialist "in remote". In the case of patients with AD this service become essential when the actors involved in the interaction are neurologists, psychiatrists, psychologists, rehabilitation specialists of a dedicated medical centre and the patient and her/his family, living in a hardly accessible remote area. Some studies (Loh, Donaldson, Flicker, Maher, & Goldswain, 2007) present development of telemedicine protocols for diagnosis of AD, in which the assessments by videoconferencing (remote) were compared with face to face (direct) ones. These studies demonstrated that there was good agreement for diagnosing AD between telemedicine and direct assessment. Moreover, cognitive assessment by means of teleconsultation appears to be a valid means to conduct neuropsychological evaluation of older adults with cognitive impairment (Cullum, Weiner, Gehrmann, & Hynan, 2006). It must be said that, because of the paucity of the sample considered, this field of research requires a larger validation;

- Teleconference, allows different health workers and all the person in charge of the AD patients, to communicate through a video link. In this case the patient isn't there or she/he comes abreast with a health worker. This type of ICT is useful to reach expertise of other super-dedicated medical centres in everywhere;

- Telereporting, in this case the procedure requires the transmission of clinical case data or medical records to other health workers, in order to obtain a second opinion or a specialist consult on the patients. In case of AD this technology is useful to send specialistic health examination reports to other seasoned professional for a second opinion;

- Telemonitoring, consists in the (continuous or at regular intervals) gathering of patient data, that can be qualitative or quantitative. In our case it is useful to follow and support AD patients and their family during the different stages of disease. In this view telemonitoring can be considered also as a treatment service, indeed the simple fact of being continuously assisted and nursed can lead AD patients and the caregivers to an improvement in their quality of life, reducing anxiety levels, having a point of reference and the awareness of being not alone.

Informative and educational services are addressed to caregivers. Some authors (Mahoney, Tarlow, & Jones, 2003; Mahoney, Tarlow, Jones, Tennstedt, & Kasten, 2001) developed a system providing caregiver stress monitoring and counseling information, personal voice-mail linkage to AD experts, a voice-mail telephone support group, and a distraction call for care recipients. Results brought out that there was a significant intervention effect as hypothesized for participants with lower mastery at baseline on bother, anxiety, and depression. Additionally, wives exhibited a significant intervention effect in the reduction of the bothersome nature of caregiving. Moreover, approximately half of the intervention group used the system regularly for two or more months. These 'adopters' were significantly older, more highly educated and reported a greater sense of management of the situation than 'non-adopters'. Adopters were much more likely than non-adopters to have been rated as highly proficient by the trainer following the technology training session

From the data presented above, telemedicine could provide an alternative option, monitored by expert health operators and the possibility for caregivers to be supported in their assistance role. Despite the depth of telemedicine pilot-studies, this remains a field of experimental researchs: in fact there are not contribution on management and implementation difficulties.

3.2 Solutions and Recommendations

3.2.1 The "Identification-Recognition-Evaluation-Application Model" for Telemedicine

Telemedicine involves technological and clinical aspects at the same time. In particular the "telemedicine in use" has to meet the healthy needs of its users. We believe that a systematic methodology can help the development of a valid telemedicine project, in which the needs of the users are at the centre.

According with sociotechnical approaches, we identify four important moments for the construction and implementation in daily clinical practice of a telemedicine model and we describe a process methodology as model for the creation of a reliable telemedicine project: the "Identification-

Recognition-Evaluation-Application Model" for telemedicine.

1. **Step:** Identification of all involved actors

In our perspective, intervention with telemedicine is a system in which numerous human actors interact each others and with technological tools.

Gherardi et al. (2004) identified several actors involved in decision making about telemedicine introduction and implementation: clinicians, technical experts, financial and project managers, politicians and users (also associations). The choices to use technological tools are not in a linear decision process because each actor has specific interests to evaluate in the design phase. To better understand the actors' interdependence, we relate the Urie Bronfenbrenner's (Bronfenbrenner, 1986) Ecological Systems Theory and its four levels of analysis: macro-, exo-, meso-, and micro-, which describe influences as intercultural, community, organizational, and interpersonal or individual on people or, in our view, on a behaviour of use. If we think telemedicine as a system in which the elements interact in a particular socio-political context, we have the idea of the complexity involved in the introduction of a new practice of care, mediated by technological tools, in an usual health care system. The analysis of the potential and limitations of technological tools, to be adopted, is too useful for evaluate the feasibility of the intervention. It is important to identify any human and non-human involved element because each can affect the success of the activity.

2. **Step:** Recognition of needs and motivations to use telemedicine

Telemedicine, as a social practice, involving people with specific thoughts and beliefs, is in a specific socio-cultural context. For each actor, identified in the previous phase, there are specific needs and motivations to use telemedicine. In the formulation of the research project is necessary to identify and to describe the healthy needs, the beliefs and the motivations of all users.

It is also important to consider financial and political aspect in an ecological system perspective. In Italy there are regional guidelines about the application of telemedicine in remote areas, in practices of home care and emergency. We focus our attention on those who will use telemedicine: patient, clinicians, technical staff and manager. All users may be involved in the design phase to select the target needs and specific technology to use. For example in the selection of tools, the new technology may not be the best to use for the target population.

The Action Research (Lewin, 1951) should be a participative methodology to involve all human actors in research planning. This method enhances the participation of all actors emphasizing their needs and suggestions about a "telemedicine-in-use". Health and technology adoption may be two controversial areas of reflection (Venkastesh & Bala,2008; Andrersen 1995). In particular, doctor-patient communication is an important topic to approach for those who come to choose telemedicine as medical practice (Miller, 2001).

3. **Step:** Analysis of barriers to use telemedicine

A prerequisite for successful telemedicine service is the use of the service (Chiu & Eysembach, 2010, p.73).

In 1999, Tanriverdi and Iacono wrote about Attewell's theory of knowledge barriers to explain why diffusion of telemedicine was low. They extended the theory and described technical, economic, organizational and behavioural knowledge barrier.

According with this perspective and with the now available scientific researches, our attention is focusing on four important aspect in the planning of a telemedicine intervention, to improve the quality of the health application. These seems the most frequent strong point or obstacles to the implementation of telemedicine in clinical every day practice.

Clinical efficacy of proposed intervention: The Telemedicine focused on needs has to adopt successful clinical interventions. In the literature, there are many summary and evaluation studies about telemedicine applications. However, it is difficult to obtain unequivocal results because the studies are few, they have small sample populations and use different technologies (e-mail, telephone, video conferencing, IVR system). In this perspective, as recommended by scientific societies, it is important to consider the guidelines, standard protocol and the usual care researches.

Use and Implementation of affordable technologies: The use of affordable technology is important for the democratic access to telemedicine service. Many technological artefacts are currently used: telephone, e-mail and many others. In our experience, more complex technological tools are expensive. It is therefore important, in the design phase, consider the economic implication for the users.

Easy learning and usability: About easy learning and usability, it is important to consider "who" should advantage from intervention. The technology has to be simple and easy to use. But users may be a family or a group, not only a person. We believe that technology have to connect people because the first need of every person is to be with others. In particular, telemedicine, as strategy of care through technology, is a tool for long-distance relationship and have to promote social network. To widen participation, each telemedicine intervention has to have a training phase to facilitate access to specific use of involved technology. Indeed the experience of technology is essential for its utilization (see Stage 3 in Figure 3).

Nonusage and dropout attrition: For Eysenbach (2005), a "science of attrition" is really important to better understand the use of e-health service. The evaluation of possible attritions is also important to planning an effective project for our target population in a specific context (Chiu et al., 2010).

4 FUTURE RESEARCH DIRECTIONS

4.1 Application of a Methodological Framework in Stages

Telemedicine project evaluation is difficult for the possible presence of clinical and/or technological barriers to use. It is interesting the integration of an health and a technological explicative models to better understand the use of telemedicine. Chiu and Eysembach's methodological framework (2010) conceptualizes the e-health use as a dynamic and continuous process divided into stages of use, as we tried to exemplify in the Figure 3.

They identified two theoretical model to better understand attrition (nonusage and dropout) in e-health service:

- Andersen's Behavioral Model of Health Service Utilization, a theoretical model for predicting and explaining health service use (Andersen, 1995);
- Venkatesh's Unified Theory of Acceptance and Use of Technology, a model for explains the intention to use information technology (Venkatesh et al., 2008).

We want to use this framework to graphically exemplify a telemedicine project (Figure 3). We believe that this division into stages of use can improve the feasibility of an intervention in the planning stage.

4.2 "Telecare for People who Care": An ICT Intervention

We applied the "Identification-Recognition-Evaluation- Application Model" in a telemedicine project for AD. Our experience is the project research "Telecare for people who care: telemedicine and Alzheimer Disease" at IRCCS Centro Neurolesi "Bonino-Pulejo" (Messina).

Figure 3. Graphic exemplification of a framework from Chiu and Eysembach (2010).

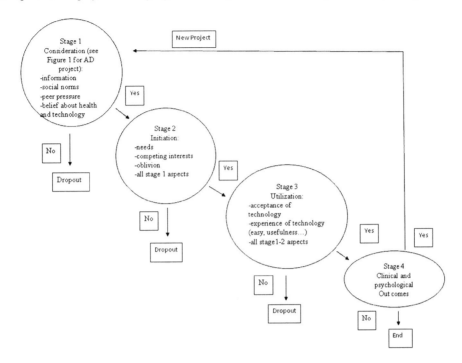

We use a longitudinal study design for a video-conference synchronous project at patient's home. In our project we identify these actors:

- AD patients and their family caregiver as users
- Psychologist and Neurologist as clinicians
- Technical staff
- Project Manager
- Financial Sponsor
- Health Policies (regional guidelines)
- Video telephone for PSTN Connection
- Set-top-box for IP Connection

Our intervention is for patients with moderate AD and their family caregivers. We focused our attention on caregiver's distress. Our hypothesis is that increased knowledge, and consequently skills, and specialist's support have a protective effect on physical and psychological health of caregivers, in particular on anxiety and depression, reducing physical and psychological care burden. We aim to promote appropriate coping strategies and self-efficacy, as moderators of stress with a domino effect on patient's health (Paerlin, 1990). For AD patient there is a weekly monitoring of vital signs, a neurological consultation and the possibility of a psychological counselling. These aspects should be the usually management of AD person.

We choose to do an integrated intervention for patients and caregivers for two reasons. The first is psychological for the importance of their relationship. The second is technical because telemedicine often involves a problem that can become a barrier to using the service: learning to use a new technological tool. Memory problems, including learning, however, are the main symptom of AD. So probably our patients get used the new tool but cannot use it alone because they have not learned how. This is one of Knowledge barrier to diffusion of telemedicine described by Tanriverdi and Iacono (1999). Using a metaphor, the caregiver often overcomes this barrier and becomes a tool that enables the relation between the patient and the clinician through the machine.

For implementation of our project is also important to understand why a caregiver and a patient should use faithfully the telemedicine service.

We have analyzed the literature on best ICT and usual treatments for this group of patients, identifying the following methods of intervention as good clinical practice:

- Monitoring of vital signs of patient and consultation with the neurologist;
- Psychological Counselling;
- Psycho-education for caregiver, about cognitive and behavioural disorder management skills.

There are a baseline and six-monthly follow-up evaluation of clinical parameters (psychological and physical).

About affordable technology, if the patients have home Internet access, they use the Set-top-box for IP Connection. If not, they use the Video telephone for PSTN Connection. IRCCS Centro Neurolesi give them technological tools through a free loan for use.

There is a technical training for the caregiver about the ICT tool. Also for this, there are numerous evaluations (at the first month and at six-monthly follow-up) of usability and the perceived comfort. To better understand the learning of patients and caregivers, the point of view of clinical and technical staff is collected.

In this section we do not describe the specific quantitative results of each outcome research, even if for the users, particularly the caregivers, the service is simple to use, useful for the learned skills, important for the perceived comfort.

The idea developed in this project is that, using the same methodology, there are many telemedicine systems that arise in the meeting of the project with the reality of users. For this reason, the quantitative analysis of the outcome must accompany the qualitative analysis of the experiences of those who daily live with telemedicine to better understand the daily possible dimension of this medical and technological practice.

CONCLUSION

AD is a primary cause of dementia among older people. AD people need for specific supports and services. The family usually has all the burden of care in high and low resource countries. Often, for health systems the care is only the "drug" even though a large literature demonstrates the need for an integrated medical, psychological and social intervention. The problem of providing an integrated face to face intervention is economical because it needs a multidisciplinary team, time and place for continued therapy over time. Actually new technologies are increasingly being used in rehabilitation and support of AD people and families. In particular, clinician-patient interaction telemedicine is the approach with the greatest potential. In this chapter, we described also a telemedicine model of implementation for AD people and their family caregivers. We do not proposed a standard applicative model but we want identify a process methodology to use telemedicine in daily life of AD people and their caregiver, using the sociotechnical framework.

We believe that all people have the Right of Health with the best practice. In our perspective, telemedicine may respond to a health need that cannot find solution in the usual care systems for the described reasons about times, places and resources. The telemedicine, overcoming the barriers of traditional clinical practice, may be a democratic way of extending the good clinical practices.

REFERENCES

Alzheimer's Disease International. (September, 21, 2010). *World Alzheimer report 2010: The global economic impact of dementia.* Alzheimer's Disease International Press. Retrieved May 10, 2010, from http://www.alz.co.uk/research/files/WorldAlzheimerReport2010.pdf.

Amirkhanyan, A. A., & Wolf, D. A. (2003). Caregiver stress and non caregiver stress: Exploring the pathways of psychiatric morbidity. *The Gerontologist, 43*(6), 817–827. doi:10.1093/geront/43.6.817

Amirkhanyan, A. A., & Wolf, D. A. (2006). Parent care and stress process: Findings from panel data. *The Journals of Gerontology. Series B, Psychological Sciences and Social Sciences, 61,* S248–S255. doi:10.1093/geronb/61.5.S248

Andersen, R. M. (1995). Revisiting a behavioral model and access to medical care: Do it matter? *Journal of Health and Social Behavior, 36,* 1–10. doi:10.2307/2137284

Bronferbrenner, U. (Ed.). (1986). *Ecologia dello sviluppo umano.* Bologna, Italy: Il Mulino Editore.

Brookmeyer, R., Johnson, E., Ziegler-Graham, K., & Arrighi, H. M. (2007). Forecasting the global burden of Alzheimer's disease. *Alzheimer's & Dementia, 3,* 186–191. doi:10.1016/j.jalz.2007.04.381

Burt, E., & Taylor, J. A. (1998). Information and communication technologies: Reshaping voluntary organizations? *Nonprofit Management & Leadership, 11*(2), 131–143. doi:10.1002/nml.11201

Callahan, C. M., Boustani, M. A., & Unverzagt, F. W. (2006). Effectiveness of collaborative care for older adults with Alzheimer disease in primary care: A randomized controlled trial. *Journal of the American Medical Association, 295,* 2148–2157. doi:10.1001/jama.295.18.2148

Censis. (Ed.). (2007). *La mente rubata, bisogni e costi sociali della malattia di Alzheimer.* Milano, Italia: FrancoAngeli Editore.

Chiu, T., & Eysembach, G. (2010). Stage of use: Consideration, initiation, utilization and outcome of an internet-mediated intervention. *Medical Informatics and Decision Making, 10,* 73–84. doi:10.1186/1472-6947-10-73

Cicourel, A. V. (1999). The interaction of cognitive and cultural models in health care delivery. In Sarangi, S., & Talk, R. S. (Eds.), *Work and institutional order: Discourse in medical, mediation and management settings* (pp. 183–224). Berlin, Germany: De Gruyter. doi:10.1515/9783110208375.2.183

Craig, J., Russell, C., Patterson, V., & Wootton, R. (1999). User satisfaction with realtime teleneurology. *Journal of Telemedicine and Telecare, 5*(4), 237–241. doi:10.1258/1357633991933774

Cullum, C. M., Weiner, M. F., Gehrmann, H. R., & Hynan, L. S. (2006). Feasibility of telecognitive assessment in dementia. *Assessment, 13*(4), 385–390. doi:10.1177/1073191106289065

Department of Economic and Social Affairs (DESA) of the United Nations. (2007). *World economic and social survey 2007: Development in an ageing world.* New York, NY: Author. Retrieved from http://www.un.org/en/development/desa/policy/wess/wess_archive/2007wess.pdf.

Eysenbach, G. (2001). What is e-health? *Journal of Medical Internet Research, 3*(2), 20–24. doi:10.2196/jmir.3.2.e20

Eysenbach, G. (2005). The law of attrition. *Journal of Medical Internet Research, 7,* 11–15. doi:10.2196/jmir.7.1.e11

Finch, T., Mort, M., May, C., & Mair, F. (2005). Telecare: Perspectives on the changing role of patients and citizens. *Journal of Telemedicine and Telecare, 11*(1), 51–53. doi:10.1258/1357633054461679

Galante, E. (2009). Rehabilitation project and tele-monitoring of patients with mildly deteriorating cognition and their caregivers. *Giornale Italiano di Medicina del Lavoro Ed Ergonomia, 31*(1 Suppl A), A64–A67.

Gaugler, J. E., Davey, A., Pearling, L. I., & Zarit, S. H. (2000). Modeling caregiver adaptation over the time: The longitudinal impact of behavior problems. *Psychology and Aging, 15*(3), 437–450. doi:10.1037/0882-7974.15.3.437

Gherardi, S., & Strati, A. (Eds.). (2004). *La telemedicina fra tecnologia e organizzazione.* Roma, Italy: Carocci.

Grisby, J., Kaehney, M. M., Sandberg, E. J., Schlenker, R. E., & Shaughnessy, P. W. (1995). Effects and effectiveness of telemedicine. *Health Care Financing Review, 17*(1), 116–131.

Hort, J., & Brien, O, J. T., Gainotti, G., et al. (2010). EFNS guidelines for the diagnosis and management of Alzheimer's disease. *European Journal of Neurology, 17,* 1236–1248. doi:10.1111/j.1468-1331.2010.03040.x

Karttunen, K., Karppi, P., & Hiltunen, A. (2011). Neuropsychiatric symptoms and quality of life in patients with very mild and mild Alzheimer's disease. *International Journal of Geriatric Psychiatry, 26,* 473–482. doi:10.1002/gps.2550

Levesque, L., Cossette, S., & Lachance, L. (1998). Predictor of psychological well-behing of primary caregivers living with a demented relatives: A 1-year follow-up study. *Journal of Applied Gerontology, 17*(2), 240–258. doi:10.1177/073346489801700211

Lewin, K. (1951). *Field theory in social science.* New York, NY: Harper &Row.

Loh, P., Donaldson, M., Flicker, L., Maher, S., & Goldswain, P. (2007). Development of a telemedicine protocol for the diagnosis of Alzheimer's disease. *Journal of Telemedicine and Telecare, 13*(2), 90–94. doi:10.1258/135763307780096159

Mahoney, D. F., Tarlow, B. J., & Jones, R. N. (2003). Effects of an automated telephone support system on caregiver burden and anxiety: Findings from the REACH for TLC intervention study. *The Gerontologist, 43*(4), 556–567. doi:10.1093/geront/43.4.556

Mahoney, D. M., Tarlow, B., Jones, R. N., Tennstedt, S., & Kasten, L. (2001). Factors affecting the use of a telephone-based intervention for caregivers of people with Alzheimer's disease. *Journal of Telemedicine and Telecare, 7*(3), 139–148. doi:10.1258/1357633011936291

May, C., Harrison, R., MacFarlane, A., Williams, T., Mair, F., & Wallace, P. (2003). Why do telemedicine systems fail to normalize as stable models of service delivery? *Journal of Telemedicine and Telecare, 9,* 25–26. doi:10.1258/135763303322196222

Miller, E. A. (2001). Telemedicine and doctor–patient communication: An analytical survey of the literature. *Journal of Telemedicine and Telecare, 7,* 1–17. doi:10.1258/1357633011936075

Neri, M., Bonati, P. A., & Pinelli, M. (2007). Biological, psychological and clinical markers of caregiver's stress in impaired elderly with dementia and age relate disease. *Archives of Gerontology and Geriatrics, 1,* 289–194. doi:10.1016/j.archger.2007.01.038

Nobili, A., Riva, E., & Tettamanti, M. (2004). The effect of a structured intervention on caregivers of patients with dementia and problem behaviors: A Randomized controlled pilot study. *Alzheimer Disease and Associated Disorders, 18,* 75–82. doi:10.1097/01.wad.0000126618.98867.fc

Pearlin, L. I., Mullan, J. T., Semple, S. J., & Skaff, M. M. (1990). Caregiving and stress process: An overview of concepts and their measures. *The Gerontologist, 30*(5), 583–594. doi:10.1093/geront/30.5.583

Raivio, M., Eloniemi-Sulkava, U., & Laakkonen, M. L. (2007). How do officially organized services meet the needs of elderly caregivers and their spouses with Alzheimer's disease? *American Journal of Alzheimer's Disease and Other Dementias*, *22*, 360–368. doi:10.1177/1533317507305178

Rajani, R., & Perry, M. (1999). The reality of medical work: The case for a new perspective on telemedicine. *Virtual Reality (Waltham Cross)*, *4*(4), 243–249. doi:10.1007/BF01421807

Robinson, S. S., Seale, D. E., Tiernan, K. M., & Berg, B. (2003). Use of telemedicine to follow special needs children. *Telemedicine Journal and e-Health*, *9*(1), 57–61. doi:10.1089/153056203763317657

Roine, R., Ohinmaa, A., & Hailey, D. (2001). Assessing telemedicine: A systematic review of the literature. *Canadian Medical Association Journal*, *165*(6), 765–771.

Rosa, E., Lussignoli, G., & Sabbatini, F. (2010). Needs of caregivers of the patients with dementia. *Archives of Gerontology and Geriatrics*, *51*, 54–58. doi:10.1016/j.archger.2009.07.008

Ryan, K. A., Weldon, A., & Huby, N. M. (2010). Caregiver support service needs for patients with mild cognitive impairment and Alzheimer disease. *Alzheimer Disease and Associated Disorders*, *24*, 171–176. doi:10.1097/WAD.0b013e3181aba90d

Schneider, J., Murray, J., Banerjee, S., & Mann, A. (1999). Eurocare: A cross sectional study of co-resident spouse for people with Alzheimer's disease factors associated with carer burden. *International Journal of Geriatric Psychiatry*, *14*, 651–661. doi:10.1002/(SICI)1099-1166(199908)14:8<651::AID-GPS992>3.0.CO;2-B

Schulz, R., O'Brien, A. T., Bookwala, J., & Fleissner, K. (1995). Psychiatric and physical morbidity effects of dementia caregiving: Prevalence, correlates and causes. *Gerontology*, *35*(6), 771–791. doi:10.1093/geront/35.6.771

Suchman, L. A. (1987). *Plans and situated actions: the problem of human-machine communication*. New York, NY: Cambridge University Press.

Tanriverdi, H., & Iacono, S. (1999). Diffusion of telemedicine: A knowledge barrier perspective. *Telemedicine Journal*, *5*(3), 223–244. doi:10.1089/107830299311989

Taylor, P. (1998). A survey of research in telemedicine. 1: Telemedicine systems. *Journal of Telemedicine and Telecare*, *4*(1), 1–17. doi:10.1258/1357633981931227

Trist, E., & Murray, H. (1993). The social engagement of social science: *Vol. II. The socio-technical perspective*. Philadelphia, PA: University of Pennsylvania Press.

Van Mierlo, L. D., Meiland, F. J. M., Van der Roest, H. G., & Dro¨es, R. M. (2012). Personalised caregiver support: Effectiveness of psychosocial interventions in subgroups of caregivers of people with dementia. *International Journal of Geriatric Psychiatry*, *27*, 1–14. doi:10.1002/gps.2694

Venkatesh, V., & Bala, H. (2008). Technology acceptance model 3 and a research agenda on interventions. *Decision Sciences*, *39*(2), 273–315. doi:10.1111/j.1540-5915.2008.00192.x

Wai-Chi Chan, S. (2010). Family caregiving in dementia: The Asian perspective of a global problem. *Dementia and Geriatric Cognitive Disorders*, *30*, 469–478. doi:10.1159/000322086

Wimo, A., Winblad, B., & Jo¨nsson, L. (2010). The worldwide societal costs of dementia: Estimates for 2009. *Alzheimer's & Dementia*, *6*, 98–103. doi:10.1016/j.jalz.2010.01.010

Yamaguchi, H., Maki, Y., & Yamagami, T. (2010). Overview of non-pharmacological intervention for dementia and principles of brain-activating rehabilitation. *Psychogeriatrics*, *10*, 206–213. doi:10.1111/j.1479-8301.2010.00323.x

Yueh-Feng Lu, Y., & Guerriero Austrom, M. (2005). Distress responses and self-care behaviors in dementia family caregivers with high and low depressed mood. *Journal of the American Psychiatric Nurses Association, 11*(4), 231–240. doi:10.1177/1078390305281422

ADDITIONAL READING

Beeber, A. S., & Zimmerman, S. (2012). Adapting the family management style framework for families caring for older adults with dementia. *Journal of Family Nursing, 18*(1), 123–145. doi:10.1177/1074840711427144

Chien, L. Y., Chu, H., Guo, J. L., Liao, Y. M., Chang, L. I., Chen, C. H., & Chou, K. R. (2011). Caregiver support groups in patients with dementia: a meta-analysis. *International Journal of Geriatric Psychiatry, 26*(10), 1089–1098. doi:10.1002/gps.2660

Cohen, C. A., Colantonio, A., & Vernich, L. (2002). Positive aspects of caregiving: Rounding out the caregiver experience. *International Journal of Geriatric Psychiatry, 17*(2), 184–188. doi:10.1002/gps.561

Cooper, C., Katona, C., Orrell, M., & Livingston, G. (2008). Coping strategies, anxiety and depression in caregivers of people with Alzheimer's disease. *International Journal of Geriatric Psychiatry, 23*(9), 929–936. doi:10.1002/gps.2007

Corbett, A., Stevens, J., Aarsland, D., Day, S., Moniz-Cook, E., & Woods, R. (2012). Systematic review of services providing information and/or advice to people with dementia and/or their caregivers. *International Journal of Geriatric Psychiatry, 27*(6), 628–636. doi:10.1002/gps.2762

Eisdorfer, C., Czaja, S. J., Loewenstein, D. A., Rubert, M. P., Arguelles, S., Mitrani, V. B., & Szapocznik, J. (2003). The effect of family therapy and technology-based intervention on caregiver depression. *The Gerontologist, 43*(4), 521–531. doi:10.1093/geront/43.4.521

Farran, C. J., Fogg, L. G., McCann, J. J., Etkin, C., Dong, X., & Barnes, L. L. (2011). Assessing family caregiver skill in managing behavioral symptoms of Alzheimer's disease. *Aging & Mental Health, 15*(4), 510–521. doi:10.1080/13607863.2010.536140

Ferri, C. P., Prince, M., & Brayne, C. (2005). Global prevalence of dementia: A Delphi consensus study. *Lancet, 366*(9503), 2112–2117. doi:10.1016/S0140-6736(05)67889-0

García-Alberca, J. M., Cruz, B., Lara, J. P., Garrido, V., Gris, E., Lara, A., & Castilla, C. (2012). Disengagement coping partially mediates the relationship between caregiver burden and anxiety and depression in caregivers of people with Alzheimer's disease. Results from the Málaga-AD study. *Journal of Affective Disorders, 136*(3), 848–856. doi:10.1016/j.jad.2011.09.026

Lauriks, S., Reinersmann, A., Van der Roest, H. G., Meiland, F. J. M., Davies, R. J., & Moelaert, F. (2007). Review of ICT-based services for identified unmet needs in people with dementia. *Ageing Research Reviews, 6*, 223–246. doi:10.1016/j.arr.2007.07.002

Llanque, S. M., & Enriquez, M. (2012). Interventions for Hispanic caregivers of patients with dementia: A review of the literature. *American Journal of Alzheimer's Disease and Other Dementias, 27*(1), 23–32. doi:10.1177/1533317512439794

Lovell, B., & Wetherell, M. A. (2011). The cost of caregiving: Endocrine and immune implications in elderly and non elderly caregivers. *Neuroscience and Biobehavioral Reviews, 35*, 1342–1352. doi:10.1016/j.neubiorev.2011.02.007

Mallen, M. J., Vogel, D. L., & Rochlen, A. B. (2005). The practical aspects of online counseling: Ethics, training, technology, and competency. *The Counseling Psychologist, 33,* 776–818. doi:10.1177/0011000005278625

McKhann, G. M., Knopman, D. S., Chertkow, H., Hyman, B. T., Jack, C. R. Jr, & Kawas, C. H. (2011). The diagnosis of dementia due to Alzheimer's disease: Recommendations from the National Institute on Aging-Alzheimer's Association workgroups on diagnostic guidelines for Alzheimer's disease. *Alzheimer's & Dementia, 7,* 263–269. doi:10.1016/j.jalz.2011.03.005

Oken, B. S., Fonareva, I., & Wahbeh, H. (2011). Stress-related cognitive dysfunction in dementia caregivers. *Journal of Geriatric Psychiatry and Neurology, 24*(4), 191–198. doi:10.1177/0891988711422524

Oremus, M., & Aguilar, S. C. (2011). A systematic review to assess the policy-making relevance of dementia cost-of-illness studies in the US and Canada. *PharmacoEconomics, 29*(2), 141–156. doi:10.2165/11539450-000000000-00000

Patterson, V., Hoque, F., Vassallo, D., Farquharson, R. M., Swinfen, P., & Swinfen, R. (2001). Store-and-forward teleneurology in developing countries. *Journal of Telemedicine and Telecare, 7*(Suppl 1), 52–53. doi:10.1258/1357633011936714

Perry, M., Drašković, I., Lucassen, P., Vernooij-Dassen, M., van Achterberg, T., & Rikkert, M. O. (2011). Effects of educational interventions on primary dementia care: A systematic review. *International Journal of Geriatric Psychiatry, 26,* 1–11. doi:10.1002/gps.2479

Pesamaa, L., Ebeling, H., Kuusimaki, M. L., Winblad, I., Isohanni, M., & Moilanen, I. (2004). Videoconferencing in child and adolescent telepsychiatry: A systematic review of the literature. *Journal of Telemedicine and Telecare, 10*(4), 187–192. doi:10.1258/1357633041424458

Poon, P., Hui, E., Dai, D., Kwok, T., & Woo, J. (2005). Cognitive intervention for community-dwelling older persons with memory problems: Telemedicine versus face-to-face treatment. *International Journal of Geriatric Psychiatry, 323,* 285–286. doi:10.1002/gps.1282

Powell, J., Chiu, T., & Eysenbach, G. (2008). A systematic review of networked technologies supporting carers of people with dementia. *Journal of Telemedicine and Telecare, 14*(3), 154–156. doi:10.1258/jtt.2008.003018

Rabinowitz, Y. G., Saenz, E. C., Thompson, L. W., & Gallagher-Thompson, D. (2011). Understanding caregiver health behaviors: Depressive symptoms mediate caregiver self-efficacy and health behavior patterns. *American Journal of Alzheimer's Disease and Other Dementias, 26*(4), 310–316. doi:10.1177/1533317511410557

Richardson, L. K., Frueh, B. C., Grubaugh, A. L., & Egede, L., & Ihai, J. D. (2009). Current directions in videoconferencing tele-mental health research. *Clinical Psychologist, 16,* 323–338.

Rigby, M., Forsstrom, J., Roberts, R., & Wyatt, J. (2001). Verifying quality and safety in health informatics services. *British Medical Journal, 323,* 552–556. doi:10.1136/bmj.323.7312.552

Robert, P. H., Verhey, F. R., Byrne, E. J., De Deyn, P. P., Nobili, F., & Riello, R. (2005). Grouping for behavioral and psychological symptoms in dementia clinical and biological aspects: Consensus paper of the European Alzheimer disease consortium. *European Psychiatry, 20,* 490–496. doi:10.1016/j.eurpsy.2004.09.031

Steffen, A. M., & Jackson, C. S. (2012). Predicting facilitators' behaviors during Alzheimer's family support group meetings. *American Journal of Alzheimer's Disease and Other Dementias, 27*(2), 114–120. doi:10.1177/1533317512441051

Van Durme, T., Macq, J., Jeanmart, C., & Gobert, M. (2012). Tools for measuring the impact of informal caregiving of the elderly: a literature review. *International Journal of Nursing Studies, 49*(4), 490–504. doi:10.1016/j.ijnurstu.2011.10.011

Van Vliet, D., de Vugt, M. E., Bakker, C., Koopmans, R. T., & Verhey, F. R. (2010). Impact of early onset dementia on caregivers: A review. *International Journal of Geriatric Psychiatry, 25*, 1091–1100. doi:10.1002/gps.2439

KEY TERMS AND DEFINITIONS

Alzheimer Disease: A neurodegenerative disease defined as progressive cognitive decline with important interferences in activities of daily living accompanied by any behavioural problems.

Caregiver: In high and low resource countries, usually, the families care for AD person. An especial family member becomes the primary caregiver, with an important assistance role.

Teleconference: Allows different health workers and all the person in charge of the AD patients, to communicate through a video link. In this case the patient isn't there or she/he comes abreast with a health worker.

Teleconsultation: Useful to obtain a medical advice or a second opinion from a health worker. It can involve not only the patient and the specialist, but also a further contact with a specialist "in remote".

Telemedicine: Information and Communication and Technologies (ICT) in medicine practice.

Telemonitoring: Consists in the (continuous or at regular intervals) gathering of patient data, that can be qualitative or quantitative.

Telereporting: The procedure requires the transmission of clinical case data or medical records to other health workers, in order to obtain a second opinion or a specialist consult on the patients.

Chapter 14
Health Services through Digital Terrestrial Television

Aldo Franco Dragoni
Università Politecnica delle Marche, Italy

ABSTRACT

This chapter defines a scenario for providing Health Services through the Digital Terrestrial Television (DTT), both for patients (monitoring health parameters) and healthy citizens. A number of services will be provided over DTT, not only by means of informative or interactive applications broadcast and installed on the set-top box, but also as transactional services through the secure return channel. However, much effort has to be spent to guarantee the usability of that new TV-based interface, which is quite different from that of a PC-based Web application.

INTRODUCTION

Western World is nowadays close to complete the transition toward the digital television, and in particular toward the Digital Terrestrial Television (DTT) (Leiva, 2006). Thanks to the presence of a modem and of a reader of smart cards, decoders can provide a new access for information and services through the secure return (telephonic) channel. The DTT software is based on the open standard called Multimedia Home Platform (MHP) (ETSI, 2003). MHP applications are written in Java and are called "Xlets" (see Morris 2005 for a complete introduction to Interactive TV Standards). They are broadcast by the TV operators inside the MPEG video stream, so they do not have to be installed on the Set Top Box (STB) and are independent from its operating system, thus being immediately available in every home. After this epochal change, Local Healthcares should not disregard the return channel of the DTT as a platform to distribute their services (as they are currently doing through the Web). This because elderly people, which are not comfortable with personal computers and the Internet, are instead used to the TV and its remote control, so it should be straightforward bringing all the important informative and interactive services over a suite of Xlets. A main problem with this project is that of ensuring the usability of such Xlets.

DOI: 10.4018/978-1-4666-2979-0.ch014

However, in our opinion, developing an Xlet to browse the Web over the return line of the DTT is quite a nonsense, since it is almost impossible to navigate the Internet through a very limited input device as the remote control (instead of the powerful couple keyboard/mouse) and with a low resolution monitor as the TV screen, but recently other researchers tried to develop a browse for the DTT (Amerini, 2010).

Furthermore, we do not believe much in monitoring health parameters of sick people through DTT, since television is an entertainment medium and it is commonly associated with fun, leisure and news, not with illness and pain, and remote controls (that must not be abandoned to fulfill the needs of the elderly) are input peripherals too much limited for complex and tricky operations.

Instead we believe that the DTT will provide a bunch of purely informative or transactional interactive services for healthy people, but also for patients released from hospitals and for the elderly in nursing homes. These services range from simple TeleTexts, with information about pharmacies and general practitioners, to advanced transactions, as medical booking and simple payments.

It has been already argued that the promise of interactive services over the Digital TV for all members of the society may remain unfulfilled, unless the usability of the new medium is adapted to the diverse characteristics of the population (Chorianopoulos, 2006) and there is a need to adapt the traditional user interfaces design and evaluation methods to the home environment (Monk 2000). It will be mandatory to assure confidentiality and authentication within sensible transactional services, and it will then be useful to permit payments over this new medium (Papa, 2010).

Being aware of all these concerns, we developed an architecture for exploiting the potential of the DTT for Healthcare Services, both for sick and healthy citizens. The idea of rendering the digital interactive television an health information platform for the future in not novel (see Gunter, 2003 and the project PANACEIA-iTV described in Maglaveras, 2003) but we provided a real scenario for many health-related services.

GENERAL ARCHITECTURE

This service platform has been originally designed to guarantee patient's monitoring and interactions with involved physicians and service operators (inspired by Maternaghan 2010)

The overall architecture consists of four main components (also see Figure 1):

1. **Patient's Control Centre:** This is the User's station at home or in a nursing home; eventually the User could be a patient that will be able to practise exercises or learn more about pathology and have a continuous monitoring sending data through an advanced patient station that transmits information collected by biomedical devices through wireless channels.

2. **Remote Clinical Centre:** This is the clinical actor of the service; during the day, or during the exercises practise, physicians at the clinical control centre can monitor patient's health status being automatically alerted in case of parameters exceeding thresholds.

3. **Broadcasting Centre:** A Local TV channel will broadcast typical programs (for example exercises like cycling, postural for cardiovascular diseases) every morning at an established hour, and the Xlet which will detect patient's vital parameters and send back them to the remote clinical centre.

4. **Service Centre:** It manages the return channel of the patients' station; it also develops, stores and send the Xlets to the broadcaster.

At home, some technological devices will eventually support continuous patient's monitor-

Figure 1. Overall human and technological infrastructure

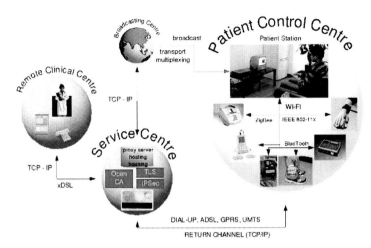

ing and will help her in getting in touch with the remote Clinical Centre. Patient's monitoring will be supported through the Patient's Station, i.e.:

1. A DVB-T decoder with Smart Card reader and modem
2. A BlueTooth dongle in order to receive data from biomedical devices
3. Accessories and biomedical devices (as the BodyGateway by STMicroelectronics or the BioHarness by Zephyr)

The decoder runs MHP-standard "Xlets" broadcast by a Local TV Network. As a typical scenario, while the TV channel will broadcast special healthcare purpose programs, the Xlet will detect data from biomedical devices, streaming them back to the Remote Clinical Centre in real-time. These applications cannot survive neither the switch-off of the patient's station nor the change of the TV channel, and they need to be re-downloaded from the "object carousel" (i.e. from the antenna) every time they are newly used. The Xlets are also able to:

• Connect to the Service Center over TCP/IP through at-home available capabilities.

• Connect to the biomedical devices in the Patient Station through USB, FireWire, or BlueTooth connections.

It will allow to collect all the information coming from the wireless devices used to monitor physiological parameters of the person as well as other data coming from wireless sensors at home to monitor environmental variables or utilities. The Xlets will be managed through an MHP-standard interactive TV remote control. For text typing it will be available a soft keypad on the lower panel of the TV screen, that will be navigated through the arrow keys of the remote control. Of course this will make it difficult to edit long texts although (Mourouzis 2007) argued that the number pad (keys 1 to 9) may be used to insert text, given an appropriate soft keyboard.

The biomedical wearable devices connected to the Set Top Box let the Xlet to:

• Monitor body functions, like taking an ECG or the breath or heart frequency, Spo2 etc.
• Monitor body activity.

The Patient Station will be connected to the Service Centre whose main tasks are:

1. Guaranteeing a secure, private, persistent and efficient Internet connection over the *return channel,*
2. Providing the "Xlets" to be multiplexed by the Broadcaster's Object Carousel into the MPEG-2 audio-video stream (thus, it is the technological actor that guarantees the functionality of the overall architecture),
3. Providing and managing the interactive Web-TV transmissions for skilled people with a broadband Internet connection,
4. Managing a customised Web portal and a suitable database for hosting/housing the medical services, through which the Remote Clinical Centre can communicate and interact with the Patient Station; that Web portal will thus have all the settings to highlight calls and requests for services and to handle the functions in an automatic way by giving the elderly as much as possible the opportunity to be self supporting.

It is the role of the Remote Clinical Center that of providing the *digital content* of the Xlets.

There are real concerns that must be addressed before the actors of the platform are comfortable to using it. We will discuss the importance of usability later, but here we want to emphasize the importance of "security". A major challenge that will be faced is the development of a platform that enables high-speed communication and easy access while maintaining confidentiality. There are different aspects of security and privacy of data such as *physical security, access controls, authentication* and *encryption* that need to be addressed. These tasks are quite in charge of the Service Centre that will adopt a Certification Authority (CA) that will deliver or recognize X.509 v3 certifies provided by Governmental Smart Cards (as the Italian Electronic Identity Card) over a Virtual Private Network grounded on TLS and IP-sec (hidden reference 2).

Special agreements have to be taken with broadcasters (basically regional or specialized national channels) in order to provide a proper broadcasting of the Xlets. The Xlets will be broadcast during appropriate TV programs. The Xlets for the elderly or patients will be of different kinds:

- **Infotainment:** People can have direct access to broadcast programs, including digital TV services from available channels.
- **Interactive services:** Bilateral communication where the User asks for specific services (external assistance, medical news, health information, etc.).
- **Infoassistance:** Information is sent by the Assistance centre periodically to support their daily life (medicine intake or other reminders).

In conclusion, the Remote Clinical Centre is the Healthcare Service Provider.

A SUITE OF XLETS FOR THE LOCAL HEALTH

Nowadays, several Public Agencies look forward offering over the DTT some of the services they are already offering through the Web. This effort is motivated by the ethical duty to reduce the digital divide in the population. Of course, the majority of elderly people is not confident with Internet or mobile Smart Phone, and it would probably prefer to have some facilities supported by the Interactive TV. This mean that the "Remote Clinical Centre" should expand its role in the DTT scenario into that of a "Local Healthcare Service Provider". Our main goal was that of bringing onto the DTT a portion of the services that where available on the WEB portal of our Local Health (hidden reference 2). We started by developing a suite of Xlets for:

- Giving information about the Local Health
- Booking radiography and laboratory examinations
- Sending and receiving emails with attached files (reports and examinations)

Since the development phase, we paid much attention to:

- The choice of the colors
- The fitting with the limited resolution of the TV screen
- A guide to the navigation
- The usability
- The contents

The TV screen has a limited range of colours w.r.t. a PC monitor, and we realized that a blue background had some advantages since almost any colour for the text is visible on a light blue background, especially the white, and the characters look more in relief. To break the monotonicity of the background we introduced some nuances in the blue

Of course, the colors of the buttons of the interface were associated to those of the corresponding buttons on the remote control. The guide in the lower part of the screen was in dark blue, to be less invasive. Generic titles and submenus were written in white, informative text in black, and the guide was written in blue. The heading was inspired by the corresponding heading on the Web portal. We looked forward a choice of colours that could be perceptible also by colorblind people. On the 14 inches TV screen we had no distortion or strain on the boundaries, but in wider TV screens there was a little molding unused by the Xlet. Interacting with an Xlet is more complex than navigating inside a pure TeleText, so an on-screen guide is necessary. The guide must be clear and concise, without technical terms. Of course, its readability increases with wide screens. Information was not excessive and the User had always a very limited number of choices, because of the constraints imposed by the remote control (which is a poor input device), but this simplicity made the interface very user friendly. The structure of the menus was deliberately trivial. We've been inspired by the menu structure of automatic telephone call centres, with no more than four branches and three menu levels, being every page always well informative about its position inside the menu tree. The branching factor was practically imposed by the standard interactive remote control, which has four coloured buttons (*red*, *green*, *yellow*, *blue*); associating them to the choice of the submenu is straightforward. It is important not to use those four colours improperly, for instance for the text or titles (we use always black or white for them).

Fonts' height was of 18 pixels or more. With MHP, texts are not tagged as in HTML, so the formatting has to be statically defined by the programmer. We developed a formatted template to be adopted as a stylesheet by the programmer, and of course the template can be freely modified.

The Xlet is started by pressing the red button on the remote control while watching the TV Channel that transmits it. After a while (which is necessary to download all the application from the Object Carousel) the main menu of the home page appears on the TV screen (Figure 2). The main information provided is about pharmacies, general practitioners and pediatricians, along with the telephone numbers of the main services of the Local Health. The left portion of the screen is reserved for general important messages.

By pressing the corresponding number it is possible to see the list of the *currently* open pharmacies (the Xlet is continuously refreshed into the Object Carousel by the Service Centre) (see Figure 3). In every section the User will have the awareness of her position inside the menu structure. By pressing the yellow button the User accesses the section "physicians", where it will be possible to find their telephone numbers, addresses and schedules. The section is divided into two subsections: "general practitioners" and "pediatricians". Each category is organized as a

Figure 2. Home page of former Xlet for the Local Health

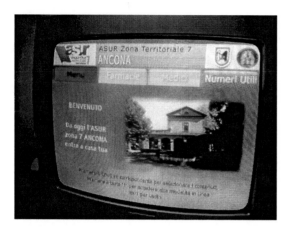

Figure 3. The section "Pharmacies"

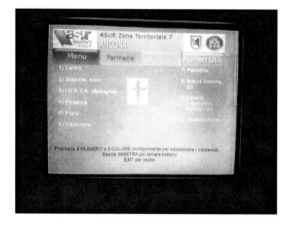

subsection with the name of the physicians ordered lexicographically. By pressing the blue button the User accesses the directory of the Local Health.

Information seen so far comes with the Xlet and is broadcast to every citizen. Other specific information can be received on demand by authenticated Users through the return channel. From the home page it is possible to get these online contents by pressing the button "1" on the remote control (Figure 4). By pressing again the button "1" the Decoder tries to connect with the Service Centre to get an IP address. To stay within a low hardware profile we performed always a "dial-up"

56Kb connection with the PPP protocol (there are open Java MHP classes to do that). The connection requires almost one minute. After connected to the Internet the User has to authenticate herself in one of these two methods:

1. By introducing her credentials through the software keypad that appears on the lower part of the screen (Figure 5),
2. By introducing her own Governmental Smart Card (see Figure 6) inside the reader of the STB.

Following the second way the subsequent SSL session uses the Public Key Infrastructure provided by the X.509 v3 certificate which resides embedded into the Smart Card. In this way we fulfil both "strong authentication" and "confidentiality", thus making it possible to perform sensible online transactions, as downloading DICOM documents (Digital Imaging and Communications in Medicine, for instance radiographic examinations and reports) or making payments. Following both the ways it will be possible to access the services made available by the Local Health through their Web portal, for instance booking medical and/or laboratory examinations. We also developed a function to manage a personal "agenda" of appointments with Local Health, also letting their owner to cancel appointments that cannot be respected in order to free the slot for other patients.

We preferred to use the on-screen keypad w.r.t. the keyboard of the remote control because elder people have difficulties with the small keys and labels of the latter. Unfortunately, even the software keypad is hard for data entry. It is necessary to move around the screen keypad by pressing the arrows keys on the remote control, but unfortunately this operation is not easy since it is difficult to watch the TV screen and the remote control simultaneously. Once the desired soft key is evidenced on the screen the User must press

Figure 4. Page to access online informative contents

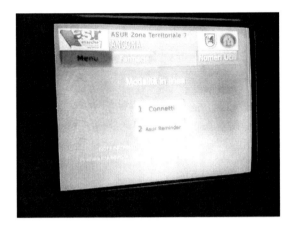

Figure 5. Authentication through data entry (without smart cards)

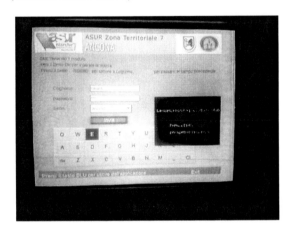

the "*OK*" button on the remote control, and so on, till the end. When the data entry is completed the User has to go to the "*return*" soft key and press "*OK*" on the remote control. That procedure is very bothering and prone to errors. We'll come back to this problem in the section "usability". Once completed, the "query" will be sent to the Service Centre that will process and send back the "answers" to the client STB.

For important operations (as the deletion of a reservation) a Pop-Up Menu of confirmation will appear. The active field for the data entry is enhanced in red in order to make it easier to

understand what kind of datum is required and in which state of the interaction protocol the User is. To simplify the data entry we choose the system to be not "case-sensitive". Every time the color of a buttons is referred, the text is written in that same color in order to facilitate the understanding.

These complex and critical operations ill-befit the state of relaxation with which you sit in front of the television, as we'll discuss later. To reduce the risk of distractions, we decided not to frame the screen so as to avoid that the User watches the TV program (in a smaller window) while s/he is performing these operations.

Security and Smart Cards

Online transactional services over the "return channel" require confidentiality and strong authentication. While we are writing, the specimens of MHP 1.1.2 about the return channel take the same recommendations of the Internet and adopt

Figure 6. (a,b) Authentication through governmental smart card

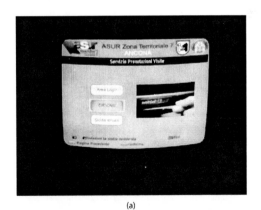

(a)

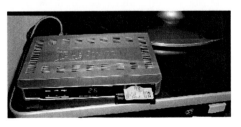

(b)

the same standard Transport Layer Security (TLS) protocol. More specifically MHP 1.1.2 forces the entire cryptographic suite RSA, MD5, SHA-1 and DES. It also specifies that authentication on the client side should be performed by passing the position of the keys to the API Java class javax.net.ssl.SSLContext through the javax.net.ssl.KeyManager.

The TLS connection requires that at least one of the certificates sent by the server belongs to those authenticated on the STB. The STB cannot connect to a telephonic number different from that of the predefined Service Centre, unless there is an explicit consensus from the User after a mandatory request from the application. The request must bring the data of the Certification Authority (i.e. the X.509v3 certificate) to authenticate the application.

Of course, Smart Cards avoid the problems of authentication (Rankl 2004, Chirico 2006). Let us sum up the current MHP specimens about Smart Cards.

1. MHP 1.0.2 and 1.0.3 did not deal with Smart Cards.
2. MHP 1.1 and 1.1.1 introduced the readers of Smart Cards (for electronic commerce) through the Open Card Framework for Embedded Devices Specification 1.2.2 (OCF); unfortunately, they didn't foresee their deployment for conditioned access.
3. MHP 1.1.2 abandoned OCF for the set of Java API called "Security and Trust Services API for Java 2 Platform, Micro Edition", (SATSA 1.0). Furthermore it adopted the same API "SATSA-APDU" used by Java in mobile networks for connecting with Smart Cards.

The "Electronic Identity Card" (CIE) and the "National Services Card" (CNS) are mass tools to access transactional services under confidentiality and strong authentication. Unfortunately,

to use them on the Internet, personal computers should be equipped with a card reader, and this peripheral is all but common. In 2005 we realized that the problem is not economic (the main Italian region, Lombardy, distributed the reader almost freely), but it is a matter of technological and practical usability; but the STB equipped with the most advanced version of MHP, would embed the card reader, thus solving the problem of putting a gate toward advanced transactional services in every home.

Usability of the Xlets

The DTT is interactive, but most of its audience is not yet ready for interactivity. Sooner or later it will be accepted but, for now, some psychological factors tend to preserve the habit of passivity against interactive television. To facilitate this change, usability plays a fundamental role (Melendreras-Ruiz 2008). The usability criteria for interactive TV applications (the MHP Xlets in the case of DTT) derive from the usability criteria of software interfaces (not only of the Web) but they must be specifically analysed as discussed in (Pemberton 2003).

Usability is defined by the International Organisation for Standardisation as *the effectiveness, efficiency and satisfaction with which certain users reach certain goals in certain contexts.* In practice, it defines the degree of ease and satisfaction of a man when using an instrument. The problem of usability arises when the designer's model of the artifact (i.e. the designer's ideas concerning the operation of the product) does not match the general user's one (i.e. the end-user's expectations about the functioning of the product). The closer the two models, the higher the usability of the artifact.

TV is still the widest medium in the World, being used by an enormous percentage of population (notwithstanding the impressive growth of the competing Internet, from 2000 to 2006 the use of the TV is also increased and reached the threshold of saturation; today the TV is watched by 93.2% of Italians). It is therefore necessary to guarantee the usability of its interactive applications. In (Nielsen 2005) the author describes the setting up of a usability lab for interactive television and considers the nature of usability in this particular context. We tried to take advantage of those observations to improve the usability of our suite of Xlets.

The audience target of the TV applications will be the widest and most uneven conceivable, and that is precisely why developers must pay particular attention to usability of their interfaces. Interacting with the TV becomes easier and more attractive if the graphics is elegant, playful, understandable and "ergonomic". Easy to use, but also efficient, entertaining and authoritative; it should have a style corresponding to the TV program and should characterize the brand of the TV network, being also coherent and constant, so that it needs not be reinterpreted each every step of a long operation. Last but not least, the graphics of interactive TV should be light in memory/band consumption and in occupation of the screen (if the User desires to watch the underlying TV program in the background or in a reduced window).

The usability criteria for interactive TV are different from those for the WEB. The latter is visualized on high-resolution displays, while interactive TV applications are shown on low resolution screens. Another important difference is that the Xlets must be interacted through a remote control, which is a far poorer input device w.r.t. the couple mouse/keyboard. The way you interact with a remote control is completely different from the way you interact with a keyboard and a mouse, and this affects the structure of the Xlet. Its interface will contain elements that characterise as far as possible the functional buttons on the remote control so as to create an intuitive connection

between what the User sees on the screen and the remote control. A final problem regards the way in which the User stands in front of the TV, which is completely different compared to how s/he faces with a personal computer. In the first case the User is seeing television comfortably seated and relaxing on a sofa (which is relatively distant from the TV and in a room where there may be other persons doing other jobs) and is not prepared to perform tasks that need concentration, while in the second case, the attention is greater and the User is concentrated to perform more challenging tasks. This means that Xlets' interfaces have to be as simple as possible, linear and with an interpretation straight and clear. The graphic design and implementation of the Xlets' will become protagonists in the near future and will affect what will be the role of digital terrestrial TV in our society. Making them as usable as possible means facilitating the dissemination and use of interactive TV allowing citizens to take full advantage by the enormous potential of that technology.

With all these concerns in mind we decided to carefully analyse the usability of our Xlet to address all the problems and redesign a new graphic interface that respects the various usability criteria and meets, wherever possible, also the requirements of accessibility. We focused our attention not on *what* the Xlet should do but on *how* it should. Hence, for the design of new graphic interface we carried on a preliminary work analysing the old interface using, wherever possible, the ten heuristic for usability and the set of guidelines for the design of software for Internet TV proposed by Jakob Nielsen.

The 10 heuristics have been originally proposed for the Web, but we tried to apply them to the interface of our Xlet taking into account the differences between the world of the Web and the interactive TV denoted in (Nielsen 2005).

The following are the result of our independent analysis.

1. Visibility of the current state of the system
   a. **Meaning:** Keeping end-users informed about the results of their actions; the system should always keep informed the Users, in reasonable time, about what's happening through adequate feedback responses.
   b. **Results:** Feedback were quite absent! Users were forced to observe changes in the interface hoping to well interpret those modifications.

2. Correspondence between the system and the real world
   a. **Meaning:** Using the language of end-users; this ensures a better understanding and retention of the contents to those visiting the system and avoids the interested User to leave the application being misled by terminology or images that are not associable to the information they're looking for.
   b. **Results:** This heuristic was almost respected; the interface presents simple textual links through coloured buttons that refer to their correspondent colored keys on the remote control.

3. Total control of the navigation by the User
   a. **Meaning:** Empowering Users to freely navigate over the information content of the system, enabling an easy access to the topics according to the expected User's needs; it is crucial to properly set links, buttons and function keys, without ambiguity of meaning and position, on the pages where Users think to find them (according to the expectations derived from the navigation in the previous pages).
   b. **Results:** The User had an acceptable control when surfing the information contents, but it was not completely clear how to make some navigation choices; there wasn't a *stable* menu to offer a synoptic of all the various functionalities, and very often the same button was associated with different features; for instance, the green button was associated with completely different functions in different sections of the Xlet; furthermore a stable menu that helps the User to navigate simpler and more quickly was not provided; moreover, the in-line help was not always directly visible or distinguishable from the normal textual information.

4. Internal and external coherence and adherence to standards commonly accepted by developers
   a. **Meaning:** Maintaining a same graphic style in all the pages to confirm the User that she is moving within the same system; for example, if a User finds a style different from that of the page just visited, she would be forced to analyse every object to verify if she is still in the same system (and if so, in which sector), or if she has gone out in error.
   b. **Results:** This heuristic was respected.

5. Care in the prevention of errors
   a. **Meaning:** Avoiding putting the User in critical situations or potential errors and ensuring her the opportunity to go back to her previous state; links and buttons must indicate clearly their functions so as not to generate false expectations; making always available functions for exiting the program or returning to the "home page".
   b. **Results:** This heuristic was almost neglected; as mentioned for the third heuristic, these messages were not understandable.

6. "Recognize" rather than "remember"

   a. **Meaning:** Designing layouts simple and schematic to facilitate the identification and consultation of information; clearly evidencing links and other factors to let Users understand what to do next, instead of remember what they did in the same situation in previous navigations.

   b. **Results:** This heuristic was almost disregarded too; the layout was problematic and it did not allow neither a sufficient understanding of what to do next, nor an easy remembering of which choices were taken in previous navigations; the layout is simple, the brand at the top and the menu navigation at the bottom remain stable and information is loaded at the centre of the page, but the problem lies in the fact that information goes to mix with the brand and menu generating confusion and not allowing an optimal visual recognition by the User.

7. Promoting flexibility and efficiency

   a. **Meaning:** Giving users the possibility to differentiate the navigation depending on their needs, experience and knowledge of the system; unskilled users, for example, like to be guided step by step, while more experienced users prefer shortcuts.

   b. **Results:** This heuristic was not applicable since the structure of the menus is not very articulated and complex.

8. Minimalist structure and graphics

   a. **Meaning:** Minimizing elements irrelevant or seldom useful; graphics too much colourful, elaborated and big, compared to the texts, are likely to put in the background the relevant information content of the page: users will be to much engaged in finding the meaning of the images and their consistency with the other elements of the page, rather than in catching the information content of the page.

   b. **Results:** Graphics and design was simple but not well organized; the experts noticed the absence of a main incisive brand, while the current one was cumbersome and difficult to understand; the main navigation menu was not stable and badly positioned; information was confused with the brand; the navigation menu was also poorly organized; the four arrows on the screen keypad did not have the same placement in the remote control and that could yield problems when pointing the objects on the screen with the remote control.

9. Provide the User with the means to recognize and repair errors

   a. **Meaning:** Writing error messages that indicate precisely the problems and suggest a constructive solution for them; for example, if a User not successfully completed some fields in a submitted form, the message acknowledging the submission should correctly report the errors so as to enable a prompt recovering and an easy resubmitting.

   b. **Results:** This heuristic was not applicable.

10. Insert help and instructions

    a. **Meaning:** Providing simple online helps; it would be better for the system to be self-explicable, but in case of necessity an online contextual help should be easy to find, small sized and focused on a list of concrete executable actions.

    b. **Results:** Help were very rare and not well defined.

In addition to the ten heuristics for usability, on its website Jakob Nielsen put an article about the Internet American TV and the future requirements for the design of TV-based usable service systems. In his article the scientist describes the main differences between the Internet TV and the Web, drawing a series of specifications for creating graphical interfaces for TV that are effectively usable.

Our claim is that the specifics proposed by Nielsen for the Internet TV are valid also for DTT, since the two platforms share the same severe limitations of use, w.r.t. the Web, namely the fact that the User is watching a relatively distant low resolution TV Set with a remote control, instead of a close high resolution monitor with a keyboard and a pointing device.

We applied the ten specific proposed by Nielsen to our Xlet for the Local Health provider (see Figure 7), and some interesting results emerged.

1. **Guideline 1:** Do not use images exceeding 544 pixels wide and 366 pixels height so as to fall in the size of the TV screen; this because the resolution of a normal TV Set (whether LCD or CRT, if it is not an High Definition screen/channel) is much smaller than that of a computer monitor.
   a. **Results:** This specification was respected even for the background image.
2. **Guideline 2:** Use images only if absolutely necessary.
   a. **Results:** In our Xlet several images were not strictly necessary, for example the picture in the home page was not functional so we eliminated it.
3. **Guideline 3:** Do not enter texts in pictures so as not to encumber legibility.
   a. **Results:** There were texts within images that made it difficult to read the corresponding links; in addition, the use of white characters on blue background made them not readable too.

4. **Guideline 4:** If it is really necessary to use a text within the images use a bold Helvetica 16p or wider.
   a. **Results:** There were texts of various size and colors that confused the User; the size of the texts were much variable and some texts were unreadable, especially those inside buttons.
5. **Guideline 5:** Do not use a layout with columns.
   a. **Results:** Specification respected.
6. **Guideline 6:** If it is strictly necessary to use the layout columns to use that to a maximum of 2 columns and be sure that they are visible in a screen 544 pixels wide.
   a. **Results:** Specification not applicable.
7. **Guideline 7:** If the size of the text exceeds the size of the page, use on-board screen navigation buttons.
   a. **Results:** The specification was partially respected since, as the size of the text exceeded that of the page, the latter was divided into smaller pages as required, but the navigation buttons for browsing were missed!
8. **Guideline 8:** Organize the contents into an hypertext with few nodes.
   a. **Results:** Specification respected.
9. **Guideline 9:** Whenever possible, keep the contents inside a single page.
   a. **Results:** Specification respected.
10. **Guideline 10:** Insert short content.
    a. **Results:** Specification almost respected.

The previous analysis revealed various flaws in the usability of our Xlet so we decided to rewrite it. We needed a design and a graphics more user-friendly, with a brand very light, immediate and complete, that would not be confused with the rest of the application. Routes of navigation must be stable and smooth, with a menu always visible. The system should give immediate feedback to the User in order to facilitate navigation. The contents

Figure 7. Home page of our former Xlet for the local health; it did not fulfil the Nielsen's guidelines for interactive TV

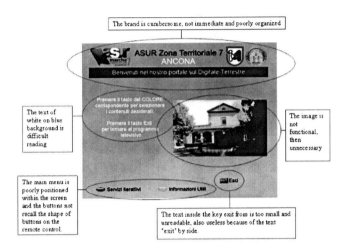

of the application should be readable simply and quickly, and only strictly necessary information should be displayed.

Before moving on to design the new interface we carried on an experimental analysis on a sample of 30 subjects there were asked to fill out a questionnaire assessment of the Xlet. The test produced data valuable for a careful statistical analysis. The measures obtained were:

- The duration of the interaction
- The achievement of the goal
- The number of mistakes
- The nature of the errors
- The degree of satisfaction of the User

All these measures entered the ANOVA test and the "Cluster Analysis"; the results obtained, compared with the evaluation performed in the initial phase, confirmed that our Xlet's user interface had serious usability problems; to perform simple actions, such as entering the Xlet, the User was taking too long. It was necessary to improve the timing of each interaction and make navigation simpler and more intuitive, creating an interface more "ergonomic". From the evaluation of usability and the results of the experimental tests

a new design for the interface were drawn. The new graphical user interface is currently (in turn) subjected to experimental testing of usability, following a cycle of refining, to obtain a product that is perfectly usable by the majority of end-users. As a general fall out of our efforts, now we are trying to reason about the definition of specific guidelines for Digital Terrestrial TV, as those developed by Jakob Nielsen for the American Internet TV.

Sending and Receiving E-Mails through the DTT

If the decoder is connected to the telephone line, it can receive an IP address from the Service Centre through some Internet Protocol as the "Point to Point Protocol" Once received the IP address, the User is *connected to the Internet*. After the WEB, the most important Internet applications is the email. We immediately thought that a light but efficient and usable client for SMTP/POP3 would be much useful for DTT. That client could be used to send/receive simple emails to/from the Local Health, both by healthy people and patients. For instance, the formers could use email for asking information or confirming appointments, the latters could receive reports of examinations or send diagnostic data collected at home (by digital portable diagnostic devices). The latter example shows that our client has two requirements other than simplicity and usability, i.e.:

- It should accept attachments according to the MIME standardization.
- It should comply the Public Key Infrastructure and accept governmental SC to achieve authentication and confidentiality for the messages and their attachments.

Figure 8 shows the flow of the encrypted email started by the patient from the STB with the Smart Card.

So, the main functions of the client are:

- Connect to POP3 servers.
- Download emails with POP3 protocol.
- Manage as simply as possible the emails and their attachments.
- Edit messages and eventually attach files.
- Encrypt the emails and their attachments through the RSA algorithm.
- Send the encrypted emails.

The client has been conceived as a sequence of pages that will be visualized or not depending on the choices of the User. Each page is a class with its own methods The interface respects the previously defined specifics and guidelines for usability of a DTT application. Figures 9-12 show the pages that the User has to interact with (for editing a new email message, attaching files to it, encrypting it, sending and decrypting the received answer from the physician).

Each page has functional buttons of the right and a legend in the bottom. The interaction schema does not change through the various pages. The User selects the buttons with the arrow keys on the remote control; once the desired button is selected, the correspondent procedure is activated by pressing the key "ok". For editing the message the software keypad appears in the lower part of the screen.

Although this is a general purpose email client, we developed it with a particular use case in mind which is described in a video on YouTube (http://youtu.be/bChsnk3qoN8). A cardiac patient makes a self-examination at home with her portable ECG and sends it as a PDF file to the STB via BlueTooth (our STB had a BlueTooth dongle at its gate RS232). The patient then sends the file to the cardiologist attached to an email (Figure

Figure 8. Encrypting emails with the governmental smart cards

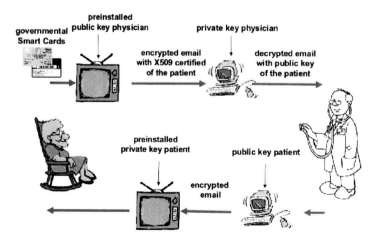

Figure 9. Improved usability of emailing for attaching homemade examinations (e.g. ECG)

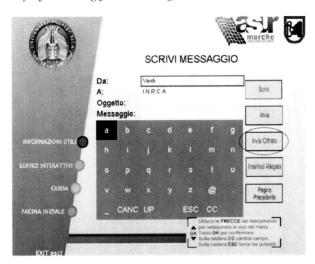

Figure 10. Selecting a preinstalled public key of a physician to send the email

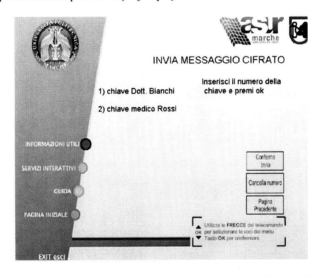

Figure 11. Receiving an email with a report (of an examination) attached and deciphering it

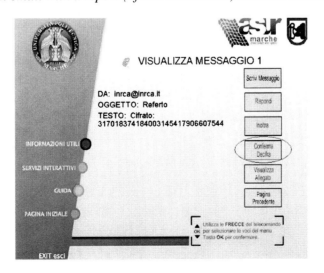

Figure 12. Selecting the (number of the) public key of a physician to decrypt the received email

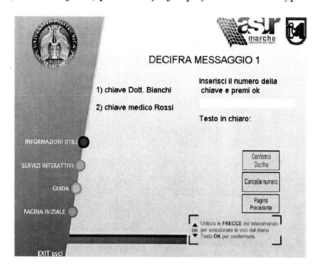

9) ciphered and authenticated through the use of her electronic identity card. After pressing the button a feedback page informs the User about the result of the operation. When the cardiologist sends back the report, the patient starts the same client to receive the email with its attached report (Figure 11). This page offers several functionalities: deciphering the email with the public key of the sender, visualizing (on the TV screen) the attachments, forwarding the email and replying it.

Payments over the DTT

Since *T-Government* includes payments, we further explored the potential of DTT by assessing the feasibility of the *T-Commerce*, i.e. the *E-Commerce* over the DTT. We tried to identify areas of weakness or strength, risks and advantages of the *T-Commerce*, whose key point w.r.t. the *E-Commerce* is still the presence of the reader of Smart Card on the STB. However, making payments over the Web is simpler since the *T-Commerce* scenario is a bit more complex. Figures 13 and 14 sketches the differences. The actors involved in the *E-Commerce* are:

1.   A buyer who purchases the goods from home

2.   An on-line shop that exposes the merchandise and sends it to the buyer

3.   The bank that handles the payments.

The purchase will be executed only if the store and the bank will be able to gain the full confidence of the buyer. To ensure proper feeling of confidence, the *E-Commerce* applications provides the seller with only the data about the clearance of goods, while the data regarding the payment (credit cards or checking accounts) are sent to the server of the bank without the intermediary of the seller. The Figure 13 shows the steps performed to complete a purchase (assuming that the user authentication has already occurred on the server of the electronic store and the goods have already been chosen):

1.   The User communicates to the store her intention to buy the goods previously selected.

2.   The store's server communicates for the first time with the bank's server reporting that someone is going to make a payment of a certain amount.

3.   The bank's server responds by delivering to the store a token for the payment session; that token will then be resubmitted by the

Figure 13. The steps for E-Commerce transaction

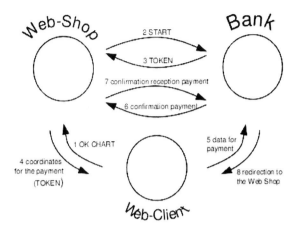

Figure 14. The steps for T-Commerce transaction

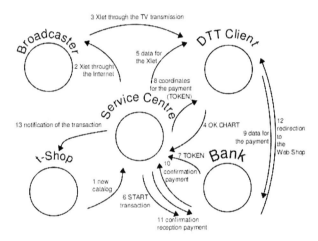

User to correctly recognize and complete the operation.

4. The shop redirects the User to the bank server delivering her the token for the payment session.

5. The User communicates for the first time with the bank's server and provides (in addition to the session token) the data for the payment, either by credit card or by bank transfer.

6. After the reception of the payment, the bank announces to the store that the User marked with the token actually paid the goods.

7. The seller responds with an "OK" signal to the information received from the bank.

8. The bank notifies the User that the transaction was successful and redirects her to the Web store for the final operations.

Data-transfer from the User and the bank is made through the HTTPS protocol. Of course this system, while avoiding the theft of sensitive data, cannot secure transactions from any fraud. In particular, there is no way of knowing if the Web shop to which we are passing the credits for a purchase has all the credentials in order. As you might guess from the diagram, there are two distinct server-side applications with only a single point of contact, which is the "token". Thus, allocating the responsibility for frauds means simply identifying at what stage the problem occurred. This separation between the bank's and the merchant's servers was strongly desired by the formers to avoid any kind of involvement in frauds organized by fake Web stores.

Teleshopping exists as long as the television itself, but the ability to *purchase* goods directly *through* the use of the TV set, while sitting on the living room, is one a main innovations introduced by Interactive TV. All problems of safety and feeling of trust related to *E-Commerce* are inherited by *T-Commerce*. We already pointed out the main differences between the Internet and the DTT, let's now add a couple of specific differences between *T-Commerce* and *E-Commerce*:

- Programming language
  - There are many programming language for *E-Commerce*; just take one of the widespread scripting languages suitable for DBMS (such as PHP, ASP or JavaScript) and almost everyone who has access to the Internet will be able to see the storefront; for the *T-Commerce* instead, language is forced: the STBs host only a customised Java Virtual Machine, so the only language used at *the client side* is a Java *with many limitations* (on the server-side language is left to the programmer of the e-store).
- Transmission channel
  - With *E-Commerce* data is transferred through the internet connection and client applications are executed after being downloaded through a Web browser; with *T-Commerce* client applications are downloaded from the air within a broadcast carousel multiplexed into an MPEG video stream.
- Actors

  - In the DTT scenario there are two more roles, the *broadcaster* and the *service centre* (this latter role could be played by one of the other actors, apart from the client).

More actors implies more complex scenarios and, hence, more risks of fraud. There are some open problems:

- Who's responsible for the security of the Xlets? (the bank, the service center, the broadcaster, the e-shop)
- Who's the owner of the Xlets? (the bank, the service center, the broadcaster, the e-shop)
- Who will pay for the damage caused by fraud?

Probably banks will want the maintain the ownership of the applications, so that nobody can interfere or even know the internal management of the transactions. But the broadcaster and the Service Center too could claim the ownership of the applications as they hosts them on their servers! In fact it is not probable that each e-shop will maintain its server for *T-Commerce* applications, so a Service Centre could take charge of hosting the server on behalf of the online store (Figure 14 shows the steps for a *T-Commerce* transaction in such a case).

Going back to our *T-government* application, we wanted to include in our Xlet a function to allow citizens to pay the fee for the Local Health service directly through the Digital TV (Figures 15 and 16). Due to administrative and political constraints our proposal was purely demonstrative, as for exploring the potential of the technology and the platform of DTT. We hypothesized that the payment could be in one of these ways:

1. Using a prepaid lodged with the Local Health
2. By Credit Card
3. By PayPal

Figure 15. First page of the payment function

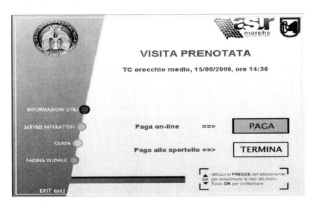

Figure 16. Choice of the method of payment

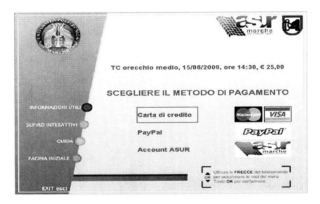

CONCLUSION

Decoders of DTT could be an interesting new access medium for health services because:

1. They are in every home.
2. They can be connected to the internet.
3. They have a card reader.
4. Their applications are broadcast transparently (along with the TV transmission) and need not to be installed.
5. They are switched-on almost 12 hour per day.
6. They are usable by elderly people that cannot use a computer.

The architecture we describe could be used for monitoring health parameters of patients at home, but we believe that DTT is more useful for providing high value healthcare services to healthy people. As a proof of concept we developed a suite of DTT applications, from simple informative to complex transactional ones, from sending and receiving secure emails with attached files to booking examinations and paying fees or tickets.

Unfortunately, during our study we have not had the chance to experience the interaction between an MHP applications and its corresponding TV program, since this kind of experiments needs the cooperation of television studios. Our suite of applications is completely unrelated from the television programs. This use of MHP applications does not fully exploit the interactive potential of DTT, which are fully employed only in a synergy with the underlying TV program that is going on the air at that time on that same channel. In our opinion, the future of interactive TV will be played at this level.

The only conclusion we can draw from our proof of concept is that, for simple and frequent online operations, interactive television can be very handy, especially for people still not familiar with the Internet and the Web.

This conclusion is not to be considered an end point, of course, but as just the first step to realize the scenario described above. It will be important the role that STB manufacturers will like to play in the project of making Digital TV a new universal access to the information society. Some important steps to be performed by producers are:

- To develop and directly connect medical devices to the STBs,
- To improve the STBs with embedded (A) DSL and Wi-Fi connections,
- To improve the usability of the remote control.

ACKNOWLEDGMENT

This work could not have been done without the effort of many students of electronic engineering and computer science from the "Università Politecnica delle Marche". So, I thank Serafino Nardini, Guido Lappa, Moreno Paolini, Fabio Maritan, Jonathan Filippini, Matteo Traù, Roberto Reinini, Alessandro Plebani, Luca Ventura, Ilaria Santini, Valentina Belfiori, Erik Marchi, Fabio Talamonti, Daniela Barigelli, Matteo Pandolfi, Riccardo Biancucci, Oscar Baffoni, Domenico Ranieri, Andrea Pace, Fabio Bracalente, Michele Bellotti and our expert in usability, Vera Stara. A special thank to Fabio Tonucci and Giuseppe Giampieri, respectively *manager* and *executive engineer* of the Information Systems Department of the the Ancona's Local Health, for having provided their laboratories, their staff, their competence and their time.

REFERENCES

Amerini, I., Ballocca, G., Becarelli, R., Borri, R., Caldelli, R., & Filippini, F. (2010). A DVB-MHP web browser to pursue convergence between digital terrestrial television and Internet. *Multimedia Tools and Applications, 50*, 381–414. doi:10.1007/s11042-009-0415-4

Barrie, G., Nicholas, D., Huntington, P., & Williams, P. (2003). Digital interactive television: Health information platform of the future? *Aslib Proceedings, 55*(5-6), 346–356.

Chirico, U. (2006). *Programmazione delle Smart Card.* Gruppo Editoriale Infomedia (in italian)

Chorianopoulos, K., & Spinellis, D. (2006). User interface evaluation of interactive TV: A media studies perspective. *Universal Access in the Information Society, 5*(2), 209–218. doi:10.1007/s10209-006-0032-1

ETSI TS 102 812 v.1.2.1. (2003). *Digital video broadcasting (DVB) – Multimedia home platform (MHP)* specification 1.1.1. Retrieved from http://www.etsi.org

Leiva, M. T. G., Starks, M., & Tambini, D. (2006). Overview of digital television switchover policy in Europe, the United States and Japan. *Info: The Journal of Policy, Regulation and Strategy for Telecommunication, Information and Media, 8*(3), 32-46. ISSN 1463-6697

Maglaveras, N., Chouvarda, I., Koutkias, V., Lekka, I., Tsakali, M., & Tsetoglou, S. … Balas, E. A. (2003). Citizen centered health and lifestyle management via interactive TV: The PANACEIA-ITV health system. *AMIA Annuual Symposium Proceedings,* (pp. 415-419).

Maternaghan, C., & Turner, K. J. (2010). A component framework for telecare and home automation. In *Proceedings of the 7th IEEE Consumer Communications and Networking Conference.*

Melendreras-Ruiz, R. (2008), ImplanTDT: Usability laboratory, real user DTT monitoring platform and MHP-based services. In *Proceedings of the 5th IEEE Consumer Communications and Networking Conference.*

Monk, A. F. (2000). User-centred design. *Proceedings of the IFIP TC9 WG9.3 International Conference on Home Oriented Informatics and Telematics, "IF at Home: Virtual Influences on Everyday Life": Information, Technology and Society,* (pp. 181-190).

Morris, S., & Smith-Chaigneau, A. (2005). *Interactive TV standards: A guide to MHP, OCAP and Java TV.* Focal Press.

Mourouzis, A., Boutsakis, E., Ntoa, S., Antona, M., & Stephanidis, C. (2007). An accessible and usable soft keyboard. *Human-Computer Interaction, 6,* 961–970.

Nielsen, J. (2005). *UseIT.* Retrieved from. http://www.useit.com

Papa, F., Livi, S., Cornacchia, M., Nicolò, E., & Sapio, B. (2010). Factors affecting the usage of payment services through digital television in Italy. *EuroITV'10 - Proceedings of the 8th International Interactive TV and Video Conference,* (pp. 209-215).

Pemberton, L., & Griffiths, R. (2003). Usability evaluation techniques for interactive television. In *Proceedings of the 10th HCII Conference.*

Rankl, W., & Effing, W. (2004). *Smart card handbook.* Wiley.

Chapter 15
Static Telecytological Applications for Proficiency Testing

Stavros Archondakis
Army Hospital, Greece

ABSTRACT

In recent years, informatics and computer sciences have changed dramatically the practice of clinical cytopathology. New types of cameras and microscopes, connected to computers made possible image capture and transmission (telecytology). The wide implementation of telemedical systems in the field of cytopathology became a necessity dictated by the need of real-time results for therapeutic decisions. A telemedical application is a valuable tool for cytopathologists in order to manage and promote inter-laboratory collaboration. The result is better cytological data management and sharing. ISO 15189:2007 for medical laboratories requires successful participation in proficiency testing programs. This chapter emphasizes on the necessity of developing a proficiency test for cytopathology labs wishing to be accredited according to ISO 15189:2007, and examines the feasibility of using low cost telemedical applications and solutions for this purpose. Furthermore, this chapter gives clear and comprehensive guidance concerning various financial, legal, professional, and ethical problems in this field.

INTRODUCTION

Accreditation is the process by which a certified organization or agency recognizes that a facility or service meets specific pre-established standards (Pantanowitz et al., 2009). ISO 15189:2007 constitutes an international accreditation standard, which can be used by medical laboratories wishing to improve their quality standards (Archondakis et

al., 2009). ISO 15189:2007 requirements consist of a group of general guidelines that will help laboratories establish and enhance their quality systems (Pantanowitz et al., 2009). There is an ongoing demand by all interested parties, such as regulators, laboratory accreditation bodies and customers for implementation of more measures that increase confidence in cytological laboratories performance.

DOI: 10.4018/978-1-4666-2979-0.ch015

According to ISO 15189:2007 requirements, one of the greatest challenges facing cytopathology laboratories today is the design and implementation of a board certified external quality control program (proficiency testing). The purpose of the adopted program should be to ensure that microscopic (cytological) findings are correctly identified and interpreted by laboratory personnel (Pantanowitz et al., 2009).

During the last three decades external control measures have been proposed for quality control and quality assurance purposes, in order to monitor and further improve cervical screening diagnostic accuracy and reliability (Husain et al., 1974; Melamed, 1976; Mitchell et al. 1988; Koss, 1989; Lundbergh 1989). External quality control includes mainly proficiency testing programs and special workshops or courses (Davey et al., 1993; Thompson, 1989; Plott et al., 1987; Valente & Schantz, 1992). Typical purposes for a special proficiency test in the field of cytopathology include:

- Evaluation of the performance of laboratories for specific tests.
- Monitoring of cytological laboratories performance.
- Identification of problems in laboratories.
- Initiation of actions for improvement.
- Establishment of the effectiveness and comparability of test or measurement methods.
- Education of participating laboratories based on the outcomes of such comparisons.
- Identification of interlaboratory differences.
- Validation of uncertainty claims.
- Production of reference materials and assessment of their suitability for use in specific procedures.

Telecytology can be defined as the process of diagnostic cytopathology performed on digital images, transferred via telecommunication networks from one site to another. Telecytological diagnosis can be achieved either with the use of cytological pictures viewed in real time from the microscope (dynamic telecytological systems), or with the use of cytological pictures that are first captured in a digital format and then transmitted to distant observers (static telecytological systems) (Weinstein et al., 1997; Georgoulakis et al., 2010).

Static image capture and transfer is the most straightforward method. It only requires the capture of cytological images via a digital camera and their transport for remote evaluation. Dynamic telecytology systems require a real-time ability to move about the specimen, focus, and change magnifications, via remote robotic or local control. In whole-slide scanning and transmission systems, entire cytology slides are captured at high resolution and the data can be transmitted and manipulated from one site to another.

Telecytology is mainly used for obtaining expert opinions on difficult cases and for educational purposes (Archondakis et al., 2009). However, little information exists about its probable use for the development of proficiency testing programs in the field of cytopathology. Most of the current studies have found a high (90%–95%) concordance between telecytological and glass slide diagnoses but they are referring to a small number of cases (Archondakis et al., 2009; Della Mea et al., 2000; Briscoe et al., 2000; Raab et al., 1996).

A digital cytological image is mainly composed of a two-dimensional array of numbers (bitmap or raster image), each element of which represents a pixel (Pantanowitz et al., 2009). Digital images size can be compressed for transmission or storage purposes via "lossless" (no loss of data) or "lossy" (some detail is lost. compression algorithms (Pantanowitz et al., 2009).

The purpose of this chapter is to examine the feasibility of developing an external quality control program for cytopathology labs wishing to be accredited according to ISO 15189:2007, by using low cost telemedical applications and solutions. Furthermore, we present our own experience from the experimental use of a low cost static telecytological system as an unofficial proficiency testing provider to all cytology labs wishing to implement external quality control policies in their everyday workflow. Finally we give clear and comprehensive guidance concerning various financial, legal, professional, and ethical problems in this field.

BACKGROUND

Quality control defines service's quality, imparting to it the credibility needed for its intended purpose, while quality assurance activities measure the degree to which desired outcomes are successful (Wiener et al., 2007). Quality control may be internal or external. Quality control in the field of cytology is mainly achieved by slide rescreening or by clinical-histological correlation of cytological diagnoses (Wiener et al., 2007). Many slide rescreening procedures have been proposed for quality assurance purposes, such as rapid reviewing of smears initially reported as negative or inadequate, rapid preview/prescreening of all smears, random rescreening, targeted rescreening of specific patient groups, seeding abnormal cases into the screening pools, retrospective rescreening of negative cytology specimens from patients with a current high grade abnormality and automated rescreening of smears initially reported as negative (Wiener et al., 2007). The laboratory manager is responsible to choose the most appropriate method for quality assurance purposes, according to the specific needs of his own laboratory (Wiener et al., 2007).

Proficiency testing (PT) is a process for checking actual laboratory performance usually by means of interlaboratory comparisons (Woodhouse et al., 1999; Cramer et al., 1991). Results from proficiency testing are an indication of a laboratory's competence and are an integral part of the assessment and accreditation process (Woodhouse et al., 1999; Cramer et al., 1991). According to ISO 15189: 2007, all accredited laboratories must conduct proficiency tests in

accordance with their normal patient testing and reporting procedures (Pantanowitz et al., 2009).

The practice of diagnostic cytopathology performed on digital images is a novel process that can be used for obtaining expert opinions on difficult cases from remote laboratories (telecytology) (Archondakis et al., 2009).

Telecytological diagnosis can be achieved either with the use of cytological pictures viewed in real time from the microscope (dynamic telecytological systems), or with the use of cytological pictures that are first captured in a digital format and then transmitted to distant observers (static telecytological systems)(Archondakis et al., 2009; Stamataki et al. 2008). The static telecytology systems have the advantage of considerably lower cost, but they only allow the capture of a selected subset of microscopic fields (Pantanowitz et al., 2009). The dynamic telecytology systems permit evaluation of the cytological material present on a slide (Yamashiro et al., 2004). These systems may be hampered by high network traffic and their high cost of purchasing and maintaining may be unaffordable by small laboratories wishing to participate in proficiency testing programs.

A small number of studies have focused, so far, on the possible role of telecytology as a tool of diagnosis and consultation in the everyday workflow (Archondakis et al., 2009).

Diagnostic concordance in telecytology is measured by diagnostic agreement and reproducibility (Stamataki et al. 2008; Pantanowitz et al., 2009). Agreement is the total or proportional number of cases in which the same diagnosis was reached between or within observers, including the part of the agreement that may be attributed to chance (Landis and Koch, 1977). Reproducibility is part of the agreement that cannot be explained purely by chance (Landis and Koch, 1977). Reproducibility is measured by the κ statistic. Within the positive κ values and in accordance with the study by Landis and Koch, the agreement was interpreted as follows: a range of 0.00– 0.20 indicated slight agreement, a range of 0.21–0.40 indicated fair agreement, a range of 0.41–0.60 indicated moderate agreement, a range of 0.61–0.80 indicated very god agreement, while a range of 0.61–0.80 indicated excellent agreement (Landis and Koch, 1977).

The use of digital images in quality control/assurance programs eliminates the need for glass slides retrieval from the laboratory's registry (at least at the point of examination), allows annotations to be added to images, enhances the ability to rapidly transmit and remotely share images electronically for several purposes (telecytology, conferences, education, quality assurance, peer review) and protects more efficiently patients anonymity (Archondakis et al., 2009).

Moreover the use of digital images for quality assurance programs is more practical and time consuming, although some additional time has to be spent during glass slides conversion to digital images.

Static telecytology systems are preferred due to their low cost by laboratories that cannot afford the high cost of buying and maintaining dynamic systems (Archondakis et al., 2009).

The limitations and diagnostic errors related to telecytology that are already mentioned by some authors may cause misinterpretation of digital images by less experienced participants (Briscoe et al., 2000). Appropriate field selection, sufficient image quality, and especially diagnostic expertise are the most crucial parameters ensuring the proper function of a static telecytological system (Archondakis et al., 2009).

The most common manifestations of interobserver discrepancy is upgrading of the telecytological diagnosis to a definitive carcinoma diagnosis or downgrading of a suspicious telecytological diagnosis to a rather benign lesion because of image deficiencies (Archondakis et al., 2009).

The author's laboratory's was the first private cytological laboratory in Greece which was officially certified according to ISO 15189:2007. In less than four years and in collaboration with colleagues from public hospitals, the laboratory has constructed an electronic library of more than 45.000 representative digital images of histologically confirmed specimens of gynaecological and non gynaecological cytology. This electronic database is currently used for interlaboratory diagnostic comparisons while the whole project is scheduled to be certified as an individual proficiency testing provider in the near future. Participants experience in making telecytological diagnoses is constantly recorded for further evaluation in the near future. Statistical parameters are continuously recorded while practical problems that may be encountered contribute to continuous self-improvement of this pilot program.

STATIC TELECYTOLOGICAL APPLICATIONS FOR PROFICIENCY TESTING PROVIDING PURPOSES IN A PRIVATE CYTOPATHOLOGY LABORATORY

In the author's laboratory, selected cytology slides with histological confirmation are retrospectively selected from the laboratory's registry or donated by cooperating cytology labs. The slides collected for the production of the digital material from the Cytology Laboratory's registries are coming from already histologically confirmed cases (Pantanowitz et al., 2009). The histological examination consists the best way cytology slides can be validated. Inadequate validation of test slides could lead to indiscriminate failure of qualified, competent personnel participating in external quality control programs (Pantanowitz et al., 2009).

The author's laboratory's managerial and technical personnel has all necessary education, resources and technical competence required. The minimum levels of qualification and experience necessary for the key positions within its organization are already defined. Contracted or additional technical personnel is not used for the time being.

The laboratory's director has authorized specific personnel to:

1. Select appropriate proficiency test items (cytology slides and digital cytological images).
2. Plan proficiency testing schemes.
3. Operate specific equipment (microscopes and cameras mounted on them).
4. Prepare, handle and distribute proficiency test items (digital cytological images).
5. Conduct statistical analysis of telecytological diagnoses.
6. Evaluate the participants diagnostic performance.
7. Give opinions and interpretations on participants telecytological diagnoses.
8. Authorize the issue of intrelaboratory comparisons reports.

The laboratory ensures that:

1. There are appropriate facilities and equipment for proficiency test item manufacturing, handling and storage.
2. There are appropriate facilities and equipment for data processing and for communications integrity.
3. The environmental conditions do not compromise the proficiency testing scheme's quality.
4. The methods and equipment used to confirm the content, homogeneity and stability of proficiency testing items (digital cytological images) are appropriately validated and maintained.
5. Processes which directly affect the quality of the proficiency testing scheme are carried out in accordance with prescribed procedures.

The laboratory maintains up-to-date records of authorizations, qualifications, training, skills, competence, and experience of all technical personnel in the professional testing scheme organization. The laboratory director is making sure that staff receive the necessary training to ensure competent performance of all activities affecting the quality of the proficiency testing scheme. The effectiveness of training activities is evaluated and described in detail.

The laboratory director ensures that there are appropriate facilities and equipment for cytology images capturing and storage, for data processing, for communications, and for retrieval of materials and records.

The laboratory director ensures that the environmental conditions do not compromise the quality proficiency testing scheme. All environmental conditions are continuously monitored.

The laboratory has also described in detail the purpose and basic design of the proficiency testing scheme, including the following information:

1. The name and address of the proficiency of each participant.
2. Criteria to be met for participation.
3. Information on what the participants are to identify during each telecytology round.
4. Requirements for the production, quality control, storage and distribution of proficiency test items (digital cytological images).
5. A description of the information provided to participants and the time schedule for the various phases of the proficiency testing scheme.
6. Any information on procedures which participants need to follow in order to perform the tests.
7. Preparation of any standardized reporting formats to be used by participants.
8. A detailed description of the statistical analysis to be used.
9. Criteria for the evaluation of performance of participants.
10. A short description of the information to be returned to participants.

11. Actions to be taken in the case of lost or damaged proficiency test items (digital cytological images).

The laboratory has access to the necessary technical expertise and experience in the field of Cytopathology and Statistics and has established an advisory group in order to:

1. Plan specific requirements.
2. Identify and resolve any difficulties expected in the preparation and maintenance of the proficiency testing scheme.
3. Prepare instructions for participants.
4. Make comments on any technical difficulties observed in previous proficiency testing rounds.
5. Provide advice in evaluating the participants performance.
6. Make comments on the results and performance of participants.
7. Respond to feedback from participants.
8. Plan and participate in technical meetings with participants.

The laboratory gives detailed instructions to all participants, concerning the following:

1. The necessity to treat digital cytological images in the same manner as the majority of routinely tested samples.
2. The procedure for viewing the digital images and writing down their final diagnosis.
3. The procedure for recording and reporting test results and associated uncertainties.

The laboratory provides expert commentary on the performance of participants with regard to the following factors:

1. Overall performance against prior expectations.
2. Variation within and between participants, and comparisons with any previous proficiency testing rounds.

3. Possible sources of error (with reference to outliers) and suggestions for improving performance.
4. Advice and educational feedback to participants as part of the continual improvement procedures of participants.

The proficiency testing reports include the following information:

1. The name and contact details for the proficiency testing provider and the coordinator.
2. The date of issue and status of the report.
3. The report number and identification of the proficiency testing scheme.
4. A description of the proficiency test items used (digital cytological images).
5. The participants' results.
6. Comments on participants' performance by the proficiency testing provider and technical advisors.
7. Statistical data and procedures used to statistically analyze the data.
8. Comments or recommendations, related to the outcomes of the proficiency testing round.

The laboratory also provides to all participants details about:

1. The application procedure.
2. The scope of the proficiency testing scheme.
3. The fees for participation.
4. The eligibility criteria for participation.
5. The confidentiality arrangements.

All information supplied by a participant to the laboratory is treated as confidential. The laboratory ensures that the identity of participants is known only to persons involved in the proficiency testing scheme. Participants can waive confidentiality for mutual assistance or for scientific discussion purposes. The laboratory implements specific policies and procedures to ensure valuable information's safety during electronic storage and transmission.

The laboratory's managerial and technical personnel is free from any commercial or financial bias that could adversely affect the quality of their work. The laboratory's managerial and technical personnel has the authority and the resources required for the implementation and improvement of the management system. The laboratory's managerial and technical personnel is also responsible to identify any departures from the management system and to initiate preventive actions. The laboratory implements specific policies and procedures to avoid personnel's involvement in any activities that might diminish confidence in its competence or impartiality. The laboratory director ensures that all employees are aware of their activities importance, provides adequate supervision to all technical staff, has appointed one quality manager for ensuring that the management system is implemented and followed at all times. Finally the laboratory director has appointed deputies for key managerial personnel.

The laboratory retains records of all data relating to each telecytology proficiency testing round for a defined period, including:

1. Instructions to participants.
2. Participants original responses.
3. Data for statistical analysis.
4. Final reports.

The laboratory periodically reviews its proficiency testing activities. More specifically, it reviews:

1. Changes in the volume and type of work.
2. Advisory group or participant feedback.
3. The outcome of recent internal or external audits.
4. Corrective and preventive actions.
5. Complaints and appeals.

The overall economic impact of applying such simple telemedical applications for quality assurance purposes is obvious. While the cost for a proficiency testing provider establishing a scheme in the field of cytopathology by using static cytological images requires about 30.000 euros, the annual cost for maintaining it does not surpass the sum of 10.000 euros. Initial subcontractors contribution to the proficiency testing scheme requires 15.000 euros for slides or digital cytological images submission, as well as for scientific collaboration. On the other hand, the cost for a proficiency testing provider establishing a scheme in the field of cytopathology by using virtual microscopy applications requires about 90.000 euros and the annual cost for maintaining it may surpass the sum of 25.000 euros. Initial subcontractors contribution to the proficiency testing scheme requires 50.000 euros for slides or digital cytological images submission, as well as for scientific collaboration.

Each individual cytology laboratory's annual participation to a proficiency testing scheme, based solely on static telemedical images may range from 400 to 600 euros, depending on each scheme's technical and scientific specifications. Static telecytology solutions reduce dramatically the expenses of postal or courier slide circulation. Even small hospitals can afford to pay annually from 400 to 600 euros for participating to a well scheduled external quality control program in the field of diagnostic cytopathology. The cost for participating in a proficiency testing scheme based on static telemedical applications is only the half of the cost for participating in a proficiency testing scheme based on virtual microscopy.

The sum required for each laboratory's participation is well spent, as it consists the most economic and feasible way for regular evaluation of the laboratories' performance. Each hospital wishing gain recognition for all diagnostic and scientific capabilities of its cytology lab personnel must encourage the participation of all doctors or screeners in a simple proficiency testing scheme based on digital images.

Regular participation to the above mentioned scheme is a valuable tool for in time identification of any kind of laboratory problems, for effective initiation of actions for improvement and for establishment of the effectiveness of cytology as a diagnostic method.

What is most important for all hospitals is that successful participation to a static telecytology external quality control program results in high quality of care and patient safety. The hospital's prestige is upgraded and the cytology laboratory's clients (doctors and patients) feel more confident and satisfied with the cytological diagnoses issued. The hospital demonstrating its commitment to quality care, is automatically raising its clients (both doctors and patients) confidence in the services provided. The image of the diagnostic services offered is automatically improved. The external recognition acquired makes the hospital more competitive, by giving access to new clients.

Participation to an external quality control program stimulates the need for continuous improvement. The digital images initially used for quality assurance purposes, can be archived to the laboratory's files for reference or educational purposes. Laboratory personnel which is already familiarized with digital images evaluation, can more easily participate in telemedical conferences, have better access to large teaching sets, take better annotations, and have in time access to critical electronic data such as radiology images.

Furthermore, the use of telemedical applications in the everyday laboratory practice may stimulate laboratory personnel to contribute to the existing or even create a new external quality control program on the basis of the existing experience on both cytological diagnosis and participation in a telemedical application for proficiency testing reasons.

Finally, we must keep in mind that all hospitals implementing such simple telemedical applications in the field of Cytopathology, have already made the first but crucial step towards accreditation of their laboratory services according to ISO 15189:2007.

Issues, Controversies, Problems

In conventional cytology, specific diagnostic criteria and pitfalls are already described. During static telecytological diagnosis, the cytopathologist has to use the same diagnostic criteria and to avoid the same pitfalls. What makes the telecytological diagnosis more demanding is uncertainty about the real specimen's adequacy or the representativity of the selected images (Archondakis et al., 2009). Static digital images suffer from representing only limited portions of the specimen and hence there is a potential bias of the image acquirer relative to the image observer. The inability of focusing and of image manipulation (contrast, brightness, and color) may cause additional problems.

Cytology slides used for digital images capture must be validated in order to make sure that the initial cytological diagnosis was correct and did not differ significantly from the final histological diagnosis.

Reporting terminology is well established for some categories of cytological specimens such as thyroid fine needle aspiration specimens and cervicovaginal smears. Still cytological diagnosis for the majority of specimens remains descriptive and no specific diagnostic categories have been established and implemented in the everyday laboratory practice. The absence of a universally accepted and adopted reporting terminology is a serious problem for the correct statistical elaboration of cytological diagnoses provided by participants in a proficiency testing scheme. A widely accepted reporting terminology would make easier the implementation of scoring systems, validating participants performance and improvement.

Participation in proficiency testing programs is still poor. Many large cytological Departments are reluctant to implement such practices as a measure of continuous improvement and quality assurance. Even when a proficiency testing program is ordered, only one or two certified cytopathologists are participating.

Last but not least, digital images storage and transmission must follow strict regulations in order to avoid any unauthorized alteration or improper use (Mun et al., 1995).Current standards of electronic medical data handling are still informative, yet the need for a secure electronic environment, especially in the field of static telecytology, continues to grow.

Solutions and Recommendations

The role of the person appointed to pictures' capture and transmission is of paramount importance for the success of a static telecytology system. In our study, the person who captures and transmits the digital images is an already certified cytopathologist with adequate experience in conventional cytological diagnosis. Less specialized personnel, such as inexperienced screeners, may endanger the acquisition of representative images from each cytological slide (Archondakis et al., 2009).

Besides histological examination, other measures for cytology slides validation must be adopted in order to avoid possible indiscriminate failure of qualified, competent personnel (Nagy et al., 2006). Such measures may be verification of cytological diagnosis by board certified, well trained, scientific personnel, establishment of specific scoring system and reporting terminology for all kinds of cytological specimens and finally capturing of a significant number of representative images by certified well trained personnel (Nagy et al.,2006).

The scoring system and reporting terminology may be simplified and possibly inappropriate and unfair for certain cytological specimens. Specific scoring systems and reporting terminologies should be established for each kind of cytological specimens in order to ensure that the cytological diagnoses reflect the clinical implications asso-

ciated with this terminology in modern practice, particularly regarding recommended follow-up (Williams et al.,2001).

Static telecytological systems are affordable by all cytopathology departments and give the opportunity to all scientific personnel to participate in proficiency testing programs, even when there is a significant time difference among participating laboratories (Raab et al., 1996).

Cytology scientific societies should focus on cytology proficiency testing particularities and define special technical aspects such as images size and analysis, suggested testing intervals, diagnostic categories and methodology used for statistical evaluation of the proficiency testing results (Nagy et al., 2006).

Laboratory management should encourage personal participation of all scientific personnel in such proficiency testing programs (Pinco et al., 2009). Laboratory management must have in mind that proficiency testing programs proffered on the basis of static digital images can improve the professional skills of the participating medical staff and make them feel more confident in their daily work.

Proficiency testing providers should ensure that the personnel appointed to pictures' capture and transmission has adequate experience in both conventional and image-based diagnosis. Previous experience in that field should be well documented and recorded (Nagy et al., 2006).

FUTURE RESEARCH DIRECTIONS

During the last decades, the absence of an integrated laboratory quality control program was making cytological diagnosis reliability subjective to various factors and self-assessment was the only way to prove each cytopathology's diagnostic proficiency.

Telecytology, when integrated into the daily workflow, can provide exceptional consultation and professional testing opportunities to distant laboratories. Static telecytology systems are preferred due to their low cost by laboratories that cannot afford the high cost of buying and maintaining dynamic systems. In any case, the cost of participation in a running telecytology program is inexpensive for small cytopathology labs (Archondakis et al., 2009; Nagy et al.,2006). Provincial hospitals where immediate scientific collaboration and support is necessary can take advantage of this great opportunity in order to improve their cytology services (Archondakis et al., 2009).

Future research must focus on the details of the implementation of a static telecytological application for proficiency testing purposes, that is, determining the required testing interval, elucidating the validation criteria applied to electronic material used for proficiency testing purposes and possibly changing the focus of the test from individuals to laboratory level testing.

The diagnostic reliability of static telecytology makes possible its use for further amelioration of the laboratory services, by producing digital educational material for use in web-based training systems (Stergiou et al.2009). These programs can improve the professional skills of the participating medical staff and make them feel more confident in their daily work (Stergiou et al., 2009).

In Greece, the accreditation of the first private cytopathology laboratory according to ISO 15189:2007 is already completed by the National Accreditation Board. Digital material from histologically confirmed cases continues to be collected in cooperation with "Saint Savvas" National Anticancer Hospital and the first static telecytology program will soon apply for accreditation as an individual proficiency testing provider. By the end of the year, this first proficiency testing program on clinical cytology is expected to have given many answers to many unresolved problems in healthcare, while scientific support and collaboration by local and distant cytology labs is expected.

CONCLUSION

Cytological images transmission and remote evaluation allow reproducible diagnoses. Diagnoses made by using static telecytological systems can be as reliable as those made by using conventional microscopy, on the condition that representative images are taken and that the standard cytological diagnostic criteria are applied.

The diagnostic reliability of telecytological systems is a sine qua non for further implementation of this method in external or internal audits and quality assurance programs. Furthermore, digital images can be used in proficiency testing programs for assessing the laboratory's medical staff diagnostic expertise. Specifically, the implementation of telecytology practices in the everyday laboratory workflow meets ISO 15189:2007 requirements.

Telecytology can be used as an economic method for the implementation of quality assurance programs in the everyday laboratory practice, provided that representative images are taken, standard diagnostic criteria are applied and the participants have already acquired sufficient experience in the evaluation of digital images. The use of static telecytology systems for proficiency testing provision is possible and the first steps towards this direction are already made in Greece.

REFERENCES

Archondakis, S., Georgoulakis, J., & Stamataki, M. (2009). Telecytology: A tool for quality assessment and improvement in the evaluation of thyroid fine-needle aspiration specimens. *Telemedicine Journal and E Health. The Official Journal of American Telemedicine Association*, *15*(7), 713–717. doi:10.1089/tmj.2009.0037

Briscoe, D., Adair, C. F., & Thompson, L. D. (2000). Telecytologic diagnosis of breast fine needle aspiration biopsies. *Acta Cytologica*, *44*, 175–180. doi:10.1159/000326357

Cramer, S. F., Roth, L. M., Ulbright, T. M., & Mills, S. E. (1991). The mystique of the mistake—With proposed standards for validating proficiency tests. *American Journal of Clinical Pathology, 96*, 774–777.

Davey, D., Nielsen, M. L., & Frable, W. J. (1993). Improving accuracy in gynecologic cytology. *Archives of Pathology & Laboratory Medicine, 117*, 1193–1198.

Della Mea, V., Cataldi, P., & Pertoldi, B. (2000). Combining dynamic and static robotic telepathology: A report on 184 consecutive cases of frozen sections, histology and cytology. *Analytical Cellular Pathology, 20*, 33–39.

Friedman, C. P., & Wyatt, J. C. (2001). Publication bias in medical informatics. *Journal of the American Medical Informatics Association, 8*, 189–191. doi:10.1136/jamia.2001.0080189

Georgoulakis, J., Archondakis, S., & Panayiotides, I. (2011). Study on the reproducibility of thyroid lesions telecytology diagnoses based upon digitized images. *Diagnostic Cytopathology, 39*, 495–499. doi:10.1002/dc.21419

Husain, O. A., Butler, E. B., & Evans, D. M. D. (1974). Quality control in cervical cytology. *Journal of Clinical Pathology, 27*, 935–944. doi:10.1136/jcp.27.12.935

Koss, L. G. (1989). The Papanicolaou test for cervical cancer detection: A triumph and a tragedy. *Journal of the American Medical Association, 261*, 737–743. doi:10.1001/jama.1989.03420050087046

Landis, J. R., & Koch, G. G. (1977). The measurement of observer agreement for categorical data. *Biometrics, 33*, 159–174. doi:10.2307/2529310

Lundbergh, G. D. (1989). Quality assurance in cervical cytology: The Papanicolaou smear. *Journal of the American Medical Association, 262*, 1672–1679. doi:10.1001/jama.1989.03430120126035

Melamed, M. R. (1976). Quality control in the cytology laboratory. *Acta Cytologica, 20*, 203–206.

Mitchell, H., Medley, G., & Drake, M. (1988). Quality control measures for cervical cytology laboratories. *Acta Cytologica, 32*, 288–292.

Mun, S. K., Esayed, A. M., & Tohme, W. G. (1995). Teleradiology/telepathology requirements and implementation. *Journal of Medical Systems, 19*, 15–164. doi:10.1007/BF02257066

Nagy, G. K., & Newton, L. E. (2006). Cytopathology proficiency testing: Where do we go from here? *Diagnostic Cytopathology, 34*, 257–264. doi:10.1002/dc.20361

Pantanowitz, L., Hornish, M., & Goulart, R. A. (2009). The impact of digital imaging in the field of cytopathology. *CytoJournal, 6*(6).

Pinco, J., Goulart, R. A., & Otis, C. N. (2009). Impact of digital image manipulation in cytology. *Archives of Pathology & Laboratory Medicine, 133*(1), 57–61.

Plott, A. E., Martin, F. J., & Cheek, S. W. (1987). Measuring screening skills in gynecologic: Results of voluntary self-assessment. *Acta Cytologica, 31*, 911–923.

Raab, S. S., Zaleski, M. S., & Thomas, P. A. (1996). Telecytology: Diagnosis accuracy in cervical-vaginal smears. *American Journal of Clinical Pathology, 105*, 599–603.

Stamataki, M., Anninos, D., & Brountzos, E. (2008). The role of liquid-based cytology in the investigation of thyroid lesions. *Cytopathology, 19*(1), 11–18.

Stergiou, N., Georgoulakis, J., & Margari, N. (2009). Using a web-based system for the continuous distance education in cytopathology. *International Journal of Medical Informatics, 78*(12), 827–838. doi:10.1016/j.ijmedinf.2009.08.007

Thompson, D. W. (1989). Canadian experience in cytology proficiency. *Acta Cytologica, 33*, 484–486.

Valente, P. T., & Schantz, H. D. (1992). Proficiency testing performance in a workshop setting: Implications for implementation of CLIA 88. *Acta Cytologica, 36*, 581.

Weinstein, L. J., Epstein, J. I., & Edlow, D. (1997). Static image analysis of skin specimens: The application of telepathology to frozen section evaluation. *Human Pathology, 28*, 22–29. doi:10.1016/S0046-8177(97)90274-4

Wiener, H. G., Klinkhamer, P., Schenck, U., & Bulten, J. (2007). Laboratory guidelines and quality assurance practices for cytology. In Arbyn, M., Anttila, A., & Jordan, J. (Eds.), *European guidelines for quality assurance in cervical cancer screening*. Luxembourg: Office of Official Publication European Union.

Williams, B. H., Mullick, F. G., & Butler, D. R. (2001). Clinical evaluation of an international static image-based telepathology service. *Human Pathology, 32*, 1309–1317. doi:10.1053/hupa.2001.29649

Woodhouse, S. L., Schulte, M. A., & Stastny, J. F. (1999). Proficient or deficient—On the razor's edge: Establishing validity in cytology proficiency testing. *Diagnostic Cytopathology, 20*, 255–256. doi:10.1002/(SICI)1097-0339(199905)20:5<255::AID-DC1>3.0.CO;2-J

Yamashiro, K., Kawamura, N., & Matsubayashi, S. (2004). Telecytology in Hokkaido Island, Japan: Results of primary telecytodiagnosis of routine cases. *Cytopathology, 15*(4), 221–227. doi:10.1111/j.1365-2303.2004.00147.x

KEY TERMS AND DEFINITIONS

Accreditation: Procedure by which an authoritative body gives formal recognition that a body or person is competent to carry out specific tasks.

Cytopathology: Medical Specialty based on microscopic evaluation of cells from various human organs.

International Organization for Standardization (ISO): A worldwide federation of national standards bodies (ISO member bodies). The work of preparing International Standards is normally carried out through ISO technical committees.

Proficiency Testing: Evaluation of participant performance against pre-established criteria by means of interlaboratory comparisons. The term may include quantitative scheme, qualitative scheme, sequential scheme, simultaneous scheme, single occasion exercise, continuous scheme, sampling or data transformation and interpretation.

Telecytology: Process of diagnostic cytopathology performed on digital images, transferred via telecommunication networks from one site to another.

Chapter 16
Telemedicine in Emergency:
A First Aid Hospital Network Experience

Vincenzo Gullà
Aditech S.R.L, Italy

Corrado Cancellotti
Hospital "High Chiascio" of Gubbio, Italy

ABSTRACT

Emergency events are always very critical to manage as in most cases there is a human life risk. Such events could become even more serious when occurring in remote areas not equipped with adequate healthcare facilities, able to manage life risk. This is the case in many rural geographical areas. In such scenarios telemedicine can play a very important and determinant role. This is mainly the basis of the experience described in the following chapter about telemedicine application in a small hospital located in the town of Branca, near Gubbio Italy. The first aid department, responsible for emergency support in a territory where distances between houses and hospital is quite important and the lack of healthcare structures and speedways connections makes it even more difficult, has decided to use telemedicine solutions to face the emergency events. The experience has shown how the use of Videocommunication based telemedicine systems has improved the service and what procedural impact the adoption of such technology has required. A brief description of the experience and highlights of the service still under experimentation will be shown in the following.

INTRODUCTION

The term "telemedicine" is a neologism arising from the composition of two terms: telematics (i.e. the set of applications derived from the integration of information technology with telecommunications, based on the exchange of data or the access to archives through the telephone network) and medicine. Telemedicine de facto involves the use of telecommunications, information and computer technologies to support the healthcare providers. Fittingly, then, telemedicine is defined as "the use of remote medical competence in the place where the need arises" and wide areas a very appropriate for such applications (see Figure 1).

Upon this principle the Branca hospital Emergency department has recently started a very new experience. The department was equipped with a

DOI: 10.4018/978-1-4666-2979-0.ch016

Figure 1. Map of the area covered by the service provision

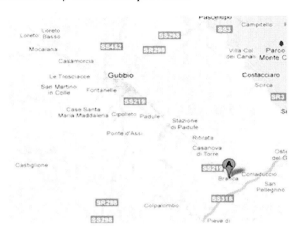

new telemedicine system able to create a two way video link with rescue crews during an emergency intervention, provide a real time medical consultation and guidelines to the onsite crew to manage the event. It is in fact a centralized system which enables the emergency physician to monitor the patient, subject to an emergency intervention directly in the ambulance or in the patient's own home, thanks to the use of video communication and mobile 3G connections. Such a system is revealed as an instrument of great value. It is optimal for supported medical resources that provide assistance to extended geographical areas but sparsely populated and the distances between the patient's home and hospital are often important (Oh, Rizo, Enkin, & Jadad, 2005; Pattichis et al., 2002).

BACKGROUND

Our experience has shown that telemedicine can provide many advantages to the NHS, to service providers, healthcare organizations, physicians and patients. With regard to the NHS, it is undeniable that the uptake of telemedicine can lead to a significant lowering of direct and indirect costs of healthcare (just think of the reduction of unnecessary administrative work, greater ratio-

nalization in the use of staff, as well as greater effectiveness in prevention). For companies and service providers or healthcare organizations, telemedicine may involve the general improvement of services and increase simplification in cooperation between specialized care centers and primary health care centers, particularly in emergencies and in acute cases, as well as the possibility of adaptation of healthcare to sudden rises of the number of patients (e.g. during earthquakes or disasters). Thus remains evident that telemedicine is able to provide medical services in remote areas, especially in cases where this is imposed by the need to eliminate the space-time distances when emergency events occur. For physicians and healthcare workers generally the use of telemedicine involves definitely an incentive to increase professionalism through systems such as Teleconsultation and videoconferencing, making it easier and cheaper to upgrade professional skills, i.e. through the exchange of texts, data research and generally increase the quality of a doctor's decision making process, being able to access more quickly and easily, to information about the patient, history and medical available resource.(Eysenbach, 2001, Currell, Urquhart, Wainwright, & Lewis, 2006).

In particular it should be noted that the use of telemedicine in healthcare must comply with the principle, valid for the adoption of all the new technologies, that it "must always be carried out in the context of a program, trying to replace the concept that the use of technology is able to rationalize processes and pathways so unquestioned, carefully planning analysis and evaluations based on experiences already gained" (Swinfen & Swinfen, 2002).

Telemedicine Systems Applied to Emergency

The system consists of a central station placed in the emergency room of the Branca hospital, operated by doctors or non-medical staffs (see Figure 2 for its architecture). The Medical Center can interact with the portable user terminals (see Figure 3) using mobile broadband 3G telecommunication links. The technological innovation introduced by the system is the use of mobile video communication. In fact, the mobile terminals are equipped with interactive video cameras that allows the doctor to see the scene of the operation, review the patients conditions, his psychophysical reaction and dialogue with the patient as if the doctor was present on the site of the event (Armstrong & Haston, 1997).

The mobile portable terminals used in our experimentation phase are equipped with all the necessary medical devices, which enable a care giver to carry out all emergency and lifesaving medical examination, allowing immediate measurements of the patient's most important vital parameters.

Figure 2. System architecture

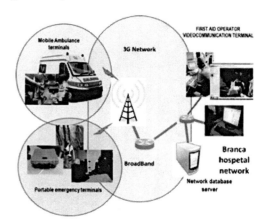

During data collection the portable terminal transmits in real time the gathered values to the first aid Medical Center terminal.

The doctor or care giver can immediately view the data displayed on the Operator station's monitor, evaluate the event and patients status, make a report, require additional on line specialist Teleconsultation, provide an immediate response or talk directly with the emergency crew and what is most important it happens all in real time. To allow an efficient monitoring of the sheen each portable station is equipped with:

- 12 lead wireless ECG device
- Wireless blood pressure measurement device
- Wireless glucometer
- Wireless SpO2 meter
- Wireless flussossimeter
- Digital Stethoscope

Figure 3. The portable telemedicine device for emergency care

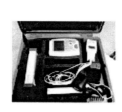 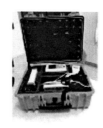 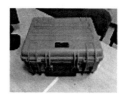

As stated above the devices have been selected in order to allow handling of the most common emergency cases and help the crew to stabilize the patient health conditions (Shanit, Cheng, & Greenbaum, 1996, Campbell et al., 1998, Goh, Lam, & Poon, 1997). See Figure 4 for electro-medical equipment used.

A similar system has been installed directly into the ambulance. In this case to facilitate the intervention of the doctor to have a complete control of the emergency site a remote controlled tilting camera has been installed on the ambulance roof (see Figure 5), having optical zoom commands, so that the doctor at the Medical Center can follow the activities of the emergency crew, see the patient and focus the image according to the needs of the case (Hebert, Paquin, & Whitten, 2007).

The Audio is guaranteed by an environmental microphone with echo suppressor, needed to eliminate annoying voice returns between the ambulance and medical staff on board the ambulance, that in emergency events is often the case to occur.

The Medical Center Station

The system composed by mobile terminals and operator stations is configured as a client server network, the operation stations software is provided with a dynamic instant presents list, showing the online status of each user and doctor station, therefore both mobile terminals and operators know in any moment who is on line (see Figure 6). The operator therefore has all the tools to put up a video call with any online terminal or any online doctor, thus allowing any operator to have a complete view of presents over the network.

The operator has access to all incoming data (as shown in Figure 7), can record and transfer the received values to other on line doctors or provide the appropriate guidelines and support to the emergency crew. It is important to have multi communication tools in order to allow specialist to view the patient and provide the appropriate report, that is made possible thanks to the multi-Videocommunication tools included in the Medical Center station.(Baer L, Elford DR, Cukor P, 2006, Mistiaen P, Poot E., 2006, Hughes-Anderson W, Rankin S, House J. 2002).

Figure 4. Electromedical equipment used

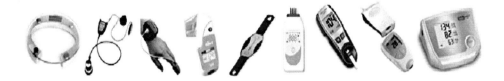

Figure 5. The ambulance equipment

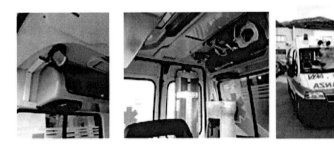

Figure 6. The videocommunication interface of the doctor station in the first aid department. Doctors and caregivers can see the sheen were the medical intervention is taking place in real time.

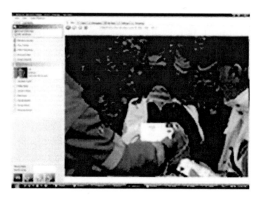

Figure 7. The operation station's GUI shows incoming vital parameters measurements from the patients

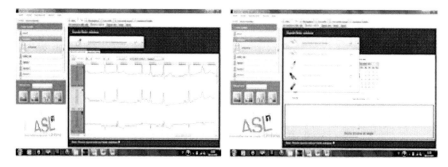

The Benefits of Telemedicine Applied to Emergency

The use so sophisticated but simple to use remote controlled systems, provides the advantage to:

- Allow to follow a patient after an emergency event, all the way during his transportation to the nearest hospital.
- Provide on the road patients information to the First Aid Department or surgery department during his transportation, allowing to save time and set up the appropriate medical teams and emergency room.
- Provide real time vital data parameters during patients transportation.

- Locally stabilize the patient and allow the remote doctor to decide whether or not to follow up transportation to the hospital, limiting access to the hospital to cases strictly necessary.

Time and resource optimization, lifesaving, case selection and access restriction, doctor is always present at the event scene, there is no doubt about the value of telemedicine adoption to emergency case. Its economic depreciation is very short and certainly the resultant benefits for both the timeliness and the improvement of quality of service are significantly higher than the investment itself (Bowersox & Cornum, 1998, Callas, Ricci, & Caputo, 2000).

Operational Flow

The adoption of new technologies into stable and tested organizations in order to avoid critical impacts must be preceded by an appropriate and efficient training and must be integrated into the daily routing activities. A similar approach has been adopted tanking in due account that the system needs a trial period before becoming a usual tool. With this in mind the team responsible to manage and run the telemedicine emergency system has proceeded in the following manner:

- An appropriate training was first dedicated to the medical and hospital staff involved in the system.
- The project was initially applied to low risk events, where the emergency crew alone and without physician on board the ambulance is called to manage events not extremely urgent (low priority green code triage).
- The medical and nursing staff may acquire the necessary knowledge and confidence to manage emergency situations of higher level and use telemedicine to daily to achieve all operational benefits.
- The Operation station was located in an 24/h surveyed emergency room where there is always doctors and nurses are present.
- The emergency crew is equipped with both portable station for home visits and equipped ambulance for on the road events.

The team in charge of the emergency telemedicine system had to define a new operational procedure granting the same healthcare safety conditions to patients and staff as for the existing procedure. In the initial phase it was decided that the two procedure be in somehow overlapped in order to cover any failure or misunderstanding that could happen in a startup stage. The following steps were approved and followed by the team:

1. Upon arrival of an emergency request and the triage defines the proper code to be green the telemedicine ambulance is alerted and the specialized crew takes the call;
2. The medical staff in charge of the Operation station is alerted, positioned on the workstation and ready to respond to the crew support request;
3. If for any reason this is not possible (unavailability of staff, network failures, software or computer crash) the ambulance crew will be advised and proceed with the normal procedure (e.i. registration of vital parameters in asynchronous mode, inform doctors about the values by phone, if necessary proceed with the transportation to the hospital);
4. The ambulance and rescue team reaches the place of the event, evaluates the situation, gives confirmation about the triage code level;
5. If the rescue team highlights the need of a medical consultation, activates the telemedicine video call and the doctors can visit the patient. The doctor after visiting the remote patient and reading the incoming vital parameters values, with eventually the measurements of the ECG will trigger the first aid department for emergency admission or decide to keep the patient home (Cancellotti & Gullà,2012, Roberts, Tayler, MacCormack, & Barwich, 2007).

Solutions and Recommendations

Even thou the service has started recently in experimental mode and the basis seem to be very promising we must underline that not enough time has been dedicated to have a real statistical significance result. It is necessary to continue testing and improving the service in a way that in the very next feature this solution will become the ordinary mode of providing emergency support to remote and urbanized areas. We have understood that there is a very strong impact to the routing daily service, due to the integration of new technologies and new procedures. There is a need to train and make the medical staff become confident with this tool, understand benefits and risks management (Saysell & Routley, 2003; Wilkes, Mohan, White, & Smith, 2004).

We are confident that in the medium short term the service can be calibrated to fit the needs of the First Aid activity. Our recommendation for the future is to continue learning how new applications deriving from telemedicine technologies adaptation, to overcome the knowledge barriers that may frighten from taken such direction and to keep in mind that today's social-health environment requires to break old paradigms and find new ways to provide healthcare service, taking advantage of the modern technologies made available by the broadband digital area. Medicine and technology must walk together to provide a better world.

One other very important aspect is the organization impact we have mentioned above. In reality our approach is to fit the new technology in the existing organization, limiting as much a possible the procedural modes to the existing ones. In practice this could be a first step but we are aware that this procedural must be adopted to the needs of a growing service, and not having any previous reference experience of such applications "remote doctor to the patients site" in emergency events, we are probably pioneering the service and we need more experience to design the service procedures.

FUTURE RESEARCH DIRECTIONS

In our short and interesting experience we are confident that this approach will provide significant cost savings and resource optimization, therefore the efforts to be addressed in the very next feature will be focused on the benefits that may be derived from an intensive use of telemedicine solutions to the emergency event managements. Hospitals and NHS may benefit from such services if this

are extended to environments where emergency events occur with higher frequency, such as nursing homes, remote healthcare structures, isolated chronicle elderly homes and so on. The possibility to virtually bring a doctor or specialist to a patient needing assistance has we now doubt a very great potential, but must be integrated into the existing service provisioning. Future research must quantify the economic benefits for the healthcare organizations and the improvement quality of life of the patients.

CONCLUSION

In conclusion, these applications, relating to telemedicine, doctors and all socio-health workers generally, representing the users of systems and service providers, need increasingly teamwork thinking and interdisciplinary collaboration, that increase the formative and culture expansion of stakeholders and interpersonal relationships. Telecommunications technologies adopted in this context provide a positive contribute to the medical profession service, in order to achieve satisfactory solution of numerous problems relating to health and social sphere, with particular reference to the need to optimize time over distances between patients and health care facilities. In this sense, Telemedicine takes on a predominant role as a tool for quick access to clinical data through remote computer technology and telecommunications, regardless of the distance between the patient, his information and the doctor can ever be. Purpose of Telemedicine is, therefore, to integrate the telematics and medical professionalism in such a way that even from remote locations or devices one can systematically benefit from specialized resources, allocate physically centralized stations. It should be noted, finally, that beyond the social importance of telemedicine, there is also the consequent economic benefits to society as a whole and, therefore, of the national health service level cost/benefit ratio: interventions in "real time" in the first rescue, protected hospital discharge, reducing hospitalization of chronically ill, providing assistance to nursing homes and elderly, reducing the "healthcare traveling" at both regional and national level, and finally the better living conditions that can provide innumerable subjects at risk, ensuring their greater safety and autonomy. All the above matched with emergency event management in the most appropriate conditions will provide new scenarios of economic and quality of life benefits.

REFERENCES

Armstrong, I. J., & Haston, W. S. (1997). Medical decision support for remote general practitioners using telemedicine. *Journal of Telemedicine and Telecare, 3*(1), 27–34. doi:10.1258/1357633971930166

Baer, L., Elford, D. R., & Cukor, P. (1997). Telepsychiatry at forty: What have we learned? *Harvard Review of Psychiatry, 5,* 7–17. doi:10.3109/10673229709034720

Bowersox, J. C., & Cornum, R. L. (1998). Remote operative urology using a surgical telemanipulator system: Preliminary observations. *Urology, 52,* 17–22. doi:10.1016/S0090-4295(98)00168-X

Callas, P. W., Ricci, M. A., & Caputo, M. P. (2006). Improved rural provider access to continuing medical education through interactive videoconferencing. *Telemedicine Journal and e-Health, 6,* 393–399. doi:10.1089/15305620050503861

Campbell, G., Loane, E., & Griffiths, R. (1998). Comparison of teleconsultations and face-to-face consultations: Preliminary results of a United Kingdom multicentre teledermatology study. *The British Journal of Dermatology, 39,* 81–87.

Currell, R., Urquhart, C., Wainwright, P., & Lewis, R. (2006). Telemedicine versus face to face patient care. *Cochrane Database of Systematic Reviews, 4,* CD002098.

Eysenbach, G. (2001). What is e-health? *Journal of Medical Internet Research, 3*(2), e20. doi:10.2196/jmir.3.2.e20

Goh, K. Y., Lam, C. K., & Poon, W. S. (1997). The impact of teleradiology on the inter-hospital transfer of neurosurgical patients. *British Journal of Neurosurgery, 11,* 52–56. doi:10.1080/02688699746708

Hebert, M. A., Paquin, M. J., & Whitten, L. (2007). Analysis of the suitability of "video-visits" for palliative home care: Implications for practice. *Journal of Telemedicine and Telecare, 13,* 74–78. doi:10.1258/135763307780096203

Hughes-Anderson, W., Rankin, S., & House, J. (2002). Open access endoscopy in rural and remote Western Australia: Does it work? *ANZ Journal of Surgery, 72,* 699–703. doi:10.1046/j.1445-2197.2002.02535.x

Leach, L. S., & Christensen, H. (2006). A systematic review of telephone-based interventions for mental disorders. *Journal of Telemedicine and Telecare, 12*(3), 122–129. doi:10.1258/135763306776738558

Mistiaen, P., & Poot, E. (2006). Telephone follow-up, initiated by a hospital-based health professional, for postdischarge problems in patients discharged from hospital to home. *Cochrane Database of Systematic Reviews, 4,* CD004510.

Oh, H., Rizo, C., Enkin, M., & Jadad, A. (2005). What is eHealth (3): A systematic review of published definitions. *Journal of Medical Internet Research, 7*(1), e1. doi:10.2196/jmir.7.1.e1

Pattichis, C. S., Kyriacou, E., & Voskarides, S. (2002). Wireless telemedicine systems: An overview. *Antennas and Propagation Magazine, 44*(2), 143–153. doi:10.1109/MAP.2002.1003651

Roberts, D., Tayler, C., MacCormack, D., & Barwich, D. (2007). Telenursing in hospice palliative care. *The Canadian Nurse, 103*, 24–27.

Saysell, E., & Routley, C. (2003). Telemedicine in community-based palliative care: Evaluation of a videolink teleconference project. *International Journal of Palliative Nursing, 9*, 489–495.

Shanit, D., Cheng, A., & Greenbaum, R. A. (1996). Telecardiology: Supporting the decision making process in general practice. *Journal of Telemedicine and Telecare, 2*(1), 7–13. doi:10.1258/1357633961929105

Swinfen, R., & Swinfen, P. (2002). Low-cost telemedicine in the developing world. *Journal of Telemedicine and Telecare, 8*(3), 63–65. doi:10.1258/13576330260440899

Wilkes, L., Mohan, S., White, K., & Smith, H. (2004). Evaluation of an after hours telephone support service for rural palliative care patients and their families: A pilot study. *The Australian Journal of Rural Health, 12*, 95–98. doi:10.1111/j.1440-1854.2004.00568.x

KEY TERMS AND DEFINITIONS

3G Telecommunication: The third generation of mobile technology allowing broadband applications over mobile phones. UMTS (Universal Mobile Telecommunications System)one of these technologies and allows data transfer at 1,8 to 3 Mbs.

First Aid: Assistance provided to patients requiring urgent healthcare support.

Multi-Videocommunication: Service that allows to video interact with more users at the same time. Typically managed by a device or software that acts as the MCU or video switching matrix.

Operation Flow: Set of actions scheduled or programmed to face in the appropriate mode any particular situation.

Specialist Teleconsultation: Is intended a visit or consultation with a specialist doctor from remote using telecommunication means such as telephony, internet ad Videocommunication.

Wireless Devices: Any electronic device that may communicate without the need of wires or physica connection. This definition includes any portable mobile phone or communication device.

Section 3

Chapter 17
Telemedicine R&D Influencing Incoming Strategies and Organization Models

Francesco Gabbrielli
Umberto I General Hospital of Rome, Department of Surgery "P. Stefanini", Rome, Italy

ABSTRACT

In the modern medicine and surgery, innovations arise from interdisciplinary work. Therefore, to analyse how telemedicine R&D is influencing strategies and organizational models in healthcare systems we have to study how ICT and robotics innovations can interact with structured healthcare services on a large scale. The problem is interdisciplinary, and the answer has to be on different levels: economical, technological, and organizational. Overall, change needs of two paradigms from telemedicine to telematic medicine and surgery and from financial strategies for saving to lean thinking for innovations. The innovation of value can be obtained when healthcare organization combines innovative telematic medicine and surgery services with utility, prices, and costs. To work on these innovations without rearranging the whole organizational flow around the future e-health service means inducing the healthcare organization to generate wastes and face unnecessary expenses attached to future healthcare processes with such high and probably unsustainable costs.

INTRODUCTION

Generally speaking the aims of research and development are clear. To research means to explore new paths and to develop means to apply new effective solutions.

Professionals working in healthcare organizations know the interaction of the research with the development processes cannot be so simple and clear. At first, we have to distinguish the application of new technologies to old therapies from new treatments performable thanks to technological innovations. Physicians are usually available to adopt new technology when it does not modify the consolidated treatment scheme. They are much less available when the technological innovations open a new treatment possibility cause of in this case they have the responsibility to abandoned a

DOI: 10.4018/978-1-4666-2979-0.ch017

well known treatment process to a new one and through new sophisticate hi-tech products not easy to manage. The ICT and Robotics industries prefer to apply technological innovations into highly standardized treatment processes which are more sure, easier and with faster return of the investment. Nevertheless, we can observe a certain progress in medical treatments anyway, but the overall results in quality and safety improvement of the healthcare services can be not so clear for patients (Scuffham, 2002; Whitten, 2002; Franzini, 2011; Ekeland, 2010; Weinstein, 2008; Schweitzer, 2012; Kohn, 2000; U.S. Food and Drug Administration, 2009).

To understand these complex organizational interactions it is useful to remember the bio-medical studies are basic research while the medical practice is essentially applicative research and for that reason in the modern Medicine and Surgery the innovations arise from interdisciplinary work rather than individual efforts (Das, 1996; Lum, 2006; Greer, 2008).

Therefore, to analyse how the Telemedicine R&D is influencing strategies and organizational models in healthcare systems we can begin to an inquiry: why in this period of great technological progresses is the ability of medical practice lower in using ICT and Robotics innovations in structured healthcare services on a large scale?

If the problem is interdisciplinary then the answer has to be on different levels.

INFLUENCING STRATEGIES AND ECONOMICS

Even if there has been any period in history a period never existed in which available resources were sufficient to satisfy the human wish to increase quality and length of life, it is real that in the last three decades the gap between healthcare expectations and resources appears disproportionately high (Klarman, 1965).

Then, all over the world, people have realised that all desired care cannot be administered to everybody, but resources have to be allocated following ethical criteria accepted by people and that at the same time are equal and effective. European politicians have chosen to invest in healthcare systems based on a cooperative spirit in order to guarantee the access to care to every citizen while saving costs at the same time.

Nevertheless, citizens are impatient owing to bureaucracy and waiting lists in public healthcare systems and they do not often realise that such limitations are a kind of hidden form of rationing. They simply perceive these systems as disorganised. To mitigate the social and economical pressures on these systems, in the last two decades several reform processes have been carried out with the aim reducing requests and increasing efficiency of healthcare services (Pink, 2003; Ikkersheim, 2012; Wyss, 2000; Hurley, 1995).

To achieve this objective in the public healthcare systems the redefinition of services using the concept of priority is considered the main action to be implemented in the experience of many countries: UK, New Zealand, Australia (Manning, 2011), Canada (Gibson, 2011), USA (Mirelman, 2012). This kind of action has led to the new criteria of filtering essential services in Holland (Tanke, 2012), or the new system of waiting list management in New Zealand (Dew, 2005).

All they are interventions made to advance from the generic model of universal care toward the selective one. Without a deep assessment of the real situation of the healthcare organizations, analyzing overall the main steps which have to be taken to create more benefits for their patients, the cost cutting based only on financial logic has the same meaning of a symptomatic cure administered without understanding the reasons of the illness. In recent years, experience has shown that, not only in management of healthcare systems, the illusion of decisive costs cutting often produced opposite results to the objectives. To copy-and-paste pre-made cost cutting solutions in different organizations can generate major problems rather than solve them (Deans, 2011; Scutchfield, 2009).

Even if different strategies for demand control in healthcare can be observed in many countries, it is clear everybody attribute great importance to the improvement of technical efficiency in hospital activity (Latifi, 2012), (Patterson, 2007). This point is considered crucial to increase the capacity of available resources used in order to maximise the care offer (Pande, 2003), (Gurman, 2012), (Young, 2011).

All these organizational issues and their technical consequences have to be faced taking into account the financial perspective as well. The importance of this link with the general economy is based on three observations: resources are scarce in proportion to human needs; resources have alternative uses; the relative importance given to what we need could be quite varied (Samuelson and Nordhaus, 2005).

Nevertheless, the first and main objective of healthcare systems is to deliver the best possible care to the patients without searching a profit if they are public, or searching a profit derived from the efficiency of the cure not on the presence of sick persons, if they are private.

In other words healthcare systems surely spend a lot of money but do not always make money. To forget these principles and evidences when analysing healthcare organizations (hospital, district, etc.) means to make the error of considering them simply like business companies. Organizations dedicated to healthcare are a special kind of companies in which often the final product is not sure. A fundamental question derived from these assumptions is: how can limited resources be allocated in the best way possible in order to satisfy people's need for health?

The answer does not lie within the economic sphere, but consists of political choices. This was effectively summed up by Fuchs (1998): "Economics is the science of means, not of ends".

Nevertheless, especially in the last two decades politicians, managers and physicians have made many efforts to modify healthcare organizations with the aim of facilitating financial solutions to increase efficiency without reducing accessibility and quality of care (Lee, 2012).

As a consequence, an amount of experiences have been reported in literature on the attempts of clinicians to study and then to validate inexpensive healthcare systems and methods (Krupinski, 2011), (Whittaker, 2012), (Shea, 2009), (Van den Brink-Muinen, 2000). At the beginning the aim was simply to reduce costs by optimizing the work organization, but in time, under the pressure exerted especially by biotechnological companies, the scientific community started to study how to exploit technological innovations in order mainly to reduce the costs of personnel through the increase of the standardization and automation of old-fashioned treatment procedures (Kahn, 2011).

Financial control together with cost/benefit analysis became first the most important parameters to judge the value of the work carried out in healthcare organizations and then the only parameter when public organizations too started to be considered like private companies.

This evolution leads healthcare systems to introduce the idea that a minimum acceptable result in disease treatments can be socially and ethically acceptable as well as economically useful to cut costs. Sciences have contributed with their achievements to give concreteness to this idea: Epidemiology first by enabling the prevention of illness, then Bio-technology, ICT and Robotics by developing mini-invasive treatments. In other words the prevention of illness is the minimum economic effort to maintain in health the majority of young active people and postpone the appearance of the most important diseases in the last decades of life and mini-invasive treatments are the most effective solution to permit an early discharge of the obligation of care towards families with the minimum expense for healthcare organizations.

In this way healthy people perceive healthcare systems to be sufficient for their needs and useful for public administration, but the perspective changes when a person is sick.

Telemedicine is a promising tool to avoid unnecessary costs and deliver effective treatments with high quality and safety (Puangmali, 2008; Leung, 2012; Schweitzer, 2012). However, it is very difficult to economically evaluate Telemedicine. Constantly changing technology, multiple applications and overall costs, inappropriateness of the conventional techniques of economic evaluation and possibly expanding indications are examples of factors that have mostly been limited to feasibility studies.

It makes little sense to talk about cost-effectiveness of telemedicine in general. It is important to be more specific about which use and in which setting, as well as to distinguish between cost-effectiveness for whom: society, health providers, professionals or patients.

If Telemedicine is going to expand, the question of reimbursement must be solved.

INFLUENCING TECHNOLOGY AND HEALTHCARE

More recently overall technological innovations, especially in Robotics and ICT (but increasingly in Nanotechnology too), have been so impressive to provide the basis for the clearing of that concept. Now they are making possible and more useful to pass towards other two paradigms:

1. From Telemedicine to Telematic Medicine and Surgery,
2. From financial strategies for saving to Lean Thinking for innovations.

These two new concepts, or better frameworks of ideas, are strictly connected to each other: the first leads us to the second. Together they are also the answer to another query: is it possible to deliver healthcare with higher levels of quality and safety while maintaining it sustainable ?

It is possible to answer if we are able to change perspective in developing medical and surgical projects and services based on ICT and Robotics: not to be simply witnesses of another technological solution in search of a clinical problem, not to employ the same old care methods using high tech products developed from marketing analysis, but new clinical methodology to administer patient treatments through technological innovations strongly based on clinical needs analysis.

This answer, this new course represents probably the most relevant implication to emerge from Telematic Medicine and Surgery innovations.

To fully understand the importance of the switchover from Telemedicine to Telematic Medicine and Surgery, let me quote Dag K.J.E. von Lubitz, brilliant innovator, pioneer of Medical Telepresence I had the honour to meet thanks to another great professional Frederic Patricelli, ICT engineer, who was the first to promote international high levels meetings on Telemedicine in Italy (L'Aquila, 2000): "Similar to virtual reality, Telemedicine became a concept so broad that it literally lost its meaning.", "Real-time medical assistance was the key element. Today, Telemedicine continues to remain largely consultative and static." These two sentences always helped me when I had doubts on the real clinical usefulness of ICT and Robotics projects dedicated to healthcare. In other words, on that occasion I learned that Telemedicine cannot represent an innovation if we lose sight of its real objectives, if we are not able to deliver adequate therapies in real time to our patients.

You can read any number of Telemedicine definitions, all invariably either too broad or too constraining. Patient data transfer, administrative issues, patient monitoring, consultation, all become part of the collective term "Telemedicine", losing distinction between the true practice of

Medicine and Surgery with their supporting activities and becoming both medical and "tele-" if the activity is executed over a distance (even if in the next room a few metres away).

Moreover, available word processing, spreadsheets, and image management software allow employees to work away from their offices, but there is nothing virtual about it. Simply, we use ICT to make possible the substitution of one environment for another. The same in Telemedicine, despite great advances in ICT, live video, Robotics and a number of commercialized sophisticated tools (someone also at low cost) we have lost a lot of time repeating the same pilot experience model on different technological prototypes without any concrete positive impact on large scale healthcare services.

In example, remote consultation through internet and dedicated software is a wonderful thing, but there is nothing new about it. Telephone, radio and fax have been used for decades to serve precisely such a purpose (Pinnock, 2005; Turk, 2010; Innes, 2006).

Nevertheless, there has been real progress in Teleradiology or Teledermatology in making correct diagnoses on patients located thousands of miles away, but this is possible only when carried out by high specialized physicians and both disciplines rely on the analysis of images rather than interaction with the live patient (Browns, 2006; Hsiao, 2008).

In healthcare systems, the two major attempts to use both the ICT and Robotics innovations to really treat patients at a distance have been Telesurgery and the Emergency and Trauma Telemedicine. These two disciplines embody both the real-time presence within the medical environment and an active interaction with it, either by means of remotely controlled devices or by effecting the required actions through voice commands using communication and viewing systems that connect the distant managing physician with the personnel in direct contact with the patient. The new

element is that the remote physician conducts medical activities as if present on the patient site. This possibility to treat the patient and to perform Robotic Surgery from a distance is the most sophisticated example of Telepresence (Eadie, 2003; Rayman, 2007; vespa, 2005; Ballantyne, 2002). If it is possible for Surgery during interventions then Telepresence can be doable also before and after for both diagnose and post-operative management and also in other medical fields, (Ellison, 2007; Umefjord, 2006; Clark, 2007).

That really means to pass from Telemedicine to Telematic Medicine and Surgery and as a consequence to practice Medicine and Surgery in new way. Moreover, the highly powerful concept of medical Telepresence can also be applied to medical training, particularly when it is based on the development of an internet-based environment providing real-time access and interactivity of the trainee with a computer assisted simulator (von Lubitz, 2003; Dankelman, 2008; Aggarwal, 2008; Sutherland, 2006).

Telemedicine has proliferated throughout much of the industrialised world, reflecting the convergence of scientific, technological, economic and social factors. Initially, Telemedicine was considered simply an enabling technology for increasing access to healthcare in remote or isolated regions, and a valuable tool for health care emergencies where swift diagnosis and treatment can be decisive (Terkelsen, 2005; Sebajang, 2006; Smith, 2005; Kirkup, 1982). Today Telematic Medicine and Surgery are seeing a greater recognition of their applicability to the entire healthcare delivery system (Ellison, 2004). Increasing access and quality of care seems to be the primary drive behind Telemedicine services deployment in Europe and in all countries in general (Beckjord, 2007; Andreassen, 2007).

Furthermore, the continuity of care can derived great advantages from Telematic Medicine and Surgery (Whitten, 2005). Home healthcare is emerging as an area of growing interest linked to elderly and chronic patient care (de-hospitalization) (Boulos, 2007). In the modern economical organization of healthcare services, after the initial stage and pilot programs (Zanaboni, 2012), Telematic Medicine and Surgery are also becoming strategic tools to decrease costs and to improve efficiency (Buntin, 2011). However, special problems and barriers are connected with the use of Telemedicine in general and they limit this positive effect. Besides these barriers, there is still a lack of assessment of Telemedicine applications and much more for Telematic Medicine and Surgery (Moffatt, 2003; Roig, 2011). The Telemedicine activity volume derived from existing projects is low, reliable cost-effective analyses are extremely difficult and rare as well as financial and economic factors are still unclear. In addition, the medical profession often resists the changes induced by the evolution from Telemedicine to Telematic Medicine and Surgery for the medical-legal issues, but probably mainly on account of needed organizational and management changes.

Telemedicine has a long history linked to the evolution of telecommunications (Strehle, 2006). In the internet era, a major impulse for Telemedicine R&D has been produced by communitarian healthcare policy, as in the European area (Stroetmann, 2007; Butter, 2008). The Exploratory Action AIM has represented a milestone for Telemedicine research funding in Europe that has continued along the successive Framework Programmes until today. An increasing activity has been produced during the last decade following the general Information and Communication Technologies revolution. A great impulse came from RDT European programmes on Health Telematics that have played a definitive role supporting Telemedicine projects in Europe. All European countries are involved in telematic healthcare projects, many of them encouraged by national or regional healthcare Authorities. Also a very important contribution has come from Structural and Regional Funds.

However, it is not clear how many and where these Telemedicine initiatives are effectively running.

Telemedicine in Europe must be considered taking into account the particular structure, funding and organizational features of the healthcare systems in each country (Roberts, 2010). The public nature of most European Healthcare Systems influences business strategies and economic status quo differently than other models. The peculiar characteristics of the healthcare sector in each country and the deep organizational changes that are currently in progress have to be taken into account. The European public healthcare systems are basically financed by taxation, but the arrangement of primary care differs from country to country. To answer to this situation the EC has already taken up some initiatives to promote the development of an information society. This process is still running and its main goal is to allow European citizens to use the most recent innovations on telecommunications and computer science, and to support an intelligent and user-friendly interaction with the information systems for the improvement of services. An important item in the field of ICT, in particular in the healthcare area, is to avoid the development of services in an un-coordinated manner.

In fact, today there are systems which are very valuable for the fulfillment of their task in specific areas, while lacking interoperability. This has negative consequences on the quality of services offered to citizens, who often has to act as system integrators (reservations, payment, medical report collection, etc.). Professionals who worked on system interoperability projects in the recent past know harmonization in data management can be a strong limit often really difficult to solve when data systems from different national or regional healthcare organizations have to be compared. How we will discuss below in this chapter regarding on Lean Thinking applied to Telematic Medicine and Surgery projects, harmonization and other issues in ICT and Robotics are not properly technical, but they origin from cultural unsuitability on R&D processes management for healthcare systems.

THE ROLE OF R&D

R&D actions was particularly aimed in the recent years to the achievement of a net-system, which has the task of allowing safe of information exchanges among various subjects, especially public institutions, in order to offer to the citizens services which really comply with their demand. The last technical evolution of this concept is the cloud computing system which makes possible to search and use data from several databases without the necessity to store them in local devices. Unfortunately many laboratories and hospitals use different units of measurement, different acronyms for the same parameters, exams or treatments, different structure of patient folders and the reports on activities-costs have quite different data structures to make hardly possible the scientific comparison of them.

We are able to transfer in few seconds a great amount of data through internet, but we have to spend quite a lot of time searching how to elaborate them because they are not harmonized at the original source. Data harmonization is not a technical problem, it is the main indicator to verify real will to share information and capability of R&D management to imagine the future of an innovation in Telematic Medicine and Surgery.

To acquire greater efficacy in R&D process, from the initial phases of a pilot project based on an innovative idea to the implementation and start-up of the new services built on the pilot experience results, means to improve services to patients with the minimum possible effort, creating durable positive effects also for the organization.

In this chapter we will try to concentrate our attention on this issue of vital importance but so often underestimated to privilege more operative phases. Logistics, services delivery, personnel management, cost cutting, all that surely utilizes the resources of the organization. It is easy to realize all these activities are different from R&D and fundamental to the healthcare organizations cause as they are complementary to the core-activity, which is to care for patients.

Nevertheless, it is important not to forget that all the same activities are also the effect, not the cause, of a distant R&D process when an innovation in patient treatment was conseived and when the decisions regarding the project development influenced the whole subsequent life of that innovation.

Even if the main objective of healthcare organizations is not to produce and sell consumer goods but to cure citizens, it can be useful to analyze examples of corporate governance of industries for the activities of development and learn what can be applicable to Telematic Medicine and Surgery R&D projects.

Not to consider this possibility for healthcare organizations and to illude oneself with technical innovations in ICT and Robotics introduced without well coordinated organizational innovations, represent two strategic mistakes. The consequences of those mistakes today will have a relevant role in future healthcare systems because it is clear that Telematic Medicine and Surgery are the main way to maintain the sustainability of a high level of quality and safety in healthcare.

A really interesting example is found in the book "The Toyota Way" by Liker (2004). In that publication, Liker analyzed the exceptional industrial development of Toyota and identified 14 management principles which were at the base of the company's success. We read the first principle was: the actions resulting in major advantages in the long term have to be always placed before those actions that give modest profits in the short term. The Toyota company showed it is possible to orient the daily work and the individual objective of the whole staff towards a unique strategic mission: to create value, for their client, company and the economy, not just to make money immediately.

To decide investments in prevention and high quality during the phases of innovation development is a cultural model of management applicable to healthcare organizations. It means investing more resources at the beginning of the development process of a new healthcare service based on technological innovations, rather than put right errors or accidents when the services are already delivered. All this is possible only when a strategic vision is maintained. Some Authors (Edmund Phelps) (Phelps, 1966) have demonstrated that companies or organizations without strategic vision in the long term are not oriented to invest in innovations and they lose competitiveness as a consequence.

This general effect is more relevant in the field of technological innovations because of the fast turn-over in product development. This becomes crucial when new therapeutic solutions are achievable through ICT and Robotics innovative products. Medical and technological studies, planning and development have to be harmonized to succeed in starting real new services proportional according to people's needs, characterised by high quality and safety.

The lack of the vision in this situation has relevant negative effects converging in losing accessibility of the care for patients, because to maintain healthcare services with poor technological innovations make their costs unsustainable and force the management to reduce their availability.

To change this negative evolution is possible but not quick. ICT and Robotics innovations can not be created through top-down processes from institutions or central organizations, but come from daily practical experiences of patients needs.

Whatever, to create innovations in treatments using clinical experience to implement new dedicated technologies is a work method well known in the medical field.

Surgeons usually follow this methodology for the development of new surgical instruments that means introducing technological innovations in treatment starting from clinical needs and using the competences of technicians. A great example of this comes from Dr. Victor P. Satinsky (Philadelphia, PA), who was one of the most innovative cardiovascular surgeons with 30 major medical innovations in operational procedures and with the invention of the Satinsky clamp, now a standard instrument used in cardiovascular surgery. It is an haemostatic clamp with a special hook-like curvature at the latter end which imitates the fingers-hand position of the surgeon when he is blocking the blood flow to suture a great vessel (Ailawadi, 2010; Kirkup, 1982).

In other words, the physician analyzed how to ameliorate his performance defining medical issue of the treatment (i.e. the haemostasis during vascular suture), he accomplished the surgical solution of that issue (i.e. to clamp vessel between two hook-like curved fingers), he worked with technicians to define the user requirements of an innovative product useful to perform the new solution better, with high quality and in safety (i.e. to define how to curve the new clamp), the technician made the innovative product prototype (i.e. Satinsky clamp prototype), the surgeon tested the new clamp and collaborated with the technicians to produce the definitive version ready also for use.

It is easy to understand the opposite process would not be possible to obtain the same Satinsky clamp. In such case we should imagine the following development process: first technicians realize that to curve the haemostatic clamp is possible and they ask the sellers of surgical clamps to whom the curved one could be sold, meanwhile the standardized production line is made. Then, technicians contact surgeons, the main clients for the marketing study, to ask them in which cases they could obtain advantages using the curved clamp. One vascular surgeon answered that in his opinion, the curved clamp could be used sometimes in vascular surgery, but it should be curved differently to imitate the hook-like position of the surgeon's fingers during the operation. The technicians at this point are compelled to give up the collaboration with the surgeon because in the production line it is not possible to modify the clamp curve.

Similar situations are illogical in the development of new clamps, but they seem usual in the development of innovations in ICT and Robotics. In reality, Telematic Medicine and Surgery development projects have often been conducted confusing research experiences generated from the intuition of a physician or an engineer with the development programs of new healthcare services based on technological innovations. The work flow can be similar but the differences in the respective objectives are the main and the first distinctive characteristic. The research experiences explore new possibilities to understand whether they are feasible or not, while the development programs try to make the innovations useful in practical applications adapting them to the organization. Therefore, for Telematic Medicine and Surgery development as well, it is necessary to assess and select new ideas from a technical and clinical point of view as well as to plan adequate strategies to introduce them into the organization in accordance with sustainability criteria.

BREAKING THE PARADIGM

The aim in the R&D processes in Telematic Medicine and Surgery cannot just be to use a technology for the first time and for one time only, but to define the utilization of innovations and disseminate them for extensive clinical use to cure patients better.

A famous example is the operation in Telesurgery performed by J. Marescaux with innovative Robotic technology. He executed a cholecistectomy from New York while the patient was in Strasbourg. Even if the intervention was successfully conducted it remained for a long period the unique experience of that kind (Marescaux, 2002). Only two years after the surgical group of M. Anvari started a pilot Telesurgery program in Canada which results on 22 patients were published only in 2007 (Anvari, 2007). The operative real-time interaction between distant surgeons on the same patient in well structured collaborative organization is still now unrealized.

The ICT and Robotics innovation are making new clinical solutions possible and Telematic Medicine and Surgery are making possible new methods and techniques of illness treatment and patient-case management. We are living in one of those particular historical periods known as "jump period" by historians. The level of sophistication in ICT and Robotics makes it possible to change the evolution of medical and surgical practice as well the progress of the whole Medicine, but it seems not sufficient to trust in the technological progress. We require contextually to modify both the delivering processes of previous healthcare services and almost always the organizational structures (hospital, district, etc.).

The most useful starting point to create the best environmental conditions to that leap forward ("jump") is to observe minutely the processes following the lessons coming from Quality Assurance methods (Groene, 2010). Then the analyzed processes can be well represented through the organizational flowchart. From this study we have the possibility to trace the flow of the activities related to the healthcare service observing with the eyes of the final users the organization and our individual actions. We can identify the differences between the healthcare service before and after the introduction of ICT and Robotics innovations. We can learn to recognize the real value in the processes through which we perform our daily work. If it is possible to recognize the value then we can also distinguish the wastes incurred in the carrying out of our activities.

It is possible to classify all work activities into three types: added-value activity (when the final users are willing to pay for it); considered necessary activity (no added-value for users but not eliminable because of legal or organizational obligations); absolutely useless activity. The last one is the most dangerous, also because it is usually hidden behind the organizational routine and it can be considered necessary or with added-value.

That is precisely what happened in the field of Telematic Medicine and Surgery innovations which were implemented for experimental projects but most often not developed as real services for patients in healthcare systems. When value is lacking the research for innovation only results in technological exercises which are too pioneer for actual use. The innovation of value can be obtained when healthcare organization combines innovative Telematic Medicine and Surgery services with utility, prices and costs. In this way, these new services can be strictly connected to the real value for patients.

To create innovations in Telematic Medicine and Surgery without rearranging the whole organizational flow around the future e-health service in order to improve value means inducing the healthcare organization to generate wastes and face unecessary expences attached to future healthcare processes with such high and probably unsustainable costs. For the same reason indiscriminate cost saving is not sufficient to maintain either high quality and safety or the accessibility of healthcare services. It is crucial to be really innovative in Telematic Medicine and Surgery to avoid indiscriminate action to prevent being overcome by activities which add little value for the patients, the organizations and ourselves.

REFERENCES

Aggarwal, R., & Darzi, A. (2008). Symposium on surgical simulation for training and certification. *World Journal of Surgery*, *32*, 139–140. doi:10.1007/s00268-007-9341-7

Ailawadi, G., Alykhan, S., Jones, N., & Jones, D. R. (2010). The legend behind cardiothoracic surgical instruments. *The Annals of Thoracic Surgery*, *89*, 1693–1700. doi:10.1016/j.athoracsur.2009.11.019

Andreassen, H. K., Bujnowska-Fedak, M. M., Chronaki, C. E., Dumitru, R. C., Pudule, I., & Santana, S. (2007). European citizens' use of E-health services: A study of seven countries. *BMC Public Health*, *7*, 53. doi:10.1186/1471-2458-7-53

Anvari, M. (2007). Remote telepresence surgery: The Canadian experience. *Surgical Endoscopy*, *21*(4), 537–541. doi:10.1007/s00464-006-9040-8

Ballantyne, G. H. (2002). Robotic surgery, telerobotic surgery, telepresence, and telementoring. Review of early clinical results. *Surgical Endoscopy*, *16*(10), 1389–1402. doi:10.1007/s00464-001-8283-7

Beckjord, E. B., Finney Rutten, L. J., Squiers, L., Arora, N. K., Volckmann, L., Moser, R. P., & Hesse, B. W. (2007). Use of the internet to communicate with health care providers in the United States: Estimates from the 2003 and 2005 Health Information National Trends Surveys (HINTS). *Journal of Medical Internet Research*, *9*(3), e20. doi:10.2196/jmir.9.3.e20

Boulos, M. N., Rocha, A., Martins, A., Vicente, M. E., Bolz, A., & Feld, R. (2007). CAALYX: A new generation of location-based services in healthcare. *International Journal of Health Geographics*, *6*(9).

Bowns, I. R., Collins, K., Walters, S. J., & McDonagh, A. J. (2006). Telemedicine in dermatology: A randomised controlled trial. *Health Technology Assessment*, *10*(43), iii-iv, ix-xi, 1-39.

Buntin, M. B., Burke, M. F., Hoaglin, M. C., & Blumenthal, D. (2011). The benefits of health information technology: A review of the recent literature shows predominantly positive results. *Health Affairs*, *30*(3), 464–471. doi:10.1377/hlthaff.2011.0178

Butter, M., Rensma, A., van Boxsel, J., Kalisingh, S., Schoone, M., & Leis, M. ... Korhonen, I. (2008). *Robotics for Heath Care, Final Report, October 2008.* European Commission, DG Information Society. Retrieved October, 3, 2008, from http://ec.europa.eu/information_society/activities/health/docs/studies/robotics_healthcare/robotics-final-report.pdf

Clark, R. A., Inglis, S. C., McAlister, F. A., Cleland, J. G., & Stewart, S. (2007). Telemonitoring or structured telephone support programmes for patients with chronic heart failure: Systematic review and meta-analysis. *British Medical Journal*, *334*(7600), 942. doi:10.1136/bmj.39156.536968.55

Dankelman, J. (2008). Surgical simulator design and development. *World Journal of Surgery*, *32*(2), 149–155. doi:10.1007/s00268-007-9150-z

Das, H., Ohm, T., Boswell, C., Paliug, E., Rodriguez, G., Steele, R., & Barlow, E. (1996). Engineering in medicine and biology society, bridging disciplines for biomedicine. *Proceedings of the 18th Annual International Conference of the IEEE, Vol. 1: Telerobotics for Microsurgery* (pp. 227-228). Pasadena, CA: California Inst. of Technol.

Deans, R., & Wade, S. (2011). Finding a balance between "value added" and feeling valued: revising models of care: The human factor of implementing a quality improvement initiative using Lean methodology within the healthcare sector. *Healthcare Quarterly*, *14*(3), 58–61.

Dew, K., Cumming, J., McLeod, D., Morgan, S., McKinlay, E., Dowell, A., & Love, T. (2005). Explicit rationing of elective services: Implementing the New Zealand reforms. *Health Policy (Amsterdam)*, *74*(1), 1–12. doi:10.1016/j.healthpol.2004.12.011

Eadie, L. H., Seifalian, A. M., & Davidson, B. R. (2003). Telemedicine in surgery. *British Journal of Surgery*, *90*(6), 647–658. doi:10.1002/bjs.4168

Ekeland, A. G., Bowes, A., & Flottorp, S. (2010). Effectiveness of telemedicine: A systematic review of reviews. *International Journal of Medical Informatics*, *79*(11), 736–771. doi:10.1016/j.ijmedinf.2010.08.006

Ellison, L. M., Nguyen, M., Fabrizio, M. D., Soh, A., Permpongkosol, S., & Kavoussi, L. R. (2007). Postoperative robotic telerounding: A multicenter randomized assessment of patient outcomes and satisfaction. *Archives of Surgery*, *142*(12), 1177–1181. doi:10.1001/archsurg.142.12.1177

Ellison, L. M., Pinto, P. A., Kim, F., Ong, A. M., Patriciu, A., & Stoianovici, D. (2004). Telerounding and patient satisfaction after surgery. *Journal of the American College of Surgeons*, *199*(4), 523–530. doi:10.1016/j.jamcollsurg.2004.06.022

Franzini, L., Sail, K. R., Thomas, E. J., & Wueste, L. (2011). Costs and cost-effectiveness of a telemedicine intensive care unit program in 6 intensive care units in a large health care system. *Journal of Critical Care*, *26*(3), 329. doi:10.1016/j.jcrc.2010.12.004

Fuchs, V. R. (1998). *Who shall live? Health, economics, and social choice.* Singapore: World Scientific. doi:10.1142/3534

Gibson, J., Mitton, C., & DuBois-Wing, G. (2011). Priority setting in Ontario's LHINs: Ethics and economics in action. *Healthcare Quarterly*, *14*(4), 35–43.

Greer, A. D., Newhook, P., & Sutherland, G. R. (2008). Human-machine interface for robotic surgery and stereotaxy. *IEEE/ ASME Transactions on MRI Compatible Mechatronic Systems*, *13*(3), 355-361. Calgary, Canada: Dept. of Clinical Neurosciences, Calgary Univ.

Groene, O., Klazinga, N., Wagner, C., Arah, O. A., Thompson, A., Bruneau, C., & Suñol, R. (2010). Investigating organizational quality improvement systems, patient empowerment, organizational culture, professional involvement and the quality of care in European hospitals: The 'Deepening our Understanding of Quality Improvement in Europe (DUQuE)' project. *BMC Health Services Research, 10*, 281.

Gurman, T. A., Rubin, S. E., & Roess, A. A. (2012). Effectiveness of mHealth behavior change communication interventions in developing countries: A systematic review of the literature. *Journal of Health Communication, 17*(1), 82–104. doi:10.1080/10810730.2011.649160

Hsiao, J. L., & Oh, D. H. (2008). The impact of store-and-forward teledermatology on skin cancer diagnosis and treatment. *Journal of the American Academy of Dermatology, 59*(2), 260–267. doi:10.1016/j.jaad.2008.04.011

Hurley, J., Birch, S., & Eyles, J. (1995). Geographically-decentralized planning and management in health care: Some informational issues and their implications for efficiency. *Social Science & Medicine, 41*(1), 3–11. doi:10.1016/0277-9536(94)00283-Y

Ikkersheim, D. E., & Koolman, X. (2012). Dutch healthcare reform: did it result in better patient experiences in hospitals? A comparison of the consumer quality index over time. *BMC Health Services Research, 12*, 76. doi:10.1186/1472-6963-12-76

Innes, M., Skelton, J., & Greenfield, S. (2006). A profile of communication in primary care physician telephone consultations: Application of the Roter Interaction Analysis System. *The British Journal of General Practice, 56*(526), 363–368.

Kahn, J. M., Hill, N. S., Lilly, C. M., Angus, D. C., Jacobi, J., & Rubenfeld, G. D. (2011). The research agenda in ICU telemedicine: A statement from the critical care societies collaborative. *Chest, 140*(1), 230–238. doi:10.1378/chest.11-0610

Kirkup, J. R. (1982). The history and evolution of surgical instruments, II origins: Function: Carriage: manufacture. *Annals of the Royal College of Surgeons of England, 64*(2), 125–132.

Klarman, H. E. (1965). *The economics of health.* New York, NY: Columbia University Press.

Kohn, L. T., Corrigan, J. M., & Donaldson, M. S. (Eds.). (2000). *To err is human: Building a safer health system. Committee on Quality of Health Care in America, Institute of Medicine.* Washington, DC: National Academy Press.

Krupinski, E. A., Patterson, T., Norman, C. D., Roth, Y., El Nasser, Z., & Abdeen, Z. (2011). Successful models for telehealth. [vii-viii]. *Otolaryngologic Clinics of North America, 44*(6), 1275–1288. doi:10.1016/j.otc.2011.08.004

Latifi, R., Dasho, E., Lecaj, I., Latifi, K., Bekteshi, F., & Hadeed, M. (2012). Beyond "initiate-build-operate-transfer" strategy for creating sustainable telemedicine programs: Lesson from the first decade. *Telemedicine Journal and e-Health, 18*(5), 388–390. doi:10.1089/tmj.2011.0263

Lee, S. Y., Weiner, B. J., Harrison, M. I., & Belden, C. M. (2012). Organizational transformation: A systematic review of empirical research in health care and other industries. *Medical Care Research Review,* Online first.

Leung, R. C. (2012). Health information technology and dynamic capabilities. *Health Care Management Review, 37*(1), 43–53. doi:10.1097/HMR.0b013e31823c9b55

Liker, J. (2004). *The Toyota way.* New York, NY: McGraw-Hill.

Lum, M. J. H., Trimble, D., Rosen, J., Fodero, K., II, King, H. H., & Sankaranarayanan, G. … Hannaford, B. (2006). Multidisciplinary approach for developing a new minimally invasive surgical robotic system. In *Proceedings of IEEE/RAS-EMBS International Conference on Biomedical Robotics and Biomechatronics* (pp. 1018-1022). Pisa, Italy: Scuola Superiore S'Anna.

Manning, J. (2011). Priority-setting processes for medicines: The United Kingdom, Australia and New Zealand. *Journal of Law and Medicine, 18*(3), 439–452.

Marescaux, J., Leroy, J., Rubino, F., Smith, M., Vix, M., Simone, M., & Mutter, D. (2002). Transcontinental robot-assisted remote telesurgery: Feasibility and potential applications. *Annals of Surgery, 235*(4), 487–492. doi:10.1097/00000658-200204000-00005

Mirelman, A., Mentzakis, E., Kinter, E., Paolucci, F., Fordham, R., & Ozawa, S. (2012). Decision-making criteria among national policymakers in five countries: A discrete choice experiment eliciting relative preferences for equity and efficiency. *Value in Health, 15*(3), 534–539. doi:10.1016/j.jval.2012.04.001

Moffatt, J. J., & Eley, D. S. (2003). Barriers to the up-take of telemedicine in Australia – A view from providers. *British Journal of Surgery, 90*(6), 647–658.

Pande, R. U., Patel, Y., Powers, C. J., D'Ancona, G., & Karamanoukian, H. L. (2003). The telecommunication revolution in the medical field: Present applications and future perspective. *Current Surgery, 60*(6), 636–640. doi:10.1016/j.cursur.2003.07.009

Patterson, V., Swinfen, P., Swinfen, R., Azzo, E., Taha, H., & Wootton, R. (2007). Supporting hospital doctors in the Middle East by email telemedicine: Something the industrialized world can do to help. *Journal of Medical Internet Research, 9*(4), e30. doi:10.2196/jmir.9.4.e30

Phelps, E. S. (1966). Models of technical progress and the golden rule of research. *The Review of Economic Studies, 33*, 133–146. doi:10.2307/2974437

Pink, G. H., & Leatt, P. (2003). The use of 'arms-length' organizations for health system change in Ontario, Canada: Some observations by insiders. *Health Policy (Amsterdam), 63*(1), 1–15. doi:10.1016/S0168-8510(01)00225-1

Pinnock, H., McKenzie, L., Price, D., & Sheikh, A. (2005). Cost-effectiveness of telephone or surgery asthma reviews: economic analysis of a randomised controlled trial. *The British Journal of General Practice, 55*(511), 119–124.

Puangmali, P., Althoefer, K., Seneviratne, L. D., Murphy, D., & Dasgupta, P. (2008). State-of-the-art in force and tactile sensing for minimally invasive surgery. *Sensors Journal, 8*(4), 371–381. doi:10.1109/JSEN.2008.917481

Rayman, R., Croome, K., Galbraith, N., McClure, R., Morady, R., & Peterson, S. (2007). Robotic telesurgery: A real-world comparison of ground- and satellite-based internet performance. *International Journal of Medical Robotics and Computer Assisted Surgery, 3*(2), 111–116. doi:10.1002/rcs.133

Roberts, A., Reponen, J., Pesola, U. M., Waterworth, E., Larsen, F., & Mäkiniemi, M. (2010). Transnational comparison: A retrospective study on e-health in sparsely populated areas of the northern periphery. *Telemedicine Journal and e-Health, 16*(10), 1053–1059. doi:10.1089/tmj.2010.0075

Roig, F., & Saigí, F. (2011). Barriers to the normalization of telemedicine in a healthcare system model based on purchasing of healthcare services using providers' contracts. *Gaceta Sanitaria, 25*(5), 397–402. doi:10.1016/j.gaceta.2011.01.004

Samuelson, P. A., & Nordhaus, W. D. (2005). *Economics.* New York, NY: McGraw-Hill.

Schweitzer, J., & Synowiec, C. (2012). The economics of eHealth and mHealth. *Journal of Health Communication, 17*(1), 73–81. doi:10.1080/10810730.2011.649158

Scuffham, P. (2002). Systematic review of cost effectiveness in telemedicine. Quality of cost effectiveness studies in systematic reviews is problematic. *British Medical Journal, 325*(7364), 598. doi:10.1136/bmj.325.7364.598

Scutchfield, F. D., Bhandari, M. W., Lawhorn, N. A., Lamberth, C. D., & Ingram, R. C. (2009). Public health performance. *American Journal of Preventive Medicine, 36*(3), 266–272. doi:10.1016/j.amepre.2008.11.007

Sebajang, H., Trudeau, P., Dougall, A., Hegge, S., McKinley, C., & Anvari, M. (2006). The role of telementoring and telerobotic assistance in the provision of laparoscopic colorectal surgery in rural areas. *Surgical Endoscopy, 20*(9), 1389–1393. doi:10.1007/s00464-005-0260-0

Shea, S., Weinstock, R. S., Teresi, J. A., Palmas, W., Starren, J., & Cimino, J. J. (2012). A randomized trial comparing telemedicine case management with usual care in older, ethnically diverse, medically underserved patients with diabetes mellitus: 5 year results of the IDEATel study. *Journal of the American Medical Informatics Association, 16*(4), 446–456. doi:10.1197/jamia.M3157

Smith, A. C., Bensink, M., Armfield, N., Stillman, J., & Caffery, L. (2005). Telemedicine and rural health care applications. *Journal of Postgraduate Medicine, 51*(4), 286–293.

Strehle, E. M., & Shabde, N. (2006). One hundred years of telemedicine: Does this new technology have a place in paediatrics? *Archives of Disease in Childhood, 91*(12), 956–959. doi:10.1136/adc.2006.099622

Stroetmann, V., Thierry, J. P., Stroetmann, K., & Dobrev, A. (2007). *Impact of ICT on patient safety and risk management, e-health for safety report October 2007. European Commission, Information Society and Media*. Luxembourg: Office for Official Publications of the European Communities.

Sutherland, L. M., Middleton, P. F., Anthony, A., Hamdorf, J., Cregan, P., Scott, D., & Maddern, G. J. (2006). Surgical simulation: A systematic review. *Annals of Surgery, 243*, 291–300. doi:10.1097/01.sla.0000200839.93965.26

Tanke, M. A., & Ikkersheim, D. E. (2012). A new approach to the tradeoff between quality and accessibility of health care. *Health Policy (Amsterdam), 105*(2-3), 282–287. doi:10.1016/j.healthpol.2012.02.016

Terkelsen, C. J., Lassen, J. F., Nørgaard, B. L., Gerdes, J. C., Poulsen, S. H., & Bendix, K. (2005). Reduction of treatment delay in patients with ST-elevation myocardial infarction: Impact of pre-hospital diagnosis and direct referral to primary percutanous coronary intervention. *European Heart Journal, 26*(8), 770–777. doi:10.1093/eurheartj/ehi100

Turk, E., Karagulle, E., Aydogan, C., Oguz, H., Tarim, A., Karakayali, H., & Haberal, M. (2011). Use of telemedicine and telephone consultation in decision-making and follow-up of burn patients: Initial experience from two burn units. *Burns, 37*(3), 415–419. doi:10.1016/j.burns.2010.10.004

Umefjord, G., Hamberg, K., Malker, H., & Petersson, G. (2006). The use of an Internet-based Ask the Doctor service involving family physicians: Evaluation by a web survey. *Family Practice, 23*, 159–166. doi:10.1093/fampra/cmi117

U.S. Food and Drug Administration. (2009). *MedSun: Medical product safety network improving patient safety by reporting problems with medical devices used in the home*. Retrieved from http://www.fda.gov/MedicalDevices/Safety/MedSun-MedicalProductSafetyNetwork/ucm205691.htm#transcript

Van den Brink-Muinen, A., Verhaak, P. F., Bensing, J. M., Bahrs, O., Deveugele, M., & Gask, L. (2000). Doctor patient communication in different European health care systems: Relevance and performance from the patients' perspective. *Patient Education and Counseling, 39*(1), 115–127. doi:10.1016/S0738-3991(99)00098-1

Vespa, P. (2005). Robotic telepresence in the intensive care unit. *Critical Care (London, England), 9*, 319–320. doi:10.1186/cc3743 von Lubitz, D. K., Carrasco, B., Gabbrielli, F., Ludwig, T., Levine, H., & Patricelli, F. (2003). Transatlantic medical education: Preliminary data on distance-based high-fidelity human patient simulation training. *Studies in Health Technology and Informatics*, *94*, 379–385.

Weinstein, R. S., Lopez, A. M., Krupinski, E. A., Beinar, S. J., Holcomb, M., & McNeely, R. A. (2008). Integrating telemedicine and telehealth: Putting it all together. *Studies in Health Technology and Informatics*, *131*, 23–38.

Whittaker, R., Merry, S., Dorey, E., & Maddison, R. (2012). A development and evaluation process for mHealth interventions: Examples from New Zealand. *Journal of Health Communication*, *17*(Suppl 1), 11–21. doi:10.1080/10810730.2011.649103

Whitten, P., & Love, B. (2005). Patient and provider satisfaction with the use of telemedicine: Overview and rationale for cautious enthusiasm. *Journal of Postgraduate Medicine*, *51*(4), 294–300.

Whitten, P. S., Mair, F. S., Haycox, A., May, C. R., Williams, T. L., & Hellmich, S. (2002). Systematic review of cost effectiveness studies of telemedicine interventions. *British Medical Journal*, *324*(7351), 1434–1437. doi:10.1136/bmj.324.7351.1434

Wyss, K., & Lorenz, N. (2000). Decentralization and central and regional coordination of health services: The case of Switzerland. *The International Journal of Health Planning and Management*, *15*(2), 103–114. doi:10.1002/1099-1751(200004/06)15:2<103::AID-HPM581>3.0.CO;2-S

Young, L. B., Chan, P. S., Lu, X., Nallamothu, B. K., Sasson, C., & Cram, P. M. (2011). Impact of telemedicine intensive care unit coverage on patient outcomes: A systematic review and meta-analysis. *Archives of Internal Medicine*, *171*(6), 498–506. doi:10.1001/archinternmed.2011.61

Zanaboni, P., & Wootton, R. (2012). Adoption of telemedicine: From pilot stage to routine delivery. *BMC Medical Informatics and Decision Making*, *12*(1). doi:10.1186/1472-6947-12-1

Chapter 18
Sensorized Garments Developed for Remote Postural and Motor Rehabilitation

Giovanni Saggio
University of Rome "Tor Vergata", Italy

Valentina Sabato
University of Rome "Tor Vergata", Italy

Roberto Mugavero
University of Rome "Tor Vergata", Italy

ABSTRACT

Every day, all around the world, millions of people request postural and/or motor rehabilitation. The rehabilitation process, also known as Tertiary Prevention, intends to be a sort of therapy to restore functionality and self-sufficiency of the patient, and regards not only millions of patients daily, but involves also a huge number of professionals in medical staffs, i.e. specialists, nurses, physiotherapists and therapists, social workers, psychologists, physiatrists. The care is given in hospitals, clinics, geriatric facilities, and with territorial home care. For the large number of patients as well as the medical staff and facilities necessary to support the appropriate postural and motor training, the monetary costs of rehabilitation is so large, it is difficult to estimate. So, every effort towards a simplification of the rehabilitation route is desirable and welcome, and this chapter covers this aspect.

INTRODUCTION

Nowadays in the world there are about 600 million of people with various types of disabilities (Fifty-Eighth World Health Assembly) with respect to a total world population of around 7 billion of persons. This number is rapidly increasing since the population growth rate, the increasing average age,

the malnutrition, the violence (especially domestic ones), the environmental degradation, the diseases (such as AIDS, malaria, Ebola,..), amputations, medical treatments, or finally because of injury reported in various type of accidents (work, road, sport, guns, etc.).

From an analysis of available statistical data on disability, it results that each country has a

DOI: 10.4018/978-1-4666-2979-0.ch018

different concept of "disabilities" and their cares. There are situations for which the disabled person is considered who doesn't have a dignified life, and therefore live in extreme poverty. Other societies consider the disability the condition for which it is not possible to work continuously, and others that define people with disabilities just who needs government support to live. Finally, some countries consider disabled only those persons with a form of physical disability or who are suffering from physically debilitating diseases like multiple sclerosis can be.

Focusing only on people with physical impairments, the 80% of them live in poverty and therefore have no care taking, and it cannot be otherwise since in the world there are only just more than 300,000 accredited physiotherapists capable of giving support to physical deficit. The percentage of disability shows a great variability between countries from 0.2 to 20.9% with respect the population, especially regarding the degree of disabilities. The average prevalence is approximately 10%, half of which 5% is from moderate to severe conditions. In the year 2000, the 70% of disabled were living in developing countries and only 3% of them were appropriately treated (WCPT Quadriennal Report 2003-2007; Takahashi et al., 2003).

Rehabilitation care cannot reach all patients and this is a problem both for developing than developed countries. In fact only 50% of States are able to provide the necessary care and the disabled population that can be medical treated is about 20% of the total. All around the world there are Nations that haven't the capability to do this at all. The distribution of physiotherapists around the world is indicative: in developing countries there is 1 physical therapist every 550,000 patients while in developed countries this ratio is only 1 every 1,400 patients (WCPT, October 2003). The point is also that a patient who claim rehabilitation need not only of therapists but also of many other medical and non-medical staff figures, as Figure 1 summarizes.

The care can be given in hospitals, clinics, geriatric facilities and with territorial home care. So, we have to consider that not only the real treatments of the patients have their costs, but also costs which come from the necessary environmental structures. In Table 1 a brief summary of setting and purpose for the rehabilitation evaluation (Ganter et al., 2005).

Let's consider some detailed examples of data regarding consistent part of the world of numerical values to be considered in rehabilitation course.

The percentage of disability in the United States of America is around the 12.1% with respect the overall population. There a disabled person is defined as who is deaf or has serious difficulty in hearing; who is blind or has serious difficulty seeing even when wearing glasses; who has serious difficulty concentrating, remembering, or making decisions because of a physical, mental, or emotional condition; who has serious difficulty walking or climbing stairs; who has difficulty dressing or bathing or has difficulty doing errands alone such as visiting a doctor's office or shopping because of a physical, mental, or emotional condition (www.bls.gov). We can guess as the 1/3 of percentage of them regards people with motor deficit.

Figure 1. People involved in patient's motor rehabilitation

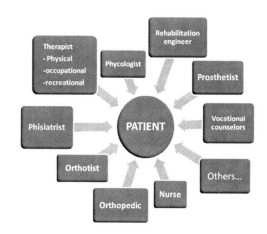

Table 1. The rehabilitation evaluation: setting and purpose

Hospital	Inpatient rehabilitation unit	Comprehensive evaluation by team
	Off-service consultation	Assessment by physician of potential for rehabilitation benefit
Clinic	General rehabilitation clinic	Comprehensive evaluation by team
		Assessment by physician of potential for rehabilitation benefit
		Limited evaluation of specific disease group (e.g., muscular dystrophy, sports injury)
	Day rehabilitation program	Comprehensive evaluation by team
	Impairment/disability clinic	Evaluation determined by requirement of referring agency (e.g., workers' compensation, social security)
	Community nursing home	Comprehensive evaluation by team
		Limited assessment by selected numbers of rehabilitation team
		Assessment by physician of potential for rehabilitation benefit
	School	Limited evaluation of physical disability
		Limited evaluation for participation in sports
	Transition living facilities	Comprehensive evaluation by team
		Limited assessment of specific problem

Table 2 shows the number of people with/without disabilities with respect the level of employment in the U.S.A., comparing the same months of the current and last year.

Reporting another example, we focus on the situation of disability in Europe, represented in the chart below (ANED, 2009), in terms of overall costs with respect to the percentage of Gross Domestic Product of each Country (see Figure 2). The overall costs are here be considered the mere rehabilitation ones and the social costs supported by the community too.

The decision to propose the situation in economic term is due to the fact that the European Union is composed of very different countries, each of one with its definition of "disability" and with its own budget and health policies (without differencing between public and private expenditure), done with respect to the Gross Domestic Product. So there are objective difficulties to compare otherwise than referring to the expenses paid for the disability conditions of European people.

The annual cost incurred pro capital is rather in the chart of Figure 3.

To try to solve the problems of disabilities, each Country assesses proper rehabilitation courses. Their management is very expensive from a monetary point of view, but also from personnel and facilities needed to carry out the health service.

As another example, let's consider the situation of the disability only in Italy (author's country), respect to a total population of around 60.6 million of people. There are about 2,830,000 disabled people, divided as follows (Ministero della Salute - Ufficio di Direzione Statistica, January 2011):

- **Patients assisted at home:** 494,204 (the 81% of them are over 65 years old);
- **Physical disabled:** 12,220 users in nursing homes, 10695 patients cared for day hospital;
- **Mobility disabled:** 21,747 patients in nursing homes (47 days in hospital on average for each patient), 4,550 patients cared for day hospital (57 days of hospitalization for each patient), 2,311,136 disabled assisted in the surgery.

Table 2. Persons with/without disabilities with respect the employed status, sex and age in USA

Employed status, sex, and age	Persons with a disability		Persons with no disability	
	May 2010	May 2011	May 2010	May 2011
TOTAL, 16 years and over				
Civilian non institutional population	26,547	27,669	210,952	211,644
Civilian labor force	5,930	5,828	147,936	147,621
Participation rate	22.3	21.1	70.1	69.7
Employed	5,060	4,917	134,437	135,11
Employed - population rate	19.1	17.8	63.7	69.7
Unemployed	870	911	13,499	12,510
Unemployment rate	14.7	15.6	9.1	8.5
Not in labor force	20,617	21,841	63,016	64,024
Men, 16 to 64 years				
Civilian labor force	2,729	2,682	75,601	75,258
Participation rate	37.5	35.3	83.1	82.5
Employed	2,282	2,218	68,019	68,474
Employed - population rate	31.3	29.2	74.7	75.1
Unemployed	448	464	7,582	6,784
Unemployment rate	16.4	17.3	10.1	9
Not in labor force	4,555	4,911	15,399	15,948
Women, 16 to 64 years				
Civilian labor force	2,381	2,280	66,472	66,109
Participation rate	30.9	29.2	71.5	70.9
Employed	2,052	1,919	60,856	60,748
Employed - population rate	26.6	24.6	65.5	65.2
Unemployed	330	360	5616.00	5,361
Unemployment rate	13.8	15.8	8.4	8.1
Not in labor force	5,321	5,531	26,452	27,107
Both sexes, 65 years and over				
Civilian labor force	820	867	5,862	6,254
Participation rate	7.1	7.1	21.7	23.0
Employed	727	780	5,561	5,889
Employed - population rate	6.3	6.4	20.6	21.6
Unemployed	93	87	301	365
Unemployment rate	11.3	10.0	5.1	5.8
Not in labor force	10,741	11,399	21,166	20,969

The expenditure which the Italian State claims for treatment and rehabilitation activities are very high: all patients hospitalized for physical rehabilitation cost 135.50 €/day, patients cared in day hospital cost 82.50 €/day, while people treated in surgery cost 38.50 €/day and finally the people cared for at home cost 47.00 €/day.

Figure 2. Invalidity in % of GDP in European countries, 2006 (all schemes, non means-tested benefits and means-tested benefits)

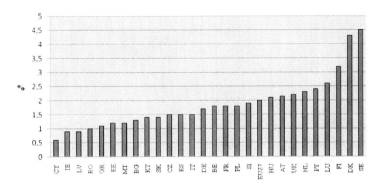

Figure 3. Tested benefit, invalidity 2006 (all schemes, non means-tested benefit and means-tested benefits)

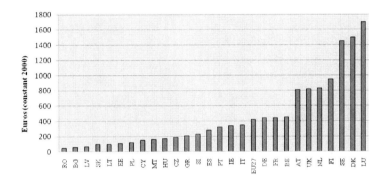

The medical and paramedical staff employed in public facilities is as follows: Orthopaedics: 681, Physiotherapists: 1,526, Speech therapists: 278, Other staff: 2,012.

The staff employed in private structures: Orthopaedics: 4,007, Physiotherapists: 14,480, Speech therapists: 2,896, Other staff: 20,685

The annual working hours for each patient are:

- **In hospital:** Orthopaedics: 21.2, Therapists: 51.1, Speech therapists: 11.1;
- **In day hospital:** Orthopaedics: 19.9, Therapists: 83.4, Speech therapists:13.8;
- **In surgery:** Doctors: 0.1, Therapists: 0.8, Speech therapists: 0.3.

These data demonstrate that rehabilitation is onerous for both the State and patients, especially because the treatment often lead to only partial motor recovery.

2. THE MEASURE OF STATIC AND DYNAMIC PATIENT'S POSTURES

After traumatic accidents, injuries, diseases, strokes, amputations and so on, a loose of partial or total motor abilities can follow. So, postural activities are compromised, but these are a pre-condition for any successful voluntary action execution (Arbib, 1981). Even a non-accidental event, such as a cosmetic surgery, with the slightest modifications (even less than 400 grams) can meaningfully affect the postural system, also if for a limited time (Bellomo et al., 2011). In all these occurrences, it is mandatory to try to return to full motor functionalities and to a convenient postural structure of the body. This can be obtained with a specific rehabilitation route, as Figure 4 schematizes.

As a starting point, a functional assessment of the patient is needed so to resolve a medical diagnosis. This stage consists in the evaluation of the historical clues and physical findings of the patient, evaluated taking into account his/her residual motor functionalities. Nurses and therapists measure, as a current practice, the patient's static postures and/or articulation's Range Of Motion (ROM) and, sometimes, joint instability and/or alignment, by manual stuff such as goniometer, reflex hammer, finger circumference gauge, Gulick anthropometric tape, plastic posture grid as reference, baseline scoliosis meter, chest calliper, inclinometer, adjustable sit and reach flexibility tester, digitometer finger motion gauge, universal protractor, and so on (in Figure 5 some examples).

These systems of measure surely occur in the preliminary stage but, quite often, they remain the only common procedures of measure, eventually adopted again if a new functional assessment is necessary (returning to functional assessment after training in Figure 4). Only for some specific cases, other more sophisticated technical measuring procedures are utilized. We refer, for instance, to patient's locomotion analysis which,

Figure 4. The rehabilitation route

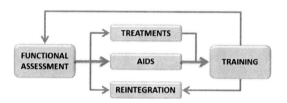

only when necessary, is performed by passive infrared cameras and/or embedded force platforms, as Figure 6 reports.

But these latter systems remain far away from be adopted as a standard rule in all circumstances, since their higher costs in terms of money, spaces and involved personnel.

Returning to the rehabilitation route, if the first stage of functional assessment reserves non negative results we can think about a reintegration of the patient in the society, otherwise treatments or aids are necessary. The treatments consist of functional recovery by means of rehabilitative procedures, or functional replacement by means of technical equipment, or functional surgery aimed at modify/replace the malfunctioning organ. On the other side, the aids are intended as technical facilities useful to allow the patient to reach the maximum possible degree of independence.

After the treatments or the aids stage, a training procedure is necessary. In fact, the patient must be educated to his/her novel condition or be re-educated to gradually return to his/her pre-trauma status of motor ability.

Figure 5. (a) Knee goniometer, (b) biplane goniometer, (c) Gollehon extendable goniometer, (d) finger goniometer, (e) digitometer finger motion gauge

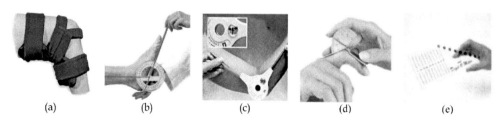

Figure 6. Platform with embedded force sensors, courtesy of ITOP

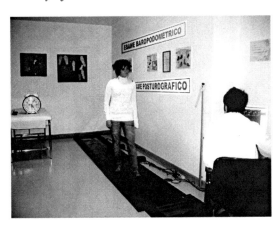

In any case, during all the rehabilitation steps, the measures play a fundamental rule, especially in clinical decision-making as already underlined and demonstrated (Giani, 2011). Furthermore, the measures can be carried on not only for the evaluation of treatment procedure, but also for a feedback to the patient, for the assessment of work capacity or, even, for research purposes. These repeated necessity to measure, claims efforts and time both from the professionals and from the patient and are, as already mentioned, performed with overcome methodologies, since anchored to manual stuff. The manual methods of measure can be highly inaccurate and can offer important disadvantages: they strictly depend on the abilities of the expert (often nurse or therapist); they can be performed only for a very limited period of time (typically few minutes or, even, seconds); necessarily the patient must be present in the medical structure (hospital, nursing home, sanitarium or what else). Furthermore, difficulties come also from the fact that ROMs present considerable variations among different persons, and factors such as age, sex, obesity, genetics can influence them. Last but not least, the patient can be asked to perform the ROM maneuver at home by him/her-self, without assistance from the examiner (these are the so called active ROM).

This is because, enabling individuals to manage daily self-care is among the most important goals undertaken by the rehabilitation staff, since such tasks relate directly to the business of living and their performance signifies a return to participation in the routines of daily life. In this occurrence, comparisons can be possible between active ROM and the measurements performed by specialists (known as passive ROM), but only if the starting position, stabilization, goniometer's alignment, and type of goniometer are strictly the same.

In addition to all the previous considerations, the mapping of the body postures/kinematics and the measured values over a period of time can be of strategic importance, again not only for rehabilitation purposes, but even for evaluating the emotional reactions a patient can present to several events, and for realizing more ergonomic stuff necessary for the rehabilitation itself, or to furnish a complete database useful for programming future interventions.

So, it becomes mandatory to reserve to the measure of patient's motor residual functionalities much more consideration and devote them more efforts respect to what has been done till now. It is now evident the importance to have the possibility to count on an alternative system of measure with the characteristic of objectivity, precision, reliability, portability (home/clinical/ other environment), economy, long term monitoring (minutes, hours till days) and ease of use even for non-specialists. The alternative system of measurements refers only to the latest years and, even if technologically enough mature, struggle to be adopted as standards. These new systems are mainly based on the latest developed sensors, and for them the electronic part plays the winning rule. Several further advantages of the new system of measure:

- The measurements can be directly presented as digit, so they can be easily read and understood;

- The measurement are expressed by electronic signals, so data can be easily directly processed and stored even in digital records specific for that particular patient;
- The measurement can be easily performed even over a long period, so data can be adopted to easily monitor the patient's long time trend;
- The measurements are not "strictly" dependent on the operator's skill.

So, we will have a look at the novel possibilities offered by the new technologies and, as a starting point, we purpose a scheme for their classification, so to offer a suggestion to be adopted as a profitable technical solution of measure for the specific patient. In addiction we will detail some solutions we developed in our laboratory.

3. CLASSIFICATION OF SYSTEMS FOR STATIC AND DYNAMIC POSTURE MEASUREMENTS

The latest technologies offer different measurement systems, more or less sophisticated, more or less expensive. To determine which are the most feasible for the purpose of obtaining objective, accurate and time protracted measure for rehabilitation purposes and for specific patients, it is convenient to classify all the current systems.

An interesting classification is based on position of the sensors and the sources (Wang, 2005; Saggio and Sbernini, 2011). Specifically, as schematized in Figure 7:

- **Outside-In Systems:** The sensors are somewhere in the world, the sources are attached to the body.
- **Inside-Out Systems:** The sensors are positioned on the body, the sources are somewhere else in the world.

Figure 7. Schematization of body posture measurement systems

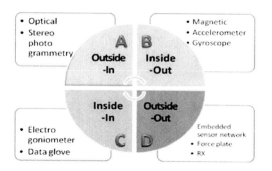

- **Inside-In Systems:** The sensors and sources are on the user's body.
- **Outside-Out Systems:** Both sensors and sources are not (directly) placed on the user's body.

The *Outside-In* Systems typically involve optical techniques with markers, which are the sources, strategically placed on the patient's body parts which are to be tracked. Cameras, which are the sensors, capture the patient's movement, and the motion of those markers can be tracked and analyzed. Examples come from the assessment of the amount and the consistency of natural motion at the trunk anatomical complex during locomotion and elementary oscillatory exercises (Benedetti, Biagi et al., 2011), biomechanical analysis in posture & gait (D'Amico et al., 2011), head-tracker device based on a light source placed on the patient's head and a CCD camera which capture the movements of the head (Lin et al., 2006), and so on.

The *Inside-Out* Systems deal with sensors attached to the body while sources are located somewhere else in the world. Examples are the systems based on accelerometers (Fiorentino et al., 2011; Mostarac et al., 2011; Silva et al., 2011), MEMS (Bifulco et al., 2011), strain gauges (Ming et al., 2009), ensemble of inertial sensors such as accelerometers, gyroscopes and magnetometers

(Benedetti, Manca et al., 2011), or IMUs which we applied to successfully measure movements of the human trunk (see Figure 8, Saggio & Sbernini, 2011).

Within this frame, same research groups and commercial companies have developed sensorized garments for all the parts of the body, over the past 10-15 years, obtaining interesting results (Post et al., 2000; Lorussi, Tognetti et al., 2005; Giorgino et al., 2009).

The *Inside-In* Systems are particularly used to track body part movements and/or relative movements between specific parts of the body, having no knowledge of the 3D world the user is in. Such systems are for sensors and sources which are for the most part realized within the same device and are placed directly on the body segment to be measured or even sewed inside the user's garment. The design and implementation of sensors that are minimally obtrusive, have low-power consumption, and that can be attached to the body or can be part of clothes, with the employ of wireless technology, allows to obtain data over an extended period of time and without significant discomfort. As an example, in the latest years innovative sensors have been the so called "bend sensors" which are mostly piezoelectric based devices, and are adopted placed directly on the human joint or trunk part under measure. Adopting them, our research group developed a version of a "data glove" (in Figure 9 three different versions), named *Hiteg glove* (*Health Involved*

Figure 8. Measured trunk movements are replicated on a PC screen

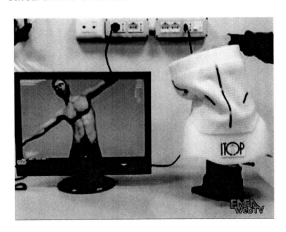

Technical Engineering Group, see paragraph 4.1.1, Saggio et al., 2009a), which is a glove provided with sensors, capable to measure all the degree of freedom of the human hand.

The *Outside-Out* Systems refer both sensors and sources not directly placed on the user's body but in the surrounding world. Let's consider, for instance, the radiology apparatus. Nowadays it is practically used for trunk movement and posture analysis. It presents the great advantage of a very high measurement accuracy since it shows directly what happens to the joints. Obviously, on the other end, it can be hazardous, for repeated X-ray exposures and needs highly skilled operators and special dedicated environment. We cannot affirm that in the radiology, sensors and sources are placed on the user's body as, in the same way,

Figure 9. (a) First, (b) second, and (c) latest version of the Hiteg glove

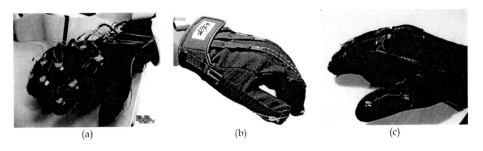

(a)   (b)   (c)

appens for non-contact sensors as microphones can be, with audio processing (for instance to measure the hearth beat), or the new Wireless Embedded Sensor Networks which consist of sensors embedded in object such as an armchair. The sensors detect the human postures and, on the basis of the recorded measures, furnish information to modify the shape of the armchair to best fit the user body, even taking into account the environment changes. A derivation of this concept was applied for adjusting cushion pressure of a wheelchair to the sitting position of the patient (Tanimoto et al., 1998), or realizing sensing devices embedded within a manually powered wheelchair to measure biomedical signals (Pinheiro at al., 2011). Other systems of the same kind were based on wireless modules integrated on forearm crutches which measure the weight applied, the tilt and the hand position of the user (Merret et al., 2010), or the measure of the respiratory effort signals using pressure sensors placed below a mattress (Holtzman et al., 2011), till the adoption of an array of embedded fiber optic pressure sensors placed under a hospital bed mattress for the detection of bouncing during sit-to-stand transfers (Arcelus et al., 2011). Clearly, this systems, as well as the others, can find applications not strictly related to measure patient's motion or postures. In fact, as a particular and curios applications, Outside-Out System was adopted to utilize the motion tracking of the hand of a surgeon as a pointing device in a surgery room (Colombo et al., 2003).

3.1. Methods

After the proposed classification, we tried to understand which is/are the system/systems among the four, that can be more interesting in order to measures of motor capability of the patients. To this aim, we conducted a survey to understand which are the most important and/or appealing requirements a measuring system must satisfy,

to discover which possible new scenarios will be opened in the next future (Saggio and Sbernini, 2011). A detailed form was submitted to 24 participants actually or potentially involved with the utilization of human measurement for motor analysis systems. In particular we interviewed 4 groups of people divided into 6 clinicians (3 spine surgeons and 3 orthopaedics), 8 bioengineers, 4 orthopaedic technicians, 6 patients with light/heavy trunk's injuries. The form is divided into four sections: the first "overall" concerns general considerations (12 questions), the second "data" (5 questions) and the third "measure" (11 questions) are devoted to acquisition and analysis of data, the last "patients" (8 questions) mostly concerns the user's point of view. Each row of the form reports a question beginning with the sentence "the importance to have …?" to which each of the 16 people are asked to reply with a weight from zero (no importance at all) to 5 (extreme importance). Table 3 reports the results, where the last four columns before the total summarize the average values obtained from each of the 4 groups of people.

To give a meaning to the form, we added each row values obtaining (12+5+11+8 questions =) 36 numeric results, and empirically (only based on our experience) we assigned a positive result only to the row sum greater than 16 (being 20 the maximum rate).

Summarizing, the most relevant parameters for the electronic measurement systems resulted to be: high portability, lightness, robustness, short calibration time, accuracy, no influence and independence from environment, no mechanical constrains, non-intrusiveness, for normal day activities, unhazardous/non-invasive and subject's acceptance.

Crossing all the results, as a conclusion we can say that the type "A" *Outside-In* Systems have a low consideration, the type "B" *Inside-Out* Systems have been positively considered with except the magnetic based solution, the type "C"

Table 3. Form submitted to 24 people involved in trunk posture measurements

	OVERALL	Clinic.	Bioeng.	Orthop.	Patients	TOT
O1	Low cost	4	3.5	3.25	2.33	13.08
O2	High porta-bility	4.5	4.25	4.5	4.67	**17.92**
O3	Lightness	3.83	3.88	4.75	4.33	**16.79**
O4	Short time to assess the measure-ment	3.67	4.13	4	3.83	15.63
O5	Easy to use	3.5	4	4.25	3.83	15.58
O6	Skilled operators, dedicated environ.	4.33	3.13	4	3.5	14.96
O7	Systems robustness	4.33	4.63	4.75	4	**17.71**
O8	Short calibration time	3.5	4	4.5	4	**16.00**
O9	Low power consump-tion	3.83	2.88	2.75	2.33	11.79
O10	Consolidat-ed technol-ogy	3.83	3.25	3.25	2.5	12.83
O11	Self consis-tency	2.67	2.25	2	1	7.92
O12	Indoor/out-door usage	3.83	4.63	3.5	3.5	15.46
	DATA	Clinic.	Bioeng.	Orthop.	Patients	TOT
D1	Low data analysis complexity/ Processing time	2.67	1.88	2.5	1.33	8.38
D2	Low num-ber of key measure-ment points	3.33	3.75	2.75	3.67	13.5
D3	Real time/ Negligible transient time	3.83	4.63	3.5	2.33	14.29
D4	High frequency sample	3.67	3.38	3	2.17	12.22
D5	No ambigu-ity	4	4.88	4.25	1.83	14.96

continued on following page

Table 3. Continued

	MEASURE	Clinic.	Bioeng.	Orthop.	Patients	TOT
M1	Repeatability/reversibility	4.83	4.13	3.75	3	15.71
M2	Accuracy	4.83	4.38	3.75	3.5	**16.46**
M3	Long term	4	4	3.75	3	14.75
M4	No sensitivity to shock	4	4	4	2.5	14.50
M5	No influence from environment	4.17	4.63	4.25	3.33	**16.38**
M6	Autonomy	3.33	3.25	4.5	3.83	14.91
M7	Immunity to noise/disturb/drift/shifts	4.67	4.25	2.75	2.5	14.17
M8	Indirect measure	3.17	2.5	2	1.5	9.17
M9	Independence from the environment	4.33	4.63	4.5	4.17	**17.63**
M10	No occlusion problems	3.67	3.75	3.5	2.17	13.09
M11	Limited to 2D or for 3D measures	4.5	4.25	3	1.33	13.08
	PATIENTS	Clinic.	Bioeng.	Orthop.	Patients	TOT
P1	No mechanical constrains	4.67	4.38	3.75	4.17	**16.96**
P2	Non intrusiveness	4.67	4	3.75	4.5	**16.92**
P3	For normal day activities	4.67	4.63	3.75	4.33	**17.38**
P4	Unhazardous/non-invasive	4.83	5	5	4.83	**19.66**
P5	Low weight/bulkiness	3.83	3.63	4	4.33	15.79
P6	Large space for movements	4.83	3.5	3.5	4	15.83
P7	Subject's acceptance	4.67	4.13	4.25	4.67	**17.72**
P8	Self-adoption	3.5	3.38	3.25	4.17	14.30

Inside-In Systems have a good consideration and finally the type "D" *Outside-Out* Systems have a great consideration if we leave out the radiology application.

So the results of our test indicates that the systems to which people look generally with more attention are hybrid, collecting the most interesting features mainly of the type "D", followed by the types "C" and finally "B" Systems. The type "A" has its importance, but restricted for applications which needs robustness and without any kind of mechanical constrains.

3.2 Technological and Economic Feasibility

It is interesting to notice that, with respect to the submitted form, for all the questioned figures in rehabilitation (clinicians, bioengineers, orthopedic technicians, patients), the "low cost" is not one of the major issue. But, as we know pretty well, it can be the first consideration, also according to our purposes here, for the realization of any kind of electronic measures. So, here we propose and discuss systems which take into account the results already discussed, but technological aspects and economic feasibility. These electronic systems must be capable to measure the human static postures, kinematics, alignments, symmetry, but we will focus especially on Range of Motions (ROMs), since these can be the most meaningful measures for the *functional assessment* step in the rehabilitation course.

Generally speaking the ROM should be checked in flexion, extension, rotation, and lateral or side bending. Going into details of the human parts, the normal ROM for shoulder are approximately 180° flexion, 45° extension, 180° abduction, 45° adduction, 55° internal rotation, 45° external rotation; ROM of the knee should be approximately 135° of flexion and 0° degrees of extension, while both internal and external rotation should be approximately 10°; when testing

ROM for the ankle, there should be at least 10° of dorsiflexion with 45° of plantar flexion; the subtalar joint (also known as the talocalcaneal joint which is a joint of the foot) should measure around 20° of inversion and 10° of eversion ROM. Regard the upper limb, the most interesting measures can be the forearm pronation and supination, the wrist flexion and extension, the wrist radial/ulnar deviation, the first, second, third, and fourth metacarpophalangeal flexion, the first, second, third, and fourth interphalangeal flexion. All the body ROM's averages are reported in an American Academy of Orthopaedic Surgeons (AAOS, 1988).

3.2.1. Hiteg Glove

Among all, initially we focused on an automatic system capable to measure movements of the hands. This is because the hands are our primary tools for interacting with the environment. Even the most significant function of the shoulder, elbow, and wrist is somewhat to position the hand in space to allow it to proceed with its functional task.

The measuring system is required to acquire data related to the ROMs of a patient's hands in a fraction of the time required by a skilled therapist, and with more repeatable results. As a comparison a skilled therapist with a mechanical goniometer can take up to two hours to perform a complete measure of the two hand's ROMs and, if the same expert with the same mechanical goniometer later re-performs the same measurements, the results are only repeatable to within five degrees in angle. The automatic system is also required to be easily usable by less skilled expert or, even, by the patient alone, without a supervision.

We satisfied the requests with the already mentioned *Hiteg glove* (www.hiteg.uniroma2.it), which summarizes the interesting properties of type "B" (*Outside-In*) and type "C" (*Inside-In*) Systems.

It is essentially a lightweight, tight-fitting, stretchable, unobtrusively, no loose-fitting glove, containing sensors capable to measure all the hand's degree of freedom. Particularly the finger joints measured are the metacarpophalangeal (MP or inner) joints, the proximal interphalangeal (PIP or middle) joints, the distal interphalangeal (DIP or outer) joints, their relative abdu-adduction movements (see Figure 10), while the other measures regard the palm, the wrist and the forearm movements and positions in space. Positioning, orientation, movements (roll, jaw, jitter) data, comes from of an ensemble of sensors, i.e. accelerometers, gyroscopes and magnetoresistances, since data recorded from one of them are correlated to the others so to compensate and reduce the measurement errors.

The analog recorded signals from the sensors are electronically conditioned, digitally converted and multiplexed to data-acquisition hardware which interfaces to a personal computer. Sensitivity of the *hiteg glove* was demonstrated to allow errors less than four degrees in angles (Saggio at al., 2009b), so a bit better than the ones produced by skilled expert of measure.

In addition to the anatomical measures obtained by the ROMs data, the *hiteg glove* can be capable to functional test measurements, i.e. to establish the times the patient needs to perform common unilateral tasks like stacking checkers, turning over cards, putting objects in a can, etc., but this aspect was not considered at this time since the rehabilitation common protocols are usually limited to

ROM and motion profiles and do not address the precision of motion (Becker and Thakor, 1988; Chao et al., 1989). In any case, in a next future, this other aspect will be covered too. In fact, the data glove was also demonstrated to be effective for functional hand assessment (Williams et al., 2000; Simone et al., 2007).

3.2.2. Trunk Measures

Another step we performed was the development of a non-invasive, light and wearable system capable to measure the human trunk movements. It is based on three-axial accelerometers and Inertial Measurement Units (IMUs), which integrate a combination of accelerometers, gyroscopes and magnetoresistances. We used a combination of sensors, because they, even if fairly diffused, suffer from drift and off-set problems. So, we implemented home-made correction algorithms capable to overcome the problems, taking into account cross-measures among the sensors.

To be confident with the realized system, we built a dummy which replicates the real human trunk movements (see Figure 11a), and a set-up to realize automatic measurements and to verify the performances of the sensors in terms of accuracy and sensitivity (see Figure 11b).

In addition we designed and realized the electronic conditioning circuitry and implemented a virtual representation of the measured movements too (see Figure 12).

Figure 10. (a) Evidence of the finger's joints, (b) flex-extension, and (c) abdu-adduction movements

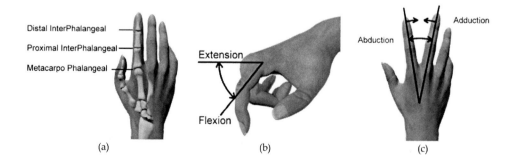

(a)   (b)   (c)

Figure 11. (a) The dummy and (b) the set-up for the automatic measurements

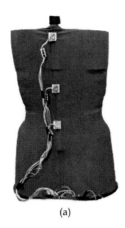
(a)

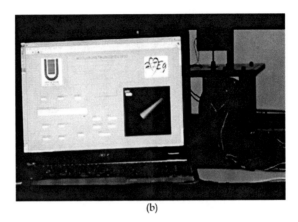
(b)

Figure 12. (a) Lateral and (b) front measured trunk movements are replicated on a pc screen

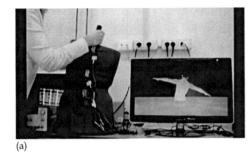
(a)

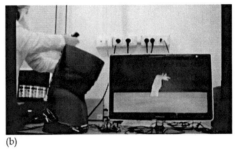
(b)

4. APPLICATIONS AT HOME

Applications at home of the previously described measurement systems can be fundamental from an economic point of view, for less time-consuming procedures, for the effectiveness of the treatment. In fact, in this manner, the number of persons and locations involved can be meaningfully reduced, there is no necessity of prepare a measurement set-up in advance, and the patient performs measurements during his/her daily common activities without bearing stressful medical sessions at the hospital. The implementation of sensors that are minimally obtrusive, have low-power consumption, and that can be attached to the body or can be part of clothes, with the employ of wireless technology, allows to obtain data over an extended period of time and without significant discomfort. Furthermore, this advantages permit to redirect

clinical assessment from the dedicated laboratory to a more real-life setting such as the home.

Again, as an example of application we will refer to the hand, since it is our first shield as a protection to fall and other kinds of mishaps, and it is one of the main part of the body to be potentially damaged by accidents. Then the motor rehabilitation highly involves the human hand, and for this aspect among the sensorized garments a fundamental rule is played by the "data glove", which is easy to don, quite comfortable since it can be made of light tissue, and does not obstruct common movements. In Figure 13 is represented the overall data acquisition system for measurements recorded by our *hiteg glove*. The glove communicates the patient's hand movements to a personal computer and an avatar replays the same recorded static and dynamic postures, so to give a visual feedback to the user.

Figure 13. (a) Set-up for data acquisition of hand movements, (b) movements are replicated in real-time on a PC screen, (c) movements can be off-line replayed

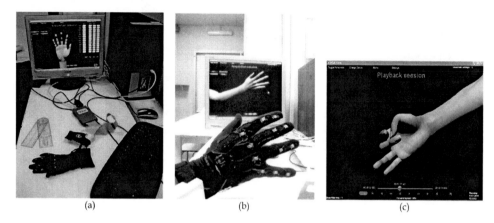

(a)　　　　　　　　　　　　(b)　　　　　　　　　　　　(c)

4.1. Virtual and Augmented Reality

The motivation of the patient can be significantly improved thanks to systems which integrates a Virtual (Holden, 2005; Saggio, Latessa et al., 2009; Saggio & Pinto, 2010) or Augmented Reality (Luo et al., 2005) scenario. The patient can visualize the movements he/she does observing a specimen avatar on a computer screen replaying his/her movements, so having non-intimidating and unambiguous suggestions. The patient can replay those movements as in a play rule, so being more motivated (Maclean et al., 2000) according to the Kemp model (Kemp, 1998). He/she can be supported by a pc-based software which records all his/her movements and classifies them so allowing a self-evaluation of the rehabilitation progresses (Saggio, Ferrari, Mugavero, patent no. PCT/IB2011/000077).

In particular a pre-imposed routine visualize qualitatively and quantitatively static and/or dynamic postures, which the user is asked to perform (for instance according to a pre-defined workload). The visualization can be realized by an ad-hoc detailed avatar on a computer screen. The quantitative information can be furnished, for instance, by simple numerical values and/or by scale indicators. The user is asked to don a wearable sensorized system useful to quantify his/her movements, of a reduced part of the body (only one hand, the knees, the neck, …) or of the total body. Sensors and transducers, electronic circuitry, wired and/or wireless system, furnish measured data to a computer (laptop, desktop, netbook, palmtop, handheld device,..). Data values can be conditioned, stored, digitalized, etc. so algorithms or analysers or classifiers (Neural Network, Support Vector Machine, Fuzzy logic etc. based) recognize and classify the postures assumed by the user. The system can provide qualitative and quantitative (numerical) values to the user to evaluate his/her motor performances, and can be capable to furnish suggestions how to improve the user's performance.

From recorded data can be possible to:

- Reproduce the real time situation.
- Analyse user's postures (static and/or dynamic) in modality: play, pause, fast forward, rewind, frame-by-frame.
- Reproduce the real situation by an avatar which can be rotated and zoomed in every possible directions.

In addiction one (or more) avatar can visually reproduce/proposes the pre-imposed routine of the static/dynamic postures the user is asked to perform, and (even superimposed) a second (or more) avatar can reproduce the real postures of the user, so he/her can easily evaluate himself/herself if his/her movements correspond to the pre-imposed ones. The pre-recorded maneuvers the patient is asked to perform are given according to a protocol furnished by the case specialist or in according to known tests e.g., Larson test, Lachman test, pivot-shift test, etc. (D'Ambrosia, 1986).

An eventual supervision of qualified personnel can be remotely furnished since all recorded data can be sent via web.

Thanks to this system, we experimented an improvement of patient's participation to the treatment, by means of actions aimed at recovering his/her best physical, cognitive, psychological and functional levels.

The great importance that sensorized garments can have for remote postural and motor rehabilitation stands for the fact that the movements are suggested without ambiguity by a "guide"-avatar (no teaching motor therapists are necessary); the patient replays the movements in a domestic environment (no room in hospitals and clinics is necessary); the sensorized garments measure the movements and reproduce them with a "ghost"-avatar superimposed to the "guide"-avatar (no physiotherapists are necessary) (see Figure 14); a pc-running software, led by classification algorithms, eventually suggests to the patients which

movements must be corrected (no medical staff in necessary and a synthesized voice can motivate the patient); all the recorded movements are remotely sent via tele-health services, as useful information to the qualified staff, who will evaluate the performances of the patient.

The example furnished by the data glove, relative to the hands, can be easily adopted for other parts of the body, or even for a full body treatment with a complete sensorized suite (see Figure 15).

The system is completed by a virtual representation of an already mentioned avatar, by a GUI (Graphic User Interface) to deal with the software, and by a database to store all the recorded data (Figure 16).

5. IMPACT FOR HOSPITAL USE

The recorded measures obtained by the previously described system can be easily provided from the house of the patient to the doctors at the hospital, thanks to a tele-medicine support, which can transmit data via internet, or via a protected connections to avoid interception of patient's sensible data. The doctors can see all the movements performed by the patient via a representation software capable

Figure 14. Training session: the movements performed by the user are visualized as "ghost" and superimposed on the avatar-teacher

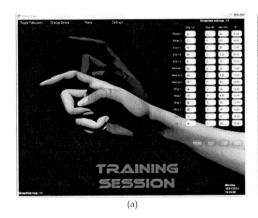
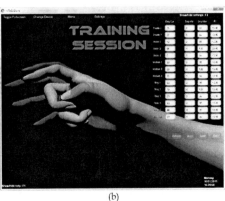

(a)   (b)

Figure 15. A complete system for a full body measurements

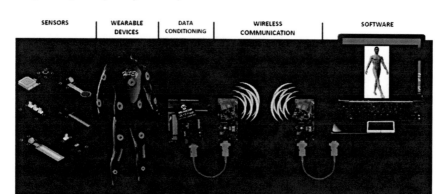

Figure 16. System completed by a 3D model, a GUI and a database

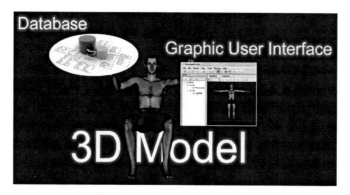

to show the avatar of the patient (see Figure 17 as an example).

The avatar can be in/out zoomed, clock-anti-clockwise rotated, translated, and parts can be even deleted, so to focus the attention to only some aspects. As an example, if the doctor is interested only on the thumb's capabilities, he/she can remove all the other fingers from the view.

All of these have a great impact for the hospital use. In fact less personnel, from medical and paramedical staff, can be involved with respect to current procedures, less hospital structures can be necessary and less time can be devoted to a unique patient. But, at the same time, results of the rehabilitation treatment can be even improved in the sense of obtaining better results with the same devoted efforts.

A pair of our hiteg gloves were adopted both for the follow-up procedures after hand's surgery so to verify the progresses of the patient, and for the rehabilitation treatments of the same patients. The procedures were adopted at the "Bel Colle" hospital in Viterbo (Italy), under the expertise medical supervision of doctors Antonio Castagnaro and Anna De Leo. The validity of the overall system and the obtained results are reported elsewhere (Castagnaro et al., 2010).

Others researchers report analogous procedures too, utilizing data gloves with more or less similar performances, in terms of sensitivity and accuracy, but sometimes adopting sensors, embedded in the glove, differing from the functioning principle with respect from ours. Also these other researchers found interesting improvement in the rehabilitation course adopting a data glove

Figure 17. Avatar representation of the patient's hand movements

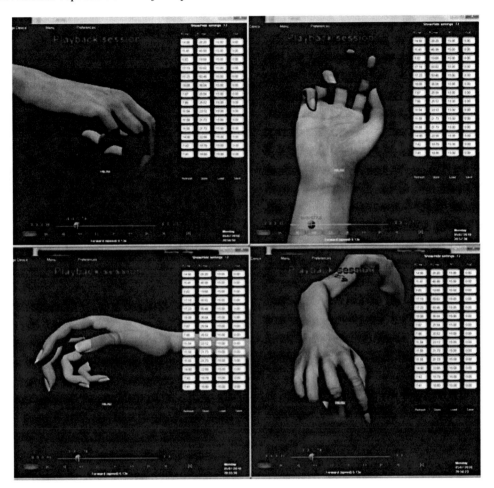

(Bonato, 2005; Lorussi, Scilingo et al., 2005; Pyk et al., 2008), and integrating it with ad-hoc created virtual reality environments (Szekely and Satava, 1999).

Of course, this is not intended to be the perfect solution to the problem of rehabilitation course and critical aspects still remain opened. In particular we refer the fact that even if the glove (or other sensorized clothes) is really comfortable to don and does not obstruct the main movements of the hand, in any case it remains an extraneous staff for the hand and it can become uncomfortable after some time. In addiction not all persons can be easily trained to this technology, as it can

happen with elderly people, or not everyone can be in the condition to use a common glove, as it can happen for people with hand's malformations. Nevertheless we consider the proposed system to be valid for the really near future.

6. OPEN SCENARIOS

Relating to our experiences, it makes sense that the measuring system has not to limit its capabilities to furnish to the operator "only" reliable measurements. We suggest that it must be completed with "added values". As a starting point it would be important to define a standardization for the measurement protocols. Nowadays each system has got its own procedure for the measure of the human hand, trunk, leg and, generally, all the parts of the human body. All teams involved in body tracking adopt procedure strictly related to proprietary protocols for commercial systems or proceed on the basis of their particular experience for self-realized systems or modified ones. So it can be hard for different research groups to share their experiences and ideas. Even the obtained measure can be difficult to compare and, over all, to validate among research groups if the results are reported on the basis of different protocols. We encountered the same problem for the Brain Computer Interface Systems, which is another of our research fields and for which we suggested to adopt the UML (Unified Modelling Language) as universal language which allows to define a protocol for method and timetable (Quitadamo et al., 2008).

Another key element we want to underline is the data "usability". Once data have been acquired it becomes fundamental to count on both a correct analytical tool and a proper representation. For a surgeon, for instance, it can make the difference to literally "see" each movement of the patient in re-play mode from any possible point of view. So we are thinking to overcome the present possibilities as the Arena graphic tool by OptiTrack or the Vicon (www.vicon.com) or the IGS-190 Technology (www.metamotion.com) applications offer, but looking for a possible future scenario of a hologram or stereogram that can report patient's motion via avatar in a real 3D space. This is what already happen in other fields as, for instance, the edutainment one (see Figure 18), in which we were involved for a project with a specialized Company (PFM Multimedia).

We suggest also that the measurement system can overcome the usual laboratory as the ones in a hospital (for rehabilitation purposes) can be. We believe that the treated systems can be usefully adopted, for instance, in psychology e psychiatry

Figure 18. Users donning special glasses see holograms of "floating planets" in the room (courtesy by PFM Multimedia Company)

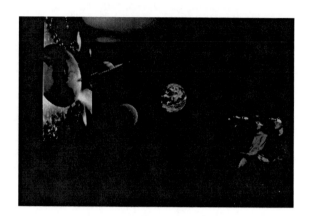

ambulatories since the body kinematic can furnish an important evaluation key for the emotional reaction a patient can present to several events. But these novel systems can be used not only to re-habilitate an existing part of the body, but also for guidance to habilitate artificially replaced parts with mechanical artifacts (see Figure 19).

A further application based on body posture measure evaluations can furnish a body mapping giving to designers a tool for realizing more er-

Figure 19. The patient can be leaned to move his/ her mechanical upper limb with the aim of the proposed systems

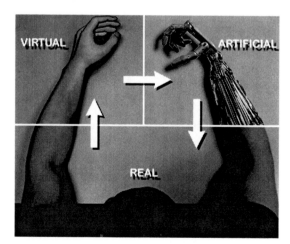

gonomic rehabilitation stuff, but also for giving information to be conveniently adopted in fields like furnishings or automotives.

But, surprisingly, it can be important to measure the postures not only of patients, but of doctors as well! In fact, our *hiteg glove* has been adopted to verify the skill of the trainee in surgery, measuring their ability to manually perform some pre-imposed tasks (see Figure 20 - Saggio, Santuosuosso et al., 2011).

Another circumstance for which the measure of the hand of surgeons can be mandatory, regards the realization of tele-surgery in a next future: the exact movements of a surgeon remotely located, can accurately drive the full potential of the hands of a robot to perform complex surgical tasks, as well as if the doctor was in the same location of the patient (see Figure 21).

CONCLUSION

Every day, all around the world, millions of people request postural and/or motor rehabilitation. This can be for really many reasons, i.e. for traumatic or connective or degenerative musculoskeletal disorders, after traumatic events such as strokes, severe cardiac disease, prolonged rest in bed, func-

Figure 20. A typical surgical gesture measured by the system

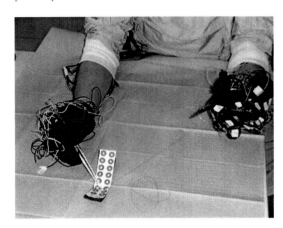

tional losses after treatment, etc. The rehabilitation process, also known as Tertiary Prevention, intends to be a sort of therapy to restore functionality and self-sufficiency of the patient. The postural and/or motor training can be necessary even to support cognitive and neurological rehabilitation request, for instance, after Traumatic Brain Injuries (TBI) due to car crashes, falls, gunshot wounds, sports. Only in the U.S., for instance, TBI affects from 500,000 to 1,900,000 persons (Rizzo et al., 1998).

The rehabilitation process regards not only millions of patients daily, but involves also a huge number of professionals in medical staffs, i.e.

Figure 21. The sensorized glove can be adopted to measure human gesture so to replicate them in a remote location to accurately drive a robot's arm

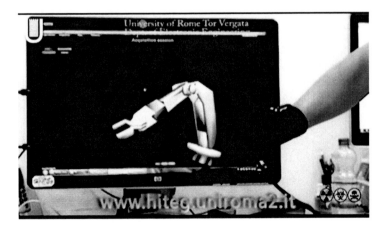

specialists, nurses, physiotherapists and therapists, social workers, psychologists, physiatrists, etc.

For the incredible number of patients, the medical staff and facilities necessary to support the appropriate postural and motor training, the monetary costs of rehabilitation is so huge to be even really difficult to estimate, but some data were given in the introduction paragraph.

Every effort towards a simplification of the rehabilitation route is really desirable and welcome. To this aim, our best efforts must have the purposes to reduce the cost, time, employees and facilities but, at the same time, increase the effectiveness of the rehabilitation. We can obtain these aims, *primum* motivating the patient (Maclean et al, 2000) according to the Kemp model (Kemp, 1988) taking into deep consideration the psychological aspects of rehabilitation (Rohe, 2005), *deinde* providing non-intimidating guides to the movements/actions suggested to perform in a domestic environment, post supplying a system which allows an self-evaluation of the rehabilitation progresses, and only as a final step remotely checking for feedback to the patient given by qualified personnel, all of these were detailed in this chapter.

Human movement analysis is not really a new science. Let's think that Giovanni Borelli is credited as being the first to make dynamic calculations of human movement even in the Renaissance period. But this science is necessarily based on systems capable to reveal human body kinematics. In this chapter a rapid overview of these systems was detailed. A classification scheme was proposed, the advantages/disadvantages of measuring systems were analysed. Finally we suggested the need of a standardization, of an universal language for protocols including time scheduling, furnished a look forward to future possibilities and novel applications of human body kinematic measure.

REFERENCES

American Academy of Orthopaedic Surgeons (Ed.). (1988). *Joint motion: Method of measuring and recording*. Edinburgh, UK: Churchill Livingstone.

Arbib, M. A. (1981). Perceptual structures and distributed motor control. In Brooks, V. B. (Ed.), *Handbook of physiology -- The nervous system II. Motor control* (pp. 1449–1480). American Physiological Society.

Arcelus, A., Goubran, R., & Knoefel, F. (2011). *Detection of bouncing during sit-to-stand transfers with sequential pressure images*. Paper presented at the IEEE International Symposium on Medical Measurements and Applications (MeMeA 2011).

Becker, J. C., & Thakor Nitish, V. (1988). A study of motion of human fingers with application to anthropomorphic designs. *IEEE Transactions on Bio-Medical Engineering, 35*(2), 110–117. doi:10.1109/10.1348

Bellomo, R. G., Iodice, P., Barassi, G., & Saggini, R. (2011). *Biomechanic measures and sense motor control of body posture after plastic surgery*. Paper presented at the IEEE International Symposium on Medical Measurements and Applications (MeMeA 2011).

Benedetti, M. G., Biagi, F., Merlo, A., Belvedere, C., & Leardini, A. (2011). *A new protocol for multi-segment trunk kinematics*. Paper presented at the IEEE International Symposium on Medical Measurements and Applications (MeMeA 2011).

Benedetti, M. G., Manca, M., Sicari, M., Ferraresi, G., Casadio, G., Buganè, F., & Leardini, A. (2011). *Gait measures in patients with and without AFO for equinus varus/drop foot*. Paper presented at the IEEE International Symposium on Medical Measurements and Applications (MeMeA 2011).

Bifulco, P., Cesarelli, M., Fratini, A., Ruffo, M., Pasquariello, G., & Gargiluo, G. (2011). *A wearable device for recording of biopotentials and body movements*. Paper presented at the IEEE International Symposium on Medical Measurements and Applications (MeMeA 2011).

Bonato, P. (2005). Advances in wearable technology and applications in physical medicine and rehabilitation. *Journal of Neuroengineering and Rehabilitation, 2*(2).

Castagnaro, A., De Leo, A., Inciocchi, S., Saggio, G., & Tarantino, U. (2010). *Nuova biotecnologia: Il guanto sensorizzato per misurare la cinesi della mano*. Paper presented at the 48° Congresso Nazionale Società Italiana Chirurgia della Mano SICM 2010, "Stato dell'arte nella chirurgia articolare del gomito, polso e mano: protesi e tecniche alternative", Savona 29 Settembre - 2 Ottobre, 2010.

Chao, E. Y. S., An, K.-N., Cooney, W. P. III, & Linscheid, R. L. (Eds.). (1989). *Biomechanics of the hand: A basic research study*. Teaneck, NJ: World Scientific Publishing Co., Inc.

D'Ambrosia, R. D. (Ed.). (1986). *Musculoskeletal disorders: Regional examination and differential diagnosis* (2nd ed.). Philadelphia, PA: Lippincott.

D'Amico, M., Bellomo, R. G., Saggini, R., & Roncoletta, P. (2011). *A 3D spine & full skeleton model for multi-sensor biomechanical analysis in posture & gait*. Paper presented at the IEEE International Symposium on Medical Measurements and Applications (MeMeA 2011).

Fiorentino, M., Uva, A. E., & Foglia, M. M. (2011). *Wearable rumble device for active asymmetry measurement and corrections in lower limb mobility*. Paper presented at the IEEE International Symposium on Medical Measurements and Applications (MeMeA 2011).

Ganter, B. K., Erickson, R. P., Butters, M. A., Takata, J. H., & Noll, S. F. (2005). Clinical evaluation. In DeLisa, J. A. (Eds.), *Physical medicine & rehabilitation: Principles and practice*. Lippincott Williams & Wilkins.

Giani, U. (2011). *Measurement, complexity and clinical decision-making*. Paper presented at the IEEE International Symposium on Medical Measurements and Applications (MeMeA 2011).

Giorgino, T., Tormene, P., Maggioni, G., Capozzi, D., Quaglini, S., & Pistarini, C. (2009). Assessment of sensorized garments as a flexible support to self-administered post-stroke physical rehabilitation. *European Journal of Physical and Rehabilitative Medicine, 45*, 75–84.

Holden, M. K. (2005). Virtual environments for motor rehabilitation [Review]. *Cyberpsychology & Behavior, 8*(3). doi:10.1089/cpb.2005.8.187

Holtzman, H., Goubran, R., & Knoefel, F. (2011). *Maximal ratio combining for respiratory effort extraction from pressure sensor arrays*. Paper presented at the IEEE International Symposium on Medical Measurements and Applications (MeMeA 2011).

Junho, S. (2005). Roadmap for e-commerce standardization in Korea. *International Journal of IT Standards and Standardization Research, 3*(2).

Kemp Bryan, J. (1988). Motivation, rehabilitation and aging: A conceptual model. *Geriatric Rehabilitation, 3*(3), 41–51.

Lin, C. S., Shi, T. H., Lin, C. H., Yeh, M. S., & Shei, H. J. (2006). The measurement of the angle of a user's head in a novel head-tracker device. *Measurements, 39*, 750–757.

Lorussi, F., Scilingo, E. P., Tesconi, M., Tognetti, A., & De Rossi, D. (2005). Strain sensing fabric for hand posture and gesture monitoring. *IEEE Transactions on Information Technology in Biomedicine, 9*(3). doi:10.1109/TITB.2005.854510

Lorussi, F., Tognetti, A., Tescioni, M., Zupone, G., Bartalesi, R., & De Rossi, D. (2005). Electroactive fabrics for distributed, confortable and interactive systems. In C. D. Nugent (Ed.), *Technology and Informatics, Vol. 117: Personalized health management systems.* IOS Press.

Luo, X., Kenyon, R., Kline, T., Waldinger, H., & Kamper, D. (2005). *An augmented reality training environment for post-stroke finger extension rehabilitation.* Paper presented at the IEEE 9th International Conference on Rehabilitation Robotics, Chicago, IL.

Maclean, N. (2000). The concept of patient motivation: A qualitative analysis of stroke professionals' attitudes. *Stroke, 33,* 444–448. doi:10.1161/hs0202.102367

Merrett, G. V., Ettabib, M. A., Peters, C., Hallett, G., & White, N. M. (2010). Augmenting forearm crutches with wireless sensors for lower limb rehabilitation. *Measurement Science & Technology, 21.*

Ming, D., Liu, X., Dai, Y., & Wan, B. (2009). *Indirect biomechanics measurement on shoulder joint moments of walker-assisted gait.* Paper presented at the IEEE Int. Conf. on Virtual Environments, Human-Computer Interfaces, and Measurement Systems, Hong Kong, China, May 11-13.

Mostarac, P., Malaric, R., Jurčević, M., Hegeduš, H., Lay-Ekuakille, A., & Vergallo, P. (2011). *System for monitoring and fall detection of patients using mobile 3-axis accelerometers sensors.* Paper presented at the IEEE International Symposium on Medical Measurements and Applications (MeMeA 2011).

Pinheiro, E., Postolache, O., & Girão, P. S. (2011). *Cardiopulmonary signal processing of users of wheelchairs with embedded sensors.* Paper presented at the IEEE International Symposium on Medical Measurements and Applications (MeMeA 2011).

Post, E. R., Orth, Russo, P. R., & Gershenfeld, N. (2000). E-broidery: Design and fabrication of textile-based computing. *IBM Systems Journal, 39*(3-4).

Pyk, P., Wille, D., Chevrier, E., Hauser, Y., Holper, L., & Fatton, I. … Eng, K. (2008). *A paediatric interactive therapy system for arm and hand rehabilitation.* Paper presented at the Virtual Rehabilitation 2008, Vancouver, Canada.

Quitadamo, L. R., Abbafati, M., Saggio, G., Marciani, M. G., Cardarilli, G. C., & Bianchi, L. (2008). *A UML model for the description of different BCI systems.* Paper presented at the 30th Annual International Conference of the IEEE Engineering in Medicine and Biology Society (EMBS 2008).

Rohe, D. E. (2005). Psychological aspects of rehabilitation. In DeLisa, J. A. (Eds.), *Physical medicine & rehabilitation: Principles and practice.* Lippincott Williams & Wilkins.

Saggio, G., Bocchetti, S., Pinto, C. A., Orengo, G., & Giannini, F. (2009a). *A novel application method for wearable bend sensors.* Paper presented at the 2nd International Symposium on Applied Sciences in Biomedical and Communication Technologies (ISABEL2009). Bratislava, Slovak Republic.

Saggio, G., Latessa, G., Bocchetti, S., Pinto, C. A., & Beck, D. (2009b). *Improving performances of data gloves based on bend sensors.* Retrieved from http://sensorprod.com/news/white-papers/dgb/index.php

Saggio, G., Latessa, G., De Santis, F., Bianchi, L., Quitadamo, L. R., Marciani, M. G., & Giannini, F. (2009). *Virtual reality implementation as a useful software tool for e-health applications.* Paper presented at the 1th IEEE International WoWMoM Workshop on Interdisciplinary Research on E-Health Services and Systems (IREHSS 2009), Kos (Greece).

Saggio, G., & Pinto, C. A. (2010). Virtuality supports reality for e-health applications. In Kim, J.-J. (Ed.), *Virtual reality* (pp. 259–284). InTech Publications. doi:10.5772/13085

Saggio, G., Santosuosso, G. L., Cavallo, P., Pinto, C. A., Petrella, M., Giannini, F., et al. (2011). *Gesture recognition and classification for surgical skill assessment.* Paper presented at the 6th IEEE International Symposium on Medical Measurements and Applications (MeMeA 2011). Bari, Italy.

Saggio, G., & Sbernini, L. (2011). *New scenarios in human trunk posture measurements for clinical applications.* Paper presented at the 6th IEEE International Symposium on Medical Measurements and Applications (MeMeA 2011). Bari, Italy.

Silva, H., Lourenco, A., Tomas, R., Lee, V., & Going, S. (2011). *Accelerometry-based study of body vibration dampening during whole-body vibration training.* Paper presented at the 6th IEEE International Symposium on Medical Measurements and Applications (MeMeA 2011). Bari, Italy.

Simone, L. K., Sundarrajan, N., Luoc, X., Jia, Y., & Kamperc, D. G. (2007). A low cost instrumented glove for extended monitoring and functional hand assessment. *Journal of Neuroscience Methods, 160,* 335–348. doi:10.1016/j.jneumeth.2006.09.021

Szekely, G., & Satava, R. M. (1999). Virtual reality in medicine. *British Medical Journal, 319.*

Takahashi, G., Millette, S., & Eftekari, T. (2003). *Exploring issue related to the qualification recognition of physical therapists.* Paper presented at the World Confederation for Physical Therapy, London (WCPT 2003).

Tanimoto, Y., Takechi, H., Nagahata, H., & Yamamoto, H. (1998). The study of pressure distribution in sitting position on cushions for patient with SCI (spinal cord injury). *IEEE Transactions on Instrumentation and Measurement, 47,* 1239–1243. doi:10.1109/19.746590

Wang, Y. (2005). *Human movement tracking using a wearable wireless sensor network.* Unpublished Master dissertation, Iowa State University. Ames, Iowa

Williams, N. W., Penrose, J. M. T., Caddy, C. M., Barnes, E., Hose, D. R., & Harley, P. (2000). A goniometric glove for clinical hand assessment. *The Journal of Hand Surgery, 25B*(2), 200–207.

Chapter 19
Virtual Carer:
A First Prototype

Aldo Franco Dragoni
Università Politecnica delle Marche, Italy

ABSTRACT

In view of the rapidly progressive increase in the average population age, "Ambient Assisted Living" (AAL) defines the actions and policies needed to promote the improvement of living conditions within domestic spaces to foster autonomy, safety, and social inclusion for the elderly or disabled. The idea is to design an innovative and comprehensive information system for AAL, an ICT-based "Virtual Caregiver," which is informed, intelligent and friendly, and which constantly monitors the health warning, informing and advising the elderly while controlling the environment and then asking for help when needed. The system will have the ability to establish interactive communication with the person but also extend it automatically outside the house in times of need. Virtual Caregiver will be able to enable the software protocols that activate the emergency phone calls to the family, medics or even first aid in emergencies.

INTRODUCTION

Aging well is one of the most important challenges of the west world. Ambient Assisted Living (AAL) is an initiative from the European Union to address that problem by reducing barriers, through ICT innovation, with the goal to lower social security costs and allow the elderly/disabled to live comfortably in their (nursing) homes (AAL 2009). The main objectives declared by the European AAL are:

- Extend the period in which people can live in their preferred environment by increasing their autonomy, self-sufficiency and mobility.
- Help maintain health and functional capacity of older people.
- Promoting lifestyles and better health for people at risk.
- Increase safety, prevent social exclusion and maintain relational network of people.
- Supporting the players, families and organizations of care.

DOI: 10.4018/978-1-4666-2979-0.ch019

- Improving the efficiency and productivity of resources in an aging society.

The themes of "good aging" and AAL activities are the focus of numerous research programs and of the new European perspective of Horizon 2020. But AAL is not just technology: it requires in all its phases, from conception to implementation and use, collaboration and effective communication between researchers, planners, industry, users, administrators, social workers and health care, in a completely new operating paradigm, challenging and stimulating.

The purpose of this article is to shed light on the key technologies involved in the design of an ICT-based innovative and comprehensive AAL-oriented information system. The hazard of being subjected to restrictions on their autonomy and independence grows rapidly over the age of sixty, and the home environment is one of the scenarios where severe limits of autonomy occur, along with independence related diseases and disabilities.

BACKGROUND

Most of the AAL projects provide ICT platforms to create and maintain an easy-to-use web-based social network for the elderly in order to stimulate their social relations. Timely information are transferred to the network on the activities and subjective state of the elderly person (e.g. presence, state of wellness, etc.) allowing for a much better-tailored and timely response, attention and care so as to improve and maintain the well-being and independence of the elderly living in their own homes and reduce healthcare costs. The AAL projects address chronic conditions such as mild cognitive impairment, and develop and test solutions to alleviate and/or prevent them. In such a way, caregivers, friends and family members have greater access to information about the person, and

those at a distance are enabled to keep in touch and share activities with their elderly family member or friend, and to know their current condition.

Despite these advances, we believe that it is necessary to find and test new services exploiting the potential of ICT to implement socially advanced and reliable services, "smart" technology-based communication and information processing that must be adapted to the needs of the elders (Weber 2005) (Weiser 1996) so that they derive real benefits in terms of autonomy and security. To illustrate what we are thinking about (at the Laboratory for Artificial Intelligence and Real Time Systems of the "Università Politecnica delle Marche," in Italy) I need to tell a personal story.

Some time ago, when my father (widow) was still alive, I experienced some difficulties which are very common in the west world, where sons live far from their old parents. My problem was that when I called my father, who lived a hundred miles from my home, he often did not answer the phone. And this happened more than once in succession so that I was forced to take the car for a long trip anxious to go and see what had happened to my father. Systematically the causes of the fact that he did not answer the phone was that, during the first phone call my father was in the garden, while the second was in the bathroom and while the third was sleeping! Paradoxically, my problems disappeared when his worse! In fact, when his health worsened, my father was forced to hire a nanny. The caretaker of my father answered the phone in his place, and kept me well informed about the health and mood of my father. She also called me when he needed something from me.

Unfortunately, in the future, the socioeconomic equilibrium of the western world will probably make it difficult for the next generations of elderly to hire personal caretakers. After this consideration, I immediately realized that almost all the informative tasks performed by the nanny could also be provided by a well designed and skilled software system! Of course it would have been a complex system that integrates various artificial intelligence technologies, from the speech synthesis and recognition, to the learning and planning of communicative acts. I tried to sketch down what were the services provided by the nanny. She:

- Noted daily biomedical signs,
- Remembered my father to take medication,
- Listened to his needs,
- Answered the phone, giving news of my father,
- Phoned me when my father needed,
- Kept company with my father and made him feel happy, even telling jokes.

Effectively, almost all these tasks could be provided by an intelligent software system and I started to think about what minimal integration of current technologies would be necessary to build our "Virtual Caregiver," that became our approach to address the objectives of the AAL initiative. This paper describes our efforts devising an infrastructure in order to make the "Virtual Caregiver" vision reality.

THE "VIRTUAL CAREGIVER"

Structure

It will focus on the system's ability to monitor and then acquire, interpret, and store the vital signs of a person. We are currently using two wearable devices: the BioHarness-Zephyr and the STMicroelectronics BodyGateway, both able to detect the main biomedical data (expecially the ECG) and send them to the Virtual Caregiver through IEEE 802.15.1 - Bluetooth. They cover most of the biomedical parameters essential for use in the project to ensure an older person's safety and service through continuous health monitoring.

However, data need to be interpreted. So it is important to map collections of data into "living scenarios" that will be given as input to the Virtual Caregiver in order to let it adopt some specific protocols of action and communication.

We believe that the Virtual Caregiver should act continuously in normal living conditions, and should be considered as a clerk or a friend, and not be associated only with pains or emergencies. However, the most important scenarios to be recognized will be those referring to specific emergency situations relating to the health and security of the assisted person in her home environment. To accomplish the task of going from pure data to descriptive scenarios we must provide our Virtual Caregiver with its own intelligence; an "Interpretative System," i.e. an inference engine that applies to the Knowledge Base (KB) consisting of all the external signals "facts" that come both from the wearable and the environment sensors (detecting temperature, open/closure of windows and door etc.) placed in various rooms.

To Interpretative System is basically implemented in Prolog, and exploits the potential of deductive and abductive paradigms. In particular we adopt an hybrid structure composed of the Java language and the language TuProlog, this latter written entirely in Java. At this stage it has proved extremely useful to build an application using different programming paradigms simultaneously.

The recognized scenario is inputted to a "Talking Head" which, for now, is a prototype based on "Lucia" which was made in January 2005 by the Institute for Cognitive Sciences and Technologies (ISTC) of the National (Italian) Research Council at Padua. "Lucia" communicates with the older person by using a system of automatic synthesis bimodal audio-visual and is able to activate other specific protocols, such as Voice-XML. This allows it to establish an interactive communication, as simply as possible with the assisted person and with her familiar and caregiver "entourage" to provide accurate information on her health status, or to request help in case of need.

Our Virtual Caregiver integrates also a chatbot (A.L.I.C.E.). It is an interface dialoguers, able to interact with the elderly in an intelligent conversation through text in natural language. The purpose of the use of a chatbot is to make it easy and immediate to exchange relevant information belonging to a specific domain. For example, information about the home environment, health information or assistance, and other details useful to the assisted person. The domain in question will be represented by appropriate files written using the meta language A.I.M.L. (Artificial Intelligence Markup Language) that represent the knowledge base used by the chatbot.

Finally it's important to integrate all components into a single logical architecture by creating points of communication between the components.

We build a software platform for simulation (simulated environment – ambient house – without the use of real sensors) to test the system's features and potential, considering all the components involved, as in (Costa 2009). Given the high flexibility of a simulation component of this type, it can represent a number of interesting scenarios that reproduce many heterogeneous situations. In this test phase it will be of great help to use the data made available by the online database PHYSIONET.ORG. This, collects data and physiological measures in a gigantic database. This is the Harvard-MIT Division of Health Sciences and Technology at its disposal this archive known as MIT - BIH Database.

DATA ACQUISITION AND INTERPRETATION

The wearable sensors (BioHarness – BodyGateway) are the main data acquisition devices of the Virtual Caregiver (see Figure 1). They should continuously monitor the health status and the proper functioning of the heart through an ECG, a respiratory rate, a temperature and an accelerometer. In particular, the BioHarness – Zephyr addresses those needs since it can detect the following vital signs: Heart Rate (BPM), Electrocardiogram (ECG), respiratory rate (RPM), Width of Breathing (mV), body posture (degrees from the horizontal axis), skin temperature ($^{\circ}$ C), acceleration of body movements (Watson 2008a).

Biomedical data must be acquired, read, interpreted and analyzed. The values sent from the sensors belong to the category of "Stream Data Packet" that is, packets sent in streaming with a period of 1008 ms (Watson 2008b). To enable communication with the device we need a standard method, as well as an economical and safe one. The current solution was the IEEE-802.15.1 Bluetooth (Gratton 2003). The communication between our system and sensor-BioHarness Zephyr is half-duplex. To implement all the functionality of receiving data from the system Carer we used the Java programming language "Java - Standard Edition SE 1.6 - JDK. In order to serve the Bluetooth protocol, Java needs to have the right tools. These are called JSR-82 and BLUECOVE. The specification defines the standard JSR-82 Java Bluetooth technology and "packages"

Figure 1. Communication of BioHarness with the virtual caregiver

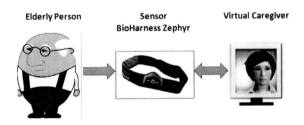

allowing the establishment and operation of Bluetooth (like L2CAP and RFCOMM) for communicating with our sensor. BLUECOVE (stack open source) is rather an implementation of J2SE JSR-82 that gives a Java client the possibility to interface with the software BLUESOLAIR Bluetooth. The latter has the main functionality of the device and can connect via Bluetooth USB Wi-Fi (Bluetooth adapter - CNET) to a computer.

The application developed in Java must be able to interface with Bluetooth devices for research use (Operation of Device Discovery) (in our case the sensor) and the service it offers (Operation Service Discovery). The specification defines two Java packages: the package javax.microedition.io allows the establishment and operation of Bluetooth (like L2CAP and RFCOMM) for communication between devices. The package also offers javax. bluetooth available application functionality and Bluetooth profiles Generic Access Profile Service Discovery Application Profile. Each package is sent and received by a sensor system of specific areas.

Each received package has to be recognised by the value of the fields msgid, STX and ETX. The latter uniquely identifies each type of data packet (General Packet Data) so as to recognize them, store them in the database and send them to the PROLOG inference engine. To store the biomedical parameters and the information from the environment we choose to use a MySQL Server 5.5, a Relational Database Management System (RDBMS). All the client side of the Data Base will then be handled by Java through the MySQL - Connector-J is a JDBC driver that belongs to.

INTERPRETATION SYSTEM

The inference engine is the heart of the Virtual Caregiver. It is the engine that allows to operate in an "intelligent" and efficient way. It analyzes, processes and interprets data from the biomedical and environmental sensors, and tries to recognize the current scenario in which act correctly through the Talking Head. In particular, the inferential system must be able to recognize abnormal situations in the point of view of the elderly (e.g. falls, illness, forgetfulness in taking medication) or within the home environment (a window or door left open). All of this is subject to a condition of extreme importance or configurability of the system. We inserted a priori the most important needs of the person (both the physical and psychological needs), and we created appropriate rules of inference, to be fired when needed. See Figure 2 for functional blocks of the Virtual Caregiver.

The interpretation system is based of well known AI techniques (particularly "abduction"), and should not be regarded as a substitute of a doctor. We do not want to replace the physician in making a diagnosis, but rather to assess from a range of collated biomedical data, the risk of generation of an abnormal situation. To do this the system of interpretation must rely on a knowledge base built from medical knowledge and based on a customized profile of the patient. Given a set of facts, the expert systems, thanks to its set of "production rules," can infer new facts (Waterman 1986). For example, suppose that a person has a problem of tachycardia; we can provide expert system based on the following facts:

1. Heart rate is higher than normal (data from the sensor BioHarness).
2. The person is not doing any physical activity (data coming from Environment Sensor).
3. The respiratory rate is higher than normal (data from the sensor BioHarness).

The expert system takes the facts and chooses a rule so formed:

```
IF ((hr > 120) AND (NOT (physical
activity) AND (respiratory rate> 20))
THEN (tachycardia).
```

Figure 2. Functional blocks of the virtual caregiver

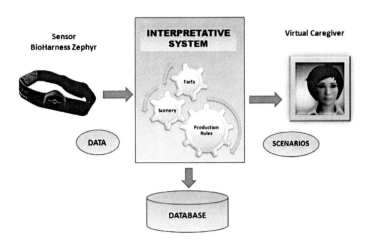

Here's an example of production rule (in Prolog) to identify another scenario of "fever":

```
fever:-
temperature (X),
heartRate (X),
restingActivity (X).
heartRate (X):-
X > = 100.
temperature(X):-
X > 38.
restingActivity:-
acceleration (X),
currentActivity (sleeping).
acceleration (X):-
X < 0.3.
notRestingActivities (X):-
acceleration (X),
currentActivity(gymnastics).
```

Java is an imperative language and hence is particularly suitable to express calculations, work with objects, sequences of commands, manage strings, although is not very suitable for "symbolic elaboration." We use Java to implement most of the features that are required for our system (virtual interactive communication, Bluetooth Manager, GUI interaction with the user, etc...) The symbolic elaboration is rather the ground of choice for the logical-deductive paradigm we've seen so far referring to Prolog. In this context we need an engine usable Prolog from Java better, which is itself a Java component, maybe available as a "jar" archive that allows easy integration and efficient interaction between the two worlds (Java and Prolog). We need a solution to allow simple and natural parameter passing in both directions: consider the flow of data from the sensor vital signs.

So we require a tool that is sufficiently lightweight and easy to use. More specifically, in the context of creating a system of interpretation, we think that Java collects, parses, and classifies all practical values from the BioHarness and the Environment sensors, and passes them to the Prolog interpreter. Prolog engine then maps values within their scenarios (Symbolic Processing) using its rules-deductive logic and then returns the information about the Java based on a given scenario. Java translates this information, and allows alarm activating opportunities for all protocols operating various graphical user interfaces or protocol Voice-XML to give advice, suggestions or alarm quickly in case of need. To implement the hybrid presented, we used TuProlog, component embedded within Java applications. TuProlog is a Prolog interpreter written entirely in Java and developed at Alma Mater Studiorum - University of Bologna and implemented by the research group based in Cesena.

COMMUNICATION WITH THE ASSISTED PERSON AND HER "ENTOURAGE"

Communication between the assisted people and the Virtual Caregiver is one of the most important aspects to consider. The interface will enable direct communication, which is friendly and easy to understand (Norman 2005). The interaction between person and our system should have the objective of supplying information on everything related to the environment and the health of the person (Norman 1986). The alarms that identify unusual or dangerous situations must be translated into verbal instructions to advise or reassure. A visual and aural communication is the best solution for the purpose of the work presented in this article. Human-Computer Interaction (HCI) gave us many implementations of interfaces. We adopted "Lucia," which is a prototype created the Institute for Cognitive Sciences and Technologies (ISTC) of the National Research Center (CNR) of Padua. This monitor anthropomorphic can faithfully reproduce the human speech using a co-articulation model, designed to make lip Lucia's more fluid and natural (see Figure 3).

Lucia is able to express emotions like anger, disgust, surprise, joy, sadness and fear, and thanks to the ELITE optoelectronic system can capture the movement of facial muscles and play in the Talking Face to make it more expressive (Magno 2007). It is clear that a monitor of this anthropomorphic type falls on a full draft Virtual Caregiver, making it an integral part. Undoubtedly the eyes and face of an assistant who remains in control and can readily assist an elderly person are needed; communication resources are important for the quantity, the subtlety and effectiveness

Figure 3. Talking head "Lucia"

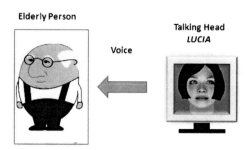

of information and guidance that can be transmitted. They are for the recipient, therefore, an invaluable aid to understand cognitive processes and memory. Lucia, is able to provide the transposition of a text written by a synthetic voice (Cosi 2002). This system adopt the "Festival" speech synthesizer (from written text, expressive and emotional) and a visible articulatory movements specific for the Italian language (a computer graphics program for the efficiency of facial surface texture). Festival is based on the technique of concatenation of speech units. This module then sends the processed data to its sound wave generation. This waveform uses the synthesis MBROLA. In the case of Lucia, MBROLA based PCM 16bit/16 KHz is used (Cosi 2008).

Out Virtual Caregiver adopt another communication media in parallel: natural language communication through a chatbot interface dialogue. The chatbot simulates a human and interacts with the user through a chat (in text). The chatbot writes, communicates with this system and answers the person's questions, or can open useful web pages. We adopted A.L.I.C.E. (Artificial Linguistic Internet Computer Entity) as one of the best chatbot open-source currently available (see Figure 4).

ALICE is based on language AIML (Artificial Intelligence Markup Language), which was created in 1995 by Dr. Richard S. Wallance. The chatbot stores a knowledge base written in AIML. The calculation engine may develop a response

Figure 4. Chatbot "ALICE"

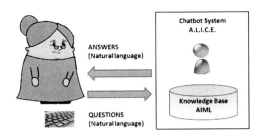

in natural language, yielding the data structure used from AIML, including an output of natural language text, due to a request by the user in natural language and always without any form of linguistic mediation. AIML language allows the definition of non-unique "Patterns" that match the generated template automatically, by drawing from the knowledge base.

Finally, we provided our Virtual Caregiver with the ability to extend communication outside the home. The solution is Voice-XML (see Figure 5). VoiceXML stands for Voice eXtensible Markup Language, and allows a communication (telephone or web communication) to be established outside of the house of the elderly (eg with the home of his family or with the web browser of the doctor), and is able to give useful information on the health of the elderly. This platform uses the full potential of systems of speech synthesis and speech recognition to build a new generation of systems able to access services via phone for now only accessible only via web. A typical application would be as depicted in the picture: in this case, the family of an elderly called the voice server via the telephone (VoiceXML 2005).

The Voice Browser interprets the Voice-XML application code developed in response to questions posed to him (the latter with logical scheme that provides questions and answers concerning the health status of the family). When the voice system provides answers containing precise figures, the voice server sends an "http request" that invokes a script or a specific Java class contained in a Web Server part of the system inside the house of elderly person. The Web server then processes the query which will be responsible for information contained in the data. The database contains

Figure 5. Voice-XML

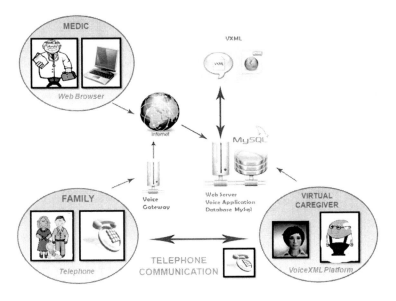

all information relating to biomedical signs and to home environment. After this operation, information and data contained in the script or Java application (Voice Application) returns control to the calling voice and the family can continue to interact with the application itself by asking more questions.

CONCLUSION

This paper describes the Virtual Caregiver project currently developing at the laboratory for Artificial Intelligence and Real Time Systems of the "Università Politecnica delle Marche." It documents the technologies needed to build this innovative ICT-based Ambient Assisted Living Tool. The Virtual caregiver goal is that of ensuring maximum autonomy to an elderly or disabled person forced to live alone at home. This was the guiding objective during the design phase. It was designed primarily for medical safety, which is ensured by acquiring the biomedical parameters of the person and therefore constantly monitoring her state of health. The implemented system uses two special wearable sensors (BioHarness-Zephyr and BodyGateway-STM) of biomedical parameters; they can detect alarm situations (fainting, falling to the ground, fever, tachycardia). To recognize all possible scenarios we needed to give to our Virtual Caregiver its own intelligence. Much time was devoted to the design of an expert system, or a system of interpretation, which can make inferences on the information content of a Knowledge Base (KB) consisting of all the signals coming from external sensors. When a particular scenario is recognized, the system delegates the Talking Head (Talking emoticons) to interact visually and vocally with the person so as to advise, warn, order or even calm. Furthermore, the Virtual Caregiver is able to establish communication with the family or with the human caregiver in cases of need. VoiceXML allows to carry on simple conversation

with the assisted person or with her "entourage" by exploiting the full potential of speech synthesis and recognition even via telephone (mobile or fixed). Finally, taking into account possible work in the future, we considered the OSGi framework (OSGI 2012). It is a model of comprehensive and dynamic programming components that could be a software solution allowing the standardization throughout the Java implementation code, in order to improve and speed-up the interaction with heterogeneous devices (sensors of all types, multimedia equipment, etc..). The Virtual Caregiver makes the use of devices inside the house as transparent as possible, and then ensures the paradigm of communication with the user more natural and faster.

REFERENCES

AAL. (2009). *Ambient assisted living - Joint programme (AAL JP) - 2008-2013*. Ambient Assisted Living. Retrieved from http://www.aal-europe.eu/

Cosi, M. (2002). Modalità e Multisensorialità nella creazione di una "Faccia Parlante" in Italiano. 2002 *Cdrom Proceedings of VIII Meeting of AIIA - AIIA 2002*, Siena, Italy, September 10-13

Cosi, P., Caldognetto Magno, E. (2008). Festival E Lucia: TTS (Text-to-speech) e IVA (Intelligent Virtual Agent) al servizio della didattica dei disabili. *Proceedings of 3rd Convegno Internazionale "Progresso e Innovazioni Tecnologiche nella riabilitazione dell'età evolutiva"* Napoli, 22 Giugno 2007.

Costa, R., Novais, P., Costa, A., & Neves, J. (2009). Memory support in ambient assisted living. *IFIP Advances in Information and Communication Technology, 307*, 745–752. doi:10.1007/978-3-642-04568-4_75

Gratton, D. (2003). *Bluetooth profiles, the definitive guide* (1st ed.). Prentice Hall.

Magno, C. E., Cosi, P., & Cavicchio, P. (2007). Interfacce multimodali per l'E-Learning. In Delogu, C. (Ed.), *Tecnologie per il weblearning: realtà e scenari* (pp. 173–183). Firenze, Italy: Florence University Press.

Norman, D. A. (1986). *User centered system design*. Hillsdale, NJ: Lawrence Erlbaum Associates.

Norman, D. A. (2005). *Emotional design*. Milano, Italy: Apogeo.

OSGI. (2012). *OSGi Alliance*. Retrieved from http://www.osgi.org

Voice, X. M. L. (2005). *VoiceXML tutorial*. Retrieved from http://www.vxml.org/

Waterman, D. A. (1986). *A guide to expert systems*. Reading, MA: Addison Wesley.

Watson, E. (2008a, January 15). *BioHarness Bluetooth API guide*. Zephyr - Technology ITD.

Watson, E. (2008b, 2 March). *General comms link specification*. Zephyr - Technology ITD.

Weber, W., Rabaey, J. M., & Aarts, E. (2005). *Ambient intelligence*. Berlin, Germany: Springer. doi:10.1007/b138670

Weiser, M. (1996). Some computer science issues in ubiquitous computing. *Communications of the ACM, 36*(7).

Chapter 20
Agent-Based Wellness Indicator

Chitsutha Soomlek
University of Regina, Canada

Luigi Benedicenti
University of Regina, Canada

ABSTRACT

An agent-based wellness indicator is an information visualization system designed to present wellness and decision-support information to individuals and their caregivers by elaborating the data provided by measuring devices utilizing the unique characteristics of software agents. The wellness indicator is constructed from an operational wellness model we developed. The model allows an automatic measuring system to calculate the wellness level for a number of indicators resulting in an overall wellness level. These results can be presented in a simple graphical format. The software has been evaluated by following the steps provided in the framework for testing a wellness visualization system. The evaluation is carried out by both general users and healthcare professionals. The results show positive feedback on various aspects of the indicator; and confirm that the wellness indicator can assist people to have a better understanding of their personal state of well-being and can support caregivers in delivering their services.

INTRODUCTION

Wellness is an important issue for both an individual and the public (Benedicenti & Soomlek, 2009; Soomlek & Benedicenti, Operational Wellness Model: A Wellness Model Designed for an Agent-Based Wellness Visualization System, 2010; Soomlek & Benedicenti, Creating a Framework for Testing Wellness Visualization Systems, 2011; Soomlek & Benedicenti, Repeatable Experimental Framework for Wellness Indi-cator Testing/Evaluation: Environmental Setup, 2012). People perform various activities, e.g., exercise regularly, nutrition control, and physical examination, to achieve the best possible state of wellness. Wellness can be achieved individually while good health may require assistance from experts. In order to have a desired level of wellness, many efforts are required. Many people utilize a portable health monitoring device and a matching application available on a smart small form factor device, since they are easy to access or buy in the

DOI: 10.4018/978-1-4666-2979-0.ch020

market. Portable health monitoring devices play an important role in assisting a person to measure and monitor certain parameters of wellness such as heart rate and blood sugar content. The measures are thus easy to obtain but difficult to interpret, and sometimes they require dedicated tools for recording and tracking purposes (Benedicenti & Soomlek, 2009). Knowing one's own wellness level is a key to maintaining or improving it. But a person must acquire specialized knowledge to interpret and contextualize most measures provided by a personal health device. Consulting with healthcare professionals does not require additional knowledge; unfortunately, there aren't enough healthcare workers compared to the number of people requiring wellness services at the time of writing (World Health Organization, 2008).

In order to improve the wellness level, it is important to understand our current conditions, our problems, risks, and what should we do to improve our state of wellbeing or which direction/approach we need to follow. There are many potential solutions to the presented problems such as training, attending a wellness improvement program, and consulting with the experts. Training allows people to have a better understanding in a certain topic; however, one training session is not enough for a person to understand everything relative to their wellness status and pursue to the right direction to improve their wellness level. In addition, training could be an expensive solution. In the United States, many companies provide worksite wellness programs to their employees with the hope of reducing healthcare costs (Hall, 2007). A comprehensive and effective wellness program could be expensive depending on what are included in the programs, i.e., approximately $US100-450 per person per year or more (Hall, 2007), but it is still cheaper than paying for health insurance (Hall, 2007). Moreover, when participating in a wellness program, a person needs motivation and personal responsibility to follow the guide in the program and, then, to be success in the long run. Consulting with the experts is the ideal solution if we have enough number of healthcare profes-

sionals to give wellness services. That is one of the reasons why telehealth and telemedicine play an important role in solving the problem. Telehealth and telemedicine do bring health services and healthcare professionals to people at distance; which is convenient and increases accessibility to medical services. In addition, telehealth services are more cost effective than face-to-face services (Persaud, et al., 2005). For example, in Nova Scotia, a study shows the patient costs for telehealth is $CAD17-70; which is cheaper than a face-to-face consultation, i.e., $CAD240-1,048 (Persaud, et al., 2005). However, there is uncertainty in the effectiveness and risks in employing the approaches, because a study shows that remote monitoring does not fewer hospitalizations and emergency department visits, and increases the death rate in elderly patients (Takahashi, et al., 2012; Kaffash, 2012).

Therefore, an alternative mechanism, that can assist people attain a better understanding of their personal state of wellbeing and to track their wellness information, is needed. The existing solutions discussed above give knowledge, instructions/suggestions, or access to healthcare services from a distance respectively, but not the combination of all. This research presents an agent-based wellness indicator as an alternative solution to the issues just identified and a complement to the existing solutions presented above. The system employs the benefits of the existing resources already provided in a hospital and other electronic resources; therefore, it does not require a highly extensive cost to be included in the existing services. The wellness indicator is designed to give people a better understanding in their wellness conditions and fast access to the relevant information, potentially help them to improve the quality of their lives. By integrating a wellness indicator system with a hospital working system, potentially assist a person to gain access to their wellness information and history, communicate to a caregiver, and present their progress to their physicians.

The wellness visualization system we built presents wellness information to people in a simple graphical format complemented by simple descriptions, suggestions and tools (Benedicenti & Soomlek, 2009; Soomlek & Benedicenti, Operational Wellness Model: A Wellness Model Designed for an Agent-Based Wellness Visualization System, 2010; Soomlek & Benedicenti, Creating a Framework for Testing Wellness Visualization Systems, 2011; Soomlek & Benedicenti, Repeatable Experimental Framework for Wellness Indicator Testing/Evaluation: Environmental Setup, 2012). The system also presents anomalies found with relevant description and suggestion. Detailed information, decision support information, and decision supporting tools are provided to healthcare professionals (Benedicenti & Soomlek, 2009; Soomlek & Benedicenti, Operational Wellness Model: A Wellness Model Designed for an Agent-Based Wellness Visualization System, 2010; Soomlek & Benedicenti, Creating a Framework for Testing Wellness Visualization Systems, 2011; Soomlek & Benedicenti, Repeatable Experimental Framework for Wellness Indicator Testing/Evaluation: Environmental Setup, 2012). Both general users and healthcare professionals can access a comprehensive display of their wellness information through either a personal computer or a small form factor device like a cellular telephone.

Wellness information of a patient is not only important to an individual, but also important to a caregiver's tasks. The healthcare professionals also gain access to the information that might not be available in the hospital, analyze data, and give suggestion to their patients. The visualization system presents a comprehensive display of wellness information with decision support information to caregivers, which potentially gives them insight and therefore assists them to provide a better wellness services to their patients.

The research presented in this chapter describes the development of the agent-based wellness visualization system, the evaluation approach used to assess its effectiveness, and the results of this assessment. We also provide some future directions based on the results.

BACKGROUND

What is Wellness?

There are a number of definitions of wellness and wellness models across the globe. They are formed from various perspectives. They are developed over time and changed by different influential factors, e.g., culture, belief, religion, etc. (Soomlek & Benedicenti, Operational Wellness Model: A Wellness Model Designed for an Agent-Based Wellness Visualization System, 2010). An individual also defines their own definition of wellness. As a result, the term wellness is very board and complex (Soomlek & Benedicenti, Operational Wellness Model: A Wellness Model Designed for an Agent-Based Wellness Visualization System, 2010). The followings are examples of definition of wellness.

In 1654, the term wellness was used for the first time by Lord Wariston (Miller, 2005). At that time, wellness is an antonym of illness and it had never been changed until the middle of the 20th century. Halbert L. Dunn officially introduced wellness as a state of being well, including good health; where "health is a state of complete physical, mental, and social well-being and not merely the absence of disease and infirmity" (Dunn, 1959). Wellness is complex, comprised of various dimensions, has different degrees, and affected by different factors such as the spirit of man. In 1975, John W. Travis presented his well-known concept of wellness (Miller, 2005). He said that wellness is highly related to personal responsibility. It is not physician's responsibility but it is the responsibility of a person to move toward high-level wellness (Miller, 2005). His improved version of wellness model was presented in 2008. The new version states that wellness is a choice made by an individual toward optimal health; a way of life designed by a person to achieve the highest potential for well-being; a process of developing awareness, health, and happiness; a balancing channels of energy received from the world around a person; an integration of body, mind, and spirit; an appreciation to everything that a person do, think, feel, and believe in; an acceptance of oneself; a non-static state; a learning process to love one's whole self; and knowing personal way to wellness (Travis, 2008). World Health Organization also defined wellness for both individual and the public as "the optimal state of health of individuals and groups. There are two focal concerns: the realization of the fullest potential of an individual physically, psychologically, socially, spiritually and economically, and the fulfillment of one's role expectations in the family, community, place of worship, workplace and other settings" (Smith, Tang, & Nutbeam, 2006).

From the examples given above, we agree with many experts that wellness is not just the state of being free from illness and disease (Soomlek & Benedicenti, Operational Wellness Model: A Wellness Model Designed for an Agent-Based Wellness Visualization System, 2010). It is complex and it does have multiple dimensions. Also, there are relationships among the dimensions of wellness. The dimensions of wellness are interrelated and integrated. Moreover, there are strong relationship between health and wellness. If we can indicate the level of wellness and influential factors for a person, it would become a powerful tool, because it is possible for the person and physician to find a way to improve the wellness level (Dunn, 1959).

Unfortunately, the existing definitions cannot be applied to an automatic measuring system (Soomlek & Benedicenti, Operational Wellness Model: A Wellness Model Designed for an Agent-Based Wellness Visualization System, 2010). Some dimensions in the existing definitions, such as spiritual and mental dimensions, cannot be evaluated by a machine at the time of writing. Also, a machine cannot process all types of inputs effectively. It is easy for an automatic measuring system to utilize objective and scale-based subjective data. However, there are many difficulties in processing conversational-based and text-based subjective data (Soomlek & Benedicenti, Operational Wellness Model: A Wellness Model Designed for an Agent-Based Wellness Visualiza-

tion System, 2010). Moreover, each of the existing definition has a certain group of dimensions of wellness. As a result, there are various methods and instruments for wellness evaluation (Soomlek & Benedicenti, Operational Wellness Model: A Wellness Model Designed for an Agent-Based Wellness Visualization System, 2010).

Wellness Inventory is an example of wellness assessment (Wellness Inventory: The Whole Person Assessment Program, 2011; Strohecker, Travis, Burdett, Kant Mishra, & Zyga). It is a questionnaire-based system that employs a predefined set of statements for wellness evaluation. Its users can have their wellness evaluated through a machine by logging into the system and answering the questions. Wellness Inventory supports limited inputs and measure wellness condition within their working definition of wellness (Wellness Inventory: The Whole Person Assessment Program, 2011; Strohecker, Travis, Burdett, Kant Mishra, & Zyga; Soomlek & Benedicenti, Operational Wellness Model: A Wellness Model Designed for an Agent-Based Wellness Visualization System, 2010). It is also obvious that the approach does not support frequent assessments, inconvenient, and time consuming (Soomlek & Benedicenti, Operational Wellness Model: A Wellness Model Designed for an Agent-Based Wellness Visualization System, 2010). Thus, a more flexible method for wellness assessment is needed. The evaluation method must correspond to the working definition of wellness as well.

As mentioned earlier that the term wellness is changed over time. The change affects the corresponding wellness model, wellness evaluation, and computer program (Soomlek & Benedicenti, Operational Wellness Model: A Wellness Model Designed for an Agent-Based Wellness Visualization System, 2010). If a graphical presentation for wellness was used, it might also need to be changed. These requirements lead us to a wellness model that is computable and flexible enough to be expanded (Soomlek & Benedicenti, Operational Wellness Model: A Wellness Model Designed for an Agent-Based Wellness Visualization System, 2010). Also, its results should be able to be presented in a graphical format to ease visual perception. Since existing wellness model do not have the required properties, the operational wellness model is created. The operational wellness model has two major parts: operational definition of wellness and operational wellness evaluation model, more information can be found in (Soomlek & Benedicenti, Operational Wellness Model: A Wellness Model Designed for an Agent-Based Wellness Visualization System, 2010).

Agent Technology

Agent technology is comprised of software agent and agent platform. A software agent is a piece of software having a certain degree of autonomy and containing various sets of operations to work on behalf of its user or another program (Gibbs, 2000; Franklin & Graesser, 1996; Green, et al., 1997). The operations can be employed to pursue the user's objectives. The user's objectives and problem domains define the capabilities and characteristics of software agents; which make each of them unique. Once an agent is launched, the agent works on its agenda until it finishes its task, decides to stop, or it is destroyed. An agent also has the ability to sense a change in an environment and acts upon the change autonomously (Gibbs, 2000; Franklin & Graesser, 1996). In addition, its actions may cause a change in the environment.

There are two types of software agents: stationary agent and mobile agent (Maes, Guttman, & Moukas, 1999). A stationary agent works at its launched location and cannot move. In contrast, a mobile agent has the ability to move to different locations on a computer network to perform designated tasks. Therefore, a mobile agent can obtain the benefits provided by different locations, e.g., gain an access to local services and data (About Aglets, 2002). A mobile agent moves an executable code to a data source instead of moving data to a program source; hence, it reduces a number of network bandwidth and communication sessions (Wong, Paciorek, & Moore, 1999). In addition,

the traditional client-server method is more time and resource consuming than the mobile agent approach because of data transfer. In order to relocate, a mobile agent requires services from a mobile agent platform at each location.

This research utilizes software agent technology because it is modular, flexible, and expandable; which are our desirable characteristics. Agent technology also gives many capabilities and benefits that cannot be easily obtained from a traditional client-server paradigm. The technology supports distributed or decentralized architecture. A decentralized architecture can relieve the problems of resource limitations and a single point of failure. In addition, distributed architecture allows a software system to work in parallel, have workload distribution, and process tasks on multiple processing units; each of which gracefully increases overall performance. Moreover, software agents can work in team to solve a more complex problem (Gibbs, 2000).

Both types of software agents require services from an agent execution environment or platform to accomplish the designated tasks. An agent platform is a software system that provides an environment or a run-time system for software agents to execute. It may also provide supporting services, a standard interface for interactions, services for creation, services for migration, services for destruction of agents, and services for non-agent-based software environments (Gibbs, 2000; Green, et al., 1997; Martens, et al., 2001). Example of agent execution environments are Aglets (About Aglets, 2002; Aglets, 2002; Chiossi, 2004; Wong, Paciorek, & Moore, 1999), Concordia (Igo Jr., 2007; Wong, Paciorek, & Moore, 1999), and TEEMA (TRLabs Execution Environment for Mobile Agents) (Gibbs, 2000; Martens, et al., 2001).

This research employs TEEMA as our agent platform since it is immediately available to the authors and there are benefits of a great deal of local experiences and resources. Plus, TEEMA is an effective and efficient software agent platform that is previously employed in many research problems. TEEMA is a Java-based mobile agent platform developed by TRLabs (Telecommunication Research and Laboratories), Regina. Java technology allows TEEMA to be platform independence. In other words, it allows an agent to be run on various types of devices. However, every device in an agent-based system must install the JVM (Java Virtual Machine) run-time environment as a requirement. Java gives various features to TEEMA such as object oriented concept, object serialization and reconstruction, networking support, and security (Wong, Paciorek, & Moore, 1999). TEEMA also provides various services such as agent creation, migration, and destruction; message handling; information logging; GUI for monitoring and controlling agents and a platform; etc.

OPERATIONAL WELLNESS MODEL

This section provides summarized information of the operational wellness model. For more details please refer to (Soomlek & Benedicenti, Operational Wellness Model: A Wellness Model Designed for an Agent-Based Wellness Visualization System, 2010).

In order to construct a wellness visualization system, the term wellness and the wellness evaluation method are needed to be clarified. The operational wellness model is a wellness model that is created for an automatic measuring system and it is also a basis for developing our wellness indicator. The model is computable, flexible and expandable. The results of the model are comparable and can be presented in graphical formats.

Concept of Wellness

In this research, the term wellness is defined as "a state of achieving best possible state of physical health and lifestyle within a person's capability" (Soomlek & Benedicenti, Operational Wellness Model: A Wellness Model Designed for an Agent-Based Wellness Visualization System, 2010).

Each person can have personal sets of wellness indicators; while each indicator has a certain target value or range. A person might not be able reach the highest level of wellness but still can achieve his desirable level of wellness; which is the case that we consider him as being well. A person having disability can be considered as being well (in certain areas), if he can manage to achieve the targets/goals of his wellness indicators. The visualization system supports a person to monitor on three sets of parameters, mainly focused on physical health, and to improve them towards his target values/ranges. The three sets of parameters are as follows:

1. **Case-based indicator:** Initial sets of clinical objective parameters that are relative to certain cases. These parameters are predefined and provided to the end-users to choose.
2. **User defined indicator:** A set of indicators defined by a user. The user can define personal indicators with target values or target ranges by following certain instructions and rules.
3. **Healthcare-professional defined indicator:** A set of indicators defined for a patient by caregivers.

Thus, the operational wellness model is flexible, customizable, and expandable. In other words, a person can have a personal set of indicators for monitoring his personal wellness level and can expand/modify it as need.

Operational Wellness Evaluation Model

The operational wellness evaluation model is constructed regarding the operational definition of wellness. In this model, both single indicator wellness and overall wellness level are measured. Single indicator wellness indicates the wellness level of an indicator. The results from a series of case-based indicators and healthcare-professional defined indicators are combined to become the overall wellness level of a person. The latest results can be compared with the previous evaluations to find the progress and trend.

The agent-based wellness visualization system employed the results from both types of wellness evaluation to visualize the state of wellbeing of a person in simple graphical formats.

AGENT-BASED WELLNESS INDICATOR

Overview

Figure 1 illustrates the overview of the agent-based wellness indicator. There are two types of users in this research: general user and healthcare professional user (Benedicenti & Soomlek, 2009; Soomlek & Benedicenti, Operational Wellness Model: A Wellness Model Designed for an Agent-Based Wellness Visualization System, 2010). A general user is a person who does not have a certain level of medical knowledge to interpret and analyze wellness information, e.g., patient. A healthcare professional user is a person who had been well trained in the medical field, therefore, has the ability to interpret, evaluate, and analyze wellness data, e.g., doctor and nurse. Both types of users can gain access to the wellness indicator system through both personal computer and mobile device; and in the future, through a television (Benedicenti & Soomlek, 2009; Soomlek & Benedicenti, Operational Wellness Model: A Wellness Model Designed for an Agent-Based Wellness Visualization System, 2010; Soomlek & Benedicenti, Creating a Framework for Testing Wellness Visualization Systems, 2011; Soomlek & Benedicenti, Repeatable Experimental Framework for Wellness Indicator Testing/Evaluation: Environmental Setup, 2012).

At the server side, there are various groups of software agents. Each group of agents acts as a service provider that provides certain services. A coordinator agent works as a service registry and a matchmaker. When a client requests for a service, the coordinator agent will check the availability of the relevant service provider, then, forward the request to it. More detailed information relative to each group of agents and supporting components will be described in the next section.

System's Components

This section describes the main components of the proof concept. Since this research focuses on information visualization, the proof of concept is developed based on the assumption of the availability of a sophisticated clinical data integration system; and therefore, wellness information is immediately available to be employed through the data integration system. Examples of data integration system and relevant techniques can be found in (Ziegler & Dittrich, Three decades of data integration—all problems solved?, 2004; Ziegler & Dittrich, Data Integration—Problems, Approaches, Perspectives, 2007; Lenzerini, 2002; Lembo, Lenzerini, & Rosati, 2002; McBrien & Poulovassilis, 2003).

Agent-Based Rule-Based System

The agent-based rule-based system is modified from Asadachatreekul's work in (Asadachatreekul, 2004). The rule-based system is responsible for making inference to the knowledge base obtaining from humans to find anomalies and simple description and suggestion for a user. The rule-based system employs forward chaining method to solve problems. This group of agents contains:

1. **Rule Agents:** Each rule agent contains a set of rules; where each rule is a part of knowledge base.
2. **MMA (Message Multiplexer Agent):** Responsible for registering and tracking Rule Agents in the rule-based system and sharing information among the registered Rule Agents.

Figure 1. System overview

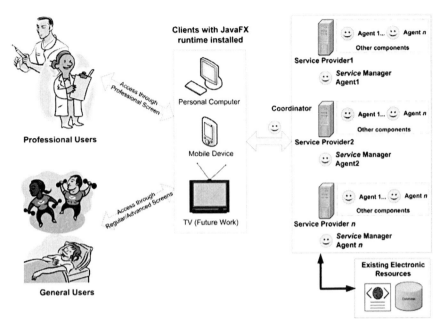

3. **Memory Agent:** Selects the best rule to be used from all fired rules.
4. **Trace Agent:** Responsible for keeping the chain of fired rules and finding the best description and suggestion for the goal.

Wellness Calculator

This group of agents is developed from the operational wellness evaluation model. There are two agents in the group:

1. **Single Wellness Calculator:** Calculates the wellness level of each indicator by utilizing the formulas in (Soomlek & Benedicenti, Operational Wellness Model: A Wellness Model Designed for an Agent-Based Wellness Visualization System, 2010).
2. **Overall Wellness Calculator:** Calculates the overall wellness level from the series of indicators in the set of case-based and healthcare professional defined indicators.

Agent-Based Statistical Tools

Agent-based statistical tools are a group of agents that provide statistical information to a user and other components in the system. The agents in this group are as follows:

1. **StatAnalyzer Agents:** A group of agents containing statistical methods. Some StatAnalyzer Agents have to work together to obtain the final result.
2. **StatAdmin Agent:** Responsible for registering and tracking StatAnalyzer Agents in the system.
3. **StatSelector Agent:** Selects statistical methods that are appropriated for retrieved data.

GUI (Graphical User Interface)

GUI presents wellness and decision support information to users. It also allows users to interact with the wellness indicator system. This research employs the knowledge gained from (Tufte, 1997) (Few, 2006; Nielson, 2005; Butow, 2007; Ware, 2004) to design the graphical presentations and user interfaces. More detailed information will be presented in the user interface design section.

Supporting Components

1. **Coordinator Agent:** Responsible for registering and tracking groups of agents providing services to both users and other components in the system. It also coordinates the GUI with the registered service providers, i.e., registered groups of agents.
2. **DataRetriever Agent:** Designed for cooperating with a data integration system. Since the proof of concept is developed based on the assumption of the availability of a sophisticated data integration system, this agent, currently, retrieves data from testing data source as requested.

User Interface Design

Since there are two types of users who have different backgrounds and requirements, the user interface is divided into two modes, i.e., regular and advanced mode (Benedicenti & Soomlek, 2009). A general user can access to both regular and advanced modes. The advanced mode allows a general user to view how his information is presented to the authorized caregivers. A healthcare professional user has advanced screens only because it is specifically designed for supporting caregivers' tasks and the information provided in this mode covers the content in the regular mode.

Moreover, the wellness indicator allows a user to access to the system through personal computer, small form factor, and, may be in the future, television; at least two versions of GUI are required. The content presented on all types of devices should be the same but on different layouts (Benedicenti & Soomlek, 2009). The main

reasons are the screen size and the limitation of those devices. In case of the small form factors, the device in this group tend to have a smaller screen, thus, the design used in large screen device may not appropriate in this case.

Figure 2 shows the overview page in the regular mode of the agent-based wellness indicator. According to Few, The top-left corner of the screen has the strongest degree of emphasis while the middle region of the screen has strong emphasis only when it is parted from its surrounding (Few, 2006). Therefore, the most important information that a general user should pay attention first after logging into the system must be placed in the strongest emphasis area, i.e., the top-left corner. We consider the current overall wellness level and the progress of wellness status of a person as a first priority, because the current overall wellness level informs the overall state of wellbeing of a person at the present and the progress shows the improvement or worsening of overall wellness condition. The "Alert" panel is also placed in the emphasis area to present a short summary of each anomaly found in an indicator. The alerts are sorted by date and severity. Color attribute is employed to differentiate the levels of severity, i.e., red-highest priority, yellow-high priority, and green-normal. More detailed information of each anomaly can be found at the "Anomalies" page or by clicking on an alert. The same criteria are applied to the advanced mode (see Figure 3) and healthcare professional's page (see Figure 4) as well. However, in the advanced mode, detailed information of each indicator is located in the emphasis area and the alerts are placed in the lower emphasis area because, by switching to the advanced mode, a user tends to find extensive information than summarized information.

Pre-attentive visual attributes, such as color attributes and form attributes (Few, 2006; Ware, 2004), are employed to create simple visual presentation, and emphasize and de-emphasize information by its priority. Gestalt principles of

Figure 2. Overview page in regular mode

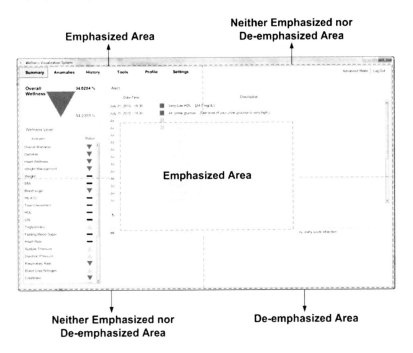

visual perception are applied to organize and group information together, and reduce non-data pixels, unnecessary decorations, and distractions (Few, 2006; Tufte, 1997). Simple graphics and display media are employed to ensure they are easy to be interpreted.

As mentioned earlier that the designs used for a larger screen device are not suitable for a small form factor device, a more appropriate GUI is required. Figure 5 illustrates the overview page designed for a general user on the left and the overview page designed for a healthcare professional user on the right. Since there is a limited space on screen, it is not possible to put all detailed information on the single screen. Therefore, the information from each panel presented on the large screen version is further prioritized. Then, the most important information of each panel is presented. In addition, the presented information can be expanded to obtain the detail in the next corresponding screen. The same idea is applied to menu bar and menu options as well. The frequently used menu options are available on the menu bar.

The rest of the menu options can be found after selecting on the "Full Menu" option.

Even though existing theories and practical guides have been applied to every version of the GUIs, the GUIs are not perfect. There is a possibility that there are unexpected errors, unexpected difficulties in using the interface, dislike objects, and distractions found by users. Therefore, usability testing should be performed to ensure that the design is usable, practical to be used, meet users' requirements, and can assist a user to accomplish their tasks.

EVALUATION

In order to ensure that the proof of concept meets all of the research goals, is usable, and can be compared to other works in the same area; an effective and efficient evaluation method is crucial. Unfortunately, there is no standard and de facto method for measuring a wellness visualization system. Therefore, we presented a method for

Figure 3. Overview page in advanced model

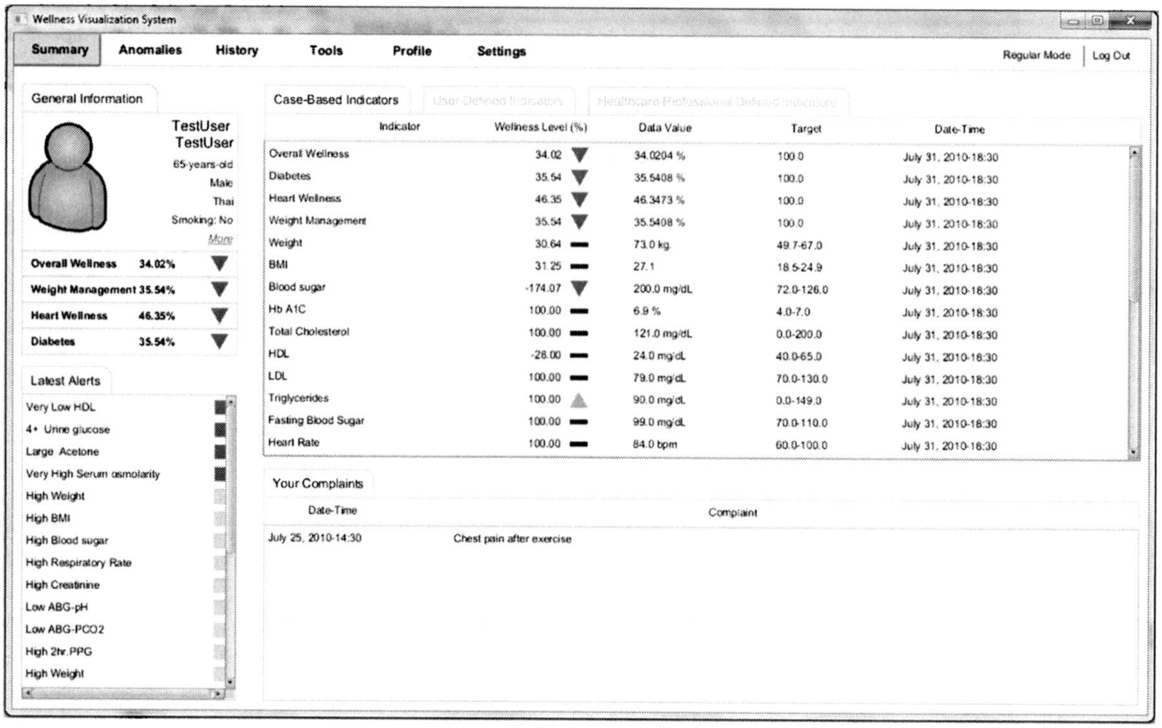

Figure 4. Overview page designed for healthcare professional users

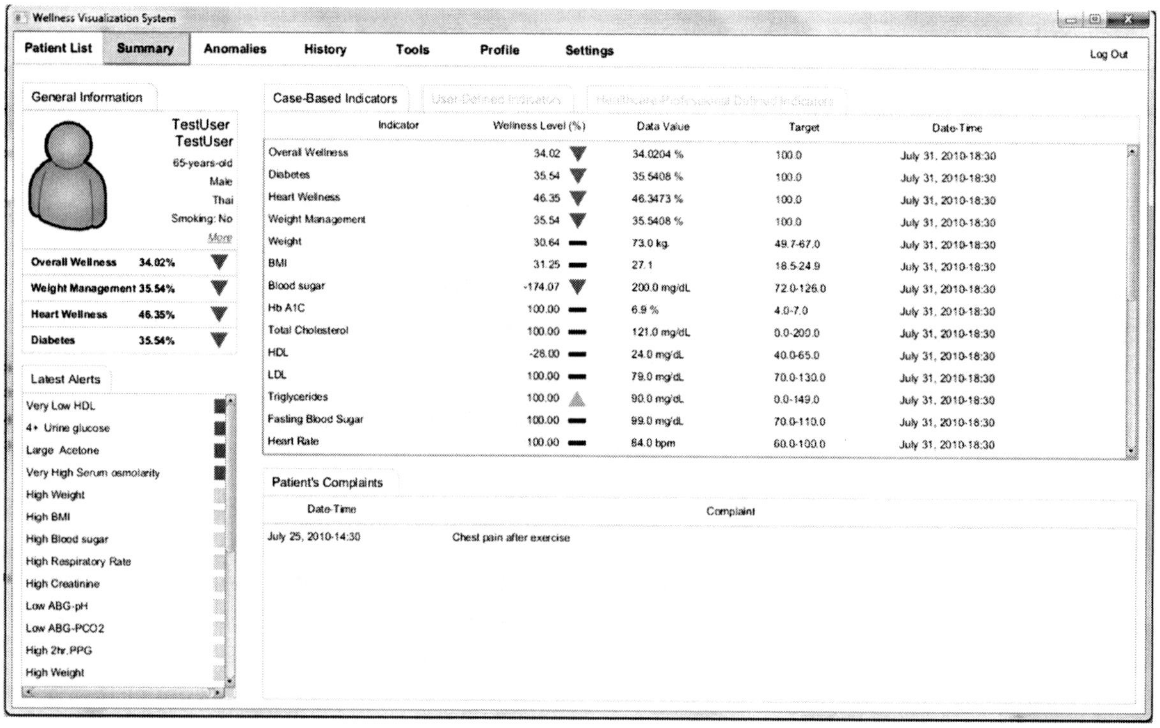

Figure 5. Mobile versions

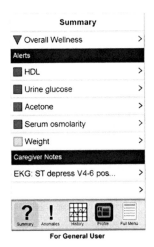
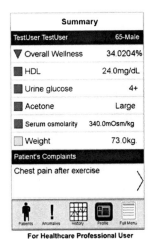

creating a framework for testing a wellness visualization system in (Soomlek & Benedicenti, Creating a Framework for Testing Wellness Visualization Systems, 2011; Soomlek & Benedicenti, Repeatable Experimental Framework for Wellness Indicator Testing/Evaluation: Environmental Setup, 2012).

Framework for Evaluating a Wellness Visualization System

This section summarized the framework for evaluating a wellness visualization system we developed.

Testing Framework

The framework is constructed by following the Goal-Question-Metric approach (Soomlek & Benedicenti, Creating a Framework for Testing Wellness Visualization Systems, 2011; Pressman, 2005; Fenton & Pfleeger, 1998). It combines the approaches used for finding a user's impression with the testing tools and methods used in software testing and usability testing (Soomlek & Benedicenti, Creating a Framework for Testing Wellness Visualization Systems, 2011). In other words, both technical-oriented and user-oriented tools/

methods are included in the framework (Soomlek & Benedicenti, Creating a Framework for Testing Wellness Visualization Systems, 2011). Technical-oriented tools/methods focus on benchmarking and technical requirements while user-oriented tools/methods involve feeling, impression, satisfaction, etc. (Soomlek & Benedicenti, Creating a Framework for Testing Wellness Visualization Systems, 2011). The framework measures a wellness visualization system in the following aspects:

- System verification
- System validation
- Verification of the system's functionalities
- Validation of the system's functionalities
- Usability of the GUI and graphical presentations
  - Useful
  - Efficient
  - Effective
  - Satisfying
  - Learnable
  - Accessible
- Accessibility
- Impression

Testing Tools/Methods

The testing tools/methods are employed in this evaluation are questionnaire, error rate evaluation, unit testing, integration testing, comparative methods, exploratory study, peer review, and system architecture analysis (Soomlek & Benedicenti, Creating a Framework for Testing Wellness Visualization Systems, 2011). Some measuring tools, such as error rate evaluation and comparative methods, require the information collected through questionnaire before full evaluation can be applied.

Two sets of questionnaires were developed to collect information from both types of users. One is designed to collect information from general users. Another one is designed to collect information from healthcare professional users. Both questionnaires contain a combination of scale, forced choices, and open-end questions; a series of tasks; and instructions. The questions are formed in regard with the testing goals. Each testing goal is created from the research's goal (Soomlek & Benedicenti, Creating a Framework for Testing Wellness Visualization Systems, 2011). The questionnaires and data collection process had been approved by the University of Regina's Ethics Board.

The questionnaire designed for a general user is divided into 6 parts. The first part collects personal and background information of a person such as gender and the user's experience towards portable health monitoring devices and e-Health systems. The data collected from section 2 and 6 are a part of the comparative methods used in this research and the two sections contain the same set of questions; please refer to (Soomlek & Benedicenti, Creating a Framework for Testing Wellness Visualization Systems, 2011) for more detailed information. In case of section 2, a volunteer has to answer the questions by employing the raw data attached with the questionnaire. For section 6, the volunteer is instructed to employ the wellness indicator to find the answers to those questions. The results from the two sections will be compared and evaluated against the testing goals. Section 3 asks a volunteer to evaluate the wellness visualization system and its functionalities based on their experience from exploring the system. The questions relative to the usability of the wellness indicator are presented in section 4. Both good and bad impressions towards the agent-based wellness visualization system are collected in section 5 of the questionnaire. The questions in section 5 allow the volunteers to express their attitude, feeling, impression, and expectation towards the wellness indicator; which assists us to create an improved version of the graphical presentation, human-computer interaction, and functionalities provided in the future.

In case of the healthcare professional user, there are five sections in the questionnaire. The first section involves personal and background information; including the experience of a volunteer in using portable health monitoring devices, electronic health record (EHR), and clinical decision support system. In section 2, a volunteer is asked to evaluate the wellness visualization system and the functionalities provided to a healthcare professional user. Section 3 requests a volunteer to evaluate the wellness indicator and its functionalities provided to his patient in regard with the experience from exploring the system as a general user. The usability is evaluated in section 4. Both good and bad impressions are collected in the last section.

Data Collection

Participant Demographics

Twenty-one general users and five healthcare professionals were volunteered to participate in this research. The volunteers were recruited within Regina area. Table 1 and 2 present the participant demographics of general users and healthcare professional users respectively.

Table 1. Participant demographics (general users)

Demographics Categories		Percent (N = 21)	Note
Gender	Male	61.9	
	Female	38.1	
Age (years)	20-29	85.7	Mean = 27.71 Std. Dev. = 5.542
	30-39	9.5	
	40-49	4.8	
Occupation	Student	85.7	
	Others	14.3	
Completed Medical Training	Yes	4.8	
	No	95.2	
Level of importance of personal wellness	Very important	28.6	
	Important	33.3	
	Somewhat	23.8	
	A little	14.3	
	Not important	0	
Having experience in using a portable health monitoring device	Yes	4.8	Frequency of usage = 1-2 times a month
	No	95.2	
Having experience in using an electronic health system	Yes	4.8	Frequency of usage = occasionally
	No	95.2	

Testing Environment

The test sessions had been performed at TRLabs, Regina and user sites. The testing environment was setup by utilizing the followings:

- PC1
  - **Processor:** Intel® Core™2 Duo CPU E6550 @2.33GHz
  - **RAM:** 2 GB
  - **Operating System:** Window XP and Windows 7 Professional (64-bit)
- PC2
  - **Processor:** Intel® Core™ i5-2557M CPU@1.70GHz
  - **RAM:** 4GB
  - **Operating System:** Windows 7 Home Premium (64-bit)
- PC3

  - **Processor:** Intel®Core™2 Duo CPU T7100@1.80GHz
  - **RAM:** 2GB
  - **Operating System:** Windows 7 Professional (64-bit)
- Mobile phone
  - **Model:** Samsung Omnia II
  - **Processor:** ARM1176 S3C6410
  - **Operating System:** Windows Mobile® 6.5 Professional
    - CE OS 5.2.21863 (Build 21863.5.0.67) ©2009 Microsoft Corporation
  - **Java:** JBlend on Windows Mobile v4.0.0, build: 20090928b
  - **JavaFX Mobile:** JavaFX 1.2, SJWC 2.2
- Wellness Indicator (Desktop versions)
  - Java ™ version 7 update 2 (64-bit), JavaFX version 2.0.2 (64-bit)

Table 2. Participant demographics (healthcare professional users)

Demographics Categories		Percent (N = 5)	Note
Gender	Male	40.0	
	Female	60.0	
Age	20-29	40.0	
	30-39	20.0	
	40-49	40.0	
Profession	Nurse	100.0	
Have you ever used a portable health monitoring device?	Yes	60.0	
	No	40.0	
How often do you use a portable health monitoring device	Everyday	20.0	
	1-2 times a week	0.0	
	1-2 times a month	20.0	
	Other	20.0	
	Never	40.0	
Have you ever use an electronic health record (EHR)?	Yes	60.0	
	No	40.0	
Do you prefer EHR or paper-based health record?	HER	80.0	
	Paper-based health record	0.0	
	No preference	20.0	
Have you ever use a clinical decision support system?	Yes	0.0	
	No	100.0	
How often do you use a clinical decision support system?	Everyday	0.0	
	1-2 times a week	0.0	
	1-2 times a month	0.0	
	Other	0.0	
	Never	100.0	

- Wellness Indicator (Mobile versions)
  - Java ™ version 6 update 19 (64-bit), JavaFX version 1.2

Evaluation Results

Results from General Users

The evaluation results presenting in this section is evaluated by general users.

1. **Comparative Method:** The objective of this test is to compare the results from before/ without using the wellness visualization system to the results from using the wellness visualization system. The hypothesis of this test is that there is no difference between the scores obtained before/without using the wellness visualization system and the scores obtained by using the wellness visualization system.

H_0: $\mu_{\text{without using wellness visualization system}} = \mu_{\text{using wellness visualization system}}$

H_1: $\mu_{\text{without using wellness visualization system}} \neq \mu_{\text{using wellness visualization system}}$

The results displayed in Tables 3-5 show that there is a significant difference between the two groups of scores, i.e. Sig. (2-tailed) < 0.05. The mean of Score1 (5.1) is lower than the mean of Score2 (13.19). That means, by using the wellness visualization system to answer the given questions, the participants gain more marks. The same group of participants received lower marks without using the wellness visualization system. The results also show that, in average, a person gain 8.095 more marks by using the wellness visualization system to answer the questions. In other words, the visualization system can assist a person to gain more knowledge relative to their personal wellness status.

2. **System and Functionalities Evaluation:** Table 6 gives overall rating of the system and its functionalities. The volunteers rated the wellness indicator as Good. The visualization system received Very Good rate on the mobile version, Good rate for the regular mode of the desktop version, and Very Good rate for the advanced mode of the desktop version; which is corresponding to the volunteers' comments. For example, *"I prefer the mobile version because it is simpler and easier to understand. The desktop version provides too much information for people who don't have medical knowledge and don't know what to do with those data."* Table 7 and Table 8 present the evaluations of the

Table 3. Paired samples statistics

	Mean	N	Std. Deviation	Std. Error Mean
Score obtained before/without using the wellness visualization system	5.10	21	2.663	.581
Score obtined by using the wellness visualization system	13.19	21	4.355	.950

Table 4. Paired samples correlations

	N	Correlation	Sig.
Score obtained before/without using the wellness visualization system & Score obtained by using the wellness visualization system	21	.141	.543

functionalities provided by the desktop version and the mobile version respectively. The mobile version received higher rating in some areas such as history and setting pages.

Moreover, the healthcare-professional defined indicator mechanism has higher rating than the other sets of indicators. As well as, the functionalities created to support the communication among caregivers and a patient, i.e., Notes from caregivers and Complaints for caregivers.

Most people stated that they were impressed by the "Alert" feature, history and progress shown, and the "Foods and Activities Diary" tool; mainly because, the three features provide decent information and allow users to track their progress over time.

3. **Responding Time and Error Rates:** All participants indicated that it took only a few seconds to get access to both versions of the GUIs. The error ratio of the desktop version is 0.238. The error ratio of the mobile version is 0.048.

4. **Usability:** According to Table 9, the overall rating for the GUIs were rated as Good. The GUIs were rated as Very Good in many aspects. The participants said this about the usability of the GUIs: "It is very impressive. It might take more than 10 minutes to get use to the system but still intuitive and impressive", "If I understand what the program is presenting, I think people in this whole world also understand.", "I find the program is very intuitive and cool. I think

Table 5. Paired samples test

	Paired Differences					t	df	Sig. (2-tailed)
	Mean	Std. Deviation	Std. Error Mean	95% Confidence Interval of the Difference				
				Lower	Upper			
Score obtined before/with-out using the wellness visualiza-tion system - Score obtained by using the wellness visualiza-tion system	-8.095	4.774	1.042	-10.268	-5.922	-7.771	20	.000

Table 6. Overall evaluations

Questions	Results (5-point Likert Scale)	Percent (N=21)
0 – Very Poor, 1 – Poor, 2 – Average, 3 – Good, 4 – Very Good		
Overall rating for the wellness visualization system based on your expectation	Good (3)	42.9
Overall rting for the desktop version	Good (3)	52.4
Overall rting for regular mode in the desktop version	Good (3)	57.1
Overall rting for advanced mode in the desktop version	Very Good (4)	47.6
Overall rating for the mobile version	Very Good (4)	52.4
Overall rating for supporting tools	Good (3)	52.4
Simplicit	Very Good (4)	38.1
Understandability	Good (3)	42.9
0 – Not a all, 1 – Somewhat, 2 – Average, 3 – Much, 4 – Very Much		
Do you like the predefined sets of case-based indicators?	Much (3)	42.9
Do you lie the user-defined indicator mechanism?	Much (3)	52.4
Do you lie the healthcare-professional defined indicator mechanism?	Much (3)	42.9
	Very Much(4)	42.9

it will provide a lot of benefits if it becomes public," and "The mobile version is really cool and convenient". Most participants indicated that the wellness visualization system is very useful and intuitive. In addition, most participants prefer the mobile version because it is simple, convenient, and does not contain too much information. A few people who prefer the desktop version said: "I like the desktop version because there are more information and things to play around."

Table 7. Functionalities provided by the desktop version

Questions	Results (5-point Likert Scale)	Percent (N=21)
0 – Not at all, 1 – Somewhat, 2 – Average, 3 – Much, 4 – Very Much		
Does the wellness visualization system immediately respond to your input?	Very Much (4)	57.1
Do you like the summary page?	Very Much (4)	57.1
Do you like the anomalies page?	Very Much (4)	57.1
Do you like the history page?	Much (3)	47.6
Do you lie the tools page?	Much (3)	38.1
	Very Much(4)	38.1
Do you like the profile page?	Very Much (4)	42.9
Do you like the setting page?	Much (3)	38.1
Do you lie the "Alert" feature?	Very Much (4)	61.9
Do you like the "Notes from caregivers" feature?	Very Much (4)	52.4
Do you like the "Complaints for caregivers" feature?	Very Much (4)	52.4
Do you like the supporting tools?	Average (2)	33.3
	Much (3)	33.3
Is the siple description of each alert useful to you?	Very Much (4)	47.6
Is the simple suggestion of each alert useful to you?	Very Much (4)	57.1
Are the links to relevant external resources useful to you?	Very Much (4)	42.9

Table 8. Functionalities provided by the mobile version

Questions	Results (5-point Likert Scale)	Percent (N=21)
0 – Not at all, 1 – Somewhat, 2 – Average, 3 – Much, 4 – Very Much		
Does the wellness visualization system immediately respond to your input?	Very Much (4)	61.9
Do you like the summary page?	Very Much (4)	71.4
Do you like the anomalies page?	Very Much (4)	57.1
Do you like the main history page?	Very Much (4)	47.6
Do you like the detail history page?	Much (3)	38.1
	Very Much(4)	38.1
Do you like the profile page?	Much (3)	38.1
	Very Much(4)	38.1
Do you like the setting page?	Very Much (4)	38.1

Our designs are not perfect. There are certain things that need to be improved. For example, many participants want the font size to be adjustable. Some people had difficulties finding sub-menu bar because it is not explicit and looks more like a decoration. One person recommended not to use symmetric triangle to present wellness status because he cannot distinguish the different between the one pointing up and the one pointing

Table 9. Usability

Questions	Results (5-point Likert Scale)	Percent (N=21)
0 – Very Poor, 1 – Poor, 2 – Average, 3 – Good, 4 – Very Good		
Overall rating for your satisfaction toward the user interface	Good (3)	52.4
Usability	Good (3)	42.9
	Very Good(4)	42.9
Usefulness	Very Good (4)	61.9
Efficiency	Very Good (4)	42.9
Effectiveness	Very good (4)	71.4
Ease of Learning	Very good (4)	47.6
Simplicity	Very good (4)	42.9
0 – Not at all, 1 – Somewhat, 2 – Average, 3 – Much, 4 – Very Much		
Is the interface easy to understand?	Much (3)	42.9
Is the inerface easy to use?	Much (3)	42.9
	Very Much(4)	42.9
Are the graphical presentations meaningful?	Very Much (4)	61.9
Do the graphical presentations reflect the meaning of relevant information?	Very Much (4)	61.9
Does the wellness visualization system give you an insight?	Very Much (4)	66.7
For the desktop version, is the presented information appropriate for the screen size?	Very Much (4)	47.6
For the mobile version, is the presented information appropriate for the screen size?	Much (3)	42.9
For the dsktop version, are the graphical presentations appropriate for the screen size?	Very Much (4)	47.6
For the mobile version, the graphical presentations appropriate for the screen size?	Very Much (4)	47.6
Is the wellness level easy to interpret?	Much (3)	47.6
Is the curent wellness status easy to understand?	Much (3)	61.9
Is the suport information, e.g. graph, trend, statistical information, and simple description useful to you?	Very Much (4)	52.4

down. To him, they are all triangle. He recommended we use arrows instead.

5. **Impression:** 19% of the volunteers had a little discomfort while using the wellness visualization system. Another 19% of the volunteers had somewhat discomfort while using the wellness indicator. The participants suggested that there should be a help button, a tooltip on each object, or a search option, such that they can find a solution when they are stuck. 66.7% of the participants completely agreed that the wellness visualization system made them feel like learning more about personal state of wellbeing and how to improve it. Only 9.5% felt stress or was too worried about their wellness status when they saw the overall wellness level moved down. One of the reasons is "I'm so young. I prefer not to know that I'm sick or unwell. If I don't see the doctor, I'm still thinking that I'm healthy. If I know that I'm not healthy, I feel sad. So, it is better for me not to know the truth." In case of the people who did not feel any stress, one said: "I think it's good to know what is wrong with you and you find it early." and "I think it is good to find problems when you are still young, so,

you can treat them and it is easier to treat them. Really, all I can see from this is the benefits." 76.2% felt more confidence, 9.5% felt somewhat more confidence, and 14.3% felt a little more confidence in realizing and learning about a state of wellbeing from the wellness visualization than from raw data and other sources, e.g., Internet and pamphlets. One said "I like the description and suggestion provided by the system because it makes me feel like having a personal doctor with me all the time. Even if I know that the information came from the knowledge base, I still be able to know what the meaning of each parameter is, what should I do or what can I do to take care of myself."

Results from Healthcare Professional Users

The evaluation results presenting in this section is evaluated by healthcare professionals.

1. **System and Functionalities Evaluation:** Table 10 presents the overall rating in various aspects evaluated by healthcare professionals. The agent-based wellness indicator was rated as Good. The participants also rated both desktop and mobile versions as Good. The system received very high score for simplicity and healthcare-professional defined indicator mechanism. Example of comments from the healthcare professionals regarding the system and functionalities are "I like it. When I want to see what the person is doing, the information is there. When I want to find the trend and history of the person, the information is there." and "The information looks very decent."

Even though the desktop and mobile versions obtained the same rating, Table 11 and Table 12 indicates that the mobile version was rated with the higher score in most areas. This is confirmed by the opinions of the participants: "I like the mobile version better, because of the font and comprehensive way of showing information." and "I like the mobile version. The desktop version is too much, I mean too much information."

2. **Responding Time and Error Rates:** All participants indicated that it took only a few seconds to get access to all versions of the GUI. The error ratio of all versions of the GUI is 0.

Table 10. Overall evaluations

Questions	Results (5-point Likert Scale)	Percent (N=5)
0 – Very Poor, 1 – Poor, 2 – Average, 3 – Good, 4 – Very Good		
Overall rating for the wellness visualization system based on your expectation	Good (3)	80.0
Overall rting for the desktop version	Good (3)	100.0
Overall rting for the mobile version	Good (3)	60.0
Overall rting for the supporting tools	Good (3)	60.0
Simplicit	Good (3)	40.0
	Very Good(4)	40.0
Understandability	Good (3)	100.0
Pre-defind sets of case-based indicators	Good (3)	80.0
User-defied indicator mechanism	Good (3)	80.0
Healthcar-professional defined indicator mechanism	Very Good (4)	100.0

Table 11. Functionalities provided by the desktop version

Questions	Results (5-point Likert Scale)	Percent (N=5)
0 – Not at all, 1 – Somewhat, 2 – Average, 3 – Much, 4 – Very Much		
Does the wellness visualization system immediately respond to your input?	Much (3)	60.0
Do you lie the patient list page?	Much (3)	80.0
Do you lie the summary page?	Much (3)	60.0
Do you lie the anomalies page?	Much (3)	60.0
Do you lie the history page?	Very Much (4)	60.0
Do you like the tools page?	Much (3)	80.0
Do you lie the profile page?	Very Much (4)	60.0
Do you like the setting page?	Very Much (4)	60.0
Do you like the "Alert" feature?	Very Much (4)	60.0
Do you like the "Notes from caregivers" feature?	Much (3)	80.0
Do you lie the "Patient's complaints" feature?	Much (3)	60.0
Do you lie the supporting tools?	Much (3)	80.0

Table 12. Functionalities provided by the mobile version

Questions	Results (5-point Likert Scale)	Percent (N=5)
0 – Not at all, 1 – Somewhat, 2 – Average, 3 – Much, 4 – Very Much		
Does the wellness visualization system immediately respond to your input?	Much (3)	60.0
Do you lie the patient list page?	Very Much (4)	60.0
Do you like the summary page?	Very Much (4)	60.0
Do you like the anomalies page?	Very Much (4)	57.1
Do you like the main history page?	Very Much (4)	60.0
Do you like the detail history page?	Very Much (4)	60.0
Do you like the profile page?	Very Much (4)	60.0
Do you like the setting page?	Very Much (4)	60.0

3. **System and Functionalities Provided to a General User:** Table 13 presents the ratings of the system and functionalities provided to patients. The wellness indicator received Good rate for all evaluations except simplicity; which obtained the highest rate. Table 14 and Table 15 present the rating of the desktop and mobile versions. Both versions received the highest rate in all evaluations.

4. **Usability:** According to Table 16, the overall rating for the GUIs were rated as Good. The GUIs were rated as Good in all aspects of usability. The participants said this about the usability of the GUIs: "The system is even more user friendly than what we are using, that one has too much column and flashing things.", "I like everything about it. I find it's good, it's nice, it's useful, but you have to keep in mind that we need to be trained before we can use the real system. But, I think I can do thing faster after I'm trained.", and "I like that you use the code. I don't have to read, just go to the right color."

Table 13. Overall evaluations of the system and functionalities provided to a general user

Questions	Results (5-point Likert Scale)	Percent (N=5)
0 – Very Poor, 1 – Poor, 2 – Average, 3 – Good, 4 – Very Good		
Overall rating for the wellness visualization system based on your expectation	Good (3)	60.0
Overall rting for the desktop version	Good (3)	80.0
Overall rting for regular mode in the desktop version	Good (3)	80.0
Overall rting for advance mode in the desktop version	Good (3)	80.0
Overall rting for the mobile version	Good (3)	60.0
Overall rting for the supporting tools	Good (3)	60.0
Simplicit	Good (3)	40.0
	Very Good(4)	40.0
Understandability	Good (3)	60.0
Pre-defind sets of case-based indicators	Good (3)	60.0
User-defied indicator mechanism	Good (3)	60.0
Healthcar-professional defined indicator mechanism	Good (3)	60.0

Table 14. Functionalities provided to a general user by the desktop version

Questions	Results (5-point Likert Scale)	Percent (N=5)
0 – Not at all, 1 – Somewhat, 2 – Average, 3 – Much, 4 – Very Much		
Does the wellness visualization system immediately respond to your input?	Very Much (4)	100.0
Do you like the summary page?	Very Much (4)	80.0
Do you like the anomalies page?	Very Much (4)	80.0
Do you like the history page?	Very Much (4)	80.0
Do you like the tools page?	Very Much (4)	80.0
Do you like the profile page?	Very Much (4)	60.0
Do you like the setting page?	Very Much (4)	80.0
Do you like the "Alert" feature?	Very Much (4)	100.0
Do you like the "Notes from caregivers" feature?	Very Much (4)	100.0
Do you like the "Patient's complaints" feature?	Very Much (4)	100.0
Do you like the supporting tools?	Very Much (4)	80.0
Do you like advance mode?	Very Much (4)	80.0
Is the simple description of each alert useful to your patients?	Very Much (4)	60.0
Is the simple suggestion of each alert useful to your patients?	Very Much (4)	60.0
Are the links to relevant external resources useful to your patients?	Very Much (4)	80.0

Table 15. Functionalities provided to a general user by the mobile version

Questions	Results (5-point Likert Scale)	Percent (N=5)
0 – Not at all, 1 – Somewhat, 2 – Average, 3 – Much, 4 – Very Much		
Does the wellness visualization system immediately respond to your input?	Very Much (4)	100.0
Do you like the summary page?	Very Much (4)	80.0
Do you like the anomalies page?	Very Much (4)	80.0
Do you like the main history page?	Very Much (4)	80.0
Do you like the detail history page?	Very Much (4)	60.0
Do you like the profile page?	Very Much (4)	60.0
Do you like the setting page?	Very Much (4)	60.0

Like general users, the participants in this group also requested for the larger font size: "I think the font is too small. So, when there is a lot of information, I can't focus. I tend to look for the part that has bigger font."

5. **Impression:** All participants agreed that the wellness visualization system can support a caregiver's tasks. Only 20% of the volunteers felt a little discomfort while using the wellness indicator system. One of the reasons is explained as follows: "You know when we use anything for the first time, we need more time to do thing [sic], but for the second round it is very easy." 60% of the participants stated that the system made they feel somewhat stress or worried about their patient's wellness status when they saw the patient's overall wellness level moved down. 60% of the participants completely agreed and 40% of the participants agreed the wellness visualization system can make their patient feels like learning more about personal state of wellbeing and how to improve it. All volunteers would like to recommend their patient to use the agent-based wellness visualization system. They said: "I think it is very useful for the patient, like they know about their own blood work. It's really ridiculous that we can't even look at our own information,

even for us the nurses have to wait for doctors to tell us that we have high cholesterol while we can read them."

APPLYING THE AGENT-BASED WELLNESS INDICATOR AND COST EVALUATION

The proof of concept had obtained good evaluation results and even compliments from the research participants in various aspects. The concept of personal wellness indicator was proved to be useful and should be employed to support both individuals and caregivers. Therefore, there is a high possibility for people to improve their state of wellbeing and for healthcare professionals to give a better wellness service to their patient, if this research is applied to existing health systems. This section explains how to apply the agent-based wellness indicator system to the central hospital organization.

As mentioned earlier since the agent-based wellness indicator is developed on the assumption of the availability of a data integration system, there is a high possibility to integrate the wellness indicator system with a central hospital organization with minimum cost. Figure 6 illustrates how to apply our approach to an existing hospital system. We assume certified electronic health record (EHR)

Table 16. Usability

Questions	Results (5-point Likert Scale)	Percent (N=5)
0 – Very Poor, 1 – Poor, 2 – Average, 3 – Good, 4 – Very Good		
Overall rating for your satisfaction toward the user interface	Good (3)	60.0
Usability	Good (3)	60.0
Usefulnes	Good (3)	60.0
Efficienc	Good (3)	60.0
Effectiveess	Good (3)	60.0
Ease of Larning	Good (3)	80.0
Simplicit	Good (3)	80.0
0 – Very oor, 1 – Poor, 2 – Average, 3 – Good, 4 – Very Good		
Is the interface easy to understand?	Much (3)	60.0
Is the inerface easy to use?	Much (3)	80.0
Are the gaphical presentations meaningful?	Very Much (4)	80.0
Do the graphical presentations reflect the meaning of relevant information?	Very Much (4)	80.0
Does the wellness visualization system give you an insight?	Very Much (4)	60.0
For the desktop version, is the presented information appropriate for the screen size?	Very Much (4)	60.0
For the mobile version, is the presented information appropriate for the screen size?	Very Much (4)	80.0
For the desktop version, are the graphical presentations appropriate for the screen size?	Very Much (4)	60.0
For the mobile version, the graphical presentations appropriate for the screen size?	Very Much (4)	80.0
Is the wellness level easy to interpret?	Very Much (4)	60.0
Is the current wellness status easy to understand?	Very Much (4)	60.0
Is the support information, e.g. graph, trend, statistical information, and simple description useful to you?	Very Much (4)	80.0
Is the support information, e.g. graph, trend, statistical information, and simple description, useful to your patient?	Very Much (4)	80.0

and clinical data integration system are already in place in a health system. Thus, it is mandatory to have an interface and authentication process to connect the data integration system with the wellness indicator. In this case, the associated costs for implementing the agent-based wellness indicator in a central hospital system are an infrastructure supporting the agent-based wellness indicator, interface, and authentication process; software licenses; maintenance costs (including the salary of staffs that are in charge of the wellness system); overhead costs (i.e., management and administrative expense, other relative services, etc.).

In case the EHR and clinical data integration system do not exist in the health system, the cost of implementing the whole system will be extremely high. According to Canada's Infoway, the Federal Government has spent $CAD52 million on architecture and standards, $CAD1,284 million on EHR, $CAD340 million on EMR (Electronic Medical Records) and integration, $CAD110 million on Telehealth, $CAD45 million on consumer health solutions, $CAD150 million on public health surveillance, and $CAD155 million on setting the future direction since 2001, in order to provide EHR system and healthcare applica-

Figure 6. Applying the agent-based wellness indicator to hospitals

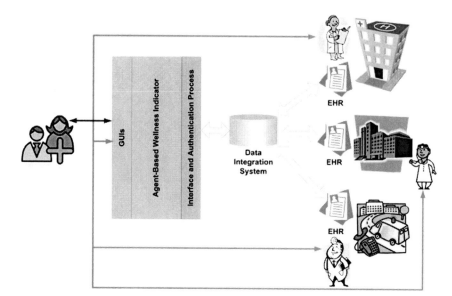

tions to Canadians (Canada Health Infoway, 2012). Even though only 50% of Canadians have their electronic health record available to their authorized health service providers, there are high benefits obtained by patients, caregivers, and Canada's hospital system. The investment already increased access to care and reduced waiting time, traveling costs, and traveling time – eliminating almost 47 million kilometers of travel (Canada Health Infoway, 2012). The approximation of benefits after it is fully implemented is $CAD1 billion per year.

For patients to obtain the full benefits from the wellness indicator system, they might have to pay for the following expenses: personal computer, mobile device, personal health monitoring devices, Internet access fees and relevant equipment, and service fees. The costs would be a one-time investment for a patient except for the Internet access fees, service fees, and maintenance costs. Moreover, by using the agent-based wellness visualization system, a person could reduce the following costs and time spent on the current health services:

1. **Number of visits:** Since a person can communicate to their caregivers through the wellness indicator system and the results obtained from sensors can be access by both types of users, the person is not required to go to a hospital when it is not necessary but they can follow the instructions and comments from their doctors, that are delivered by the wellness indicator system. The same practice can be applied to a discharged patient as well. A doctor can analyze the recovery status of a patient and decide whether the person has to come back for further examination or can continue with the current recovery process at home.

2. **Traveling cost and time:** When the number of visit is reduced, the cost for traveling to a health service location and the time spent on traveling to the location and waiting in a queue are also reduced.

3. **Health insurance:** As mentioned earlier that the agent-based wellness visualization system can give a better understanding in personal wellness status to a person, there is a high possibility that the person will take a better care of himself/herself and

therefore increase his/her state of wellbeing. When a person achieves the desirable level of wellness, that person is in his/her best possible state of physical health and lifestyle. Therefore, it might not necessary for that person to pay for a premium health insurance package. A cheaper one might be sufficient.

The benefit provided by the wellness visualization system to an individual can be calculated as follows:

Annual cost benefit = (cost per visit + traveling cost per visit)*reduced number of visit + reduced cost paid to health insurance

Where, reduced number of visit = number of visit from previous year - number of visit in this year, and reduced cost paid to health insurance = amount paid to health insurance from last year - amount paid to health insurance in this year

For example, let the cost per visiting a hospital be $60; the traveling cost per visit be $40; the number of visits from last year be 5 times; the number of visits in this year be 2 times; the amount paid to health insurance from last year be $250; and the amount paid to health insurance in this year be $200. Thus, the person has saved (60+40)*3+50 = $350 in one year by using the agent-based wellness indicator.

CONCLUSION AND FUTURE WORK

A high state of wellbeing is desirable. We developed the concept of personal wellness indicator to support this need and to solve the existing problems. The proof of concept was developed and evaluated in various aspects. The proof of concept of this research can give a better understanding of wellness to an individual, can assist caregivers'

tasks and it is useful, usable, and worth recommending to a patient. Even though the wellness visualization system has received high scores in various evaluations, it has to be improved to eliminate the difficulties and distractions found during the testing sessions and to fulfill the requirements and suggestions obtained from the users. The participants' comments are considered as our future direction for enhancing the proof of concept as well as the full implementation.

In order to perform a full implementation on a central hospital system, it is mandatory to have an infrastructure supporting the agent-based wellness indicator, an interface for communication, and an authentication process. If the hospital does not have EHR and is not connected to the central data integration system, implementing the concept of personal wellness indicator requires extra work and the cost of full implementation could be extremely high.

Patients might have to invest on personal computer, mobile device, personal health monitoring devices, Internet access fees and relevant equipment, and service fees to get access to the wellness indicator system to gain benefits from the system. The investment's payback however is in term of costs, time, a better standing in personal wellness and may lead to a higher state of wellbeing.

REFERENCES

About Aglets. (2002, March 14). IBM research. Retrieved July 30, 2012, from http://www.research. ibm.com/trl/aglets/about_e.htm

Aglets. (2002, March 14). IBM research. Retrieved July 30, 2012, from http://www.research.ibm. com/trl/aglets/

Anspaugh, D. J., Hamrick, M. H., & Rosato, F. (1994). *Wellness: Concepts and applications.* St. Louis, MO: Mosby.

Asadachatreekul, S. (2004). *An agent-based distributed inference engine for expert system construction*. Regina, Canada: University of Regina, Faculty of Graduate Studies and Research.

Benedicenti, L., & Soomlek, C. (2009). An agent-based modeling system for wellness. In Paranjape, R., & Sadanand, A. (Eds.), *Multi-agent systems for healthcare simulation and modeling: Applications for system improvement* (pp. 137–163). Hershey, PA: IGI Global. doi:10.4018/978-1-60566-772-0.ch008

Broyles, R. W. (2006). *Fundamentals of statistics in health administration*. Sudbury, MA: Jones and Bartlett.

Butow, E. (2007). *User interface design for mere mortals* (Hernandez, M. J., Ed.). 1st ed.). Addison-Wesley Professional.

Canada Health Infoway. (2012). *2012-2013 summary corperate plan*. Canada Health Infoway.

Chen, C. (1999). *Information visualisation and virtual environments*. London, UK: Springer.

Chiossi, C. (2004, October 6). *Aglets*. Retrieved July 30, 2012, from http://aglets.sourceforge.net/

Chow, S.-C. (2003). *Encyclopedia of biopharmaceutical statistics*. New York, NY: Marcel Dekker.

Dannheisser, L. M., & Rosenbaum, J. M. (2005). *What's wrong with me? The frustrated patients' guide to getting an accurate diagnosis*. New York, NY: McGraw-Hill.

Darkins, A. W., & Cary, M. A. (2000). *Telemedicine and telehealth: Principles, policies, performance, and pitfalls* (1st ed.). New York, NY: Springer Publishing Co.

Dunn, H. L. (1959). High-level wellness for man and society. *American Journal of Public Health and the Nation's Health*, *49*(6), 786–792. doi:10.2105/AJPH.49.6.786

Fenton, N. E., & Pfleeger, S. L. (1998). *Software metrics: A rigorous and practical approach* (2nd ed.). PWS Publishing Company.

Few, S. (2006). *Information dashboard design: The effective visual communication of data* (1st ed.). O'Reilley Media, Inc.

Franklin, S., & Graesser, A. (1996). Is it an agent, or just a program? A taxonomy for autonomous agents. *Proceedings of the Third International Workshop on Agent Theories, Architectures, and Languages*. Springer-Verlag. Retrieved from http://www.agent.ai/doc/upload/200302/fran96_1.pdf

Gibbs, C. (2000). *TEEMA reference guide version 1.0*. Regina, Canada: TRLabs, Regina.

Goolsby, M. J., & Grubbs, L. (2006). *Advanced assessment: Interpreting findings and formulating differential diagnoses*. Philadelphia, PA: F.A. Davis Company.

Green, S., Hurst, L., Nangle, B., Cunningham, P., Somers, F., & Evans, R. (1997, May). *Agent technology: An overview*. Dublin, Ireland: Department of Computer Science, Trinity College Dublin. Retrieved July 27, 2006, from https://www.cs.tcd.ie/research_groups/aig/iag/pubreview/chap2/chap2.html

Hackos, J. T., & Redish, J. C. (1998). *User and task analysis for interface design*. New York, NY: John Wiley & Sons, Inc.

Hall, D. (2007). *How much does a good wellness program cost?* Clackamas, OR: Wellsource, Inc. Retrieved June 25, 2012, from http://www.google.ca/url?sa=t&rct=j&q=wellness%20improvement%20program%20price&source=web&cd=2&ved=0CGEQFjAB&url=http%3A%2F%2Fwww.wellsource.com%2Fsite%2Fdownload%2Fasset%2F16%2F10%2F92%2Fc569ea541b1e4b1f39957cf6aa5f1478&ei=wtLoT9rkO6ec2QXDvpHmCg&usg=AFQj

Hersh, W. R. (2003). *Information retrieval: A health and biomedical perspective*. New York, NY: Springer.

Ichimura, T., & Yoshida, K. (2004). *Knowledge-based intelligent systems for healthcare*. Adelaide, Australia: Advanced Knowledge International.

Ichimura, T., & Yoshida, K. (2004). *Knowledge-based intelligent systems for healthcare* (Howlett, R. J., & Jain, L. C., Eds.). 1st ed., *Vol. 7*). Adelaide, Australia: Advanced Knowledge International Pty Ltd.

Igo, F. J., Jr. (2007, September 12). *Concordia*. Mitsubishi Electric Research Laboratories. Retrieved July 30, 2012, from http://www.merl.com/projects/concordia/

Kaffash, J. (2012, April 20). *Telemedicine 'trebles death rate' in elderly patients*. Retrieved June 26, 2012, from http://www.pulsetoday.co.uk/news-article-content/-/article_display_list/13803303/telemedicine-trebles-death-rate-in-elderly-patients

Kirkwood, B. R., & Sterne, J. A. (2003). *Essential medical statistics*. Malden, MA: Blackwell Science.

Lembo, D., Lenzerini, M., & Rosati, R. (2002). Source inconsistency and incompleteness in data integration. *Proceeding of the 2002 International Workshop on Description Logics (DL2002)*, Toulouse.

Lenzerini, M. (2002). Data integration: A theoretical perspective. *Proceeding of the 21st ACM SIGMOD-SIGACT-SIGART Symposium Principle of Database Systems*, Madison, Wisconsin.

Maes, P., Guttman, R., & Moukas, A. (1999, March). Agent that buy and sell:Transforming commerce as we know it. *Communications of the ACM, 42*(3), 81–91. doi:10.1145/295685.295716

Maheu, M. M., Whitten, P., & Allen, A. (2001). *E-Health, telehealth, and telemedicine: A guide to start-up and success* (1st ed.). San Francisco, CA: Jossey-Bass.

Martens, R., Hu, W., Liu, A., Mahovsky, J., Saenchai, K., Schauenberg, T., et al. (2001). *TEEMA TRLabs execution environment for mobile agents*. Telecommunication Research and Laboratories (TRLabs) Regina. Regina, Canada: Telecommunication Research and Laboratories (TRLabs) Regina.

Matthews, D., & Farewell, V. T. (2007). *Using and understanding medical statistics*. Basel, Switzerland: Karger.

McBrien, P., & Poulovassilis, A. (2003). Data integration by bi-directional schema transformation rules. *Proceeding of the 19th International Conference Data Eng. (ICDE'03)*.

Miller, J. W. (2005). Wellness: The history and development of a concept. *Spektrum Freizeit, 1*, 84–102.

Nielson, J. (2005, April 11). *Medical usability: How to kill patients through bad design*. Retrieved July 8, 2009, from http://www.useit.com/alertbox/20050411.html

Persaud, D. D., Jreige, S., Skedgel, C., Finley, J., Sargeant, J., & Hanlon, N. (2005, March 1). An incremental cost analysis of telehealth in Nova Scotia from a societal perspective. *Journal of Telemedicine and Telecare, 11*(2), 77–84. doi:10.1258/1357633053499877

Petrie, A., & Sabin, C. (2005). *Medical statistics at a glance*. Malden, MA: Blackwell.

Preim, B., & Bartz, D. (2007). *Visualization in medicine: Theory, algorithms, and applications* (1st ed.). Amsterdam, The Netherlands: Elsevier.

Pressman, R. S. (2005). *Software engineering: A practitioner's approach* (6th ed.). McGraw-Hill.

Rao, C. R., Wegman, E. J., & Solka, J. L. (2005). *Data mining and data visualization*. Amsterdam, The Netherlands: Elsevier North Holland.

Raskin, J. (2000). *The humane interface: New direction for designing interactive systems* (1st ed.). Reading, MA: Addison Wesley.

Rosson, M. B., & Carroll, J. M. (2002). *Usability engineering: Scenario-based development of human-computer interaction* (1st ed.). San Fancisco, CA: Academic Press.

Shortliffe, E. H., & Barnett, G. O. (2001). Medical data: Their acquisition, storage, and use. In E. H. Shortliffe, & L. E. Perreault (Eds.), *Medical informatics: Computer applications in health care and biomedicine* (2nd ed.). New York, NY: Springer Science+Business Media, Inc.

Smith, B. J., Tang, K. C., & Nutbeam, D. (2006, September 7). WHO health promotion glossary: New terms. *Health Promotion International Advance Access, 21*, 340–345. doi:10.1093/heapro/dal033

Soomlek, C., & Benedicenti, L. (2010). Operational wellness model: A wellness model designed for an agent-based wellness visualization system. The Second International Conference on eHealth, Telemedicine, and Social Medicine (eTELEMED2010). St. Maarten.

Soomlek, C., & Benedicenti, L. (2011). Creating a framework for testing wellness visualization systems. *The Third International Conference on eHealth, Telemedicine, and Social Medicine (eTELEMED2011)*. Guadeloupe.

Soomlek, C., & Benedicenti, L. (2012). *Repeatable experimental framework for wellness indicator testing/evaluation: Environmental setup*. The Fourth International Conference on eHealth, Telemedicine, and Social Medicine (eTELEMED2012), Valencia.

Spence, R. (2001). *Information visualization*. Harlow, UK: Addison-Wesley.

Spiegelhalter, D. J., & Myles, J. P. (2004). *Bayesian approaches to clinical trials and health-care evaluation*. Chichester, UK: John Wiley & Sons. doi:10.1002/0470092602

Strohecker, J., Travis, J. W., Burdett, B., Kant Mishra, S., & Zyga, M. (n.d.). *Wellness inventory: The whole person assessment program*. HealthWorld Online. Retrieved June 18, 2012, from http://www.mywellnesstest.com/index_wt.asp?UID=&Id=

Takahashi, P. Y., Pecina, J. L., Upatising, B., Chaudhry, R., Shah, N. D., & Houten, H. V. (2012, May 28). A randomized controlled trial of telemonitoring in older adults with multiple health issues to prevent hospitalizations and emergency department visits. *Archives of Internal Medicine, 172*(10), 773–779. doi:10.1001/archinternmed.2012.256

Tan, J. (2005). *E-health care information systems: An introduction for students and professionals* (1st ed.). San Francisco, CA: Jossey-Bass.

Travis, J. W. (2008, May 6). Beyond ordinary wellness: A roadmap to high-level wellness. Durack, Australia: National Wellness Institute of Australia Inc. Retrieved June 24, 2012, from http://www.wellnessaustralia.org/NWIA%20Travis%20forum%20may%202008.pdf

Tufte, E. R. (1997). *The visual display of quantitative information* (15th ed.). Connecticut: Graphics Press.

Velde, R. V., & Degoulet, P. (2003). *Clinical information systems: A component-based approach* (Hannah, K. J., & Ball, M. J., Eds.). 1st ed.). New York, NY: Springer-Verlag Inc.

Ware, C. (2004). *Information visualization: Perception for design* (Card, S., Grudin, J., & Nielsen, J., Eds.). 2nd ed.). San Francisco, CA: Morgan Kaufman.

Wellness Inventory: The Whole Person Assessment Program. (2011). Wellness Inventory. Retrieved June 18, 2012, from http://www.wellpeople.com/index_wp.asp?UID=&Id

Wong, D., Paciorek, N., & Moore, D. (1999). Java-based mobile agents. *Communications of the ACM*, *42*(3). Retrieved from http://portal.acm.org/citation.cfm?id=295717 doi:10.1145/295685.295717

World Health Organization. (2008, September 10). *WHOSIS: WHO statistical information system*. Retrieved May 31, 2012, from http://apps.who.int/whosis/data/Search.jsp?indicators=%255bIndicator%255d.Members%253e

Young, F. W., Valero-Mora, P. M., & Friendly, M. (2006). *Visual statistics: Seeing data with dynamic interactive graphics*. Hoboken, NJ: Wiley-Interscience. doi:10.1002/9781118165409

Young, K. M. (2000). *Informatics for healthcare professionals* (1st ed.). Philadelphia, PA: F.A. Davis Company.

Ziegler, P., & Dittrich, K. R. (2004). Three decades of data integration—All problems solved? *18th IFIP World Computer Congress (WCC 2004)*, (p. 12). Toulouse.

Ziegler, P., & Dittrich, K. R. (2007). Data integration—Problems, approaches, perspectives. In J. Krogstie, A. L. Opdahl, & S. Brinkkemper (Eds.), *Conceptual modelling in information systems engineering* (pp. 39-58). Berlin, Germany: Springer. Retrieved from http://www.springerlink.com/content/tu6g43697442742n/

ADDITIONAL READING

Anspaugh, D. J., Hamrick, M. H., Anspaugh, F. D., & J., D. (1994). *Wellness: Concepts and applications*. St. Louis, MO: Mosby.

Broyles, R. W. (2006). *Fundamentals of statistics in health administration*. Sudbury, MA: Jones and Bartlett.

Chen, C. (1999). *Information visualisation and virtual environments*. London, UK: Springer.

Chow, S.-C. (2003). *Encyclopedia of biopharmaceutical statistics*. New York, NY: Marcel Dekker.

Dannheisser, L. M., & Rosenbaum, J. M. (2005). *What's wrong with me? The frustrated patients' guide to getting an accurate diagnosis*. New York, NY: McGraw-Hill.

Darkins, A. W., & Cary, M. A. (2000). *Telemedicine and telehealth: Principles, policies, performance, and pitfalls* (1st ed.). New York, NY: Springer Publishing Co.

Goolsby, M. J., & Grubbs, L. (2006). *Advanced assessment: Interpreting findings and formulating differential diagnoses*. Philadelphia, PA: F.A. Davis Company.

Hackos, J. T., & Redish, J. C. (1998). *User and task analysis for interface design*. New York, NY: John Wiley & Sons, Inc.

Hersh, W. R. (2003). *Information retrieval: A health and biomedical perspective*. New York, NY: Springer.

Ichimura, T., & Yoshida, K. (2004). *Knowledge-based intelligent systems for healthcare*. Adelaide, Australia: Advanced Knowledge International.

Ichimura, T., & Yoshida, K. (2004). *Knowledge-based intelligent systems for healthcare* (Howlett, R. J., & Jain, L. C., Eds.). 1st ed., *Vol. 7*). Adelaide, Australia: Advanced Knowledge International Pty Ltd.

Kirkwood, B. R., & Sterne, J. A. (2003). *Essential medical statistics*. Malden, MA: Blackwell Science.

Maheu, M. M., Whitten, P., & Allen, A. (2001). *E-health, telehealth, and telemedicine: A guide to start-up and success* (1st ed.). San Francisco, CA: Jossey-Bass.

Petrie, A., & Sabin, C. (2005). *Medical statistics at a glance*. Malden, MA: Blackwell.

Preim, B., & Bartz, D. (2007). *Visualization in medicine: Theory, algorithms, and applications* (1st ed.). Amsterdam, The Netherlands: Elsevier.

Rao, C. R., Wegman, E. J., & Solka, J. L. (2005). *Data mining and data visualization*. Amsterdam, The Netherlands: Elsevier North Holland.

Raskin, J. (2000). *The humane interface: New direction for designing interactive systems* (1st ed.). Reading, MA: Addison Wesley.

Rosson, M. B., & Carroll, J. M. (2002). *Usability engineering: Scenario-based development of human-computer interaction* (1st ed.). San Francisco, CA: Academic Press.

Shortliffe, E. H., & Barnett, G. O. (2001). Medical data: Their acquisition, storage, and use. In E. H. Shortliffe, & L. E. Perreault (Eds.), *Medical informatics: Computer applications in health care and biomedicine* (2nd ed.). New York, NY: Springer Science+Business Media, Inc.

Spence, R. (2001). *Information visualization*. Harlow, NY: Addison-Wesley.

Spiegelhalter, D. J., & Myles, J. P. (2004). *Bayesian approaches to clinical trials and health-care evaluation*. Chichester, UK: John Wiley & Sons. doi:10.1002/0470092602

Tan, J. (2005). *E-health care information systems: An introduction for students and professionals* (1st ed.). San Francisco, CA: Jossey-Bass.

Velde, R. V., & Degoulet, P. (2003). *Clinical information systems: A component-based approach* (Hannah, K. J., & Ball, M. J., Eds.). 1st ed.). New York, NY: Springer-Verlag Inc.

Young, F. W., Valero-Mora, P. M., & Friendly, M. (2006). *Visual statistics: Seeing data with dynamic interactive graphics*. Hoboken, NJ: Wiley-Interscience. doi:10.1002/9781118165409

Young, K. M. (2000). *Informatics for healthcare professionals* (1st ed.). Philadelphia, PA: F.A. Davis Company.

Chapter 21
Life Style Evaluation by Accelerometer

Laura Stefani
University of Florence, Italy

Irene Scacciati
University of Florence, Italy

Gabriele Mascherini
University of Florence, Italy

Giorgio Galanti
University of Florence, Italy

ABSTRACT

The assessment of the Spontaneous Motor Activity (SMA) of the life style (LS) is fundamental to establish the daily Physical Activity (PA) dose as therapy. The recent employment the accelerometer (AiperMotion 440 PC – Aipermon GmBH – Germany), can immediately distinguish "active" from "sedentary" subjects providing a larger adhesion to the exercise program. The study aims to verify the role of the accelerometer. 28 obese-hypertensive were evaluated either by the questionnaire or by the accelerometer. A larger sedentary LS in the population investigated was found by the accelerometer respect of questionnaire. After three months of regular physical exercise, the body compositions parameters, investigated principally, resulted to be improved. The accelerometer determines a real and objective visualization of the LS expressed as PAL resulting on a direct early improvement of the parameters strongly related with the cardiovascular risk. The results support the educational role of the employ of the accelerometer.

DOI: 10.4018/978-1-4666-2979-0.ch021

ACCELEROMETER FOR LIFE STYLE EVALUATION: THE EDUCATIONAL ROLE IN A GROUP OF OBESE-HYPERTENSIVE SUBJECTS

Introduction

The daily evaluation of the life style is the first step to start with the" Exercise as prescription "that represents a new and helpful therapy in several kinds of patients. Particularly in subjects at high risk level, a correct investigation of the daily Spontaneous Physical Activity (SPA) in term of time, frequency, intensity and kind of exercise can play a relevant role to plan the "exercise as prescription" program (Lee, 2010; Brown & Siahpush, 2007). It has been proved that a correct life style is associated to a progressive reduction of acute events and increase of survival. It is reasonable to think that and adequate life style can also produce a reduction social costs mainly in terms of drugs and also costs social assistance. The necessity to distinguish sedentary from non-sedentary subjects (Historical leisure activity questionnaire, 1997), a longer period of registration by an accelerometer, can verify the effective SPA and quantify the time spends to practice exercise at different level of intensity (Bravata, et al., 2007; Bassett et al., 2010). It is note that the poor recognition of physical inactivity may be in fact an important barrier to improve the healthy behavior change (Ronda, Van Asserrna, & Brug, 2001). Respect of simple questionnaire, where the information of the life style are often summarized, the accelerometer can discover the presence of several "daily sedentary behaviors " and therefore can play an educational role promoting an improvement of the own LS (Klem et al., 1997; Melanson et al., 2004; Tudor –Locke et al., 2001). Particularly in case of ambulatory patients, where the main goal is to reduce the cardiovascular risks, the accelerometer, for its peculiar small size and easy employment, can be considered to better visualize the effective exposure to sedentary life style. It is reasonable to think that this kind of approach, applied at the onset of a program of exercise as therapy and whose intensity is often at the beginning difficult to establish, can be helpful toward a stronger of and objective realization of the real characteristics of own LS (Bravata et al., 2007; Tudor-Locke & Basset Jr., 2004). The aim of the manuscript is to highlights the role of accelerometer in identifying sedentary behaviors and also to quantify the immediate positive impact on the improvement of the main anthropometrics and body composition parameters. For this reason an investigation in a cohort of subjects at high risk level as overweight hypertensive subjects has been conducted. In consequence of this application, this popular tool, normally induce to motivate their Physical Activity (PA).

BACKGROUND

The use of wearable systems to measure physical activity are recently involved in several chronic disease (Beaglehole et al., 2007; Yach et al., 2004) in order to reduce the progression of these illness and to avoid the sedentarism. If the exercise is considered to play a relevant role in the management of the chronic diseases, in a parallel a valid outcome to measure of physical activity is in fact important in reducing the developing of chronic disease and delay the premature mortality at any age (Chodzko-Zajko et al., 2009). Several tools are available for measuring physical activity and literature supports the use of the accelerometer to better evidentiate the basic physical function instead of simple questionnaire. The oral investigation can contain a subjective judgment which leads to estimation of the daily habits. A recent development is the use of wearable motion sensing technology for studying human movement (Myers et al., 1993, de Bruin et al., 2008) based on a miniaturized motion sensors, widely approved in old people. The application and the clinical relevance to assess the PA of this system in chronic disease is currently absent.

MAIN FOCUS OF THE CHAPTER

The aim of the present investigation is to verify the clinical relevance and the feasibility of applying wearable motion sensing technology in individuals at high cardiovascular risk, demonstrating the special property and validity for a daily employment of the accelerometer in this context. However it is note as the quality of life assessment using wearable systems include "Accelerometers, pedometers, or activity monitors." Some controversies are now open among the role and the position of these systems for a long term monitor during the free living conditions.

Issues, Controversies, Problems

From a literature overview, it results as the three different applications cannot be considered completely overlapped (Talbot et al. 2003; de Blok et al. 2006; Bjorgaas et al., 2008; Knols et al., 2010; Crouter et al., 2003; Corder et al., 2007) in consequence of the fact that pedometers allows a report with the numbers of steps, encouraging the daily PA while accelerometers, as a combination of both systems, is a measure of energy consumption. None of them, with the exclusion of the more advanced system are able to evaluate the measurement of postural transition movement in terms of exercise. This feature is particularly of interest in case of obese subjects where the life style investigation needs to be more precise. Another controversy has been reported in some studies and it regards the adherence problem to wear or to wear the devices in the proper position (Toda et al., 1998; Keyserling et al., 2002). It has been also remarked as the intensity of the exercise can reduce the validity of the collection of the exams.

The present investigation on a special population of overweight and hypertensive subjects is also addressed to verify the positive impact of the accelerometer for an immediate and long term physical activity monitor, with a good acquisition of the data for a laboratory analysis system.

Protocol Study

A cohort of 28 hypertensive and overweight patients (14 male, 14 female,) were enrolled for exercise–prescription program planned at Sport Medicine Center at the University of Florence-Italy. They all gave their informal consent to approve and participate to the protocol study. All the subjects were submitted to a general check up in order to verify the absence of cardiovascular acute symptom as chest pain, contraindicating a regular physical activity.

They were aged 57 ± 12.88 y, showing a Body Mass Index (BMI) values compatible with an overweight pattern. All were affected by mild-hypertension, as the ESC-AHA classification (Mancia & De Backer, 2007) reports, and all under pharmacological treatment including ace-inhibitors or Calcium-antagonist drugs. The own LS perception of the subjects was investigated by a questionnaire. It consisted on an interview conducted singularly for every subject enrolled during the first check up and before to start with the exercise program. The questionnaire collected data about the occupation, leisure time activity (watching TV, reading, cycling, planning indoor games), smoking behavior, regular alcohol consumption, physical activity and dietary habits. In addition to evaluate physical activity, as programmed daily exercise and including for example fast walk or jogging, it was particularly important to verify the rate (i.e. 1, 2 3. o r more times a week) and also approximately the duration time, expressed in minutes, dedicated to this one. From the information obtained, the subjects were classified as "sedentary or active" attributing to the first group a correspondent amount of the daily physical activity lower than 2 METS, while in case of subject more active the limit was up to 3-4 MET. In addition to the questionnaire, the exploration of LS was completed also by the accelerometer (AiperMotion 440 PC – Aipermon GmBH –Germany) report. It was positioned on the waist of the patient, asking the subject to wear the device for almost 6 days with the exclusion of the night time. After this period the data obtained from the accelerometer registration were downloaded to a laptop computer for the analysis of the SPA: more than 3 hours a week represents the threshold point to distinguish sedentary from active subjects, however several other parameters were analyzed: the Physical Activity Level (PAL: definite as EE/ resting Energy Expenditure), medium daily distance and intensity of the PA expressed as slow (up to 3 Km/h) or fast (up to 5/km/h) walk, and also the number of total daily steps. The daily PA, expressed as physical activity level (PAL) was further classified as "low walking "(LW), "fast walking" (FW) and jogging.

The exercise prescribed was established following the AHA, ACC guidelines by a Cardio Pulmonary Test (CPT) estimating the Energy Expenditure (EE).The physical exercise prescribed was programmed up to the 60% of the VO2 max for at least 3 times in a weak.

The BIA (Bioelectrical Impedance Analysis-Akern/STA/BIA –Italy) was used to measure the body compositions parameters at the beginning (T0) and after 3 months (T3) of physical exercise.

The parameters analyzed included the (FM) Fat Mass, (TBW) Total Body Water, Extra Cellular Water (ECW), Intra Cellular Water (ICW), and the Angle Phase (AP). The anthropometrics parameters were the (BMI) Body Mass Index, Waist Circumference (WC), Hip Circumference (HC) and the ration between them.

Statistical Analysis

Statistical analysis was performed using the SPSS 13.0package for Windows XP. All data are expressed as mean± Standard Deviation (SD). All the data were compared by T-Student test for paired data. A probability value (p) of < 0.05 was considered statistically significant.

Results

For the LS analysis, respect of the questionnaire (Table 1) where only 10/28 subjects resulted to be sedentary, the accelerometer showed a predominantly inactive LS (PAL = 1.56±0.14) in all. The PAL (Physical Activity Level) observed by the accelerometer was 1.56±0.14, medium daily distance was 6289.34±2536.18 m. The amount of inactive LS time during 6 days (Figure 1 Time, minutes and hours, of physical activity spents at different intensity level), consisted on 51±7.48 hours; while the hours of exercise corresponding to3 METs were 21.9±6.22, the time of exercise at 3-4.5 METs was 10.88±4.11 hours, and the minutes spent for jogging were 73.54±8.66. The time of hours

Table 1. Questionnaire investigation

Activity Self Perception									
10 Sedentary	12 Moderate Active		6 Active						
Occupational Activity			Leisure Time Activity						
10 Pensioners 6 House-wife	7 Sedentary Work	5 Active Work	12 Watching TV/ Reading	2 Modeling	4 Gardening	6 Walking	1 Gymnastic	2 Cycling	1 Evening Sport

Figure 1. Weekly and daily physical activity level

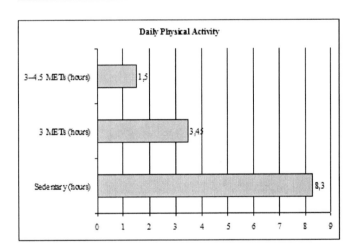

corresponding to the different daily PA degree were 8h 30 min in case of sedentary, 3h 45 min for slow walk, 1h 50 min for fast walk. The number of the daily steps was around 9522.44±3987.15 in all the subjects analyzed. The daily calories spent were 878.6±302.09 (Table 2). After three months of exercise the BMI was significantly reduced (Figure 2, T0=29.58±8.33; T3=28.7±8.75 P<0.05). A trend toward a reduction was observed (Table 3) also for the FM (T0= 25.88±10.6; T3= 23.11±7.98), the WC (T0= 101±14; T3= 94.66±14), the HC (T0= 107±6.88; T3= 100.9±2) the TBW (T0= 48.9±8.9; T3= 41.24±9.55) and

ICW (T0= 24.01±6.32; T3= 22.92±6.13) (Figure 3 Total Body Water, Intracellular ed Extracellular water distribution in all the subjects at the onset (T0) and after 3 months of physical exercise (T3)). The AP values maintain (Table 3) within the normal range (T0= 7.55±1.6; T3= 6.67±1.24). A trend to a slight reduction was observed in the mean values of the Systolic and diastolic blood pressure (T0= 129.65±12.02/78.11±7.35; T3= 123.23±9.66/73.57±4.88). An inverse relationship (R=-0.31) between PAL and the BMI results has been found.

Table 2. Physical activity level expressed as daily and weekly duration time

Physical Activity (in duration of time during 6 days)					
Sedentary (hours)	3 METs (hours)	3–4.5 METs (hours)	Jogging (minutes)		PAL
51±7.48	21.9±6.22	10.88±4.11	73.54±8.66		1.56±0.14
Physical Activity (in duration of time per day)					
Sedentary (min)	3 METs (min)	3–4.5 METs (min)	Distance (m)	Steps	Calories Spent (kcal)
8h 30 min	3h 45 min	1h 50 min		9522.44±3987.15	878.6±302.09

Figure 2. Weight and BMI media values of the overweight-hypertensive group at T0 and T3

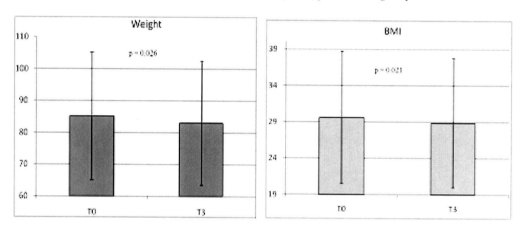

Table 3. Anthropometrics and body composition parameters of the obese-overweight subjects analyzed

Obese-overweight 15 male - 7female (57.48 ± 12.77 y)	T 0	T 3	P value
Fat Mass (kg)	25.88±10.6	23.11±7.98	NS
Waist Circunference (cm)	101±14	94.66±14	NS
Hip Circunference (cm)	107±6.88	100.9±2	NS
Total Body Water (l)	48.9±8.9	41.24±9.55	NS
Intra Cellular Water (l)	24.01±6.32	22.92±6.13	NS
Angle Phase (degrees)	7.55±1.6	6.67±1.24	NS
Weight (kg)	85.13 ± 20.10	83.01 ± 19.49	0.026
BMI	29.58 ±8.33	28.7±8.75	0.021
BSP	129.65±12.02	= 123.23±9.66	NS
BDP	78.11±7.35	73.57±4.88	NS

Figure 3. Total body water and intracellular-extraceullular water distribution

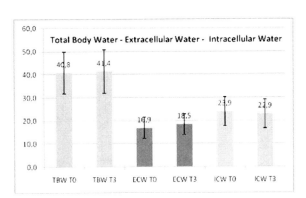

Discussion

Correct LS is the first step to start with an adequate "Exercise Prescription. This phase is anyway the most complicate evaluation for the difficulties to objective the numerous kinds of physical activities in term of EE. The accurate LS is normally associated to a reduction of the global cardiovascular risk (Lee, 2010; Chodzko-Zajko, et al., 2009), however the awareness of the presence of a predominant sedentary behaviors is not commonly easily demonstrable (Ronda, Van Asserrna, & Brug, 2001). Before starting with a regular training program, the necessity to evaluate the SPA to plan the daily physical activity is mandatory (Bravata et al., 2007; Bassett et al., 2010; Melanson et al., 2004). Normally the exclusive employment of the "questionnaire", (Historical leisure activity questionnaire, 1997) can address to a wrong and incomplete evaluation of the own LS giving few data about the type, the intensity of the exercises practiced (as walking, jogging beck.) The inevitable tendency to underestimate the PAL that is in fact often associated to a high BMI values. More recently the employment of the accelerometers is growing in general population, in patients and also among the healthy subjects. It is reasonable to think that all these subjects can take benefit from the regular employment of this tool, in terms of reduction of global risk of morbidity for their disease and also in terms of drugs and

assistance costs, both strongly related with their life style. The data obtained demonstrate that the accelerometer can typify (Bravata et al., 2007; Bassett et al.; Tudor –Locke et al., 2001), much more than the simple questionnaire, the presence of the " sedentary behaviors" and in addition can investigate the intensity, time and the kind of exercise practiced. The information related to the SPA result in fact in a good definition of the LS that is in many cases misunderstood. The identification of the presence of a predominant moderate PAL in a group at high risk level, can therefore play a relevant role to encourage to start with a " more adequate" PA program in subjects were the balancing of the moderate vs intense exercise is in agreement with the recent ACSM Guidelines (de Bruin et al., 2008). All the values obtained have an inverse relationship with the intensity of the PA. This special and relevant aspect cannot be evaluated by a simple questionnaire. According to the recent literature (Talbot, 2003), the results demonstrate also the role of the accelerometer, to determine direct improvement in a short time of the parameters strongly related with the cardiovascular risk. In conclusion the data support the global educational role in this context of the employment of the accelerometer, which could be considered as an additional tool for the periodical assessment of the LS changes in order to enhance the empowerment on the exercise prescription.

FUTURE RESEARCH DIRECTIONS

Complete studies have underline the relevance of the positive intervention of the accelerometer as wearable tool to measure physical activity in several chronic diseases like arthritis or diabetes (Talbot et al., 2003; Toda, 1998)) demonstrating a progressive increase of the daily activity(Talbot, L.A. et al., 2003) This aspect could be of special interest mainly for the patients affected by perferical arteriopaty where exclusively the supervision exercise has been in literature investigated. Non data are in fact available on the possible impact of the regular exercise when it is monitorized by the accelerometer only. The effective difficulty to follow an exercise program as therapy for the presence of the pain at the lower arts, represents one of the most important limit of the exercise as prescription therapy in this kind of patients. The daily employment of an accelerometer could be proposed to overcame this aspect.

CONCLUSION

Clinical Applications of the Accelerometers: General Considerations

The accelerometers represent actually important tools to distinguish sedentarism from physical activity and to measure moderate and vigorous intensity of PA. The easy system of application allows the possibility of a large employment in general population and also in patients affected by chronic disease where the exercise as prescription program can be applied. An immediate benefit derived from a evaluation in real time of the life style is represented by the correct perception of the own daily PA

It is expectable that the application in hospital and other regions will be in future developed to encourage and enhance the collaboration with the doctors of the territory involved in a larger system of the evaluation of the life style in the general population.

The result obtained in the present investigation strongly highlights this aspect giving significance and feasibility to a possible large application to this system.

REFERENCES

Bassett, D. R. (2000). Validity and reliability issues in objective monitoring of physical activity. *Research Quarterly for Exercise and Sport, 71*(2), 30–36.

Bassett, D. R., Wyatt, H., Thompson, H., & Peters, J. (2010). Pedometer-measured physical activity and health behaviors in US adults. *Medicine and Science in Sports and Exercise, 42*(10), 1819–1825. doi:10.1249/MSS.0b013e3181dc2e54

Bauldoff, G. S., Hoffman, L. A., Zullo, T. G., & Sciurba, F. C. (2002). Exercise Maintenance following pulmonary rehabilitation: Effect of distractive stimuli. *Chest, 122*, 948–954. doi:10.1378/chest.122.3.948

Beaglehole, R., Ebrahim, S., Reddy, S., Voute, J., & Leeder, S. (2007). Prevention of chronic diseases: A call to action. *Lancet, 370*, 2152–2157. doi:10.1016/S0140-6736(07)61700-0

Bjorgaas, M. R., Vik, J. T., Stolen, T., Lydersen, S., & Grill, V. (2008). Regular use of pedometer does not enhance beneficial outcomes in a physical activity intervention study in type 2 diabetes mellitus. *Metabolism: Clinical and Experimental, 57*, 605–611. doi:10.1016/j.metabol.2007.12.002

Bravata, D. M., Smith-Spangler, C., & Sundaram, V. (2007). Using pedometers to increase physical activity and improve health: A systematic review. *Journal of the American Medical Association, 298*(19), 2296–2304. doi:10.1001/jama.298.19.2296

Bravata, D. M., Spangler, C. S., Sundaram, V., Gienger, A. L., Lin, N., & Lewis, R. (2007). Using pedometers to increase physical activity and improve health. *Journal of the American Medical Association, 19*(298), 2296–2304. doi:10.1001/jama.298.19.2296

Brown, A., & Siahpush, M. (2007). Risk factors for overweight and obesity: Results from the 2001 National Health Survey. *Public Health, 121*(8), 603–613. doi:10.1016/j.puhe.2007.01.008

Cheitilin, M. D., Armstrong, W. F., & Aurigemma, G. R. (2003). ACC/AHA/ASE 2003 guideline update for the clinical application of echocardiography: A report of the American College of Cardiology, American Heart Association Task Force on Practice Guidelines. *Journal of the American Society of Echocardiography, 16*(10), 1091–1110. doi:10.1016/S0894-7317(03)00685-0

Chodzko-Zajko, W. J., Proctor, D. N., Fiatarone Singh, M. A., Minson, C. T., Nigg, C. R., Salem, G. J., & Skinner, J. S. (2009). American College of Sports Medicine position stand. Exercise and physical activity for older adults. *Medicine and Science in Sports and Exercise, 41*, 1510–1530. doi:10.1249/MSS.0b013e3181a0c95c

Corder, K., Brage, S., & Ekelund, U. (2007). Accelerometers and pedometers: Methodology and clinical application. *Current Opinion in Clinical Nutrition and Metabolic Care, 10*, 597–603. doi:10.1097/MCO.0b013e328285d883

Crouter, S. E., Schneider, P. L., Karabulut, M., & Bassett, D. R. Jr. (2003). Validity of 10 electronic pedometers for measuring steps, distance, and energy cost. *Medicine and Science in Sports and Exercise, 35*, 1455–1460. doi:10.1249/01.MSS.0000078932.61440.A2

de Blok, B. M., de Greef, M. H., ten Hacken, N. H., Sprenger, S. R., Postema, K., & Wempe, J. B. (2006). The effects of a lifestyle physical activity counseling program with feedback of a pedometer during pulmonary rehabilitation in patients with COPD: A pilot study. *Patient Education and Counseling, 61*, 48–55. doi:10.1016/j.pec.2005.02.005

de Bruin, E. D., Hartmann, A., Uebelhart, D., Murer, K., & Zijlstra, W. (2008). Wearable systems for monitoring mobility-related activities in older people: A systematic review. *Clinical Rehabilitation, 22*, 878–895. doi:10.1177/0269215508090675

Donnelly, S. N., Blair, S. N., Jakicic, J. M., & Manore, M. M. (2009). ACSM position stand: Special communication: Appropriate physical activity intervention strategies for weight loss and prevention of weight regain for adults. *Medicine and Science in Sports and Exercise, 41*(2), 459–471. doi:10.1249/MSS.0b013e3181949333

Historical, L. A. Q. (1997)...*Medicine and Science in Sports and Exercise, 29*, 43–45.

Johnson, F., Cooke, L., Croker, H., & Wardle, J. (2008). Changing perceptions of weight Great Britain: Comparison of two population surveys. *British Medical Journal, 337*, 494. doi:10.1136/bmj.a494

Keyserling, T. C., Samuel-Hodge, C. D., Ammerman, A. S., Ainsworth, B. E., Elasy, T. A., & Henriquez-Roldan, C. F. (2002). A randomized trial of an intervention to improve self-care behaviors of African-American women with type 2 diabetes: Impact on physical activity. *Diabetes Care, 25*(9), 1576–1583. doi:10.2337/diacare.25.9.1576

Klem, M. L., Wing, R. R., McGuire, M. T., Seagle, H. M., & Hill, J. O. (1997). A descriptive study of individuals successful at long-term maintenances of substantial weight loss. *The American Journal of Clinical Nutrition, 66*(2), 239–246.

Knols, R. H., de Bruin, E. D., Shirato, K., Uebelhart, D., & Aaronson, N. K. (2010). Physical activity interventions to improve daily walking activity in cancer survivors. *BMC Cancer, 10,* 406:1-406:10.

Lee, I.-M. (2010). Physical activity and cardiac protection. *Exercise is. Medicine, 9*(4), 214–219.

Mancia, G., & De Backer, G. (2007). The Task Force for the Management of Arterial Hypertension of the European Society of Hypertension (ESH) and of the European Society of Cardiology (ESC). *European Heart Journal, 28,* 462–1536. doi:doi:10.1093/eurheartj/ehm236

Melanson, E. L., Knoll, J. R., & Bell, M. L. (2004). Commercially available pedometers: Consideration for accurate step counting. *Preventive Medicine, 39*(2), 361–368. doi:10.1016/j.ypmed.2004.01.032

Myers, A. M., Holliday, P. J., Harvey, K. A., & Hutchinson, K. S. (1993). Functional performance measures: Are they superior to self-assessments? *Journal of Gerontology, 48,* M196–M206. doi:10.1093/geronj/48.5.M196

Ronda, G., Van Asserrna, P., & Brug, J. (2001). Stages of change, psychological factors and awareness of physical activity levels in the Netherlands. *Health Promotion International, 16,* 305–314. doi:10.1093/heapro/16.4.305

Talbot, L. A., Gaines, J. M., Huynh, T. N., & Metter, E. J. (2003). A home-based pedometer-driven walking program to increase physical activity in older adults with osteoarthritis of the knee: A preliminary study. *Journal of the American Geriatrics Society, 51,* 387–392. doi:10.1046/j.1532-5415.2003.51113.x

Toda, Y., Toda, T., Takemura, S., Wada, T., Morimoto, T., & Ogawa, R. (1998). Change in body fat, but not body weight or metabolic correlates of obesity, is related to symptomatic relief of obese patients with knee osteoarthritis after a weight control program. *The Journal of Rheumatology, 25.*

Tudor-Locke, C., & Basset, D. R. Jr. (2004). How many steps /day are enough? Preliminary pedometers indices, for public health. *Sports Medicine (Auckland, N.Z.), 34*(1), 1–8. doi:10.2165/00007256-200434010-00001

Tudor-Locke, C., & Lutes, L. (2009). Why do pedometers work? A reflection upon the factors related to successfully increasing physical activity. *Sports Medicine (Auckland, N.Z.), 39,* 981–993. doi:10.2165/11319600-000000000-00000

Tudor–Locke, C. E., Ainsworth, B. E., Whitt, M. C., Thompson, R. W., Addy, C. L., & Jones, D. (2001). The relationship between pedometer-determined ambulatory activity and body composition variables. *International Journal of Obesity, 25*(11), 1571–1578. doi:10.1038/sj.ijo.0801783

Yach, D., Hawkes, C., Gould, C. L., & Hofman, K. J. (2004). The global burden of chronic diseases: Overcoming impediments to prevention and control. *Journal of the American Medical Association, 291,* 2616–2622. doi:10.1001/jama.291.21.2616

Chapter 22
Implementation of Telecytology in Georgia

Ekaterine Kldiashvili
Georgian Telemedicine Union, Georgia

ABSTRACT

The field of e-Health is rapidly evolving. The new models and protocols of application of info-communication technologies for healthcare purposes are developed. Despite of obvious advantages and benefits, practical application of e-Health and its possibilities in everyday practice are slow. Much progress has been made around the world in the field of digital imaging and virtual slides. But in Georgia, telecytology is still in evolving stages. It revolves around static telecytology. It has been revealed that the application of easy available and adaptable technology together with the improvement of the infrastructure conditions is the essential basis for telecytology. This is a very useful and applicable tool for consulting on difficult cases. Telecytology has significantly increased knowledge exchange and thereby ensured a better medical service. The chapter aims description of practical application of telecytology under conditions of Georgia.

INTRODUCTION

Telecytology is a branch of telemedicine that consists in the exchange of microscopy digital images through telecommunication with the purposes of diagnosis, consultation, research and/or education. The concept of telecytology to provide diagnostic services to remote locations was first described in the USA in 1968, when monochrome images were transmitted in real time using a dedicated point to point microwave link. In little more than a decade telecytology has developed from the prototype commercial system first described in 1986 to today's multimedia computers which can be purchased 'off the shelf' at very low prices and can be used as the basis of telecytology systems (Furness, 1997). There are technological concerns which may prevent the acceptance of telecytology by cytologists and thus hinder its application within the routine environment. Some cytologists believe that telecytology is too expensive and that it does not have a useful role in routine cytology.

DOI: 10.4018/978-1-4666-2979-0.ch022

Others have doubted if computer monitors can be used for making a diagnosis, although results have shown no significant difference between a cytologist's performance using a microscope and using a digital image (Coleman, 2009). Many of the concerns expressed about the use of telecytology are not derived from knowledge. There is a need to involve as many cytologists as possible in the use of these systems, particularly cytologists working in routine services roles. Many cytologists believe that fast access to expert opinion is the key to reducing the numbers of diagnostic errors, which have been estimated at up to 5%. Although most of these are not necessarily critical to the patient, some could be.

There is a very clear need for the expanded application of information technology (IT) in healthcare. Clinical workflow still depends largely on manual, paper-based medical record systems, which is economically inefficient and produces significant variances in medical outcomes (Banta, 2003; Detmer, 2000; Detmer, 2001).

Quality assurance programs in cytology are one of the most important methods to maintain and improve the diagnostic acumen of cytotechnologists and cytologists, but there are difficulties in carrying out such programs. A long turnaround time for the circulation of glass slides is a major drawback. It is well known, that it is prolonged in the case of large number of participants and widely spread institutions. The use of photographed slides has been a partial, but unsatisfactory solution because of costs and delays in preparation. Nowadays digital images acquire more and more importance for morphology practice.

BACKGROUND

It is well known, that telecytology may be static (store and forward), dynamic (real-time), or hybrid. Store and forward telecytology is a less efficient method but there have been isolated reports of a concordance of as high as 95-100% between glass slide and telecytology diagnosis (Rocha et al, 2009; Raab et al, 1996). It has limitations because of the disjointed nature of the images, and the diagnostic errors incurred with this method have been attributed to inappropriate field selection by the submitting cytologist. Dynamic telecytology using fully motorized robotic systems, through cost-prohibitive, has revolutionized the field, and a concordance rate of 99-100% has been reported between telecytology and light microscopy diagnosis. The fully motorized robotic systems are a cost-prohibitive for Georgia, but they are used very routinely in other locations, especially in countries with middle and high incomes. Hybrid systems use virtual slides (so called whole slide images – WSI) and in various studies the diagnostic efficacy was shown. The 'virtual slides' are entirely digitalized glass slides at a very high resolution and can be viewed by multiple cytologists and without any loss of resolution.

The applications of telecytology, like those of telemedicine can be classified into four major groups: primary opinion (first diagnosis on a case), second opinion (expert opinion about a case), third opinion (expert group opinion/discussion about a case) and distance learning. The most frequently use case of telecytology is the second opinion. In remote and rural areas where because of economic reasons, one cannot afford to have a competent cytologist, telecytology is considered to be a boon. eLearning in cytology has also gained acceptance. Telecytology has been used for research applications, distance education, remote consultations with astounding success (Coleman, 2009; Rocha et al, 2009; Weinstein et al, 2009).

Georgia is not lagging far behind in the field of telecytology. The first telecytology consultation was done in 2003. Since then a number of distance consultations were implemented.

Digital images acquire more and more importance for morphology practice. They can be easily captured by the conventional digital camera, so by the specific hardware (slide scanner, robotic microscope and etc.). By application of digital images the distance consultations in cytology became reality and are implemented routinely. Most studies reviewing digital images and their application for telecytology have focused on usage of robotic microscopes and online microscopy. Other studies have evaluated the use of digital images of slides (Rocha et al, 2009; Weinstein et al, 2009; Mencarelli et al, 2008). There is no previous study examining the application of digital images for implementation of quality assurance programs.

Medical information system (MIS) is at the heart of IT implementation policies in healthcare systems around the world (Detmer, 2001; Dixon et al, 2008). Most of these policies are based on beliefs about the positive value of MIS rather than on the available empirical evidence; as a result, policy documents comprise aspirational statements rather than detailed and realistic expectations.

It is obvious and well known that the field of healthcare informatics is rapidly evolving. The new models and protocols of MIS are developed. They are based on implementation of profiles such as HL7 and DICOM. Despite of obvious advantages and benefits, practical application of MIS in everyday practice is slow. Research and development projects are ongoing in several countries around the world to develop MIS: examples include Canada, Australia, England, the United States, and Finland. MIS is used primarily for setting objectives and planning patient care, documenting the delivery of care, and assessing the outcomes of care. It includes information regarding patient needs during episodes of care provided by different healthcare professionals. The amount and quality of information available to healthcare professionals in patient care has an impact on the outcomes of patient care and the continuity of care. The information included in MIS has some functions in the decision-making process in patient care. It also supports decision making in management and in health policy (Van Ginneken, 2002; Clamp et al, 2007). There is no

previous study examining the application of MIS for online quality assurance programs in cytology.

Therefore, this chapter presents the implementation of telecytology under the conditions of Georgia.

TELECYTOLOGY IN GEORGIA: ACTIVITIES, RESULTS, AND ACHIEVEMENTS

For the aim to realize telecytology in effective and comprehensive mode the different models and schema of organization of cytology second opinion consultation has been tested. At the beginning the telecytology consultation server has been allocated, set up and installed. The main services available on the server were Simple Machines Forum (distance consultations) and Moodle (eLearning). Using the basic methodology: idea-analysis-conception-implementation-test/deployment the server was established under the premise 'keep it small, safe and simple'. The technology should be available soon and as easy as it is possible with very low technical requirements. It is well known, that within the scope of telecytology, distance consultation is an important sub area, where several cases can be discussed with experts all over the world. The main idea for distance consultation tool was the possibility to create a case by a team completed by Georgian and/or international healthcare professionals and medical doctors. For the purpose to organize distance cytology consultation in the most effective and comprehensive degree preparation of each case was supervised by responsible person. This process includes preparation of case, its uploading at server and notification of experts by email. Therefore, distance consultation implements individual management of incoming requests. Each case contains description (text data – the resume of medical history) and illustrations (microphotographs). All cases were reviewed by board-certified cytologists. The conventional light microscope and 2.0 USB digital eyepiece camera of resolution 2048x1536 pixels have been used for virtual slides preparation. The essential data were stored on the server and they are viewable by every authorized group and/or individual. The only software required is the widely used browser (e.g. Internet Explorer). The authorized user can comment the case and recommend the questions and requests. To ensure the case discussion the responsible person replied to consultants and moderate elaboration of the final diagnosis. After finalization the case is stored on the server and can be viewed by the registered users. For quality control mechanism implementation each consultant subjectively assessed the image quality. This was to be graded on a four-tier scale, with a score of 1 being the lowest score (poor) and a score of 4 being the highest score (excellent) according to the following criteria:

1. Images are of such poor quality that no diagnosis can be ascertained from such images via telecytology.
2. Loss of high-quality resolution precludes an accurate diagnosis via telecytology.
3. Images are of high enough quality as to render a diagnosis via telecytology.
4. Images are of excellent quality.

The service was available as for Georgian so for international healthcare professionals and medical doctors. This was useful and suitable web-based secure service. Simple Machines Forum (www.simplemachines.org) was used for organization of distance consultations. The Simple Machines Forum is the only one that contains the possibility to attach files to a thread.

Since beginning telecytology activity in Georgia has been strongly interlaced with education of healthcare personnel. A learning management system is a software application and/or web-based technology which are used to plan, implement, and access a specific learning process. Typically, learning management system provides an instruc-

tor with a method to create and deliver content, monitor student participation, and access student performance. A learning management system may also provide students with the ability to use interactive features such as threaded discussions, video conferencing and discussion forums. There are several learning management systems. The Moodle (www.moodle.org) was determined as the most suitable and appropriate tool. Moodle is a software package for the production of internet-based courses and websites. It is provided freely as Open Source software (under the GNU Public License). The word Moodle was originally an acronym for Modular Object-Oriented Dynamic Learning Environment, which is mostly useful to programmers and education theorists. It's also a verb describing the process of lazily meandering through something. As such it applies both to the way Moodle has been developed and to the way a student or teacher might approach studying or teaching an online course. Moodle will run on any computer that can run popular programming language PHP designed to be embedded inside Hyper Text Markup Language (HTML) to build dynamic web pages or update them from databases and can support many types of database. It is used for creation, implementation and management of own educational programs. As Simple Machines Forum so Moodle are Open Source software, available under the GNU Public License.

The telecytology consultation server has been implemented for distance consultation of clinical cytology cases and presentation of educational cases. Since July 2006 up to February 2008 140 cases were created (see Table 1). The images have been captured by the 2.0 USB digital eyepiece camera mounted at light microscope (Karl Zeiss) of resolution 2048x1536 pixels. The brightness and contrast of images were adjusted by Adobe Photoshop. The average number of images per case was 4 (95 cases, 67, 86%). An average number of consultants per case were 3 (105 cases, 75%). In 135 cases (96, 43%) the first comment was made in less than 12 hours. In 92 cases (65, 71%) the

Table 1. Cases from July 2006-February 2008

Total number of cases	140
The average number of images per case	4 (95 cases, 67,86%)
The average number of consultants per case	3 (105 cases, 75%)
First comment made in less than 12 hours	135 cases (96,43%)
The primary diagnosis has been confirmed as a result of second opinion consultation	92 cases (65,71%)
The diagnosis has been corrected as a result of telecytology consultation	25 cases (17,86%)
Additional laboratory investigations has been suggested	10 cases (7,14%)
Cases insufficient for telecytology consultation	13 cases (9,29%)

primary diagnosis has been confirmed as a result of remote cytology consultation. In 25 cases (17, 86%) the diagnosis has been corrected as a result of telecytology consultation. In 10 cases (7, 14%) additional laboratory investigations has been suggested. In 13 cases (9,29%) the images were of poor quality, insufficient for telecytology consultation.

The server has been implemented for introduction of Pap-smear technique and 2001 Bethesda System for reporting cervico-vaginal cytologic diagnosis in Georgia too. Microscopic image capturing again has been performed by application of 2.0 USB digital eyepiece camera with resolution 2048x1536 pixels. The brightness and contrast of images were adjusted by Adobe Photoshop. During 5 months (February-June, 2008) there were discussed 300 cases (see Table 2). The primary diagnosis has been worked out by local cytologist. The average number of images for each case was 8 (172 cases, 57,3%). An average number of consultants was 2 per each case (231 cases, 77%) presented their comments or diagnosis. In 87 cases (29%) the first comment was made in less than 8 hours (a single working day) and only in 3 cases (1%) the final diagnosis was reported in 12 hours. In 270 cases (90%) the primary diagnosis has been confirmed as a result of telecytology consultation. A definite final diagnosis with clinically unimportant discrepancies was achieved in 25 cases (8,3%). In 5 cases (1,67%) the diagnosis has been corrected as a result of

telecytology consultation. 220 cases (73,33%) have been submitted by four different persons from three different locations. Web-based transmission has been applied for sending cases.

Quality control mechanism has been implemented for all cases. These cases were related to cancer (mainly breast and cervical cancer) diagnostic.

eLearning tool realized by application of Moodle has been implemented for creation, implementation and management of own educational programs. 15 programs have been realized. 14 programs (93.33%) have been implemented for realization of Continuous Medical Education (CME) of healthcare professionals and medical doctors distantly. The average number of teachers per CME program was 5 (12 programs, 85,71%). The average number of pupils per CME program was 25 (9 programs, 64,29%). Educational cases for review and consultation have been implemented in 14 CME programs (100%). The average number of educational cases per CME program was 15 (10 CME programs, 71,43%). 1 program (6,67%) from above mentioned 15s has been dedicated for actual tasks of Pap-smear technique and Bethesda system.

Healthcare information technology models are constantly evolving as the industry expands. Medical information system (MIS) is a comprehensive solution that automates the clinical, administrative and supply-chain functions. It enables healthcare

Table 2. Cases from February 2008- June 2008

Total number of cases	300
The average number of images per case	8 (172 cases, 57,3%)
The average number of consultants per case	2 (231 cases, 77%)
First comment made in less than 8 hours	87 cases (29%)
The final diagnosis was reported in 12 hours	3 cases (1%)
The primary diagnosis has been confirmed as a result of second opinion consultation	270 cases (90%)
The cases with a definite final diagnosis with clinically unimportant discrepancies	25 cases (8,3%)
The cases with corrected diagnosis as a result of telecytology consultation	5 cases (1,67%)
Cases submitted by different persons from different locations	220 cases (73,33%)

providers to improve their operational effectiveness, to reduce costs and medical errors and to enhance quality of care (Clamp et al, 2007). The aim of MIS was and is as simple as relevant: to contribute to and ensure a high-quality, efficient patient care. The relevance of 'good' MIS for high-level quality of care is obvious. Without having appropriate access to relevant data, practically no decisions on diagnostic, therapeutic or other procedures can be made.

MIS has been launched in Georgia in October, 2008. Its primary goal is patient management. However, the system is also targeted at creating a unified information space in the framework of the wider medical organization. Since first practical application of the MIS arose the idea to use it for telecytology too. Our goal was to review and study the application of MIS for telecytology under the conditions of Georgia. This was a pilot study.

The MIS has been created with .Net technology and SQL database architecture. It involves a multi-user web-based approach. This ensures local (intranet) and remote (internet) access of the system and management of databases. .Net technology can be installed on computers running Microsoft Windows operating systems. It includes a large library of coded solutions to common programming problems. .Net technology is a Microsoft offering and is intended for usage by most new applications created for the Windows

platform (see Figure 1 for the application and user interface scheme). Version 3.0 of the .Net technology included with Windows Server 2008 has been used for creation of MIS. The medical information system is object-oriented software. It is realizing client-server concept. Its architecture provides a secure, robust and extensible system for managing multiple medical terminals within a centralized depository. The medical information system has a flexible architecture that can run on numerous combinations. The recommended server operating requirement is: Windows Server 2003. Hardware recommended requirements are the following: memory – 1 GB, disk space – 1 GB. Internet Explorer 6.0+ and/or Mozila Firefox 2.0+ can be used as client browsers. The medical information system was started to create in December 2007, and the draft version was released in April 2008. After some tests and corrections, the application of ready-for-use version of the medical information system started in October 2008.

The medical information system consists of three key modules:

1. Administration and configuration module,
2. Working module for medical personnel,
3. Reporting module.

The administration and configuration module is dedicated for setting up users' basic rights. It

Figure 1. Software application and user interface scheme

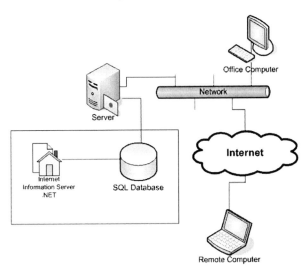

allows users registration or blocking, defining, and configuring of their rights. All medical forms (consultation, clinical investigation, diagnosis, prescription, treatment, etc.) are generated by this module. It is a database for staff too. Each employee is provided by a unique code, alongside with gathering biographical and professional data. Using the working module, medical history can be generated, edited, and updated by medical personnel (see Table 3). At generation, a unique code is given to medical history. It consists of text and multimedia files – images, video, and invoice. Planning of patient visits and schedule of staff are also implemented by this module. Medical history and medical forms (consultation, examination report, etc.) can be fully or partially exported by the reporting module. The documents can be exported in various file formats, including pdf, rtf, and jpg. This module also implements statistical analysis of medical data (patient's age, sex, diagnosis, date of investigation, treatment parameters, etc.). It can be used for quality control of medical services.

Since March 2010 up to January 2011 100 cases in cytology were cared by application of medical information system. These were cases of gynecological cytology. All slides were conventional PAP tests. The slides were photographed with the 2.0 USB digital eyepiece microscope camera with resolution 3.0 MP. The images had resolution 2048x1536 pixels. An average number of images per case were 5 (88 cases, 88%). Each series of images per case began with a general view, followed by higher magnification of diagnostically interesting and actual areas. Cytologist selected these areas. The images were captured by laboratory personnel trained in the use of the camera. The images were stored in a personal computer. They were adjusted by using of Adobe Photoshop. This manipulation has been done by laboratory personnel. It means the correction of image contrast and brightness. Adjusted images were uploaded to corresponding electronic medical record. All 100 electronic medical records were marked as cases for telecytology consultation. For security reasons telecytology experts have been registered as users at medical information system. Four Georgian certified cytologists were selected as experts for second opinion consultations. Cases selected for telecytology were listed at MIS home page.

For implementation of quality control mechanism each telecytology expert subjectively assessed the image quality. The ratings of image sharpness and quality were given using a 4 level

Table 3. Modules of the medical information system

Function / Module	Users registration	Users blocking	Users right definition and configuration	Generation of medical history	Edition / update of medical history	Schedule of staff	Data export	Data statistical analysis
Administration and configuration module	X	X	X	-	-	-	-	-
Working module for medical personnel	-	-	-	X	X	X	–	–
Reporting module	-	-	-	-	-	-	X	X

scale: 1 – "excellent", 2 – "good", 3 – "fair", 4 – "poor". An average number of consultants per case were 3 (86 cases, 86%). In 94 cases (94%) the first comment was made in less than 8 hours. In 96 cases (96%) the primary diagnosis has been confirmed as a result of telecytology consultation. In 3 cases (3%) the diagnosis has been corrected. In 1 case (1%) the images were of poor quality, insufficient for remote cytology consultation (Table 4.).

Overall, 97.5% of the cases were rated as having excellent or good image sharpness and contrast, with 2.5% being rated as fair and poor. With respect to image color, 95% of the images were rated as excellent or good, with only 5% being rated as fair and poor. There was a high positive correlation ($r = 0.83$) between color, sharpness and contrast ratings. Images with excellent or good

ratings generally received excellent or good color ratings. There were relatively low correlations between color ($r = 0.27$) and sharpness/contrast ($r = 0.32$) ratings and the decision confidence values.

For the online quality assurance program in cytology we randomly selected 100 gynecological cytology cases (benign – 54; atypical squamous cells of undetermined significance (ASCUS) – 24; low-grade squamous intraepithelial lesion (LSIL) – 7; high-grade squamous intraepithelial lesion (HSIL) – 15). The randomization has been done by application of the Research Randomizer. This is a free service offered to students and researchers interested in conducting random assignment and random sampling. This service is available at www.randomizer.org. Cases were diagnosed routinely by 3 certified cytologists with an ex-

Table 4. March 2010-January 2011 cases

Total number of cases	100
The average number of images per case	5 (88 cases, 88%)
The average number of consultants per case	3 (86 cases, 86%)
First comment made in less than 8 hours	94 cases (94%)
The primary diagnosis has been confirmed as a result of second opinion consultation	96 cases (96%)
The cases with corrected diagnosis as a result of telecytology consultation	3 cases (3%)
The cases with images of poor quality, insufficient for telecytology consultation	1 case (1%)

perience of work with digital images and usage of medical information system who provided cytology diagnoses. All participating cytologists have more than 7 years of cytology and up to 2 years experience to work with digital images and medical information system. The most worrisome cells or groups in each case were selected and marked by all participating cytologists. These areas were photographed with 2.0 USB digital eyepiece microscope camera with resolution 3.0 by cytologist. The images had a resolution 2048x1536 pixels. The mean number of selected fields and digital images for each case were 5 (range 5-7) and 20 (range 18-22), respectively. Each series of images began with a general view (magnification x40), followed by higher magnification (x100) of diagnostically interesting areas as directed by the cytologist. The images were stored in a personal computer and uploaded at medical information system (MIS) together with necessary medical data. The upload to the medical information system was done 100% successful. There was no image distortion identifiable after the upload process. Created cases were labeled "QA".

100 electronic medical records (EMRs) with cytology diagnosis, illustrated by images and labeled "QA" were created. Email notifications that cases are available for review have been sent to cytologists who already diagnosed these cases in routine manner after creation of the EMRs. These cytologists have been registered as users at MIS.

Diagnoses of "QA" cases were recorded in 4 categories: (1) benign; (2) ASCUS; (3) LSIL; (4) HSIL (Table 5). Additional information, including comments on adequacy of images, total time required for review and problems encountered in diagnosing "QA" cases, and whether there was a need for low-magnification digital images, was recorded by each participating cytologist.

Diagnoses of "QA" cases correspond with initial diagnoses made in routine manner. The mean diagnostic time was 125.8 minutes (range 115-142 minutes) for glass slides and 47.3 minutes (range 38-62 minutes) for "QA" cases. Low magnification (x40) of digital images was recorded as not necessary by all participating cytologists. The inability to focus at different levels to examine the architectural and cellular details of overlapping cellular groups was recorded as an impediment to diagnosis in "QA" cases (Table 6).

Solutions and Recommendations

Perspectives and strategies for telecytology are currently evolving, as emerging operative requirements would allow self-sustainable large scale exploitation while recent technological developments are available to support integrated and cost-effective solutions to such requirements. However, as far as we know few telecytology services have proceeded to large scale exploitation, even after successful technological demonstration phases. Telecytology is the most important for the ensuring the safe medical care.

Use of telecytology consultation is appearing to have many advantages over conventional light microscopy. The International Union Against Cancer (UICC) has estimated that at least in 5-10% of cancer cases a cytologist need consultation during routine work because of uncertainty. Sending glass slides or paraffin blocks by mail or courier for experts in the field, is a time consuming way

Table 5. Diagnosis according to the Bethesda system

Cytology diagnosis according the Bethesda system	Number of cases
NILM – Negative for intraepithelial lesion or malignancy	54
ASCUS – Atypical squamous cells of undetermined significance	24
LSIL – Low grade squamous intraepithelial lesion	7
HSIL – High grade squamous intraepithelial lesion	15

Table 6. Diagnoses of "QA" cases vs. routine diagnoses

Parameters	Routine diagnostic	"QA" cases
Number of cases diagnosed NILM	54	54
Number of cases diagnosed ASCUS	24	24
Number of cases diagnosed LSIL	7	7
Number of cases diagnosed HSIL	15	15
The mean diagnostic time	125.8 min	47.3 min
The necessity of low magnification (x40)	yes	no
The problems with examination of overlapping cellular groups	no	yes

especially in critical specimens for cytologists working alone in distant hospitals with no facilities for intradepartmental consultation. Besides, the probability of loss and damage are always present. Today, telecytology in the forms of static and dynamic seems to be the basic solution for this major problem. Conventional cytology with glass slide has many limitations. For example they may be easily broken, their stain is unstable and could fade with time, the tissue mount can bubble and dry out and finally certain procedure such as fluorescent stains are not stable more than few days. In this situation it seems that the best replacement for conventional slide cytology is telecytology, which never change in appearance as long as the data integrity is maintained. It is also a good approach for eLearning and already is used widely for this purpose. However, in the spite of mentioned points, telecytology in Georgia is not popular. In this chapter we wanted to evaluate the position of telecytology in Georgia. This is used only for consultation in limited centers and only in the form of static telecytology because of the limitations in equipment, bandwidth and high cost of internet connections, low foreign language ability and computer literacy among healthcare professionals. Another reason is the tendency of centralization of cytology service in Georgia. Medical information systems as well as electronic medical records are not widely realized in the country. It shall be emphasized, that the most part of laboratories in Georgia are equipped by the conventional light microscopes

of Soviet age. The special attention requires the quality of internet in Georgia, the internet connection in regions isn't fast and uninterrupted. In such situation centralization of cytology service in Georgia means movement of patient from region to the capital for the aim to obtain the best possible care and not a transmission of the extract from the medical history illustrated by the virtual slides. It has been revealed that education and clear guidelines for cytologist is essential before starting telecytology. This tool is the most important thing which should be taken into account in the future planning. Because beside the benefits telecytology has no sampling error and all the things it needs are a microscope and a digital camera. We shall say that implementation of telecytology needs continuous education of cytologists to change their opinion about use of this tool in their routine works and taking into account the benefits of replacing conventional cytology by telecytology.

Healthcare IT models are constantly evolving as the industry expands. The medical information system is a comprehensive solution that automates the clinical, administrative, and supply-chain functions. It enables healthcare providers to improve their operational effectiveness, to reduce costs and medical errors, and to enhance quality of care. The aim of the medical information system was and is as simple as relevant: to contribute to and ensure a high-quality, efficient patient care. The relevance of "good" medical information system for high-level quality of care is obvious. Without having appropriate access to relevant data, practically no decisions on diagnostic, therapeutic, or other procedures can be made. In such a situation, consequences will be fatal for patients. The medical information system has been launched in Georgia. The draft version was available since August 2008. After some tests the necessary corrections and editions have been made and the working version is available since October 2008. The medical information system is used by the medical center "Neoclinic" since October 2008 and by the medical laboratory "Neolab" since May 2010. Both medical organizations are located in the capital of Georgia, Tbilisi. Its primary goal is patient management. However, the system also targeted at creating a unified information space in the framework of the wider medical organization.

It is obvious, that digital imaging can be used in many areas of anatomic pathology, including the photography of gross and microscopic findings in both surgical and autopsy pathology. It is practical and cost-effective and provides many advantages over traditional morphology practices. Digital imaging also is the first step toward opening the door to many future applications and improved diagnostic, educational, and quality assurance activities. It is obvious, that digital imaging is rapidly becoming an integral part of the healthcare activities in many hospitals and clinics around the world. In many cases it accounts for over 50% of all e-health activities. There are many advantages of using digital images for quality assurance in cytology. The major advantage is rapid turnaround time. Transmission of digital images through the internet undoubtedly is faster than the conventional method of circulating glass slides, especially when the availability of cytologic smears is limited compared with that of histologic material. Slow turnaround of glass slides during quality assurance exercises is a serious problem. It is reality that glass slides were circulated among more than 20 institutions throughout the country. This exercise alone took

at least 3 months. Sometimes participants have to attend the meeting without viewing the slides.

The use of digital images ensures the assessment of identical fields, avoiding the problem posed by differences in field selection. The main aim in cytology quality assurance programs is to test participants' ability to make the correct decision on a specific abnormal finding rather than the ability to screen an entire slide. Thus, digital images circumvent the problem of field selection and assess interpretation. The time that would be spent for searching the slide for abnormal cells is eliminated. In the present study, the mean diagnostic time was reduced by more than half for "QA" cases (47.3 minutes) compared with glass slides (125.8 minutes).

It should be noted and emphasized, that the main aim in cytology quality assurance programs is to test participants' ability to make correct decision on a specific pathology finding. It is well known, that the specialty of cytology, the analysis of cellular morphology and architecture for the presence and nature of pathology, is involved in the care of virtually every patient who seeks medical attention. In a typical medical center studies have indicated that 70% of the clinical data in the electronic medical record are from cytology. Significantly, clinical decision support programs are highly dependent on cytology data. Much of the analysis performed in the cytology lab is visual; therefore cytology imaging has become an important and growing area of medical imaging environment. However, cytology imaging presents a number of unique challenges. Some of these challenges include the fact that cytology image quality is a function of many processes (many of which are outside the traditional realm of imaging). For example, image quality is a function of the processing of cellular group(s), the staining of the slide, and the ability of the microscope to form a clear, in focus image worthy of capturing. These functions and tasks are unified and standardized. Therefore the selection of the diagnostically important area is the routine procedure during screening of the entire slide and can be easily and effectively performed by the certified cytologist. The most important is the ability to correctly diagnose the concrete pathology finding. This ability usually correlates with a professional experience and development of this skill is the task of the cytology quality assurance programs.

Cost savings is another advantage. Implementation of quality assurance programs in cytology by usage of digital images reduces the expenses of postal or courier slide circulation and the cost and delays of photography slide preparation. Easy and continuous access to the case material from the medical information system is yet another advantage over glass slides, which have to be returned to the owner institution. After the quality assurance exercise, the digital images are still available for reference and teaching purposes. These advantages, together with the acceptable levels of diagnostic accuracy and reproducibility, strongly support the use of medical information system and digital images for cytology quality assurance programs (Table 7).

As it was noted above, the practical application of the medical information system in Georgia started in October 2008. It is successfully used for:

- **Clinical decision support:** Provides users with tools to acquire, manipulate, apply, and display appropriate information to aid in making accurate, timely, and evidence-based clinical decisions.

- **EMRs:** Contain information about patients, from personal details (such as name, age, address, and sex) to details of every aspect of care given by the clinic (ranging from routine visits to major operations).

- **Training and research:** Patient information is available to medical personnel for training and research in e-health and telemedicine.

By the term "EMR" we describe a computerized legal medical record created in the clinic. Usually, however, the term "electronic health record" (also electronic patient record or computerized patient record) is used. EMRs are a part of the medical information system that allows storage, retrieval, and manipulation of data. This is an evolving concept defined as a longitudinal collection of electronic health information about individual patients or populations. Such records may included a whole range of data in comprehensive or summary form, including demographical data, medical history, medication and allergies, immunization status, laboratory test results, radiology images, and billing information. In accordance with our model, EMRs are generated and maintained within clinic. This is a complete record that allows managing and follow-up workflow in healthcare settings and to increase patient safety through evidence-based decision support, quality management, and outcome reporting. EMRs can be continuously updated. A centralized data server is used for EMR's storage.

Table 7. Cytology quality assessment, traditional vs. online programs

Parameter	Cytology quality assurance program in traditional mode	Online cytology quality assurance program
Cost saving	No	Yes
Time effectiveness	No	Yes
Long term accessibility of the case	No	Yes

It has been revealed, that the MIS has yielded significant benefits.

- **Easy access to patient data:** The system provides convenient access to medical records at all points of clinic. Internet-based access improves the ability to remotely access such data.
- **Structured information:** The data captured in clinical information system is well organized. Relevant information can be easily maintained and quickly found. The medical information system reduces the likelihood of mistakes arising from illegible writing too.
- **Safe and secure exchange of medical data:** This task is highly important in the case of organization of teleconsultations and online tumor boards.

Despite of such benefits, there are still barriers that prevent the medical information system from being rolled out in every healthcare organization across Georgia.

- **Initial cost of acquisition:** High price of the basic infrastructure is a stumbling block for many healthcare organizations.
- **Privacy and security:** There are still huge concerns in the healthcare industry about the privacy of patient data on computer systems and how to keep such information secure.
- **Clinician resistance:** Clinicians usually have 10-20 minutes to see their patients and if their use of a medical information system takes up more time than before, it leads to resistance.
- **Integration of legacy systems:** As elsewhere, this poses a stiff challenge for many organizations in Georgia.

Before practical application of the medical information system, education and training of staff is essential. The system is a very useful and easy-for-use tool. It ensures a situation where healthcare professionals spend more time for creating knowledge from medical information than managing of medical information. Further, medical information system holds the potential to reduce medical errors.

Today, application of digital images in cytology seems to be basic solution for organization of quality assurance programs. Conventional cytology with glass slide has many limitations. For example, they may be easily broken; their stain is unstable and could fade with time, and etc. In such situation, the best replacement for conventional slide cytology is digital imaging. The appearance never changes as long as the data integrity is maintained. However, despite of mentioned advantages, digital imaging in Georgia is not popular. In this study we evaluated the application of the medical information system and digital images for implementation of online cytology quality assurance programs under conditions of Georgia. It has been revealed that the mentioned system can be easily and effectively applied as a platform for online cytology quality assurance programs. The data from the present study support the use of digital images for implementation of online cytology quality assurance programs too. Diagnostic concordance was high (100%) for "QA" cases. The data revealed no differences between routine diagnostic versus diagnostic with digital images, supporting the reliability of using digital images displayed on a computer monitor to render accurate diagnoses and undergo online cytology quality assurance programs. It should be noted, however, that although there was a relatively large number of cases in this study, there were only three cytologists. The study would have had more power if there had been more cytologists.

Image quality was generally rated as excellent to good (98%). One interesting finding was that neither diagnostic decision nor diagnostic confidence was highly correlated with ratings of color, sharpness, or with viewing time. The present study illustrates that digital image include potentially eliminating the need for glass slides (at least at the point of examination), allowing annotation to be added to images, and the ability to rapidly transmit and remotely share images electronically. As it was noted above, low magnification (x40) of digital images was recorded as not necessary by all participating cytologists. The inability to focus at different levels to examine the architectural and cellular details of overlapping cellular groups was recorded as an impediment to diagnosis in "QA" cases. It has been proposed to obtain several images focusing different levels of overlapping cellular groups. This might be a solution for examination of the architectural and cellular details of such groups.

We can separate out two main groups of theories, which we can call micro and macro. At the micro level, the MIS and digital image technology might influence behavior in organization through, for example, improved scheduling, better clinical and administrative communications, and localized structural change. These are three possible programme theories in Pawson's method. Another theory is that modern electronic services appear to work in more subtle ways as well, for example by aiding education and learning on the job. The key general point here is that there is no agreed set of theories, or mechanisms, whereby MIS influence clinical or administrative work.

Macro effects arise as a consequence of a network operating across many sites, rather than just one. Commercial ventures such as Amazon and eBay provide compelling examples of this kind of network effect, exploiting economies of scope and scale to offer lower prices than shops for books, CDs, and other goods. The mechanisms whereby network services might exert their effects

in organizational settings have not been extensively researched, but it seemed reasonable to expect to find papers examining them, giving the central place of electronic networking in information technology policies around the world.

We found four main programme theories, namely that MIS may affect patient outcomes (directly), clinician or administrator work patterns, the time costs of undertaken specific tasks (e.g. entering data into patient records), and costs and cost savings. Similarly, we identified a number of variables that MIS might be expected to influence, namely:

- Reduction in medical error rates.
- Reduction in preventable adverse drug event rates.
- Standardization of care (through use of defined protocols and clinical decision support).
- Improved efficiency of care delivery (through automation of manual tasks; reduction in illegibility; reduced turnaround time, scheduling).
- Improved quality of care (through faster access to information; release of time from administrative task to clinical care), and
- Cost savings (e.g. reduction in hospital length of stay).

FUTURE RESEARCH DIRECTIONS

Telemedicine services are rapidly becoming an integral part in many hospitals and clinics around the world. In many programs, telepathology and telecytology account for over 50% of all teleconsultations. Most studies of telepathology and telecytology have focused on usage of robotic microscopes and online microscopy. Other studies have evaluated the use of digital images of slides. Often diagnostic accuracy tends to be high, but image quality is judged to be poor. Given these equivocal results, the methods of obtaining still images as well as the adjustment of images (which usually means improvement of contrast and brightness) need to be investigated. We aimed to compare the diagnostic concordance of a cytology diagnoses based on routine diagnostic with a diagnoses based on digital images acquired using a digital eyepiece microscope camera and displayed on a computer monitor. We tried to evaluate the effectiveness of application of digital images for telecytology diagnostic under the conditions of Georgia too.

420 gynecological cytology cases have been reviewed and diagnosed by one of four certified cytologists experienced in the examination of conventional cytology smears. Each cytologist examines all 420 cases and rendered a single diagnosis. Diagnoses of these cases were recorded in 5 categories: (1) benign; (2) ASCUS; (3) ASC-H (4) LSIL; (5) HSIL (Table 8). After the routine cytology investigation the slides of all cases were photographed with the 2.0 USB digital eyepiece microscope camera with resolution 3.0 MP. The images had a resolution 2048 x 1536 pixels. Up to five images were obtained for each case. Each series of images began with a general view, followed by higher magnification of diagnostically interesting areas as directed by the cytologist. In the actual telecytology situation, the digital images would be taken by the referring cytologist. In our study the digital images were taken by the laboratory personnel trained in the use of the digital eyepiece microscope camera. The images were transferred and stored in a personal computer. The contrast and brightness of images were adjusted

by using of Adobe Photoshop. Brief patient story (age, sex, clinical diagnosis and etc.) derived from the patient's printed medical record was added into each case file. Only patient history information was included to the case. Any reference to actual diagnosis, patient name and etc. has been omitted. The 420 cases were randomized and numbered for presentation order during the study.

Approximately 100 days after all 420 cases had been diagnosed routinely, the same four cytologists reviewed the digital images presented on the computer. Patient history was noted prior to viewing the images for each case. A single diagnosis was rendered for each case. Subjective ratings of image sharpness and quality were given using a 4 level scale: 1 – "excellent", 2 – "good", 3 – "fair", 4 – "poor". Viewing time was recorded by a study coordinator using a stopwatch, beginning when the first image of a case appeared on the computer monitor, and ending when the cytologist rendered a diagnosis. The cytologists were restricted to 40 minutes viewing sessions. Each cytologist evaluated all 420 digital records, which included the images obtained from cases which routine evaluation he/she had performed.

For the analysis, the routine diagnoses have been defined as the correct diagnoses. Diagnostic decisions based on digital images have been divided into two groups. Matches were those cases for which the decisions for the digital image corresponded to diagnoses rendered through routine diagnostic. If the digital image diagnosis did not match diagnose elaborated through routine diagnostic, the case has been classified as a mismatch (i.e., incorrect decision).

Table 8. All 420 cases according to Bethesda scale

Cytology diagnosis according the Bethesda system	Number of cases
NILM – Negative for intraepithelial lesion or malignancy	345
ASCUS – Atypical squamous cells of undeterminated significance	42
ASC-H – Atypical squamous cells, cannot exclude HSIL (High grade squamous intraepithelial lesion	17
LSIL – Low grade squamous intraepithelial lesion	9
HSIL – High grade squamous intraepithelial lesion	7

Diagnostic concordance was measured by calculating the percentage of correctly matching routine diagnoses versus digital images based diagnoses each cytologist had for all 420 gynecological cytology cases (Table 9). The four cytologists had 94%, 93%, 92% and 97% correctly matching decisions, with 6%, 7%, 8% and 3% mismatches respectively. No statistically significant differences ($p<0.001$) between cytologists in terms of percent correct decisions has been revealed. Intra-observer variation was analyzed to determine the degree to which each cytologist's diagnosis using the digital images agreed with their own routine diagnosis. The agreement levels were 97% (n = 260 cases), 99% (n=60 cases), 91% (n=60 cases), 95% (n= 40 cases) for cytologists 1, 2, 3 and 4 respectively.

Overall, 97% of the cases were rated as having excellent or good image sharpness and contrast, with 3% being rated as fair and poor. With respect to image color, 96% of the images were rated as excellent or good, with only 4% being rated as fair and poor.

On average, it took 15.8 minutes to render a diagnosis. The minimum viewing time was 7 minutes and maximum was 22 minutes. Overall, 75% of the cases were diagnosed in less than 18 minutes. An additional 15% were diagnosed in less than 25 minutes, and 10% took longer than 30 minutes to diagnose.

The possibilities of the medical information system presented in the present article are of course not only view that can be taken. The most important and perspective application of the medical information system is the creation of the unified and comprehensive system of virtual healthcare in the country, region and etc. This can be viewed as the realization of the concept of the virtual organization and the successful application of cloud computing. It is proposed, that the cloud is a next-generation Internet – "The Cloud" is not an alternative to "The Internet". It is rather a set of additional protocols and services that build on Internet protocols and services to support the creation and use of computation and data enriched environments. Any resource that is "on the Cloud" is also by definition "on the Net".

The most important and perspective application of the medical information system is the possibility to realize e-health and telemedicine routinely in every medical organization. By this education of medical staff at a distance, so called distance education (eLearning) can be realized in the most effective and comprehensive mode routinely. It is plausible, that the medical information systems as well as implementation of cloud computing and virtual organization technology are the tasks of the future development of e-health and telemedicine. We believe that, the question how technology will change our world is not any more relevant. The answer to this question is obvious. Advanced technologies such as computer, diagnostic imaging, robotics, voice-activating machines, and remote controls have changed hospitals and operating theatres in hospitals around the world. But there is the urgent necessity to develop the unified platform for joining these technologies. This will stipulate the development of healthcare sector. The implementation of quality assurance programs in cytology by application of digital images and the

Table 9. Diagnostic concordance

Cytologist	NILM, %	ASCUS, %	ASC-H, %	LSIL, %	HSIL, %
1	93 %	90 %	88 %	85 %	84 %
2	95 %	92 %	91 %	80 %	87 %
3	95 %	96 %	95 %	89 %	90 %
4	99 %	98 %	98 %	95 %	97 %

possibilities of the medical information system is the excellent example of the process of developing of a unified, resilient and easy to use platform for realization and routine application of technologic solutions. Furthermore, it should be taken in mind, that the application of the medical information system will ensure the realization of the following competencies:

- Patient centered care,
- Work on inter-disciplinary teams,
- Employ evidenced-based practices,
- Apply quality improvement techniques, and
- Utilize the resources and possibilities of IT.

While all five these competences are extremely important, the utilization of the resources and possibilities of IT as an important element of implementation of the medical information system and ensuring of healthcare development can effectively:

- Reduce the medical errors,
- Helps manage the knowledge and information and support the decisions making process based on evidence based practice guidelines,
- Ensures better communication between healthcare providers and patient,
- Advance the goals of redesigning the healthcare systems.

As a result, the core competencies help implement new evidence-based healthcare protocols, ensure quality of medical service and support the notion, that every citizen of the world need to receive the best possible existing care.

Most MIS focused studies are concerned with medications, and there are very few studies concerned with MIS for laboratory and imaging tests. The majority of studies showed a reduction of medication errors to varying degrees. The evi-

dence base on MIS is disappointing. This is partly because the number of good published papers is small, but more because it provides policy makers and practitioners with the thinnest of gruels. There is little sign of the clear evidence that realist syntheses strive form i.e. evidence about what works, where, and why. The papers we identified tend to support two theories of change. They support the view that MIS can have a direct impact on behavior and that it can influence processes, particularly communication patterns and the quality of communications (generally positively). The evidence in the literature was disappointing, especially in light of the fact that policy in the USA is driving towards widespread uptake, seemingly on a very weak evidence base. We failed to find studies which shed any useful light on any other possible mechanisms whereby MIS influence behavior at the micro level, demonstrated effects on patient outcomes. Perhaps most strikingly, we found no technologically sound evidence about cost changes associated with MIS. We also failed to find any good papers on "macro" effects. There is now good evidence that modern electronic networks generate economies of scope and scale in other contexts, but there do not appear to have been any such studies on MIS.

The weakness of the evidence base is due in part to the study designs used by health services research teams. The designs reflect deep assumptions about the ways in which MIS influence health-care processes; specifically that it is possible and desirable to capture the cost and effects of an MIS by studying it in a single setting. The good studies were able to demonstrate a causal link between MIS and work processes by using experimental study designs, where comparisons were made between processes with and without the MIS. As a result, though, these studies had small units of analysis, e.g. pediatric primary care, a clinical laboratory – where direct relationships between MIS and their effects on work patterns or communications could be observed.

The corollary of this point is that we did not find any studies which captured the costs and effects of the MIS "in the round". It is possible to imagine studies which would do this, for example by gathering evidence about the impact of a MIS at several points along a care pathway, such that the sum of the costs and effects at the different points would provide a reasonable proxy of the total impact of a MIS on a service. In order to be clear which programme theories lead to change and which do not, these studies would need to have an observational component, i.e. evidence would be collected that directly tests the different theories of change proposed for MIS. As we have noted, it would also be possible to study the macro effects of MIS. These approaches could be used to determine which of the various programme theories reported in the literature is accurate and we would know for the first time what works, where and why.

CONCLUSION

We concluded that telecytology is a very useful and applicable tool for consulting on difficult cytology cases and can be established with very few technical equipment and software. It has significantly increased knowledge exchange, decentralization of pathology service and thereby ensured a better medical service, while simultaneously saving a lot of time and money over the previous practices.

We evaluated the application of medical information system for telepathology consultations in Georgia. It has been revealed, that mentioned system can be easily and effectively applied for remote consultations in pathology. We concluded that medical information system is a useful and applicable tool for distance consultations on difficult cases. It significantly increases knowledge exchange and thereby ensures a better medical service.

Telecytology can be conducted using a variety of technologies with varying levels of image quality and cost. The data from our studies support the use of digital images for diagnosis. Diagnostic concordance was quite high for all four cytologists. The data revealed no significant differences between routine diagnostic versus digital images based diagnostic, supporting the reliability of using digital images displayed on a computer monitor to render accurate diagnoses. It should be noted, however, that although there was a relatively large number of cases in this study, there were only four cytologists. The study would have had more power if there had been more cytologists.

Image quality was generally rated as excellent to good. One interesting finding was that neither diagnostic decision nor diagnostic confidence was highly correlated with ratings of color, sharpness, or with viewing time. The present data illustrates that digital image based diagnostic is a viable means for cytology diagnostic and can be easily applied for rural and/or regional medical centers. The advantages of digital images include potentially eliminating the need for glass slides (at least at the point of examination), allowing annotation to be added to images, and the ability to rapidly transmit and remotely share images electronically for several purposes (telecytology, conferences, education, quality assurance, peer review). In Georgia, digital images are currently utilized in telecytology, training and education (e.g. online digital atlases and eLearning cycles).

Our study revealed that digital images are a suitable substitute for online cytology quality assurance programs. Medical information system is a useful platform for implementation of online cytology quality assurance programs. But it should be also noted, that perspectives and strategies for medical information system and its practical application in routine work of the medical organization are currently evolving, as emerging operative requirements would allow self-sustainable large scale exploitation while recent technological developments are available to support integrated and cost-effective solutions to such requirements. However, as far as we know few pilot projects have proceeded to large scale exploitation, even after successful technological demonstration phases. Main exploitation drawbacks, problems and deficiencies have been:

1. Partial solutions approach instead of integrated total approach to healthcare assistance needs,
2. Lack of economical drive and consequently no self-sustainability for large scale exploitation,
3. Insufficient H24 (24 hours /day 365 days/ year) medical support,
4. Insufficient networking approach for medical operators and scientific /clinical structures.

The medical information system is the most important background for the ensuring the safe and effective medical care through the appropriate organization of medical information storage and exchange. But instead of management of medical data and clinical workflow by itself the medical information system has the potential for offering the worldwide medical community the following qualitative and quantitative improvements:

- Distance consultations and follow up.
- Opening up new ways for education and training of medical personnel.
- Overall improvement of service by regional centralization of resources.
- Effectiveness and efficiency in a management of actions related to reduction of waiting times for consultations.
- Effective and adequate quality assurance programs.

The medical information system is able to reduce healthcare costs in the following ways:

- Reduction of operating costs through centralization and optimization of resources (expertise, laboratories, and etc.).
- Reduction in travel cost and time for specialists visiting other hospitals and centers for consulting.
- Reduction in costs for training and updating, improvement of specialists' qualifications through eLearning and access to medical databases.

The medical information system introduces added value and a positive impact at social, economic and cultural levels. As a result, it is initiating to have an important influence on many aspects of medical service in countries with low and middle income.

REFERENCES

Banta, D. (2003). The development of health technology assessment. *Health Policy (Amsterdam)*, *63*, 121–132. doi:10.1016/S0168-8510(02)00059-3

Chatman, C. (2010). How cloud computing is changing the face of health care information technology. *Journal of Health Care Compliance*, *12*(3), 37–70.

Clamp, S., & Keen, J. (2007). Electronic health records: Is the evidence base any use? *Journal of Medical Informatics and Internet Medicine*, *32*, 5–10. doi:10.1080/14639230601097903

Coleman, R. (2009). Can histology and pathology be taught without microscopes? The advantages and disadvantages of virtual histology. *Journal Acta Histochemica*, *111*(1), 1–4. doi:10.1016/j.acthis.2008.09.003

Detmer, D. (2000). Information technology for quality health care: a summary of United Kingdom and United States experiences. *Quality in Health Care, 9*, 181–189. doi:10.1136/qhc.9.3.181

Detmer, D. (2001). Transforming health care in the internet era. *World Hospitals and Health Services, 37*, 2.

Dixon, R., & Stahl, J. (2008). Virtual visits in a general medicine practice: A pilot study. *Telemedicine and e-Health, 14*(6), 525-530.

Furness, P. N. (1997). The use of digital images in pathology. *The Journal of Pathology, 183*, 15–24. doi:10.1002/(SICI)1096-9896(199711)183:3<253::AID-PATH927>3.0.CO;2-P

Haughton, J. (2011). Year of the underdog: Cloud-based EHRs. *Health Management Technology, 32*(1), 9.

Hayrinen, K., Saranto, K., & Nykanen, P. (2008). Definition, structure, content, use and impacts of electronic health records: A review of the research literature. *International Journal of Medical Informatics, 77*, 291–304. doi:10.1016/j.ijmedinf.2007.09.001

Horbinski, C., & Wiley, C. A. (2009). Comparison of telepathology systems in neuropathological intraoperative consultations. *Journal of Neuropathology, 19*(2), 317–322.

Hufnagl, P., & Schluns, K. (2008). Virtual microscopy and routine diagnostics: A discussion paper. *The Journal of Pathology, 29*(2), 250–254. doi:10.1007/s00292-008-1093-0

Kabachinski, J. (2011). What's the forecast for cloud computing in healthcare? *Biomedical Instrumentation & Technology, 45*(2), 146–150. doi:10.2345/0899-8205-45.2.146

Kayser, K., Hoshang, S. A., Metze, K., Goldmann, T., Vollmer, E., & Radziszowski, D. (2008). Texture- and object-related automated information analysis in histological still images of various organs. *Journal of Analytical and Quantitative Cytology and Histology, 30*(6), 323–335.

Kobb, R., & Lane, R., & Stallings, D. (2008). E-learning and tele-health: Measuring your success. *Telemedicine and e-Health, 14*(6), 576-579.

Lane, K. (2006). Telemedicine news. *Telemedicine and e-Health, 12*(5), 507-511.

Lareng, L. (2002). Telemedicine in Europe. *European Journal of Internal Medicine, 13*, 1–13. doi:10.1016/S0953-6205(01)00188-1

Leong, F. J., Graham, A. K., & Schwarzmann, P. (2000). Clinical trial of telepathology as an alternative modality in breast histopathology quality assurance. *Journal of Telemedicine and E-Health, 6*, 373–377. doi:10.1089/15305620050503834

Mencarelli, R., Marcolongo, A., & Gasparetto, A. (2008). Organizational model for a telepathology system. *Journal of Diagnostic Pathology, 15*(3), S7.

Merell, R., & Doarn, C. (2008). Is it time for a telemedicine breakthrough? *Telemedicine and e-Health, 14*(6), 505-506.

Moore, D., Green, J., Jay, S., Leist, J., & Maitland, F. (1994). Creating a new paradigm for CME: Seizing opportunities within the health care revolution. *The Journal of Continuing Education in the Health Professions, 14*, 4–31. doi:10.1002/chp.4750140102

Moura, A., & Del Giglio, A. (2000). Education via internet. *Revista da Associação Médica Brasileira, 46*(1), 47–51.

Nannings, B., & Abu-Hanna, A. (2006). Decision support telemedicine systems: A conceptual model and reusable templates. *Telemedicine and e-Health, 12*(6), 644-654.

Pak, H. (2007). Telethinking. *Telemedicine and e-Health, 13*(5), 483-486.

Raab, S. S., Zaleski, M. S., & Thomas, P. A. (1996). Telecytology: Diagnostic accuracy in cervical-vaginal smears. *American Journal of Clinical Pathology, 105*, 599–603.

Riva, G. (2000). From tele-health to e-health: Internet and distributed virtual reality in health care. *Journal of CyberPsychology & Behavior, 3*(6), 989–998. doi:10.1089/109493100452255

Riva, G. (2002). The emergence of e-health: Using virtual reality and the internet for providing advanced healthcare services. *International Journal of Healthcare Technology and Management, 4*(1/2), 15–40. doi:10.1504/IJHTM.2002.001127

Rocha, R., Vassallo, J., Soares, F., Miller, K., & Gobbi, H. (2009). Digital slides: Present status of a tool for consultation, teaching, and quality control in pathology. *Journal of Pathology – Research and Practice, 205*(11), 735-41.

Rosenthal, A., Mork, P., Li, M. H., Stanford, J., Koester, D., & Reynolds, P. (2010). Cloud computing: A new business paradigm for biomedical information sharing. *Journal of Biomedical Informatics, 43*(2), 342–353. doi:10.1016/j.jbi.2009.08.014

Sloot, P., Tirado-Ramos, A., Altintas, I., Bubak, M., & Boucher, C. (2006). From molecule to man: Decision support in individualized E-Health. *Computer, 39*(11), 40–46. doi:10.1109/MC.2006.380

Van Ginneken, A. M. (2002). The computerized patient record: Balancing effort and benefit. *International Journal of Medical Informatics, 65*, 97–119. doi:10.1016/S1386-5056(02)00007-2

Weinstein, R. S., Graham, A. R., Richte, L. C., Barker, G. P., Krupinski, E. A., & Lopez, A. M. (2009). Overview of telepathology, virtual microscopy, and whole slide imaging: Prospects for the future. *Journal of Human Pathology, 40*(8), 1057–1069. doi:10.1016/j.humpath.2009.04.006

KEY TERMS AND DEFINITIONS

Digital Imaging: Also known as digital image acquisition; the creation of digital images.

Ehealthe-Health: An emerging field in the intersection of medical informatics, public health and business, referring to health services and information delivered or enhanced through the Internet and related technologies.

Elearning: An approach to facilitate or enhance education by electronic means such as email, computers, or the Internet.

Electronic Medical Record: A computerized medical record.

Internet: Is a global system of interconnected computer networks that interchange data by packet switching using the standardized Internet Protocol Suite (TCP/IP).

Medical Information System: The software which is used for management of medical data and generates electronic medical record.

Telecytology: A branch of telemedicine that consists in the exchange of microscopy digital images through telecommunication with the purposes of diagnosis, consultation, research and/or education.

Telemedicine: The rapid access to shared and remote medical expertise by means of telecommunications and information technologies, no matter where the patient or relevant information is located.

Compilation of References

A Salud Program. (2011). *Diabetes health, CVS Pharmacy begins free health screenings in communities nationwide.*

AAL. (2009). *Ambient assisted living - Joint programme (AAL JP) - 2008-2013.* Ambient Assisted Living. Retrieved from http://www.aal-europe.eu/

About Aglets. (2002, March 14). IBM research. Retrieved July 30, 2012, from http://www.research.ibm.com/trl/aglets/about_e.htm

Aggarwal, R., & Darzi, A. (2008). Symposium on surgical simulation for training and certification. *World Journal of Surgery, 32*, 139–140. doi:10.1007/s00268-007-9341-7

Agha, Z., Schapira, R. M., & Maker, A. H. (2002). Cost effectiveness of telemedicine for the delivery of outpatient pulmonary care to a rural population. *Telemedicine and E-Health, 8*(3), 281–291. doi:10.1089/15305620260353171

Aglets. (2002, March 14). IBM research. Retrieved July 30, 2012, from http://www.research.ibm.com/trl/aglets/

Ahern, D. K., Kreslake, J. M., & Phalen, J. M. (2006). What is ehealth: Perspectives on the evolution of ehealth research. *Journal of Medicine on the Internet, 8*(1), 4. Retrieved from http://www.jmir.org/2006/1/e4/

Ailawadi, G., Alykhan, S., Jones, N., & Jones, D. R. (2010). The legend behind cardiothoracic surgical instruments. *The Annals of Thoracic Surgery, 89*, 1693–1700. doi:10.1016/j.athoracsur.2009.11.019

Alboliras, E. T., Berdusis, K., Fisher, J., Harrison, R. A., Benson, D. W. Jr, & Webb, C. L. (1996). Transmission of full-length echocardiographic images over ISDN for diagnosing congenital heart disease. *Telemedicine Journal: The Official Journal of the American Telemedicine Association, 2*(4), 251–258.

Allen, A., & Hayes, J. (1994). Patient satisfaction with telemedicine in a rural clinic. *American Journal of Public Health, 84*(10), 1693. doi:10.2105/AJPH.84.10.1693

Alzheimer's Disease International. (September, 21, 2010). *World Alzheimer report 2010: The global economic impact of dementia.* Alzheimer's Disease International Press. Retrieved May 10, 2010, from http://www.alz.co.uk/research/files/WorldAlzheimerReport2010.pdf.

American Academy of Orthopaedic Surgeons (Ed.). (1988). *Joint motion: Method of measuring and recording.* Edinburgh, UK: Churchill Livingstone.

American Telemedicine Association. (2012). *Telemedicine defined.* Retrieved from http://www.americantelemed.org/i4a/pages/index.cfm?pageid=3333

Amerini, I., Ballocca, G., Becarelli, R., Borri, R., Caldelli, R., & Filippini, F. (2010). A DVB-MHP web browser to pursue convergence between digital terrestrial television and Internet. *Multimedia Tools and Applications, 50*, 381–414. doi:10.1007/s11042-009-0415-4

Amirkhanyan, A. A., & Wolf, D. A. (2003). Caregiver stress and non caregiver stress: Exploring the pathways of psychiatric morbidity. *The Gerontologist, 43*(6), 817–827. doi:10.1093/geront/43.6.817

Amirkhanyan, A. A., & Wolf, D. A. (2006). Parent care and stress process: Findings from panel data. *The Journals of Gerontology. Series B, Psychological Sciences and Social Sciences, 61*, S248–S255. doi:10.1093/geronb/61.5.S248

Andersen, R. M. (1995). Revisiting a behavioral model and access to medical care: Do it matter? *Journal of Health and Social Behavior, 36*, 1–10. doi:10.2307/2137284

Andreassen, H. K., Bujnowska-Fedak, M. M., Chronaki, C. E., Dumitru, R. C., Pudule, I., & Santana, S. (2007). European citizens' use of E-health services: A study of seven countries. *BMC Public Health*, *7*, 53. doi:10.1186/1471-2458-7-53

Anker, S., Koehler, F., & Abraham, W. (2011). Telemedicine and remote management of patients with heart failure (Heart Failure 4). *Lancet*, *378*, 731–739. doi:10.1016/S0140-6736(11)61229-4

Anspaugh, D. J., Hamrick, M. H., & Rosato, F. (1994). *Wellness: Concepts and applications*. St. Louis, MO: Mosby.

Anvari, M. (2007). Remote telepresence surgery: The Canadian experience. *Surgical Endoscopy*, *21*(4), 537–541. doi:10.1007/s00464-006-9040-8

Arbib, M. A. (1981). Perceptual structures and distributed motor control . In Brooks, V. B. (Ed.), *Handbook of physiology -- The nervous system II. Motor control* (pp. 1449–1480). American Physiological Society.

Arcelus, A., Goubran, R., & Knoefel, F. (2011). *Detection of bouncing during sit-to-stand transfers with sequential pressure images*. Paper presented at the IEEE International Symposium on Medical Measurements and Applications (MeMeA 2011).

Archondakis, S., Georgoulakis, J., & Stamataki, M. (2009). Telecytology: A tool for quality assessment and improvement in the evaluation of thyroid fine-needle aspiration specimens. *Telemedicine Journal and E Health . The Official Journal of American Telemedicine Association*, *15*(7), 713–717. doi:10.1089/tmj.2009.0037

Armstrong, I. J., & Haston, W. S. (1997). Medical decision support for remote general practitioners using telemedicine. *Journal of Telemedicine and Telecare*, *3*(1), 27–34. doi:10.1258/1357633971930166

Asadachatreekul, S. (2004). *An agent-based distributed inference engine for expert system construction*. Regina, Canada: University of Regina, Faculty of Graduate Studies and Research.

Asamoah-Odei, E., de Backer, H., Dologuele, N., Embola, I., Groth, S., & Horsch, A. (2007). eHealth for Africa – Opportunities for enhancing the contribution of ICT to improve health services. *European Journal of Medical Research*, *12*(Suppl. 1), 1–38.

Ashby, S., Nyenwe, E., Tidewell, J., Nouer, S., & Kitabchi, A. (2011). Improving diabetes care via telemedicine: Lessons from the Addressing Diabetes in Tennessee (ADT) project. *Diabetes Care, March*.

Audit Commission. (2004). *Assistive technology: Independence and well-being*. National Report No. 4.

Baer, L., Elford, D. R., & Cukor, P. (1997). Telepsychiatry at forty: What have we learned? *Harvard Review of Psychiatry*, *5*, 7–17. doi:10.3109/10673229709034720

Baker, E., Ford, R., Newell, M., & Schmitz, D. (2007). *Idaho family physician rural work force assessment pilot study*. Idaho Department of Health and Welfare, June 2007.

Ballantyne, G. H. (2002). Robotic surgery, telerobotic surgery, telepresence, and telementoring. Review of early clinical results. *Surgical Endoscopy*, *16*(10), 1389–1402. doi:10.1007/s00464-001-8283-7

Banta, D. (2003). The development of health technology assessment. *Health Policy (Amsterdam)*, *63*, 121–132. doi:10.1016/S0168-8510(02)00059-3

Barrie, G., Nicholas, D., Huntington, P., & Williams, P. (2003). Digital interactive television: Health information platform of the future? *Aslib Proceedings*, *55*(5-6), 346–356.

Bashshur, R., & Shannon, G. (2009). *National telemedicine initiatives: Essential to healthcare reform*. Telemedicine and e-Health, July/August. doi:10.1089/tmj.2009.9960

Bassett, D. R. (2000). Validity and reliability issues in objective monitoring of physical activity. *Research Quarterly for Exercise and Sport*, *71*(2), 30–36.

Bassett, D. R., Wyatt, H., Thompson, H., & Peters, J. (2010). Pedometer-measured physical activity and health behaviors in US adults. *Medicine and Science in Sports and Exercise*, *42*(10), 1819–1825. doi:10.1249/MSS.0b013e3181dc2e54

Bauldoff, G. S., Hoffman, L. A., Zullo, T. G., & Sciurba, F. C. (2002). Exercise Maintenance following pulmonary rehabilitation: Effect of distractive stimuli. *Chest*, *122*, 948–954. doi:10.1378/chest.122.3.948

Beaglehole, R., Ebrahim, S., Reddy, S., Voute, J., & Leeder, S. (2007). Prevention of chronic diseases: A call to action. *Lancet*, *370*, 2152–2157. doi:10.1016/S0140-6736(07)61700-0

Becker, J. C., & Thakor Nitish, V. (1988). A study of motion of human fingers with application to anthropomorphic designs. *IEEE Transactions on Bio-Medical Engineering, 35*(2), 110–117. doi:10.1109/10.1348

Beckjord, E. B., Finney Rutten, L. J., Squiers, L., Arora, N. K., Volckmann, L., Moser, R. P., & Hesse, B. W. (2007). Use of the internet to communicate with health care providers in the United States: Estimates from the 2003 and 2005 Health Information National Trends Surveys (HINTS). *Journal of Medical Internet Research, 9*(3), e20. doi:10.2196/jmir.9.3.e20

Bella, S., Murgia, F., Tozzi, A. E., Cotognini, C., & Lucidi, V. (2009). Five years of telemedicine in cystic fibrosis disease. *La Clinica Terapeutica, 160*(6), 457–460.

Bellomo, R. G., Iodice, P., Barassi, G., & Saggini, R. (2011). *Biomechanic measures and sense motor control of body posture after plastic surgery.* Paper presented at the IEEE International Symposium on Medical Measurements and Applications (MeMeA 2011).

Belmont, J. M., & Mattioli, L. F. (2003). Accuracy of analog telephonic stethoscopy for pediatric telecardiology. *Pediatrics, 112*(4), 780–786. doi:10.1542/peds.112.4.780

Belmont, J. M., Mattioli, L. F., Goertz, K. K., Ardinger, R. H. Jr, & Thomas, C. M. (1995). Evaluation of remote stethoscopy for pediatric telecardiology. *Telemedicine Journal: The Official Journal of the American Telemedicine Association, 1*(2), 133–149.

Benedetti, M. G., Biagi, F., Merlo, A., Belvedere, C., & Leardini, A. (2011). *A new protocol for multi-segment trunk kinematics.* Paper presented at the IEEE International Symposium on Medical Measurements and Applications (MeMeA 2011).

Benedetti, M. G., Manca, M., Sicari, M., Ferraresi, G., Casadio, G., Buganè, F., & Leardini, A. (2011). *Gait measures in patients with and without AFO for equinus varus/drop foot.* Paper presented at the IEEE International Symposium on Medical Measurements and Applications (MeMeA 2011).

Benedicenti, L., & Soomlek, C. (2009). An agent-based modeling system for wellness . In Paranjape, R., & Sadanand, A. (Eds.), *Multi-agent systems for healthcare simulation and modeling: Applications for system improvement* (pp. 137–163). Hershey, PA: IGI Global. doi:10.4018/978-1-60566-772-0.ch008

Bhat, D., Upponi, A., Rakecha, A., & Thomson, J. (2010). Evaluating safety, effectiveness, and user satisfaction of home international normalized ratio monitoring service: Experience from a tertiary pediatric cardiology unit in the United Kingdom. *Pediatric Cardiology, 31*(1), 18–21. doi:10.1007/s00246-009-9535-x

Bifulco, P., Cesarelli, M., Fratini, A., Ruffo, M., Pasquariello, G., & Gargiluo, G. (2011). *A wearable device for recording of biopotentials and body movements.* Paper presented at the IEEE International Symposium on Medical Measurements and Applications (MeMeA 2011).

Bischoff, R., Robinson, W., & Swinton, J. (2009). Telehealth and rural depression: Physician and patient perspectives. *Families, Systems & Health, 27*(2), 172–182. doi:10.1037/a0016014

Bjorgaas, M. R., Vik, J. T., Stolen, T., Lydersen, S., & Grill, V. (2008). Regular use of pedometer does not enhance beneficial outcomes in a physical activity intervention study in type 2 diabetes mellitus. *Metabolism: Clinical and Experimental, 57*, 605–611. doi:10.1016/j.metabol.2007.12.002

Black, A. D., Car, J., Pagliari, C., Anandan, C., Cresswell, K., & Bokun, T. (2011). The impact of ehealth on the quality and safety of health care: A systematic overview. *PLoS Medicine, 8*(1). doi:10.1371/journal.pmed.1000387

Blumenthal, D., & Tavenner, M. (2010). The "meaningful use" regulation for electronic health records. *The New England Journal of Medicine, 363*, 501–504. doi:10.1056/NEJMp1006114

Bonato, P. (2005). Advances in wearable technology and applications in physical medicine and rehabilitation. *Journal of Neuroengineering and Rehabilitation, 2*(2).

Boulos, M. N., Rocha, A., Martins, A., Vicente, M. E., Bolz, A., & Feld, R. (2007). CAALYX: A new generation of location-based services in healthcare. *International Journal of Health Geographics, 6*(9).

Bove, E. L., Ohye, R. G., & Devaney, E. J. (2004). Hypoplastic left heart syndrome: Conventional surgical management. *Seminars in Thoracic and Cardiovascular Surgery. Pediatric Cardiac Surgery Annual, 7*, 3–10. doi:10.1053/j.pcsu.2004.02.003

Bowers, B., Nolet, K., Roberts, T., & Esmond, S. (2009). Implementing change in long term care . In Nolet, K., Roberts, T., & Esmond, S. (Eds.), *Implementing change in long-term care* (pp. 1–129).

Bowersox, J. C., & Cornum, R. L. (1998). Remote operative urology using a surgical telemanipulator system: Preliminary observations. *Urology, 52*, 17–22. doi:10.1016/S0090-4295(98)00168-X

Bowns, I. R., Collins, K., Walters, S. J., & McDonagh, A. J. (2006). Telemedicine in dermatology: A randomised controlled trial. *Health Technology Assessment, 10*(43), iii-iv, ix-xi, 1-39.

Bowonder, B., Bansal, B., & Giridhar, A. (2005). Telemedicine platform: A case study of Apollo Hospitals telemedicine project. *International Journal of Services, Technical and Management, 6*(3-5).

Boxer, R. (2009). *Telehealth can enable convenient, high-quality and affordable care for children and their families.*

Bravata, D. M., Spangler, C. S., Sundaram, V., Gienger, A. L., Lin, N., & Lewis, R. (2007). Using pedometers to increase physical activity and improve health. *Journal of the American Medical Association, 19*(298), 2296–2304. doi:10.1001/jama.298.19.2296

Briscoe, D., Adair, C. F., & Thompson, L. D. (2000). Telecytologic diagnosis of breast fine needle aspiration biopsies. *Acta Cytologica, 44*, 175–180. doi:10.1159/000326357

Bronferbrenner, U. (Ed.). (1986). *Ecologia dello sviluppo umano*. Bologna, Italy: Il Mulino Editore.

Brookmeyer, R., Johnson, E., Ziegler-Graham, K., & Arrighi, H. M. (2007). Forecasting the global burden of Alzheimer's disease. *Alzheimer's & Dementia, 3*, 186–191. doi:10.1016/j.jalz.2007.04.381

Broome, J. (1978). Trying to value a life. *Journal of Public Economics, 9*, 91. doi:10.1016/0047-2727(78)90029-4

Brown, A., & Siahpush, M. (2007). Risk factors for overweight and obesity: Results from the 2001 National Health Survey. *Public Health, 121*(8), 603–613. doi:10.1016/j.puhe.2007.01.008

Broyles, R. W. (2006). *Fundamentals of statistics in health administration*. Sudbury, MA: Jones and Bartlett.

Brugada, P. (2006). What evidence do we have to replace in-hospital implantable cardioverter defibrillator follow-up? *Clinical Research in Cardiology; Official Journal of the German Cardiac Society, 95*(Suppl 3), 3–9. doi:10.1007/s00392-006-1302-x

Bull, C., Yates, R., Sarkar, D., Deanfield, J., & de Leval, M. (2000). Scientific, ethical, and logistical considerations in introducing a new operation: A retrospective cohort study from paediatric cardiac surgery. *British Medical Journal, 320*(7243), 1168–1173. doi:10.1136/bmj.320.7243.1168

Buntin, M. B., Burke, M. F., Hoaglin, M. C., & Blumenthal, D. (2011). The benefits of health information technology: A review of the recent literature shows predominantly positive results. *Health Affairs, 30*(3), 464–471. doi:10.1377/hlthaff.2011.0178

Burt, E., & Taylor, J. A. (1998). Information and communication technologies: Reshaping voluntary organizations? *Nonprofit Management & Leadership, 11*(2), 131–143. doi:10.1002/nml.11201

Butow, E. (2007). *User interface design for mere mortals* (Hernandez, M. J., Ed.). 1st ed.). Addison-Wesley Professional.

Butter, M., Rensma, A., van Boxsel, J., Kalisingh, S., Schoone, M., & Leis, M. … Korhonen, I. (2008). *Robotics for Heath Care, Final Report, October 2008*. European Commission, DG Information Society. Retrieved October, 3, 2008, from http://ec.europa.eu/information_society/activities/health/docs/studies/robotics_healthcare/robotics-final-report.pdf

Callahan, C. M., Boustani, M. A., & Unverzagt, F. W. (2006). Effectiveness of collaborative care for older adults with Alzheimer disease in primary care: A randomized controlled trial. *Journal of the American Medical Association, 295*, 2148–2157. doi:10.1001/jama.295.18.2148

Callas, P. W., Ricci, M. A., & Caputo, M. P. (2006). Improved rural provider access to continuing medical education through interactive videoconferencing. *Telemedicine Journal and e-Health, 6*, 393–399. doi:10.1089/15305620050503861

Camarinha-Matos, L. M., & Afsarmanesh, H. (2002). Design of a virtual community infrastructure for elderly care . In Camarinha-Matos, I. M. (Ed.), *Collaborative business ecosystems and virtual enterprises.*

Campbell, G., Loane, E., & Griffiths, R. (1998). Comparison of teleconsultations and face-to-face consultations: Preliminary results of a United Kingdom multicentre teledermatology study. *The British Journal of Dermatology*, *39*, 81–87.

Campbell, M., Fitzpatrick, R., Haines, A., Kinmonth, A., Sandercock, P., & Spiegelhalter, D. (2000). Framework for design and evaluation of complex interventions to improve health. *British Medical Journal*, *321*, 694–696. doi:10.1136/bmj.321.7262.694

Canada Health Infoway. (2011). Welcome to infoway's resource centre. Retrieved October 24, 2011, from https://www.infoway-inforoute.ca/lang-en/working-with-ehr/resource-centre

Canada Health Infoway. (2012). *2012-2013 summary corperate plan*. Canada Health Infoway.

Carlson, M. (2006). Recommendations from the Heart Rhythm Society Task Force on Device Performance Policies and Guidelines. *Heart Rhythm*, *3*(10), 1250–1273. doi:10.1016/j.hrthm.2006.08.029

Casey, F. A. (1999). Telemedicine in paediatric cardiology. *Archives of Disease in Childhood*, *80*(6), 497–499. doi:10.1136/adc.80.6.497

Castagnaro, A., De Leo, A., Inciocchi, S., Saggio, G., & Tarantino, U. (2010). *Nuova biotecnologia: Il guanto sensorizzato per misurare la cinesi della mano*. Paper presented at the 48° Congresso Nazionale Società Italiana Chirurgia della Mano SICM 2010, "Stato dell'arte nella chirurgia articolare del gomito, polso e mano: protesi e tecniche alternative", Savona 29 Settembre - 2 Ottobre, 2010.

Censis. (Ed.). (2007). *La mente rubata, bisogni e costi sociali della malattia di Alzheimer*. Milano, Italia: FrancoAngeli Editore.

Chao, E. Y. S., An, K.-N., Cooney, W. P. III, & Linscheid, R. L. (Eds.). (1989). *Biomechanics of the hand: A basic research study*. Teaneck, NJ: World Scientific Publishing Co., Inc.

Chatman, C. (2010). How cloud computing is changing the face of health care information technology. *Journal of Health Care Compliance*, *12*(3), 37–70.

Chaudhry, S., Mattera, J., Curtis, J., Sperlus, J., Herrin, J., & Lin, Z. (2010). Telemonitoring in patients with heart failure. *The New England Journal of Medicine*, *363*(24), 2301–2309. doi:10.1056/NEJMoa1010029

Cheitilin, M. D., Armstrong, W. F., & Aurigemma, G. R. (2003). ACC/AHA/ASE 2003 guideline update for the clinical application of echocardiography: A report of the American College of Cardiology, American Heart Association Task Force on Practice Guidelines. *Journal of the American Society of Echocardiography*, *16*(10), 1091–1110. doi:10.1016/S0894-7317(03)00685-0

Chen, C. (1999). *Information visualisation and virtual environments*. London, UK: Springer.

Chiossi, C. (2004, October 6). *Aglets*. Retrieved July 30, 2012, from http://aglets.sourceforge.net/

Chirico, U. (2006). *Programmazione delle Smart Card*. Gruppo Editoriale Infomedia (in italian)

Chiu, P., & Hedrick, H. L. (2008). Postnatal management and long-term outcome for survivors with congenital diaphragmatic hernia. *Prenatal Diagnosis*, *28*(7), 592–603. doi:10.1002/pd.2007

Chiu, T., & Eysembach, G. (2010). Stage of use: Consideration, initiation, utilization and outcome of an internet-mediated intervention. *Medical Informatics and Decision Making*, *10*, 73–84. doi:10.1186/1472-6947-10-73

Chodzko-Zajko, W. J., Proctor, D. N., Fiatarone Singh, M. A., Minson, C. T., Nigg, C. R., Salem, G. J., & Skinner, J. S. (2009). American College of Sports Medicine position stand. Exercise and physical activity for older adults. *Medicine and Science in Sports and Exercise*, *41*, 1510–1530. doi:10.1249/MSS.0b013e3181a0c95c

Chorianopoulos, K., & Spinellis, D. (2006). User interface evaluation of interactive TV: A media studies perspective. *Universal Access in the Information Society*, *5*(2), 209–218. doi:10.1007/s10209-006-0032-1

Chow, S.-C. (2003). *Encyclopedia of biopharmaceutical statistics*. New York, NY: Marcel Dekker.

Cicourel, A. V. (1999). The interaction of cognitive and cultural models in health care delivery . In Sarangi, S., & Talk, R. S. (Eds.), *Work and institutional order: Discourse in medical, mediation and management settings* (pp. 183–224). Berlin, Germany: De Gruyter. doi:10.1515/9783110208375.2.183

Clamp, S., & Keen, J. (2007). Electronic health records: Is the evidence base any use? *Journal of Medical Informatics and Internet Medicine*, *32*, 5–10. doi:10.1080/14639230601097903

Clark, R. A., Inglis, S. C., McAlister, F. A., Cleland, J. G., & Stewart, S. (2007). Telemonitoring or structured telephone support programmes for patients with chronic heart failure: Systematic review and meta-analysis. *British Medical Journal*, *334*(7600), 942. doi:10.1136/bmj.39156.536968.55

Cleland, J. C. F. (2006). *The Trans-European Network –Home care management system study: An investigation of the effect of telemedicine on outcomes in Europe*. DIS Manage Health Outcomes 2006.

Clinfowiki. (2010). *Physician resistance as a barrier to implement clinical information systems*. Retrieved from clinfowiki.org/wiki/index.php/Physician_resistance_as_a_barrier_to_implement_clinical_information_systems

Cloutier, A. (2000). Distance diagnosis in pediatric cardiology: A model for telemedecine implementation. *Telemedicine Today*, *8*(3), 20–21.

Cloutier, A., & Finley, J. (2004). Telepediatric cardiology practice in canada. Telemedicine Journal and e-Health . *The Official Journal of the American Telemedicine Association*, *10*(1), 33–37. doi:10.1089/153056204773644553

Coleman, R. (2009). Can histology and pathology be taught without microscopes? The advantages and disadvantages of virtual histology. *Journal Acta Histochemica*, *111*(1), 1–4. doi:10.1016/j.acthis.2008.09.003

Commission of the European Communities. (2008). *COM(2008) 689: Communication from the Commission to the European Parliament, the Council, the European economic and social Committee and the Committee of the Regions on telemedicine for the benefit of patients, healthcare systems and society*. Retrieved November 4, 2008, from http://www.epractice.eu/

Congenital Cardiac Audit Database. (2009). Congenital heart disease website. Retrieved from http://www.ccad.org.uk/002/congenital.nsf/WMortality?Openview

Continua Health Alliance. (2009). *Connected health vision, personal telehealth overview*. Retrieved October 24, 2011, from http://www.continuaalliance.org/connected-health-vision.html

Corder, K., Brage, S., & Ekelund, U. (2007). Accelerometers and pedometers: Methodology and clinical application. *Current Opinion in Clinical Nutrition and Metabolic Care*, *10*, 597–603. doi:10.1097/MCO.0b013e328285d883

Cosi, M. (2002). Modalità e Multisensorialità nella creazione di una "Faccia Parlante" in Italiano. 2002 *Cdrom Proceedings of VIII Meeting of AIIA - AIIA 2002*, Siena, Italy, September 10-13

Cosi, P., Caldognetto Magno, E. (2008). Festival E Lucia: TTS (Text-to-speech) e IVA (Intelligent Virtual Agent) al servizio della didattica dei disabili. *Proceedings of 3rd Convegno Internazionale "Progresso e Innovazioni Tecnologiche nella riabilitazione dell'età evolutiva"* Napoli, 22 Giugno 2007.

Costa, R., Novais, P., Costa, A., & Neves, J. (2009). Memory support in ambient assisted living. *IFIP Advances in Information and Communication Technology*, *307*, 745–752. doi:10.1007/978-3-642-04568-4_75

Cotton, J. L., Gallaher, K. J., & Henry, G. W. (2002). Accuracy of interpretation of full-length pediatric echocardiograms transmitted over an integrated services digital network telemedicine link. *Southern Medical Journal*, *95*(9), 1012–1016.

Courtney, K. L. (2008). Needing smart home technologies: the perspectives of older adults in continuing care retirement communities. *Informatics in Primary Care*, *16*, 195–201.

Craig, J., Russell, C., Patterson, V., & Wootton, R. (1999). User satisfaction with realtime teleneurology. *Journal of Telemedicine and Telecare*, *5*(4), 237–241. doi:10.1258/1357633991933774

Cramer, S. F., Roth, L. M., Ulbright, T. M., & Mills, S. E. (1991). The mystique of the mistake—With proposed standards for validating proficiency tests. *American Journal of Clinical Pathology*, *96*, 774–777.

Cross, M. (2006). Will connecting for health deliver its promises? *British Medical Journal*, *332*(7541), 599–601. doi:10.1136/bmj.332.7541.599

Crouter, S. E., Schneider, P. L., Karabulut, M., & Bassett, D. R. Jr. (2003). Validity of 10 electronic pedometers for measuring steps, distance, and energy cost. *Medicine and Science in Sports and Exercise*, *35*, 1455–1460. doi:10.1249/01.MSS.0000078932.61440.A2

Cullum, C. M., Weiner, M. F., Gehrmann, H. R., & Hynan, L. S. (2006). Feasibility of telecognitive assessment in dementia. *Assessment*, *13*(4), 385–390. doi:10.1177/1073191106289065

Currell, R., Urquhart, C., Wainwright, P., & Lewis, R. (2006). Telemedicine versus face to face patient care. *Cochrane Database of Systematic Reviews*, *4*, CD002098.

Currier, G., & Kshetri, N. (2011). *Baseline mobile, two keys to successful cloud computing, cloud computing in developing economies: Drivers, effects and policy measures. PTC 2010*. Greensboro: University of North Carolina.

Cystic Fibrosis Foundation. (1994). *Microbiology and infectious disease in Cystic Fibrosis: V*. Bethesda, MD: Author.

Cystic Fibrosis Foundation. (1997). *Clinical practice guidelines for cystic fibrosis*. Bethesda, MD: Author.

D'Amico, M., Bellomo, R. G., Saggini, R., & Roncoletta, P. (2011). *A 3D spine & full skeleton model for multi-sensor biomechanical analysis in posture & gait*. Paper presented at the IEEE International Symposium on Medical Measurements and Applications (MeMeA 2011).

Dahl, L. B., Hasvold, P., Arild, E., & Hasvold, T. (2002). Heart murmurs recorded by a sensor based electronic stethoscope and e-mailed for remote assessment. *Archives of Disease in Childhood*, *87*(4), 297–301. doi:10.1136/adc.87.4.297

D'Ambrosia, R. D. (Ed.). (1986). *Musculoskeletal disorders: Regional examination and differential diagnosis* (2nd ed.). Philadelphia, PA: Lippincott.

Dankelman, J. (2008). Surgical simulator design and development. *World Journal of Surgery*, *32*(2), 149–155. doi:10.1007/s00268-007-9150-z

Dannheisser, L. M., & Rosenbaum, J. M. (2005). *What's wrong with me? The frustrated patients' guide to getting an accurate diagnosis*. New York, NY: McGraw-Hill.

Dario, C., Dunbar, A., Feliciani, F., Garcia-Barbero, M., Giovannetti, S., & Graschew, G. (2005). Opportunities and challenges of ehealth and telemedicine via satellite. *European Journal of Medical Research*, *10*(Suppl. 1), 1–52.

Darkins, A., Ryan, P., Kobb, R., Foster, L., Edmonson, E., Wakefield, B., et al. (2008). Care coordination/home telehealth: The systematic implementation of health informatics, telehealth, and disease management to support the care of veteran patients with chronic conditions. *Telemedicine and e-Health*, *14*(10), 1118-26.

Darkins, A. W., & Cary, M. A. (2000). *Telemedicine and telehealth: Principles, policies, performance, and pitfalls* (1st ed.). New York, NY: Springer Publishing Co.

Das, H., Ohm, T., Boswell, C., Paliug, E., Rodriguez, G., Steele, R., & Barlow, E. (1996). Engineering in medicine and biology society, bridging disciplines for biomedicine. *Proceedings of the 18th Annual International Conference of the IEEE, Vol. 1: Telerobotics for Microsurgery* (pp. 227-228). Pasadena, CA: California Inst. of Technol.

Davalos, M. E., French, M. T., Budrick, A. E., & Simmons, S. C. (2009). Economic evaluation of telemedicine: Review of the literature and research guidelines for benefit-cost analysis. *Telemedicine and eHealth*, *15*(10), 933-948.

Davey, D., Nielsen, M. L., & Frable, W. J. (1993). Improving accuracy in gynecologic cytology. *Archives of Pathology & Laboratory Medicine*, *117*, 1193–1198.

Davis, S., Jones, M., & Kisling, J. (2001). Comparison of normal infants and infants with cystic fibrosis using forced expiratory flows breathing air and heliox. *Pediatric Pulmonology*, *31*, 17–23. doi:10.1002/1099-0496(200101)31:1<17::AID-PPUL1002>3.0.CO;2-8

de Blok, B. M., de Greef, M. H., ten Hacken, N. H., Sprenger, S. R., Postema, K., & Wempe, J. B. (2006). The effects of a lifestyle physical activity counseling program with feedback of a pedometer during pulmonary rehabilitation in patients with COPD: A pilot study. *Patient Education and Counseling*, *61*, 48–55. doi:10.1016/j.pec.2005.02.005

de Bruin, E. D., Hartmann, A., Uebelhart, D., Murer, K., & Zijlstra, W. (2008). Wearable systems for monitoring mobility-related activities in older people: A systematic review. *Clinical Rehabilitation, 22*, 878–895. doi:10.1177/0269215508090675

De Tullio, R., Dottorini, M., et al. (2004). La telemedicina in Pneumologia: I risultati di un questionario in Italia. *Rassegna di Patologia dell'Apparato Respiratorio, 19*, 11–17.

Deans, R., & Wade, S. (2011). Finding a balance between "value added" and feeling valued: revising models of care: The human factor of implementing a quality improvement initiative using Lean methodology within the healthcare sector. *Healthcare Quarterly, 14*(3), 58–61.

Decreto del Presidente della Repubblica. (10 novembre 1997). *Regolamento contenente i criteri e le modalità per la formazione, l'archiviazione e la trasmissione di documenti con strumenti informatici e telematici. A norma dell'articolo 15, comma 2, della legge 15 marzo 1997, n. 59.*

Della Mea, V. (2001). What is e-Health: The death of telemedicine? *Journal of Medicine on the Internet, 3*(2), 22. Retrieved 2001 from http://www.jmir.org/2001/2/e22/

Della Mea, V., Cataldi, P., & Pertoldi, B. (2000). Combining dynamic and static robotic telepathology: A report on 184 consecutive cases of frozen sections, histology and cytology. *Analytical Cellular Pathology, 20*, 33–39.

Dellifraine, J. L., & Dansky, K. H. (2008). Home-based telehealth: A review and meta-analysis. *Journal of Telemedicine and Telecare, 14*(2), 62–66. doi:10.1258/jtt.2007.070709

Department of Economic and Social Affairs (DESA) of the United Nations. (2007). *World economic and social survey 2007: Development in an ageing world.* New York, NY: Author. Retrieved from http://www.un.org/en/development/desa/policy/wess/wess_archive/2007wess.pdf.

Department of Health and Ageing. AU. (2009). *HealthConnect evaluation.* Retrieved October 24, 2011, from http://www.health.gov.au/internet/main/Publishing.nsf/Content/B466CED6B6B1D799CA2577F30017668A/$File/HealthConnect.pdf

Department of Health. (2005). *Building telecare in England.* London, UK: Author.

Department of Health. (2012a). *A concordat between the Department of Health and the telehealth and telecare industry.* London, UK: Author.

Department of Health. (2012b). *COPD commissioning toolkit: A resource for commissioners.* London, UK: Author.

Department of Health. UK. (2004). *Improving chronic disease management.* Retrieved October 24, 2011, from http://www.dh.gov.uk/en/Publicationsandstatistics/Publications/PublicationsPolicyAndGuidance/DH_4075214

Detmer, D. E. (2003). Building the national health information infrastructure for personal health, health care services, public health, and research. *BMC Medical Informatics and Decision Making, 3*(1). eHealth ERA - Towards the Establishment of a European eHealth Research Area. (2007). *Report eHealth priorities and strategies in European countries.* Retrieved October 24, 2011, from http://www.ehealth-era.org/index.htm

Detmer, D. (2000). Information technology for quality health care: a summary of United Kingdom and United States experiences. *Quality in Health Care, 9*, 181–189. doi:10.1136/qhc.9.3.181

Detmer, D. (2001). Transforming health care in the internet era. *World Hospitals and Health Services, 37*, 2.

Dew, K., Cumming, J., McLeod, D., Morgan, S., McKinlay, E., Dowell, A., & Love, T. (2005). Explicit rationing of elective services: Implementing the New Zealand reforms. *Health Policy (Amsterdam), 74*(1), 1–12. doi:10.1016/j.healthpol.2004.12.011

Dhillon, D., & Redington, A. N. (2002). Hypoplastic left heart syndrome. In Anderson, R. H., Baker, E. J., Macartney, F. J., Rigby, M. L., Shinebourne, E. A., & Tynan, M. (Eds.), *Paediatric cardiology* (2nd ed., pp. 1191–1211). Edinburgh, UK: Churchill Livingstone.

Diamandis, P., & Kotler, S. (2012). *Abundance: The future is better than you think.* New York, NY: Free Press, Simon & Schuster, Inc.

Dixon, R., & Stahl, J. (2008). Virtual visits in a general medicine practice: A pilot study. *Telemedicine and e-Health, 14*(6), 525-530.

Donnelly, S. N., Blair, S. N., Jakicic, J. M., & Manore, M. M. (2009). ACSM position stand: Special communication: Appropriate physical activity intervention strategies for weight loss and prevention of weight regain for adults. *Medicine and Science in Sports and Exercise, 41*(2), 459–471. doi:10.1249/MSS.0b013e3181949333

Dowie, R., Mistry, H., Rigby, M., Young, T. A., Weatherburn, G., & Rowlinson, G. (2009). A paediatric telecardiology service for district hospitals in South-East England: An observational study. *Archives of Disease in Childhood, 94*(4), 273–277. doi:10.1136/adc.2008.138495

Dowie, R., Mistry, H., Young, T. A., Franklin, R. C., & Gardiner, H. M. (2008). Cost implications of introducing a telecardiology service to support fetal ultrasound screening. *Journal of Telemedicine and Telecare, 14*(8), 421–426. doi:10.1258/jtt.2008.080401

Drummond, M., Sculpher, M., Torrence, G., O'Brien, B., & Stoddart, G. (Eds.). (2005b). Methods for the economic evaluation of health care programmes (3rd ed.). Oxford, UK: Oxford University Press: Farrell, P. M., Lai, H. J., Li, Z., Kosorok, M. R., Laxova, A., Green, C. G., et al. (2005). Evidence on improved outcomes with early diagnosis of cystic fibrosis through neonatal screening: Enough is enough! The Journal of Pediatrics, 147(3 Suppl), S30-6.

Drummond, M., Sculpher, M., Torrence, G., O'Brien, B., & Stoddart, G. (Eds.). (2005a). *Methods for the economic evaluation of health care programmes* (3rd ed.). Oxford, UK: Oxford University Press.

Dunn, H. L. (1959). High-level wellness for man and society. *American Journal of Public Health and the Nation's Health, 49*(6), 786–792. doi:10.2105/AJPH.49.6.786

Eadie, L. H., Seifalian, A. M., & Davidson, B. R. (2003). Telemedicine in surgery. *British Journal of Surgery, 90*(6), 647–658. doi:10.1002/bjs.4168

Ekeland, A. G., Bowes, A., & Flottorp, S. (2010). Effectiveness of telemedicine: A systematic review of reviews. *International Journal of Medical Informatics, 79*(11), 736–771. doi:10.1016/j.ijmedinf.2010.08.006

Ekeland, A. G., Bowes, A., & Flottorp, S. (2012). Methodologies for assessing telemedicine: A systematic review of reviews. *International Journal of Medical Informatics, 81*, 1–11. doi:10.1016/j.ijmedinf.2011.10.009

Ellison, L. M., Nguyen, M., Fabrizio, M. D., Soh, A., Permpongkosol, S., & Kavoussi, L. R. (2007). Post-operative robotic telerounding: A multicenter randomized assessment of patient outcomes and satisfaction. *Archives of Surgery, 142*(12), 1177–1181. doi:10.1001/archsurg.142.12.1177

Ellison, L. M., Pinto, P. A., Kim, F., Ong, A. M., Patriciu, A., & Stoianovici, D. (2004). Telerounding and patient satisfaction after surgery. *Journal of the American College of Surgeons, 199*(4), 523–530. doi:10.1016/j.jamcollsurg.2004.06.022

Ellis, T. (2008). *Evaluation of the whole system demonstrators - An overview of the key features.* Department of Health.

Emont, S., & Emont, N. (2007). *Advancing eHealth opportunities and challenges for health e-technologies initiative (HETI) NPO, findings for interviews and surveys of opinion leaders and stakeholders.* Princeton, NJ: Robert Wood Johnson Foundation.

ETSI TS 102 812 v.1.2.1. (2003). *Digital video broadcasting (DVB) – Multimedia home platform (MHP)* specification 1.1.1. Retrieved from http://www.etsi.org

European Commission. (2007). *Accelerating the development of the eHealth market in Europe: eHealth Taskforce report 2007.* Retrieved October 24, 2011, from http://ec.europa.eu/enterprise/policies/innovation/policy/lead-market-initiative/ehealth/index_en.htm

European Commission. (2008). *Telemedicine for the benefit of patients, healthcare systems and society.* COM(2008) 689.

European Commission. (2011). Ageing well in the information society action plan. Retrieved October 24, 2011 from http://ec.europa.eu/information_society/activities/einclusion/policy/ageing/action_plan/index_en.htm

European Science Foundation. (2010). *A holistic citizen-centric vision for information and communication technologies to support personal health.* Declaration by the members of the European Science Foundation Exploratory Workshop on Social Care Informatics and Holistic Health Care, Keele University, UK, July 2010. Social Care Informatics meets Health Care Informatics. Retrieved October 24, 2011, from http://iig.umit.at/dokumente/n29.pdf

Eysenbach, G. (2001). What is e-health? *Journal of Medical Internet Research, 3*(2). doi:10.2196/jmir.3.2.e20

Eysenbach, G. (2005). The law of attrition. *Journal of Medical Internet Research, 7*, 11–15. doi:10.2196/jmir.7.1.e11

F.M. (2011). *Sanità, in Italia la spesa IT non decolla.* Retrieved May 3, 2011, from http://www.corrierecomunicazioni.it/

Federanziani, Centre for Economic and International Studies (Ceis) of University of Tor Vergata (Rome), Università Cattolica Sacro Cuore. (2009). *Compendio SIC – Sanità in cifre 2009.* Retrieved from http://www.sanitaincifre.it

Feliciani, F. (2003). Medical care from space: Telemedicine. *ESA Bulletin, 114.*

Fenton, N. E., & Pfleeger, S. L. (1998). *Software metrics: A rigorous and practical approach* (2nd ed.). PWS Publishing Company.

Ferrucci, L., et al. (2001). Linee-Guida sull'Utilizzazione della Valutazione Multidimensionale per l'Anziano Fragile nella Rete dei Servizi. *Giornale di Gerontologia, 49*(Suppl. 11)

Few, S. (2006). *Information dashboard design: The effective visual communication of data* (1st ed.). O'Reilley Media, Inc.

Figueredo, M. V. M., & Dias, J. S. (2004). Mobile telemedicine system for home care and patient monitoring. In *Annual International Conference of the IEEE Engineering in Medicine and Biology Society* (pp. 3387-3390). Piscataway, NJ: IEEE Service Center.

Finch, T., Mort, M., May, C., & Mair, F. (2005). Telecare: Perspectives on the changing role of patients and citizens. *Journal of Telemedicine and Telecare, 11*(1), 51–53. doi:10.1258/1357633054461679

Finkelstein, S. M., Wielinski, C. L., & Kujawa, S. J. (1992). The impact of home monitoring and daily diary recording on patient status in cystic fybrosis. *Pediatric Pulmonology, 12*, 3–10. doi:10.1002/ppul.1950120104

Finkelstein, S., Speedie, S., Demiris, G., Veen, M., & Lundgren, J. (2004). Telehomecare: Quality, perception, satisfaction. *Telemedicine Journal and e-Health, 10*(2), 122–128. doi:10.1089/tmj.2004.10.122

Finley, J. P., Human, D. G., Nanton, M. A., Roy, D. L., Macdonald, R. G., & Marr, D. R. (1989). Echocardiography by telephone--Evaluation of pediatric heart disease at a distance. *The American Journal of Cardiology, 63*(20), 1475–1477. doi:10.1016/0002-9149(89)90011-8

Finley, J. P., Sharratt, G. P., Nanton, M. A., Chen, R. P., Bryan, P., & Wolstenholme, J. (1997). Paediatric echocardiography by telemedicine-Nine years' experience. *Journal of Telemedicine and Telecare, 3*(4), 200–204. doi:10.1258/1357633971931165

Finley, J. P., Warren, A. E., Sharratt, G. P., & Amit, M. (2006). Assessing children's heart sounds at a distance with digital recordings. *Pediatrics, 118*(6), 2322–2325. doi:10.1542/peds.2006-1557

Fiorentino, M., Uva, A. E., & Foglia, M. M. (2011). *Wearable rumble device for active asymmetry measurement and corrections in lower limb mobility.* Paper presented at the IEEE International Symposium on Medical Measurements and Applications (MeMeA 2011).

Fisher, J. B., Alboliras, E. T., Berdusis, K., & Webb, C. L. (1996). Rapid identification of congenital heart disease by transmission of echocardiograms. *American Heart Journal, 131*(6), 1225–1227. doi:10.1016/S0002-8703(96)90103-9

Flume, P. A., O'Sullivan, B. P., & Robinson, K. A. (2007). Cystic fibrosis pulmonary guidelines: Chronic medication for maintenance of lung health. *American Journal of Respiratory and Critical Care Medicine, 176*, 957–969. doi:10.1164/rccm.200705-664OC

Forbess, J. M. (2003). Pre-stage II mortality after the Norwood operation: Addressing the next challenge. *The Journal of Thoracic and Cardiovascular Surgery, 126*(5), 1257–1258. doi:10.1016/S0022-5223(03)01040-7

Fragasso, G., Cuko, A., Spoladore, R., Montano, C., Palloshi, A., & Silipigni, C. (2007). Validation of remote cardiopulmonary examination in patients with heart failure with a videophone-based system. *Journal of Cardiac Failure, 13*(4), 281–286. doi:10.1016/j.cardfail.2007.01.008

Fragasso, G., De Benedictis, M., Palloshi, A., Moltrasio, M., Cappelletti, A., & Carlino, M. (2003). Validation of heart and lung teleauscultation on an internet-based system. *The American Journal of Cardiology, 92*(9), 1138–1139. doi:10.1016/j.amjcard.2003.07.015

Franklin, S., & Graesser, A. (1996). Is it an agent, or just a program? A taxonomy for autonomous agents. *Proceedings of the Third International Workshop on Agent Theories, Architectures, and Languages.* Springer-Verlag. Retrieved from http://www.agent.ai/doc/upload/200302/fran96_1.pdf

Franzini, L., Sail, K. R., Thomas, E. J., & Wueste, L. (2011). Costs and cost-effectiveness of a telemedicine intensive care unit program in 6 intensive care units in a large health care system. *Journal of Critical Care, 26*(3), 329. doi:10.1016/j.jcrc.2010.12.004

Fried, L. P., Borhani, N. O., Enright, P., Furberg, C. D., Gardin, J. M., & Kronmal, R. A. (1991). The Cardiovascular Health Study: design and rationale. *Annals of Epidemiology, 1*(3), 263–276. doi:10.1016/1047-2797(91)90005-W

Fried, L. P., Tangen, C. M., Walston, J., Newman, A. B., Hirsch, C., & Gottdiener, J. (2001). Frailty in older adults: Evidence for a phenotype. Cardiovascular Health Study Collaborative Research Group. *The Journals of Gerontology. Series A, Biological Sciences and Medical Sciences, 56*(3), 146–156. doi:10.1093/gerona/56.3.M146

Friedman, C. P., & Wyatt, J. C. (2001). Publication bias in medical informatics. *Journal of the American Medical Informatics Association, 8,* 189–191. doi:10.1136/jamia.2001.0080189

Fuchs, V. R. (1998). *Who shall live? Health, economics, and social choice.* Singapore: World Scientific. doi:10.1142/3534

Furness, P. N. (1997). The use of digital images in pathology. *The Journal of Pathology, 183,* 15–24. doi:10.1002/(SICI)1096-9896(199711)183:3<253::AID-PATH927>3.0.CO;2-P

Galante, E. (2009). Rehabilitation project and tele-monitoring of patients with mildly deteriorating cognition and their caregivers. *Giornale Italiano di Medicina del Lavoro Ed Ergonomia, 31*(1Suppl A), A64–A67.

Ganter, B. K., Erickson, R. P., Butters, M. A., Takata, J. H., & Noll, S. F. (2005). Clinical evaluation . In DeLisa, J. A. (Eds.), *Physical medicine & rehabilitation: Principles and practice.* Lippincott Williams & Wilkins.

Gartner. (2009). *eHealth for a healthier Europe! – Opportunities for a better use of healthcare resources.* Swedish Presidency of the European Union. Retrieved October 24, 2011, from http://www.regeringen.se/sb/d/574/a/129815

Gaugler, J. E., Davey, A., Pearling, L. I., & Zarit, S. H. (2000). Modeling caregiver adaptation over the time: The longitudinal impact of behavior problems. *Psychology and Aging, 15*(3), 437–450. doi:10.1037/0882-7974.15.3.437

Gensini, G. (2010) Manifesto Italiano della medicina telematica. *Giornate nazionali di studio in medicina telematica.*

Georgoulakis, J., Archondakis, S., & Panayiotides, I. (2011). Study on the reproducibility of thyroid lesions telecytology diagnoses based upon digitized images. *Diagnostic Cytopathology, 39,* 495–499. doi:10.1002/dc.21419

Ghanayem, N. S., Cava, J. R., Jaquiss, R. D., & Tweddell, J. S. (2004). Home monitoring of infants after stage one palliation for hypoplastic left heart syndrome. *Seminars in Thoracic and Cardiovascular Surgery. Pediatric Cardiac Surgery Annual, 7,* 32–38. doi:10.1053/j.pcsu.2004.02.017

Ghanayem, N. S., Hoffman, G. M., Mussatto, K. A., Cava, J. R., Frommelt, P. C., & Rudd, N. A. (2003). Home surveillance program prevents interstage mortality after the Norwood procedure. *The Journal of Thoracic and Cardiovascular Surgery, 126*(5), 1367–1377. doi:10.1016/S0022-5223(03)00071-0

Ghanayem, N. S., Tweddell, J. S., Hoffman, G. M., Mussatto, K., & Jaquiss, R. D. (2006). Optimal timing of the second stage of palliation for hypoplastic left heart syndrome facilitated through home monitoring, and the results of early cavopulmonary anastomosis. *Cardiology in the Young, 16*(1), 61–66. doi:10.1017/S1047951105002349

Gherardi, S., & Strati, A. (Eds.). (2004). *La telemedicina fra tecnologia e organizzazione.* Roma, Italy: Carocci.

Giani, U. (2011). *Measurement, complexity and clinical decision-making.* Paper presented at the IEEE International Symposium on Medical Measurements and Applications (MeMeA 2011).

Gibbs, C. (2000). *TEEMA reference guide version 1.0.* Regina, Canada: TRLabs, Regina.

Gibson, J., Mitton, C., & DuBois-Wing, G. (2011). Priority setting in Ontario's LHINs: Ethics and economics in action. *Healthcare Quarterly, 14*(4), 35–43.

Giorgino, T., Tormene, P., Maggioni, G., Capozzi, D., Quaglini, S., & Pistarini, C. (2009). Assessment of sensorized garments as a flexible support to self-administered post-stroke physical rehabilitation. *European Journal of Physical and Rehabilitative Medicine, 45*, 75–84.

Goh, K. Y., Lam, C. K., & Poon, W. S. (1997). The impact of teleradiology on the inter-hospital transfer of neurosurgical patients. *British Journal of Neurosurgery, 11*, 52–56. doi:10.1080/02688699746708

Goolsby, M. J., & Grubbs, L. (2006). *Advanced assessment: Interpreting findings and formulating differential diagnoses*. Philadelphia, PA: F.A. Davis Company.

Gramegna, L., Tomasi, C., Gasparini, G., Scaboro, G., Zanon, F., & Boaretto, G. (2012). In-hospital follow-up of implantable cardioverter defibrillator and pacemaker carriers: Patients' inconvenience and points of view. A four-hospital Italian survey. *Journal of the Working Groups on Cardiac Pacing, Arrhythmias, and Cardiac Cellular Electrophysiology of the European Society of Cardiology, 14*(3), 345–350. doi:10.1093/europace/eur334

Grant, B. (2006). *The development of telemedicine systems applicable to the diagnosis and monitoring of children with congenital heart disease*. MD: Queen's University Belfast.

Gratton, D. (2003). *Bluetooth profiles, the definitive guide* (1st ed.). Prentice Hall.

Green, S., Hurst, L., Nangle, B., Cunningham, P., Somers, F., & Evans, R. (1997, May). *Agent technology: An overview*. Dublin, Ireland: Department of Computer Science, Trinity College Dublin. Retrieved July 27, 2006, from https://www.cs.tcd.ie/research_groups/aig/iag/pubreview/chap2/chap2.html

Greenes, R. A., & Shortliffe, E. H. (1990). Medical informatics: An emerging academic discipline and institutional priority. *Journal of the American Medical Association, 263*(8), 1114–1120. doi:10.1001/jama.1990.03440080092030

Greer, A. D., Newhook, P., & Sutherland, G. R. (2008). Human-machine interface for robotic surgery and stereotaxy. *IEEE/ ASME Transactions on MRI Compatible Mechatronic Systems, 13*(3), 355-361. Calgary, Canada: Dept. of Clinical Neurosciences, Calgary Univ.

Grigsby, J., Brega, A., & Devore, P. (2005). The evaluation of telemedicine and health services research. *Telemedicine Journal and e-Health, 11*(3), 317–328. doi:10.1089/tmj.2005.11.317

Grisby, J., Kaehney, M. M., Sandberg, E. J., Schlenker, R. E., & Shaughnessy, P. W. (1995). Effects and effectiveness of telemedicine. *Health Care Financing Review, 17*(1), 116–131.

Groene, O., Klazinga, N., Wagner, C., Arah, O. A., Thompson, A., Bruneau, C., & Suñol, R. (2010). Investigating organizational quality improvement systems, patient empowerment, organizational culture, professional involvement and the quality of care in European hospitals: The 'Deepening our Understanding of Quality Improvement in Europe (DUQuE)' project. *BMC Health Services Research, 10*, 281.

Groves, R., & Medtronic. (2007). *Sprint Fidelis® lead patient management recommendations*. Letter Appendix A Oct.

Gulla, V. (2004). *Broadband in Europe: Markets and trends*. Paper presented at the WCIT 2004, Information Technology Conference - Athens 19-21 May 2004.

Gulla, V. (2005). *The telemedicine market: A fast growing technology*. Paper presented at the E-Merging/E-Learning Conference, Dubai 19-21 Nov. 2005.

Gulla, V. (2007). *Tele-medicine is a driver for quality of life improving broadband application*. Paper presented at the 3rd Croatian & International Congress on Telemedicine and e-Health, June 2007

Gulla, V. (2008). Telemedicine potential business models . In Pillai, M. V. (Ed.), *Telemedicine concepts and applications*.

Gulla, V. (2009). How can tele-medicine benefit from broadband technologies? In Khoumbati, K., Dwivedi, Y. K., & Srivastava, A. (Eds.), *Handbook of research on advances in health informatics and electronic healthcare applications: Global adoption and impact of information communication technologies.* Hershey, PA: IGI Global. doi:10.4018/978-1-60566-030-1.ch006

Gurman, T. A., Rubin, S. E., & Roess, A. A. (2012). Effectiveness of mHealth behavior change communication interventions in developing countries: A systematic review of the literature. *Journal of Health Communication, 17*(1), 82–104. doi:10.1080/10810730.2011.649160

Hackos, J. T., & Redish, J. C. (1998). *User and task analysis for interface design.* New York, NY: John Wiley & Sons, Inc.

Hägglund, M., Chen, R., & Koch, S. (2011). Modeling shared care plans using CONTsys and openEHR to support shared home care of elderly. *Journal of the American Medical Informatics Association, 18*(1), 66–69. doi:10.1136/jamia.2009.000216

Hägglund, M., Henkel, M., Zdravkovic, J., Johannesson, P., Rising, I., Krakau, I., & Koch, S. (2010). A new approach for goal-oriented analysis of healthcare processes. *Studies in Health Technology and Informatics, 160*, 1251–1255.

Hägglund, M., Scandurra, I., & Koch, S. (2010). Scenarios to capture work processes in shared homecare - From analysis to application. *International Journal of Medical Informatics, 79*(6), e126–e134. doi:10.1016/j.ijmedinf.2008.07.007

Hailey, D., Ohinmaa, A., & Roine, R. (2004). Published evidence on the success of telecardiology: A mixed record. *Journal of Telemedicine and Telecare, 10*(1), 36–38. doi:10.1258/1357633042614195

Hall, D. (2007). *How much does a good wellness program cost?* Clackamas, OR: Wellsource, Inc. Retrieved June 25, 2012, from http://www.google.ca/url?sa=t&rct=j&q=wellness%20improvement%20program%20price&source=web&cd=2&ved=0CGEQFjAB&url=http%3A%2F%2Fwww.wellsource.com%2Fsite%2Fdownload%2Fasset%2F16%2F10%2F92%2Fc569ea541b1e4b1f39957cf6aa5f1478&ei=wtLoT9rkO6ec2QXDvpHmCg&usg=AFQj

Hanan, J., & Cronin, K. (2011). *Helping nurse managers effectively lead change.* Madison, WI: Howick Associates.

Harnett, B. (2006). Telemedicine systems and telecommunications. *Journal of Telemedicine and Telecare, 12*(1), 4–15. doi:10.1258/135763306775321416

Haughton, J. (2011). Year of the underdog: Cloud-based EHRs. *Health Management Technology, 32*(1), 9.

Hauser, R. G., Hayes, D. L., & Epstein, A. E. (2006). Multicenter experience with failed and recalled implantable cardioverter-defibrillator pulse generators. *Heart Rhythm, 3*(6), 640–644. doi:10.1016/j.hrthm.2006.02.011

Hauser, R. G., & Kallinen, L. (2004). Deaths associated with implantable cardioverter defibrillator failure and deactivation reported in the United States Food and Drug Administration manufacturer and user facility device experience database. *Heart Rhythm, 1*(4), 399–405. doi:10.1016/j.hrthm.2004.05.006

Hayrinen, K., Saranto, K., & Nykanen, P. (2008). Definition, structure, content, use and impacts of electronic health records: A review of the research literature. *International Journal of Medical Informatics, 77*, 291–304. doi:10.1016/j.ijmedinf.2007.09.001

Hebert, M. A., Paquin, M. J., & Whitten, L. (2007). Analysis of the suitability of "video-visits" for palliative home care: Implications for practice. *Journal of Telemedicine and Telecare, 13*, 74–78. doi:10.1258/135763307780096203

Hersh, W. R. (2003). *Information retrieval: A health and biomedical perspective.* New York, NY: Springer.

Hersh, W. R., Wallace, J. A., Patterson, P. K., Shapiro, S. E., Kraemer, D. F., & Eilers, G. M. (2001). Telemedicine for the Medicare population: Pediatric, obstetric, and clinician-indirect home interventions. *Evidence Report/technology Assessment, 24*, 1–32.

Hickey, K. T., Reiffel, J., Sciacca, R. R., Whang, W., Biviano, A., & Baumeister, M. (2010). The utility of ambulatory electrocardiographic monitoring for detecting silent arrhythmias and clarifying symptom mechanism in an urban elderly population with heart failure and hypertension: Clinical implications. *Journal of Atrial Fibrillation, 1*(12), 663–674. doi:10.4022/jafib.v1i12.567

Higgs, G. (1999). Investigating trends in rural health outcomes: A research agenda. *Geoforum, 30*(3), 203–221. doi:10.1016/S0016-7185(99)00021-4

Hillestad, R., & Bigelow, J. (2011). *Can HIT lower costs and raise quality?* Santa Monica, CA: Rand Health, Health Information Technology.

Hintz, S. R., Kendrick, D. E., Vohr, B. R., Poole, W. K., Higgins, R. D., & National Institute of Child Health and Human Development Neonatal Research Network. (2005). Changes in neurodevelopmental outcomes at 18 to 22 months' corrected age among infants of less than 25 weeks' gestational age born in 1993-1999. Pediatrics, 115(6), 1645-1651.

Historical, L. A. Q. (1997).. . *Medicine and Science in Sports and Exercise, 29*, 43–45.

Holden, M. K. (2005). Virtual environments for motor rehabilitation [Review]. *Cyberpsychology & Behavior, 8*(3). doi:10.1089/cpb.2005.8.187

Holtzman, H., Goubran, R., & Knoefel, F. (2011). *Maximal ratio combining for respiratory effort extraction from pressure sensor arrays.* Paper presented at the IEEE International Symposium on Medical Measurements and Applications (MeMeA 2011).

Hook, J., Pearlstein, J., Samarth, A., & Cusack, C. (2009). *AHRQ reports that there are more than a million medical injuries and over 100,000 deaths due the medication errors.* Melbourne, Australia: State Government of Victoria.

Horbinski, C., & Wiley, C. A. (2009). Comparison of telepathology systems in neuropathological intraoperative consultations. *Journal of Neuropathology, 19*(2), 317–322.

Hort, J., & Brien, O, J. T., Gainotti, G., et al. (2010). EFNS guidelines for the diagnosis and management of Alzheimer's disease. *European Journal of Neurology, 17*, 1236–1248. doi:10.1111/j.1468-1331.2010.03040.x

Hsiao, J. L., & Oh, D. H. (2008). The impact of store-and-forward teledermatology on skin cancer diagnosis and treatment. *Journal of the American Academy of Dermatology, 59*(2), 260–267. doi:10.1016/j.jaad.2008.04.011

Hufnagl, P., & Schluns, K. (2008). Virtual microscopy and routine diagnostics: A discussion paper. *The Journal of Pathology, 29*(2), 250–254. doi:10.1007/s00292-008-1093-0

Hughes-Anderson, W., Rankin, S., & House, J. (2002). Open access endoscopy in rural and remote Western Australia: Does it work? *ANZ Journal of Surgery, 72*, 699–703. doi:10.1046/j.1445-2197.2002.02535.x

Hurley, J., Birch, S., & Eyles, J. (1995). Geographically-decentralized planning and management in health care: Some informational issues and their implications for efficiency. *Social Science & Medicine, 41*(1), 3–11. doi:10.1016/0277-9536(94)00283-Y

Husain, O. A., Butler, E. B., & Evans, D. M. D. (1974). Quality control in cervical cytology. *Journal of Clinical Pathology, 27*, 935–944. doi:10.1136/jcp.27.12.935

Ichimura, T., & Yoshida, K. (2004). *Knowledge-based intelligent systems for healthcare* (Howlett, R. J., & Jain, L. C., Eds.). 1st ed., *Vol. 7*). Adelaide, Australia: Advanced Knowledge International Pty Ltd.

Igo, F. J., Jr. (2007, September 12). *Concordia.* Mitsubishi Electric Research Laboratories. Retrieved July 30, 2012, from http://www.merl.com/projects/concordia/

Ikkersheim, D. E., & Koolman, X. (2012). Dutch health-care reform: did it result in better patient experiences in hospitals? A comparison of the consumer quality index over time. *BMC Health Services Research, 12*, 76. doi:10.1186/1472-6963-12-76

Inglis, S., Clark, R., McAlister, F., Ball, J., Lewinter, C., & Cullington, D. (2010). Structured telephone support or telemonitoring programmes for patients with chronic heart failure. *Cochrane Database of Systematic Reviews, 8*.

Innes, M., Skelton, J., & Greenfield, S. (2006). A profile of communication in primary care physician telephone consultations: Application of the Roter Interaction Analysis System. *The British Journal of General Practice, 56*(526), 363–368.

Jacklin, P. B., Roberts, J. A., Wallace, P., Haines, A., Harrison, R., & Barber, J. A. (2003). Virtual outreach: Economic evaluation of joint teleconsultations for patients referred by their general practitioner for a specialist opinion. *British Medical Journal, 327*(7406), 84. doi:10.1136/bmj.327.7406.84

Johnson, F., Cooke, L., Croker, H., & Wardle, J. (2008). Changing perceptions of weight Great Britain: Comparison of two population surveys. *British Medical Journal, 337*, 494. doi:10.1136/bmj.a494

Jones, S., & Edwards, R. T. (2010). Diabetic retinopathy screening: A systematic review of the economic evidence. *Diabetic Medicine, 27*(3), 249–256. doi:10.1111/j.1464-5491.2009.02870.x

Joseph, V., West, R., Shickle, D., Keen, J., & Clamp, S. (2011). Key challenges in the development and implementation of Telehealth projects. *Journal of Telemedicine and Telecare, 17*(2), 71–77. doi:10.1258/jtt.2010.100315

Junho, S. (2005). Roadmap for e-commerce standardization in Korea. *International Journal of IT Standards and Standardization Research, 3*(2).

Justo, R., Smith, A. C., Williams, M., Van der Westhuyzen, J., Murray, J., & Sciuto, G. (2004). Paediatric telecardiology services in queensland: A review of three years' experience. *Journal of Telemedicine and Telecare, 10*(1), 57–60. doi:10.1258/1357633042614258

Kabachinski, J. (2011). What's the forecast for cloud computing in healthcare? *Biomedical Instrumentation & Technology, 45*(2), 146–150. doi:10.2345/0899-8205-45.2.146

Kaffash, J. (2012, April 20). *Telemedicine 'trebles death rate' in elderly patients*. Retrieved June 26, 2012, from http://www.pulsetoday.co.uk/newsarticle-content/-/article_display_list/13803303/telemedicine-trebles-death-rate-in-elderly-patients

Kahn, J. M., Hill, N. S., Lilly, C. M., Angus, D. C., Jacobi, J., & Rubenfeld, G. D. (2011). The research agenda in ICU telemedicine: A statement from the critical care societies collaborative. *Chest, 140*(1), 230–238. doi:10.1378/chest.11-0610

Karttunen, K., Karppi, P., & Hiltunen, A. (2011). Neuropsychiatric symptoms and quality of life in patients with very mild and mild Alzheimer's disease. *International Journal of Geriatric Psychiatry, 26*, 473–482. doi:10.1002/gps.2550

Kayser, K., Hoshang, S. A., Metze, K., Goldmann, T., Vollmer, E., & Radziszowski, D. (2008). Texture- and object-related automated information analysis in histological still images of various organs. *Journal of Analytical and Quantitative Cytology and Histology, 30*(6), 323–335.

Kemp Bryan, J. (1988). Motivation, rehabilitation and aging: A conceptual model. *Geriatric Rehabilitation, 3*(3), 41–51.

Keyserling, T. C., Samuel-Hodge, C. D., Ammerman, A. S., Ainsworth, B. E., Elasy, T. A., & Henriquez-Roldan, C. F. (2002). A randomized trial of an intervention to improve self-care behaviors of African-American women with type 2 diabetes: Impact on physical activity. *Diabetes Care, 25*(9), 1576–1583. doi:10.2337/diacare.25.9.1576

Kirkley, D., & Stein, M. (2004). *Nursing economics, nurses and clinical technology sources of resistance and strategies for success*.

Kirkup, J. R. (1982). The history and evolution of surgical instruments, II origins: Function: Carriage: manufacture. *Annals of the Royal College of Surgeons of England, 64*(2), 125–132.

Kirkwood, B. R., & Sterne, J. A. (2003). *Essential medical statistics*. Malden, MA: Blackwell Science.

Klapan, I. (2005). *Telemedicine*. Zagreb, Croatia: Telemedicine Association Zagreb.

Klarman, H. E. (1965). *The economics of health*. New York, NY: Columbia University Press.

Kleiboer, A. G. (2010). Monitoring symptoms at home: what methods would cancer patients be comforable using? *Quality of Life Research, 19*, 965–968. doi:10.1007/s11136-010-9662-0

Klem, M. L., Wing, R. R., Mc Guire, M. T., Seagle, H. M., & Hill, J. O. (1997). A descriptive study of individuals successful at long-term maintenances of substantial weight loss. *The American Journal of Clinical Nutrition, 66*(2), 239–246.

Knols, R. H., de Bruin, E. D., Shirato, K., Uebelhart, D., & Aaronson, N. K. (2010). Physical activity interventions to improve daily walking activity in cancer survivors. *BMC Cancer, 10*, 406:1-406:10.

Kobb, R., & Lane, R., & Stallings, D. (2008). E-learning and tele-health: Measuring your success. *Telemedicine and e-Health, 14*(6), 576-579.

Kohn, L. T., Corrigan, J. M., & Donaldson, M. S. (Eds.). (2000). *To err is human: Building a safer health system. Committee on Quality of Health Care in America, Institute of Medicine.* Washington, DC: National Academy Press.

Koss, L. G. (1989). The Papanicolaou test for cervical cancer detection: A triumph and a tragedy. *Journal of the American Medical Association, 261,* 737–743. doi:10.1001/jama.1989.03420050087046

Krupinski, E. A., Patterson, T., Norman, C. D., Roth, Y., El Nasser, Z., & Abdeen, Z. (2011). Successful models for telehealth. [vii-viii]. *Otolaryngologic Clinics of North America, 44*(6), 1275–1288. doi:10.1016/j.otc.2011.08.004

Landis, J. R., & Koch, G. G. (1977). The measurement of observer agreement for categorical data. *Biometrics, 33,* 159–174. doi:10.2307/2529310

Lane, K. (2006). Telemedicine news. *Telemedicine and e-Health, 12*(5), 507-511.

Lareng, L. (2002). Telemedicine in Europe. *European Journal of Internal Medicine, 13,* 1–13. doi:10.1016/S0953-6205(01)00188-1

Latifi, R., Dasho, E., Lecaj, I., Latifi, K., Bekteshi, F., & Hadeed, M. (2012). Beyond "initiate-build-operate-transfer" strategy for creating sustainable telemedicine programs: Lesson from the first decade. *Telemedicine Journal and e-Health, 18*(5), 388–390. doi:10.1089/tmj.2011.0263

Lauterborn, J. (2011). *Technology assessment and requirements analysis helps put medical facilities back on track.* United States Army Online.

Lazarus, A. (2007). Remote, wireless, ambulatory monitoring of implantable pacemakers, cardioverter defibrillators, and cardiac resynchronization systems: Analysis of a worldwide database. *Pacing and Clinical Electrophysiology, 30,* S2–S12. doi:10.1111/j.1540-8159.2007.00595.x

Leach, L. S., & Christensen, H. (2006). A systematic review of telephone-based interventions for mental disorders. *Journal of Telemedicine and Telecare, 12*(3), 122–129. doi:10.1258/135763306776738558

Lee, S. Y., Weiner, B. J., Harrison, M. I., & Belden, C. M. (2012). Organizational transformation: A systematic review of empirical research in health care and other industries. *Medical Care Research Review,* Online first.

Lee, I.-M. (2010). Physical activity and cardiac protection. *Exercise is . Medicine, 9*(4), 214–219.

Leiva, M. T. G., Starks, M., & Tambini, D. (2006). Overview of digital television switchover policy in Europe, the United States and Japan. *Info: The Journal of Policy, Regulation and Strategy for Telecommunication, Information and Media, 8*(3), 32-46. ISSN 1463-6697

Lembo, D., Lenzerini, M., & Rosati, R. (2002). Source inconsistency and incompleteness in data integration. *Proceeding of the 2002 International Workshop on Description Logics (DL2002),* Toulouse.

Lenzerini, M. (2002). Data integration: A theoretical perspective. *Proceeding of the 21st ACM SIGMOD-SIGACT-SIGART Symposium Principle of Database Systems,* Madison, Wisconsin.

Leong, F. J., Graham, A. K., & Schwarzmann, P. (2000). Clinical trial of telepathology as an alternative modality in breast histopathology quality assurance. *Journal of Telemedicine and E-Health, 6,* 373–377. doi:10.1089/15305620050503834

Leung, R. C. (2012). Health information technology and dynamic capabilities. *Health Care Management Review, 37*(1), 43–53. doi:10.1097/HMR.0b013e31823c9b55

Levesque, L., Cossette, S., & Lachance, L. (1998). Predictor of psychological well-behing of primary caregivers living with a demented relatives: A 1-year follow-up study. *Journal of Applied Gerontology, 17*(2), 240–258. doi:10.1177/073346489801700211

Lewin, K. (1951). *Field theory in social science.* New York, NY: Harper &Row.

Lewin, M., Xu, C., Jordan, M., Borchers, H., Ayton, C., & Wilbert, D. (2006). Accuracy of paediatric echocardiographic transmission via telemedicine. *Journal of Telemedicine and Telecare, 12*(8), 416–421. doi:10.1258/135763306779378636

Liker, J. (2004). *The Toyota way.* New York, NY: McGraw-Hill.

Lin, C. S., Shi, T. H., Lin, C. H., Yeh, M. S., & Shei, H. J. (2006). The measurement of the angle of a user's head in a novel head-tracker device. *Measurements*, *39*, 750–757.

Lo, B., Thiemjarus, S., King, R., & Yang, G.-Z. (2005). Body sensor network – A wireless sensor platform for pervasive healthcare monitoring. *Proceedings of the International Conference on Pervasive Computing.*

Loane, M. A., Bloomer, S. E., Corbett, R., Eedy, D. J., Hicks, N., & Lotery, H. E. (2000). A randomized controlled trial to assess the clinical effectiveness of both realtime and store-and-forward teledermatology compared with conventional care. *Journal of Telemedicine and Telecare*, *6*(Suppl 1), S1–S3. doi:10.1258/1357633001933952

Loh, P., Donaldson, M., Flicker, L., Maher, S., & Goldswain, P. (2007). Development of a telemedicine protocol for the diagnosis of Alzheimer's disease. *Journal of Telemedicine and Telecare*, *13*(2), 90–94. doi:10.1258/135763307780096159

Lorussi, F., Tognetti, A., Tescioni, M., Zupone, G., Bartalesi, R., & De Rossi, D. (2005). Electroactive fabrics for distributed, confortable and interactive systems. In C. D. Nugent (Ed.), *Technology and Informatics, Vol. 117: Personalized health management systems*. IOS Press.

Lorussi, F., Scilingo, E. P., Tesconi, M., Tognetti, A., & De Rossi, D. (2005). Strain sensing fabric for hand posture and gesture monitoring. *IEEE Transactions on Information Technology in Biomedicine*, *9*(3). doi:10.1109/TITB.2005.854510

Lum, M. J. H., Trimble, D., Rosen, J., Fodero, K., II, King, H. H., & Sankaranarayanan, G. ... Hannaford, B. (2006). Multidisciplinary approach for developing a new minimally invasive surgical robotic system. In *Proceedings of IEEE/RAS-EMBS International Conference on Biomedical Robotics and Biomechatronics* (pp. 1018-1022). Pisa, Italy: Scuola Superiore S'Anna.

Lundbergh, G. D. (1989). Quality assurance in cervical cytology: The Papanicolaou smear. *Journal of the American Medical Association*, *262*, 1672–1679. doi:10.1001/jama.1989.03430120126035

Luo, X., Kenyon, R., Kline, T., Waldinger, H., & Kamper, D. (2005). *An augmented reality training environment for post-stroke finger extension rehabilitation*. Paper presented at the IEEE 9th International Conference on Rehabilitation Robotics, Chicago, IL.

Mabo, P., Victor, F., Bazin, P., Ahres, S., Babuty, D., & Da Costa, A. (2011). A randomized trial of long-term remote monitoring of pacemaker recipients (the COMPAS trial). *European Heart Journal*, *33*(9), 1105–1111. doi:10.1093/eurheartj/ehr419

Maclean, N. (2000). The concept of patient motivation: A qualitative analysis of stroke professionals' attitudes. *Stroke*, *33*, 444–448. doi:10.1161/hs0202.102367

Maes, P., Guttman, R., & Moukas, A. (1999, March). Agent that buy and sell: Transforming commerce as we know it. *Communications of the ACM*, *42*(3), 81–91. doi:10.1145/295685.295716

Maglaveras, N., Chouvarda, I., Koutkias, V., Lekka, I., Tsakali, M., & Tsetoglou, S. ... Balas, E. A. (2003). Citizen centered health and lifestyle management via interactive TV: The PANACEIA-ITV health system. *AMIA Annuual Symposium Proceedings*, (pp. 415-419).

Magno, C. E., Cosi, P., & Cavicchio, P. (2007). Interfacce multimodali per l'E-Learning . In Delogu, C. (Ed.), *Tecnologie per il weblearning: realtà e scenari* (pp. 173–183). Firenze, Italy: Florence University Press.

Magrabi, F., Lovell, N. H., & Henry, R. L. (2005). Designing home telecare: A case study in monitoring cystic fibrosis. *Telemedicine Journal and e-Health*, *11*, 707–719. doi:10.1089/tmj.2005.11.707

Maheu, M. M., Whitten, P., & Allen, A. (2001). *E-Health, telehealth, and telemedicine: A guide to start-up and success* (1st ed.). San Francisco, CA: Jossey-Bass.

Mahoney, D. F., Tarlow, B. J., & Jones, R. N. (2003). Effects of an automated telephone support system on caregiver burden and anxiety: Findings from the REACH for TLC intervention study. *The Gerontologist*, *43*(4), 556–567. doi:10.1093/geront/43.4.556

Mahoney, D. M., Tarlow, B., Jones, R. N., Tennstedt, S., & Kasten, L. (2001). Factors affecting the use of a telephone-based intervention for caregivers of people with Alzheimer's disease. *Journal of Telemedicine and Telecare*, *7*(3), 139–148. doi:10.1258/1357633011936291

Mancia, G., & De Backer, G. (2007). The Task Force for the Management of Arterial Hypertension of the European Society of Hypertension (ESH) and of the European Society of Cardiology (ESC). *European Heart Journal*, *28*, 462–1536. doi:doi:10.1093/eurheartj/ehm236

Manning, J. (2011). Priority-setting processes for medicines: The United Kingdom, Australia and New Zealand. *Journal of Law and Medicine*, *18*(3), 439–452.

Marescaux, J., Leroy, J., Rubino, F., Smith, M., Vix, M., Simone, M., & Mutter, D. (2002). Transcontinental robot-assisted remote telesurgery: Feasibility and potential applications. *Annals of Surgery*, *235*(4), 487–492. doi:10.1097/00000658-200204000-00005

Marino, B. S. (2002). Outcomes after the Fontan procedure. *Current Opinion in Pediatrics*, *14*(5), 620–626. doi:10.1097/00008480-200210000-00010

Martens, R., Hu, W., Liu, A., Mahovsky, J., Saenchai, K., Schauenberg, T., et al. (2001). *TEEMA TRLabs execution environment for mobile agents*. Telecommunication Research and Laboratories (TRLabs) Regina. Regina, Canada: Telecommunication Research and Laboratories (TRLabs) Regina.

Maternaghan, C., & Turner, K. J. (2010). A component framework for telecare and home automation. In *Proceedings of the 7th IEEE Consumer Communications and Networking Conference*.

Matthews, D., & Farewell, V. T. (2007). *Using and understanding medical statistics*. Basel, Switzerland: Karger.

Mattioli, L., Goertz, K., Ardinger, R., Belmont, J., Cox, R., & Thomas, C. (1992). Pediatric cardiology: Auscultation from 280 miles away. Kansas Medicine . *The Journal of the Kansas Medical Society*, *93*(12), 326, 347–350.

Mattoscio, N., & Colantonio, E. (2003). La valutazione contingente quale strumento per la determinazione di un ticket prestazionale. *Il Risparmio, 3.*

May, C., Finch, T., Mair, F., Ballini, L., Dowrick, C., & Eccles, M. (2007). Understanding the implementation of complex interventions in health care: the normalization process model. *BMC Health Services Research*, *7*(148).

May, C., Harrison, R., & Finch, T. (2003). Understanding the normalisation of telemedicine services through qualitative evaluation. *Journal of the American Medical Informatics Association*, *10*, 596–604. doi:10.1197/jamia.M1145

May, C., Harrison, R., MacFarlane, A., Williams, T., Mair, F., & Wallace, P. (2003). Why do telemedicine systems fail to normalize as stable models of service delivery? *Journal of Telemedicine and Telecare*, *9*, 25–26. doi:10.1258/135763303322196222

McBrien, P., & Poulovassilis, A. (2003). Data integration by bi-directional schema transformation rules. *Proceeding of the 19th International Conference Data Eng. (ICDE'03).*

McConnell, M. E., Steed, R. D., Tichenor, J. M., & Hannon, D. W. (1999). Interactive telecardiology for the evaluation of heart murmurs in children. *Telemedicine Journal: The Official Journal of the American Telemedicine Association*, *5*(2), 157–161.

McCrossan, B. A. (2008). *Questmark*. Personal communication.

McCrossan, B. A. (2009). *Little hearts matter*. Personal communication.

McCrossan, B. A. (2009). *Tiny life*. Personal communication.

McCrossan, B. A. (2009). *The role of telemedicine in paediatric cardiology. Unpublished Medical Doctorate*. Belfast, Belfast: Queen's University.

McCrossan, B. A., Sands, A. J., Kileen, T., Cardwell, C. R., & Casey, F. A. (2011). Fetal diagnosis of congenital heart disease by telemedicine. *Archives of Disease in Childhood. Fetal and Neonatal Edition*, *96*(6), F394–F397. doi:10.1136/adc.2010.197202

McElhinney, D. B., & Wernovsky, G. (2001). Outcomes of neonates with congenital heart disease. *Current Opinion in Pediatrics*, *13*(2), 104–110. doi:10.1097/00008480-200104000-00003

McLean, S., Chandler, D., Nurmatov, U., Liu, J., Pagliari, C., & Car, J. (2010). *Telehealthcare for asthma (review). The Cochrane Collaboration.* John Wiley & Sons, Ltd.

McLean, S., Nurmatov, U., Liu, J. L., Pagliari, C., Car, J., & Sheikh, A. (2011). Telehealthcare for chronic obstructive pulmonary disease. *Cochrane Database of Systematic Reviews, 7,* CD007718.

McLean, T. R., & McLean, P. B. (2007). Is a black market in telemedicine on the horizon? *International Journal of Medical Robotics and Computer Assisted Surgery, 3*(4), 291–296. doi:10.1002/rcs.167

MD PnP. (2009). *Advancing the adoption of medical device plug-and-play interoperability to improve patient safety and healthcare efficiency. Center for Integration of Medicine and Innovative Technology, Partners Healthcare.* Massachusetts General Hospital, National Academic Press.

Melamed, M. R. (1976). Quality control in the cytology laboratory. *Acta Cytologica, 20,* 203–206.

Melanson, E. L., Knoll, J. R., & Bell, M. L. (2004). Commercially available pedometers: Consideration for accurate step counting. *Preventive Medicine, 39*(2), 361–368. doi:10.1016/j.ypmed.2004.01.032

Melendreras-Ruiz, R. (2008), ImplanTDT: Usability laboratory, real user DTT monitoring platform and MHP-based services. In *Proceedings of the 5th IEEE Consumer Communications and Networking Conference.*

Mencarelli, R., Marcolongo, A., & Gasparetto, A. (2008). Organizational model for a telepathology system. *Journal of Diagnostic Pathology, 15*(3), S7.

Merell, R., & Doarn, C. (2008). Is it time for a telemedicine breakthrough? *Telemedicine and e-Health, 14*(6), 505-506.

Merrett, G. V., Ettabib, M. A., Peters, C., Hallett, G., & White, N. M. (2010). Augmenting forearm crutches with wireless sensors for lower limb rehabilitation. *Measurement Science & Technology, 21.*

Meystre, S. (2005). The current state of telemonitoring: A comment on the literature. *Telemedicine Journal and e-Health, 11,* 63–69. doi:10.1089/tmj.2005.11.63

Michailidis, G. D., Simpson, J. M., Karidas, C., & Economides, D. L. (2001). Detailed three-dimensional fetal echocardiography facilitated by an internet link. Ultrasound in Obstetrics & Gynecology . *The Official Journal of the International Society of Ultrasound in Obstetrics and Gynecology, 18*(4), 325–328. doi:10.1046/j.0960-7692.2001.00520.x

Miller, E. A. (2001). Telemedicine and doctor–patient communication: An analytical survey of the literature. *Journal of Telemedicine and Telecare, 7,* 1–17. doi:10.1258/1357633011936075

Miller, J. W. (2005). Wellness: The history and development of a concept. *Spektrum Freizeit, 1,* 84–102.

Ming, D., Liu, X., Dai, Y., & Wan, B. (2009). *Indirect biomechanics measurement on shoulder joint moments of walker-assisted gait.* Paper presented at the IEEE Int. Conf. on Virtual Environments, Human-Computer Interfaces, and Measurement Systems, Hong Kong, China, May 11-13.

Ministero della salute, Dipartimento della qualità. (2011). *Sicurezza dei pazienti e gestione del rischio clinico: Manuale per la formazione degli operatori sanitari.* Retrieved from http://www.salute.gov.it/imgs/C_17_pubblicazioni_640_allegato.pdf

Mirelman, A., Mentzakis, E., Kinter, E., Paolucci, F., Fordham, R., & Ozawa, S. (2012). Decision-making criteria among national policymakers in five countries: A discrete choice experiment eliciting relative preferences for equity and efficiency. *Value in Health, 15*(3), 534–539. doi:10.1016/j.jval.2012.04.001

Mishan, E. J. (1971). Evaluation of life and limb: A theoretical approach. *The Journal of Political Economy, 79,* 687. doi:10.1086/259784

Mistiaen, P., & Poot, E. (2006). Telephone follow-up, initiated by a hospital-based health professional, for post-discharge problems in patients discharged from hospital to home. *Cochrane Database of Systematic Reviews, 4,* CD004510.

MIT. (2010). *Healthcare business models and operations strategy: A comparative study of Cleveland Clinic and CVS Minute Clinic 15.768: Operations management in the services sector.* Cambridge, MA: MIT.

Mitchell, H., Medley, G., & Drake, M. (1988). Quality control measures for cervical cytology laboratories. *Acta Cytologica, 32*, 288–292.

Mitchell, J. (1999). *From telehealth to e-health: the unstoppable rise of e-health*. Canberra, Australia: National Office for the Information Technology.

Mitchell, J. (2000). Increasing the cost-effectiveness of telemedicine by embracing e-health. *Journal of Telemedicine and Telecare, 1*(6), 16–19. doi:10.1258/1357633001934500

Miyasaka, K., Suzuki, Y., Sakai, H., & Kondo, Y. (1997). Interactive communication in high-technology home care: Videophones for pediatric ventilatory care. *Pediatrics, 99*(1), E1. doi:10.1542/peds.99.1.e1

Moffatt, J. J., & Eley, D. S. (2003). Barriers to the up-take of telemedicine in Australia – A view from providers. *British Journal of Surgery, 90*(6), 647–658.

Mohon, R. T., Wagener, J. S., & Abman, S. H. (1993). Relationship of genotype to early pulmonary function in infants with cystic fibrosis identified through neonatal screening. *The Journal of Pediatrics, 122*, 550–555. doi:10.1016/S0022-3476(05)83534-6

Monitor Group and the Financial Times. (2011). *Telemedicine market shares, strategies, and forecasts, worldwide, 2010 to 2016*. Cambridge, MA: Author.

Monk, A. F. (2000). User-centred design. *Proceedings of the IFIP TC9 WG9.3 International Conference on Home Oriented Informatics and Telematics, "IF at Home: Virtual Influences on Everyday Life": Information, Technology and Society*, (pp. 181-190).

Moore, D., Green, J., Jay, S., Leist, J., & Maitland, F. (1994). Creating a new paradigm for CME: Seizing opportunities within the health care revolution. *The Journal of Continuing Education in the Health Professions, 14*, 4–31. doi:10.1002/chp.4750140102

Moreno, L., Dale, S., Chen, A., & Magee, C. (2009). Costs to Medicare of the informatics for diabetes education and telemedicine (IDEATel) home telemedicine demonstration: Findings from an independent evaluation. *Diabetes Care, 32*(7), 1202–1204. doi:10.2337/dc09-0094

Morris, S., & Smith-Chaigneau, A. (2005). *Interactive TV standards: A guide to MHP, OCAP and Java TV*. Focal Press.

Mostarac, P., Malaric, R., Jurčević, M., Hegeduš, H., Lay-Ekuakille, A., & Vergallo, P. (2011). *System for monitoring and fall detection of patients using mobile 3-axis accelerometers sensors*. Paper presented at the IEEE International Symposium on Medical Measurements and Applications (MeMeA 2011).

Moura, A., & Del Giglio, A. (2000). Education via internet. *Revista da Associação Médica Brasileira, 46*(1), 47–51.

Mourouzis, A., Boutsakis, E., Ntoa, S., Antona, M., & Stephanidis, C. (2007). An accessible and usable soft keyboard. *Human-Computer Interaction, 6*, 961–970.

Mulholland, H. C., Casey, F., Brown, D., Corrigan, N., Quinn, M., & McCord, B. (1999). Application of a low cost telemedicine link to the diagnosis of neonatal congenital heart defects by remote consultation. *Heart (British Cardiac Society), 82*(2), 217–221.

Mun, S. K., Esayed, A. M., & Tohme, W. G. (1995). Teleradiology/telepathology requirements and implementation. *Journal of Medical Systems, 19*, 15–164. doi:10.1007/BF02257066

Murgia, F., Cilli, M., Renzetti, E., Popa, N., Romano, T., Alghisi, F., & Bella, S. (2010). Valutazione economica del telemonitoraggio domiciliare in malattie polmonari croniche. *La Clinica Terapeutica, 162*(2), e43–e48.

Murphy, R. L., Block, P., Bird, K. T., & Yurchak, P. (1973). Accuracy of cardiac auscultation by microwave. *Chest, 63*(4), 578–581. doi:10.1378/chest.63.4.578

Murray, E., May, C., Mair, F., & Rocket Science, U. K. Ltd. (2010). *E-health implementation toolkit (e-HIT): A guide for senior managers to implement e-health initiatives in the NHS*. UCL, SDO, University of Glasgow, Newcastle University.

Myers, A. M., Holliday, P. J., Harvey, K. A., & Hutchinson, K. S. (1993). Functional performance measures: Are they superior to self-assessments? *Journal of Gerontology, 48*, M196–M206. doi:10.1093/geronj/48.5.M196

Naccarella, F., Sun, L., Zhou, S., et al. (2012). *2012 Beijing Workshop in collaboration with Embassy of Italy*. Euro China Society for Health Research and Dao Health Care Management Company.

Nace, D. K., & Gartland, J. (2011). *Providing accountability: Accountable care concepts for providers*. Relay Health. Retrieved October 24, 2011 from http://healthsystemcio.com/white-papers/providing-accountability-aco-concepts-for-providers/

Nagy, G. K., & Newton, L. E. (2006). Cytopathology proficiency testing: Where do we go from here? *Diagnostic Cytopathology*, *34*, 257–264. doi:10.1002/dc.20361

Nannings, B., & Abu-Hanna, A. (2006). Decision support telemedicine systems: A conceptual model and reusable templates. *Telemedicine and e-Health*, *12*(6), 644-654.

National Health Service. (n.d.). Paediatric cardiology. Retrieved March 12, 2012, from http://www.nhscareers.nhs.uk/details/Default.aspx?Id=593

National Institute for Health and Clinical Excellence. (2008). *Guide to the methods of technology appraisal*. London, UK: National Institute for Health and Clinical Excellence.

Neri, M., Bonati, P. A., & Pinelli, M. (2007). Biological, psychological and clinical markers of caregiver's stress in impaired elderly with dementia and age relate disease. *Archives of Gerontology and Geriatrics*, *1*, 289–194. doi:10.1016/j.archger.2007.01.038

NHS - Medical Careers. (2009). Paediatric cardiology. Retrieved from http://www.medicalcareers.nhs.uk/SpecialtyPages/Medicine/Paediatriccardiology/Pages/default.aspx

Nielsen, J. (2005). *UseIT*. Retrieved from. http://www.useit.com

Nielson, J. (2005, April 11). *Medical usability: How to kill patients through bad design*. Retrieved July 8, 2009, from http://www.useit.com/alertbox/20050411.html

Nobili, A., Riva, E., & Tettamanti, M. (2004). The effect of a structured intervention on caregivers of patients with dementia and problem behaviors: A Randomized controlled pilot study. *Alzheimer Disease and Associated Disorders*, *18*, 75–82. doi:10.1097/01.wad.0000126618.98867.fc

Norman, D. A. (1986). *User centered system design*. Hillsdale, NJ: Lawrence Erlbaum Associates.

Norman, D. A. (2005). *Emotional design*. Milano, Italy: Apogeo.

Nucita, A., Bernava, G. M., Bartolo, M., Di Pane Masi, F., Peroni, M., Pizzimenti, G., & Palombi, L. (2009). A global approach to the management of EMR (Electronic Medical Records) of patients with HIV/AIDS in Sub-Saharan Africa: The experience of DREAM Software. *BMC Journal of Medical Informatics and Decision Making*, *9*(42).

Nuti, F. (1998). *Introduzione all'economia sanitaria e alla valutazione economica delle decisioni sanitarie* (Giappichelli, G., Ed.). Torino.

OECD-NSF. (2011). *Building a smarter health and wellness future*. Summary of main workshop messages, Washington, 15-16 February 2011. Retrieved October 24, 2011 from http://www.oecd.org/sti/smarterhealth

Oh, H., Rizo, C., Enkin, M., Jadad, A., Powell, J., & Pagliari, C. (2005). What is eHealth (3): A systematic review of published definitions. *Journal of Medical Internet Research*, *7*(e1). doi:10.2196/jmir.7.1.e1

Ohman, A., Stromvall-Larsson, E., Nilsson, B., & Mellander, M. (2012). Pulse oximetry home monitoring in infants with single-ventricle physiology and a surgical shunt as the only source of pulmonary blood flow. Cardiology in the Young, online before print, 1-7.

OSGI. (2012). *OSGi Alliance*. Retrieved from http://www.osgi.org

Paediatric and Congenital Cardiac Services Review Group. (2003). *Report of the paediatric and congenital cardiac services review group*. London, UK: Department of Health.

Pagliari, C., Sloan, D., Gregor, P., Sullivan, F., Detmer, D., & Kahan, J. (2005). What is eHealth (4): A scoping exercise to map the field. *Journal of Medical Internet Research*, *7*(e9). doi:10.2196/jmir.7.1.e9

Pak, H. (2007). Telethinking. *Telemedicine and e-Health*, *13*(5), 483-486.

Palombi, L., Bernava, G. M., Nucita, A., Giglio, P., Liotta, G., & Nielsen-Saines, K. (2012). Predicting trends in HIV-1 sexual transmission in sub-Saharan Africa through the drug resource enhancement against AIDS and malnutrition model: Antiretrovirals for reduction of population infectivity, incidence and prevalence at the district level. *Clinical Infectious Diseases*, *55*(2), 268–275. doi:10.1093/cid/cis380

Pande, R. U., Patel, Y., Powers, C. J., D'Ancona, G., & Karamanoukian, H. L. (2003). The telecommunication revolution in the medical field: Present applications and future perspective. *Current Surgery*, *60*(6), 636–640. doi:10.1016/j.cursur.2003.07.009

Pantanowitz, L., Hornish, M., & Goulart, R. A. (2009). The impact of digital imaging in the field of cytopathology. *CytoJournal*, *6*(6).

Papa, F., Livi, S., Cornacchia, M., Nicolò, E., & Sapio, B. (2010). Factors affecting the usage of payment services through digital television in Italy. *EuroITV'10 - Proceedings of the 8th International Interactive TV and Video Conference*, (pp. 209-215).

Paré, G., Jaana, M., & Sicotte, C. (2007). Systematic review of home telemonitoring for chronic diseases: The evidence base. *Journal of the American Medical Informatics Association*, *14*(3), 269–277. doi:10.1197/jamia.M2270

Patterson, V., Swinfen, P., Swinfen, R., Azzo, E., Taha, H., & Wootton, R. (2007). Supporting hospital doctors in the Middle East by email telemedicine: Something the industrialized world can do to help. *Journal of Medical Internet Research*, *9*(4), e30. doi:10.2196/jmir.9.4.e30

Pattichis, C. S., Kyriacou, E., & Voskarides, S. (2002). Wireless telemedicine systems: An overview. *Antennas and Propagation Magazine*, *44*(2), 143–153. doi:10.1109/MAP.2002.1003651

Paul, D. L. (2004). A field study of the effect of interpersonal trust on virtual collaborative relationship performance. *Management Information Systems Quarterly*, *28*(2), 183–227.

Paul, J. H., Patrick, Y. K. C., Olivia, R. L. S., & Kar Yan, T. (1999). Examining the technology acceptance model using physician acceptance of telemedicine technology. *Journal of Management Information Systems*, *16*(2), 91.

Pawar, P., Jones, V., Van Beijnum, B., & Hermaens, H. (2012). A framework for the comparison of mobile patient monitoring system. *Journal of Biomedical Informatics*, *45*, 544–556. doi:10.1016/j.jbi.2012.02.007

Pearlin, L. I., Mullan, J. T., Semple, S. J., & Skaff, M. M. (1990). Caregiving and stress process: An overview of concepts and their measures. *The Gerontologist*, *30*(5), 583–594. doi:10.1093/geront/30.5.583

Pearlstein, H., Samarth, J., & Cusack, A. (2008). *Using barcode medication to improve quality and safety. Findings from the AHRQ health IT portfolio. Prepared by the AHRQ National Resource Center for Health IT under contract # 290-0023-EF*. Rockville, MD: Agency for Healthcare Research and Quality.

Pech, E. (2004). *Making innovation happen*. Technical paper produced by Detecon, Inc.

Pema, G. (2010). Telemedicine comes into its own. *International Business Times, 4*.

Pemberton, L., & Griffiths, R. (2003). Usability evaluation techniques for interactive television. In *Proceedings of the 10th HCII Conference*.

Perednia, D. A., & Allen, A. (1995). Telemedicine technology and clinical applications. *Journal of the American Medical Association*, *273*(6), 483–488. doi:10.1001/jama.1995.03520300057037

Perings, C., Bauer, W. R., Bondke, H. J., Mewis, C., James, M., & Bocker, D. (2011). Remote monitoring of implantable-cardioverter defibrillators: Results from the reliability of IEGM online interpretation (RIONI) study. *Journal of the Working Groups on Cardiac Pacing, Arrhythmias, and Cardiac Cellular Electrophysiology of the European Society of Cardiology*, *13*(2), 221–229. doi:10.1093/europace/euq447

Persaud, D. D., Jreige, S., Skedgel, C., Finley, J., Sargeant, J., & Hanlon, N. (2005, March 1). An incremental cost analysis of telehealth in Nova Scotia from a societal perspective. *Journal of Telemedicine and Telecare*, *11*(2), 77–84. doi:10.1258/1357633053499877

Petrie, A., & Sabin, C. (2005). *Medical statistics at a glance*. Malden, MA: Blackwell.

Phelps, E. S. (1966). Models of technical progress and the golden rule of research. *The Review of Economic Studies*, *33*, 133–146. doi:10.2307/2974437

PHI. (2003). Long term care financing and the long-term care workforce crisis: Causes and solutions. *Citizens for Long-Term Care*, 1-42.

Pinco, J., Goulart, R. A., & Otis, C. N. (2009). Impact of digital image manipulation in cytology. *Archives of Pathology & Laboratory Medicine*, *133*(1), 57–61.

Pinheiro, E., Postolache, O., & Girão, P. S. (2011). *Cardiopulmonary signal processing of users of wheelchairs with embedded sensors*. Paper presented at the IEEE International Symposium on Medical Measurements and Applications (MeMeA 2011).

Pink, G. H., & Leatt, P. (2003). The use of 'arms-length' organizations for health system change in Ontario, Canada: Some observations by insiders. *Health Policy (Amsterdam)*, *63*(1), 1–15. doi:10.1016/S0168-8510(01)00225-1

Pinnock, H., McKenzie, L., Price, D., & Sheikh, A. (2005). Cost-effectiveness of telephone or surgery asthma reviews: economic analysis of a randomised controlled trial. *The British Journal of General Practice*, *55*(511), 119–124.

Plott, A. E., Martin, F. J., & Cheek, S. W. (1987). Measuring screening skills in gynecologic: Results of voluntary self-assessment. *Acta Cytologica*, *31*, 911–923.

Polisena, J., Coyle, D., Coyle, K., McGill, S., Polisena, J., & Coyle, D. (2009). Home telehealth for chronic disease management: A systematic review and an analysis of economic evaluations. *International Journal of Technology Assessment in Health Care*, *25*(3), 339–349. doi:10.1017/S0266462309990201

Post, E. R., Orth, Russo, P. R., & Gershenfeld, N. (2000). E-broidery: Design and fabrication of textile-based computing. *IBM Systems Journal*, *39*(3-4).

Preim, B., & Bartz, D. (2007). *Visualization in medicine: Theory, algorithms, and applications* (1st ed.). Amsterdam, The Netherlands: Elsevier.

Pressman, R. S. (2005). *Software engineering: A practitioner's approach* (6th ed.). McGraw-Hill.

Puangmali, P., Althoefer, K., Seneviratne, L. D., Murphy, D., & Dasgupta, P. (2008). State-of-the-art in force and tactile sensing for minimally invasive surgery. *Sensors Journal*, *8*(4), 371–381. doi:10.1109/JSEN.2008.917481

Pyk, P., Wille, D., Chevrier, E., Hauser, Y., Holper, L., & Fatton, I. … Eng, K. (2008). *A paediatric interactive therapy system for arm and hand rehabilitation*. Paper presented at the Virtual Rehabilitation 2008, Vancouver, Canada.

Que, C., Cullinan, P., & Geddes, D. (2006). Improving rate of decline of FEV1 in young adults with cystic fibrosis. *Thorax*, *61*, 155–157. doi:10.1136/thx.2005.043372

Quitadamo, L. R., Abbafati, M., Saggio, G., Marciani, M. G., Cardarilli, G. C., & Bianchi, L. (2008). *A UML model for the description of different BCI systems*. Paper presented at the 30th Annual International Conference of the IEEE Engineering in Medicine and Biology Society (EMBS 2008).

Qureshi, S. A. (2008). Requirements for provision of outreach paediatric cardiology service. London, UK: British Congenital cardiac Association.

Raab, S. S., Zaleski, M. S., & Thomas, P. A. (1996). Telecytology: Diagnostic accuracy in cervical-vaginal smears. *American Journal of Clinical Pathology*, *105*, 599–603.

Raivio, M., Eloniemi-Sulkava, U., & Laakkonen, M. L. (2007). How do officially organized services meet the needs of elderly caregivers and their spouses with Alzheimer's disease? *American Journal of Alzheimer's Disease and Other Dementias*, *22*, 360–368. doi:10.1177/1533317507305178

Rajani, R., & Perry, M. (1999). The reality of medical work: The case for a new perspective on telemedicine. *Virtual Reality (Waltham Cross)*, *4*(4), 243–249. doi:10.1007/BF01421807

Rajan, S., & Saiman, L. (2002). Pulmonary infections in patients with cystic fibrosis. *Seminars in Respiratory Infections*, *17*, 47–56. doi:10.1053/srin.2002.31690

Ramsey, B. W., & Boat, T. F. (1994). Outcome measures for clinical trials in cystic fibrosis: Summary of a cystic fibrosis consensus conference. *The Journal of Pediatrics*, *124*, 177–192. doi:10.1016/S0022-3476(94)70301-9

Ramsey, B. W., Farrell, P. M., & Pencharz, P. (1992). Nutritional assessment and management in cystic fibrosis: A consensus report. The Consensus Committee. *The American Journal of Clinical Nutrition, 55*(1), 108–116.

Randolph, G. R., Hagler, D. J., Khandheria, B. K., Lunn, E. R., Cook, W. J., & Seward, J. B. (1999). Remote telemedical interpretation of neonatal echocardiograms: Impact on clinical management in a primary care setting. *Journal of the American College of Cardiology, 34*(1), 241–245. doi:10.1016/S0735-1097(99)00182-5

Rankl, W., & Effing, W. (2004). *Smart card handbook.* Wiley.

Rao, C. R., Wegman, E. J., & Solka, J. L. (2005). *Data mining and data visualization.* Amsterdam, The Netherlands: Elsevier North Holland.

Raskin, J. (2000). *The humane interface: New direction for designing interactive systems* (1st ed.). Reading, MA: Addison Wesley.

Rayman, R., Croome, K., Galbraith, N., McClure, R., Morady, R., & Peterson, S. (2007). Robotic telesurgery: A real-world comparison of ground- and satellite-based internet performance. *International Journal of Medical Robotics and Computer Assisted Surgery, 3*(2), 111–116. doi:10.1002/rcs.133

Raymond, B. (2005). The Kaiser Permanente IT transformation. *Healthcare Financial Management, 59*(1), 62–66.

Reece, R. (2008). *MediaHealth leaders: The physician culture and resistance to change.* Health Leader Media Council.

Report Linker. (2010). *Telemedicine market shares, strategies, and forecasting worldwide.* Report Linker.

Res, J. C. J., Theuns, D., & Jordaens, L. (2006). The role of remote monitoring in the reduction of inappropriate implantable cardioverter defibrillator therapies. *Clinical Research in Cardiology; Official Journal of the German Cardiac Society, 95*(Suppl 3), 17–21. doi:10.1007/s00392-006-1304-8

Rigby, M., Hill, P., Koch, S., & Keeling, D. (2011). Social care informatics as an essential part of holistic health care: A call for action. *International Journal of Medical Informatics, 80*(8), 544–554. doi:10.1016/j.ijmedinf.2011.06.001

Riva, G. (2000). From tele-health to e-health: Internet and distributed virtual reality in health care. *Journal of CyberPsychology & Behavior, 3*(6), 989–998. doi:10.1089/109493100452255

Riva, G. (2002). The emergence of e-health: Using virtual reality and the internet for providing advanced healthcare services. *International Journal of Healthcare Technology and Management, 4*(1/2), 15–40. doi:10.1504/IJHTM.2002.001127

Roberts, A., Reponen, J., Pesola, U. M., Waterworth, E., Larsen, F., & Mäkiniemi, M. (2010). Transnational comparison: A retrospective study on e-health in sparsely populated areas of the northern periphery. *Telemedicine Journal and e-Health, 16*(10), 1053–1059. doi:10.1089/tmj.2010.0075

Roberts, D., Tayler, C., MacCormack, D., & Barwich, D. (2007). Telenursing in hospice palliative care. *The Canadian Nurse, 103,* 24–27.

Robinson, S. S., Seale, D. E., Tiernan, K. M., & Berg, B. (2003). Use of telemedicine to follow special needs children. *Telemedicine Journal and e-Health, 9*(1), 57–61. doi:10.1089/153056203763317657

Rocha, R., Vassallo, J., Soares, F., Miller, K., & Gobbi, H. (2009). Digital slides: Present status of a tool for consultation, teaching, and quality control in pathology. *Journal of Pathology – Research and Practice, 205*(11), 735-41.

Rohe, D. E. (2005). Psychological aspects of rehabilitation . In DeLisa, J. A. (Eds.), *Physical medicine & rehabilitation: Principles and practice.* Lippincott Williams & Wilkins.

Roig, F., & Saigí, F. (2011). Barriers to the normalization of telemedicine in a healthcare system model based on purchasing of healthcare services using providers' contracts. *Gaceta Sanitaria, 25*(5), 397–402. doi:10.1016/j.gaceta.2011.01.004

Roine, R., Ohinmaa, A., & Hailey, D. (2001). Assessing telemedicine: A systematic review of the literature. *Canadian Medical Association Journal, 165*(6), 765–771.

Rojas, S. V., & Gagnon, M. P. (2008). A systematic review of the key indicators for assessing telehomecare cost-effectiveness. *Telemedicine and e-Health, 14*(9).

Ronda, G., Van Asserrna, P., & Brug, J. (2001). Stages of change, psychological factors and awareness of physical activity levels in the Netherlands. *Health Promotion International, 16*, 305–314. doi:10.1093/heapro/16.4.305

Rosa, E., Lussignoli, G., & Sabbatini, F. (2010). Needs of caregivers of the patients with dementia. *Archives of Gerontology and Geriatrics, 51*, 54–58. doi:10.1016/j.archger.2009.07.008

Rosen, S. (1994). The quantity and quality of life: A conceptual framework. In Kenkel, D., Tolley, G., & Fabian, R. (Eds.), *Valuing health for policy: An economic approach* (p. 221). Chicago, IL: University of Chicago Press.

Rosenthal, A., Mork, P., Li, M. H., Stanford, J., Koester, D., & Reynolds, P. (2010). Cloud computing: A new business paradigm for biomedical information sharing. *Journal of Biomedical Informatics, 43*(2), 342–353. doi:10.1016/j.jbi.2009.08.014

Rossi Mori, A., Mazzeo, M., & D'Auria, S. (2009). deploying connected health among the actors on chronic conditions. *European Journal of ePractice, 8*(1). Retrieved October 24, 2011, from http://www.epractice.eu/files/European%20Journal%20epractice%20Volume%208_1.pdf

Rossi Mori, A., & Freriks, G. (2005). A European perspective on the cultural and political context for EHR deployment . In Kolodner, R. M., Demetriades, J. E., & Christopherson, G. A. (Eds.), *Health-e-people: Transformation to person-centered health systems.* Springer Verlag.

Rosson, M. B., & Carroll, J. M. (2002). *Usability engineering: Scenario-based development of human-computer interaction* (1st ed.). San Fancisco, CA: Academic Press.

Roth, A., Korb, H., Gadot, R., Kalter, E., Roth, A., & Korb, H. (2006). Telecardiology for patients with acute or chronic cardiac complaints: The 'SHL' experience in Israel and Germany. *International Journal of Medical Informatics, 75*(9), 643–645. doi:10.1016/j.ijmedinf.2006.04.004

Royal College of Paediatrics and Child Health. (2009). Cardiology training for paediatric SpRs. Retrieved from www.rcph.ac.uk/publications/education_and_training_documents/cardiology_for_paeds_march2005.pdf

Royal College of Physicians. (2009). Consultant physicians working with patients: The duties, responsibilities and practice of physicians in general medicine and the specialties - Paediatric cardiology. Retrieved from http://www.rcplondon.ac.uk/pubs/contents/39318d3e-4efb-49d6-994b-761892064f03.pdf

Ryan, K. A., Weldon, A., & Huby, N. M. (2010). Caregiver support service needs for patients with mild cognitive impairment and Alzheimer disease. *Alzheimer Disease and Associated Disorders, 24*, 171–176. doi:10.1097/WAD.0b013e3181aba90d

Sable, C. (2002). Digital echocardiography and telemedicine applications in pediatric cardiology. *Pediatric Cardiology, 23*(3), 358–369. doi:10.1007/s00246-001-0199-4

Sable, C. (2003). Telemedicine applications in pediatric cardiology. *Minerva Pediatrica, 55*(1), 1–13.

Sable, C. A., Cummings, S. D., Pearson, G. D., Schratz, L. M., Cross, R. C., & Quivers, E. S. (2002). Impact of telemedicine on the practice of pediatric cardiology in community hospitals. *Pediatrics, 109*(1), E3. doi:10.1542/peds.109.1.e3

Sable, C., Roca, T., Gold, J., Gutierrez, A., Gulotta, E., & Culpepper, W. (1999). Live transmission of neonatal echocardiograms from underserved areas: Accuracy, patient care, and cost. *Telemedicine Journal: The Official Journal of the American Telemedicine Association, 5*(4), 339–347.

Saggio, G., & Sbernini, L. (2011). *New scenarios in human trunk posture measurements for clinical applications.* Paper presented at the 6th IEEE International Symposium on Medical Measurements and Applications (MeMeA 2011). Bari, Italy.

Saggio, G., Bocchetti, S., Pinto, C. A., Orengo, G., & Giannini, F. (2009a). *A novel application method for wearable bend sensors.* Paper presented at the 2nd International Symposium on Applied Sciences in Biomedical and Communication Technologies (ISABEL2009). Bratislava, Slovak Republic.

Saggio, G., Latessa, G., Bocchetti, S., Pinto, C. A., & Beck, D. (2009b). *Improving performances of data gloves based on bend sensors.* Retrieved from http://sensorprod.com/news/white-papers/dgb/index.php

Saggio, G., Latessa, G., De Santis, F., Bianchi, L., Quitadamo, L. R., Marciani, M. G., & Giannini, F. (2009). *Virtual reality implementation as a useful software tool for e-health applications.* Paper presented at the 1th IEEE International WoWMoM Workshop on Interdisciplinary Research on E-Health Services and Systems (IREHSS 2009), Kos (Greece).

Saggio, G., Santosuosso, G. L., Cavallo, P., Pinto, C. A., Petrella, M., Giannini, F., et al. (2011). *Gesture recognition and classification for surgical skill assessment.* Paper presented at the 6th IEEE International Symposium on Medical Measurements and Applications (MeMeA 2011). Bari, Italy.

Saggio, G., & Pinto, C. A. (2010). Virtuality supports reality for e-health applications . In Kim, J.-J. (Ed.), *Virtual reality* (pp. 259–284). InTech Publications. doi:10.5772/13085

Samuelson, P. A., & Nordhaus, W. D. (2005). *Economics.* New York, NY: McGraw-Hill.

Sano, S., Ishino, K., Kado, H., Shiokawa, Y., Sakamoto, K., & Yokota, M. (2004). Outcome of right ventricle-to-pulmonary artery shunt in first-stage palliation of hypoplastic left heart syndrome: A multi-institutional study. *The Annals of Thoracic Surgery, 78*(6), 1951–1958. doi:10.1016/j.athoracsur.2004.05.055

Sarfaraz, S., Sund, Z., & Jarad, N. (2010). Real-time, once-daily monitoring of symptoms and FEV1 in cystic fibrosis patients – A feasibility study using a novel device. *Clinical Respiration Journal, 4*(2), 74–82. doi:10.1111/j.1752-699X.2009.00147.x

Saysell, E., & Routley, C. (2003). Telemedicine in community-based palliative care: Evaluation of a videolink teleconference project. *International Journal of Palliative Nursing, 9*, 489–495.

Scalvini, S., Vitacca, M., & Paletta, L. (2004). Telemedicine: A new frontier for effective healthcare services. *Monaldi Archives for Chest Disease, 61*, 226–233.

Schneider, J., Murray, J., Banerjee, S., & Mann, A. (1999). Eurocare: A cross sectional study of co-resident spouse for people with Alzheimer's disease factors associated with carer burden. *International Journal of Geriatric Psychiatry, 14*, 651–661. doi:10.1002/(SICI)1099-1166(199908)14:8<651::AID-GPS992>3.0.CO;2-B

Schoenfeld, M. H., Compton, S. J., & Hardwin Mead, R. (2004). Remote monitoring of implantable cardioverter defibrillators: A prospective analysis. *Pacing and Clinical Electrophysiology, 27*, 757–763. doi:10.1111/j.1540-8159.2004.00524.x

Schoenfeld, M. H., & Reynolds, D. W. (2005). Sophisticated remote implantable cardioverter-defibrillator follow-up: A status report. *Pacing and Clinical Electrophysiology, 28*, 235–240. doi:10.1111/j.1540-8159.2005.09554.x

School of Management del Politecnico delle Milano. (2011). *Quarto Rapporto dell'Osservatorio ICT in Sanità: L'innovazione in cerca d'autore.* Retrieved from http://www.osservatori.net/

Schulz, R., O'Brien, A. T., Bookwala, J., & Fleissner, K. (1995). Psychiatric and physical morbidity effects of dementia caregiving: Prevalence, correlates and causes. *Gerontology, 35*(6), 771–791. doi:10.1093/geront/35.6.771

Schweitzer, J., & Synowiec, C. (2012). The economics of eHealth and mHealth. *Journal of Health Communication, 17*(1), 73–81. doi:10.1080/10810730.2011.649158

Scottish Centre for Telehealth and Telecare. (2010). *Scottish Centre for Telehealth strategic framework 2010 – 2012.* Retrieved October 24, 2011, from http://www.sctt.scot.nhs.uk/strategy.html

Scuffham, P. (2002). Systematic review of cost effectiveness in telemedicine. Quality of cost effectiveness studies in systematic reviews is problematic. *British Medical Journal, 325*(7364), 598. doi:10.1136/bmj.325.7364.598

Scutchfield, F. D., Bhandari, M. W., Lawhorn, N. A., Lamberth, C. D., & Ingram, R. C. (2009). Public health performance. *American Journal of Preventive Medicine, 36*(3), 266–272. doi:10.1016/j.amepre.2008.11.007

Sebajang, H., Trudeau, P., Dougall, A., Hegge, S., McKinley, C., & Anvari, M. (2006). The role of telementoring and telerobotic assistance in the provision of laparoscopic colorectal surgery in rural areas. *Surgical Endoscopy, 20*(9), 1389–1393. doi:10.1007/s00464-005-0260-0

Setyono, A., Alam, M. J., & Al-Saqour, R. A. (2010). Design of multimedia messaging service for mobile telemedicine system. *International Journal of Network and Mobile Technologies, 1*(1), 15–21.

Shanit, D., Cheng, A., & Greenbaum, R. A. (1996). Telecardiology: Supporting the decision making process in general practice. *Journal of Telemedicine and Telecare*, 2(1), 7–13. doi:10.1258/1357633961929105

Sharma, S., Parness, I. A., Kamenir, S. A., Ko, H., Haddow, S., & Steinberg, L. G. (2003). Screening fetal echocardiography by telemedicine: Efficacy and community acceptance. *Journal of the American Society of Echocardiography: Official Publication of the American Society of Echocardiography*, 16(3), 202–208. doi:10.1067/mje.2003.46

Shea, S., Weinstock, R. S., Teresi, J. A., Palmas, W., Starren, J., & Cimino, J. J. (2012). A randomized trial comparing telemedicine case management with usual care in older, ethnically diverse, medically underserved patients with diabetes mellitus: 5 year results of the IDEATel study. *Journal of the American Medical Informatics Association*, 16(4), 446–456. doi:10.1197/jamia.M3157

Shea, S., Weinstock, R., Teresi, J., Palmas, W., Starren, J., & Cimino, J. (2009). A randomised trial comparing telemedicine case management with usual care in older, ethnically diverse, medically underserved patients with diabetes mellitus: 5 year results of the IDEATel study. *Journal of the American Medical Informatics Association*, 16(4), 446–456. doi:10.1197/jamia.M3157

Sheikh, A., McLean, S., Cresswell, K., Pagliari, C., Pappas, Y., Car, J., et al. (2011). *The impact of ehealth on the quality and safety of healthcare: An updated systematic overview and synthesis of the literature: Final report for NHS Connecting for Health Evaluation programme* (p. 772). London, UK: The University of Edinburgh; and Imperial College.

Shortliffe, E. H., & Barnett, G. O. (2001). Medical data: Their acquisition, storage, and use. In E. H. Shortliffe, & L. E. Perreault (Eds.), *Medical informatics: Computer applications in health care and biomedicine* (2nd ed.). New York, NY: Springer Science+Business Media, Inc.

Siaplaaouras, S., Buob, A., & Neuberger, H. R. (2006). Femote detection of incessant slow VT with an ICD capable of home monitoring. *Europace*, 6(8), 512–514. doi:10.1093/europace/eul050

Siau, K. (2003). Health care informatics. *IEEE Transactions on Information Technology in Biomedicine*, 7(1), 1–7. doi:10.1109/TITB.2002.805449

Sicotte, C., Lehoux, P., Van Doesburg, N., Cardinal, G., & Leblanc, Y. (2004). A cost-effectiveness analysis of interactive paediatric telecardiology. *Journal of Telemedicine and Telecare*, 10(2), 78–83. doi:10.1258/135763304773391503

Silva, H., Lourenco, A., Tomas, R., Lee, V., & Going, S. (2011). *Accelerometry-based study of body vibration dampening during whole-body vibration training*. Paper presented at the 6th IEEE International Symposium on Medical Measurements and Applications (MeMeA 2011). Bari, Italy.

Simone, L. K., Sundarrajan, N., Luoc, X., Jia, Y., & Kamperc, D. G. (2007). A low cost instrumented glove for extended monitoring and functional hand assessment. *Journal of Neuroscience Methods*, 160, 335–348. doi:10.1016/j.jneumeth.2006.09.021

Singh, M., & Das, R. (2010). Utility of telemedicine for children in India. *Indian Journal of Pediatrics*, 77(1), 73–75. doi:10.1007/s12098-009-0292-x

Sloot, P., Tirado-Ramos, A., Altintas, I., Bubak, M., & Boucher, C. (2006). From molecule to man: Decision support in individualized E-Health. *Computer*, 39(11), 40–46. doi:10.1109/MC.2006.380

Smith, A. C. (2007). Telepaediatrics. *Journal of Telemedicine and Telecare*, 13(4), 163–166. doi:10.1258/135763307780908021

Smith, A. C., Bensink, M., Armfield, N., Stillman, J., & Caffery, L. (2005). Telemedicine and rural health care applications. *Journal of Postgraduate Medicine*, 51(4), 286–293.

Smith, A. C., Scuffham, P., & Wootton, R. (2007). The costs and potential savings of a novel telepaediatric service in queensland. *BMC Health Services Research*, 7, 35. doi:10.1186/1472-6963-7-35

Smith, B. J., Tang, K. C., & Nutbeam, D. (2006, September 7). WHO health promotion glossary: New terms. *Health Promotion International Advance Access*, 21, 340–345. doi:10.1093/heapro/dal033

Smith, D. L. (2005). The influence of financial factors on the deployment of telemedicine. *Journal of Health Care Finance, 32*(1), 16–27.

Soomlek, C., & Benedicenti, L. (2010). Operational wellness model: A wellness model designed for an agent-based wellness visualization system. The Second International Conference on eHealth, Telemedicine, and Social Medicine (eTELEMED2010). St. Maarten.

Soomlek, C., & Benedicenti, L. (2011). Creating a framework for testing wellness visualization systems. *The Third International Conference on eHealth, Telemedicine, and Social Medicine (eTELEMED2011).* Guadeloupe.

Soomlek, C., & Benedicenti, L. (2012). *Repeatable experimental framework for wellness indicator testing/evaluation: Environmental setup.* The Fourth International Conference on eHealth, Telemedicine, and Social Medicine (eTELEMED2012), Valencia.

Spence, R. (2001). *Information visualization.* Harlow, UK: Addison-Wesley.

Spiegelhalter, D. J., & Myles, J. P. (2004). *Bayesian approaches to clinical trials and health-care evaluation.* Chichester, UK: John Wiley & Sons. doi:10.1002/0470092602

Stamataki, M., Anninos, D., & Brountzos, E. (2008). The role of liquid-based cytology in the investigation of thyroid lesions. *Cytopathology, 19*(1), 11–18.

Stasik, C. N., Gelehrter, S., Goldberg, C. S., Bove, E. L., Devaney, E. J., & Ohye, R. G. (2006). Current outcomes and risk factors for the norwood procedure. *The Journal of Thoracic and Cardiovascular Surgery, 131*(2), 412–417. doi:10.1016/j.jtcvs.2005.09.030

Stensland, J., Speedie, S. M., Ideker, M., House, J., & Thompson, T. (1999). The relative cost of outpatient telemedicine services. *Telemedicine Journal: The Official Journal of the American Telemedicine Association, 5*(3), 245–256.

Stergiou, N., Georgoulakis, J., & Margari, N. (2009). Using a web-based system for the continuous distance education in cytopathology. *International Journal of Medical Informatics, 78*(12), 827–838. doi:10.1016/j.ijmedinf.2009.08.007

Steventon, A., Bardsley, M., Billings, J., Dixon, J., Doll, H., & Hirani, S. (2012). Effect of telehealth on use of secondary care and mortality: findings from the Whole System Demonstrator cluster randomised trial. *British Medical Journal, 344*(e3874). doi:10.1136/bmj.e3874

Stone, J. (2010). Long-term care (LTC): Financing overview and issues for congress. *Congressional Research Service*, 1-22.

Strehle, E. M., & Shabde, N. (2006). One hundred years of telemedicine: Does this new technology have a place in paediatrics? *Archives of Disease in Childhood, 91*(12), 956–959. doi:10.1136/adc.2006.099622

Stroetmann, K. A., Jones, T., Dobrev, A., & Stroetmann, V. N. (2008). *eHealth is worth it: The economic benefits of implemented eHealth solutions at ten European sites.* European Commission. Retrieved from http://www.ehealth-impact.org

Stroetmann, V., Thierry, J. P., Stroetmann, K., & Dobrev, A. (2007). *Impact of ICT on patient safety and risk management, e-health for safety report October 2007. European Commission, Information Society and Media.* Luxembourg: Office for Official Publications of the European Communities.

Strohecker, J., Travis, J. W., Burdett, B., Kant Mishra, S., & Zyga, M. (n.d.). *Wellness inventory: The whole person assessment program.* HealthWorld Online. Retrieved June 18, 2012, from http://www.mywellnesstest.com/index_wt.asp?UID=&Id=

Suchman, L. A. (1987). *Plans and situated actions: the problem of human-machine communication.* New York, NY: Cambridge University Press.

Sutherland, L. M., Middleton, P. F., Anthony, A., Hamdorf, J., Cregan, P., Scott, D., & Maddern, G. J. (2006). Surgical simulation: A systematic review. *Annals of Surgery, 243*, 291–300. doi:10.1097/01.sla.0000200839.93965.26

Swinfen, R., & Swinfen, P. (2002). Low-cost telemedicine in the developing world. *Journal of Telemedicine and Telecare, 8*(3), 63–65. doi:10.1258/13576330260440899

Swinton, J. J. (2009). Telehealth and rural depression: Physician and patient perspectives. *American Psychological Association, 27*(2), 172-182.

System of Systems. (2011). *Wikipedia*. Retrieved from http://en.wikipedia.org/wiki/System_of_systems

Szekely, G., & Satava, R. M. (1999). Virtual reality in medicine. *British Medical Journal, 319.*

Takahashi, G., Millette, S., & Eftekari, T. (2003). *Exploring issue related to the qualification recognition of physical therapists.* Paper presented at the World Confederation for Physical Therapy, London (WCPT 2003).

Takahashi, P. Y., Pecina, J. L., Upatising, B., Chaudhry, R., Shah, N. D., & Houten, H. V. (2012, May 28). A randomized controlled trial of telemonitoring in older adults with multiple health issues to prevent hospitalizations and emergency department visits. *Archives of Internal Medicine, 172*(10), 773–779. doi:10.1001/archinternmed.2012.256

Talbot, L. A., Gaines, J. M., Huynh, T. N., & Metter, E. J. (2003). A home-based pedometer-driven walking program to increase physical activity in older adults with osteoarthritis of the knee: A preliminary study. *Journal of the American Geriatrics Society, 51,* 387–392. doi:10.1046/j.1532-5415.2003.51113.x

Tanimoto, Y., Takechi, H., Nagahata, H., & Yamamoto, H. (1998). The study of pressure distribution in sitting position on cushions for patient with SCI (spinal cord injury). *IEEE Transactions on Instrumentation and Measurement, 47,* 1239–1243. doi:10.1109/19.746590

Tan, J. (2005). *E-health care information systems: An introduction for students and professionals* (1st ed.). San Francisco, CA: Jossey-Bass.

Tanke, M. A., & Ikkersheim, D. E. (2012). A new approach to the tradeoff between quality and accessibility of health care. *Health Policy (Amsterdam), 105*(2-3), 282–287. doi:10.1016/j.healthpol.2012.02.016

Tanriverdi, H., & Iacono, S. (1999). Diffusion of telemedicine: A knowledge barrier perspective. *Telemedicine Journal, 5*(3), 223–244. doi:10.1089/107830299311989

Tao, W. (2005). *IP broadband access network construction.* Network Marketing Department Technical paper produced by Huawei Technologies Co., Ltd.

Taylor, P. (1998). A survey of research in telemedicine. 1: Telemedicine systems. *Journal of Telemedicine and Telecare, 4*(1), 1–17. doi:10.1258/1357633981931227

Terkelsen, C. J., Lassen, J. F., Nørgaard, B. L., Gerdes, J. C., Poulsen, S. H., & Bendix, K. (2005). Reduction of treatment delay in patients with ST-elevation myocardial infarction: Impact of pre-hospital diagnosis and direct referral to primary percutanous coronary intervention. *European Heart Journal, 26*(8), 770–777. doi:10.1093/eurheartj/ehi100

The European Files. (2010). *The telemedicine challenge in Europe.* The European Files.

The Joint Commission. (2008). *Guiding principles for the development of the hospital of the future.* Retrieved October 24, 2011, from http://www.jointcommission.org/topics/default.aspx?k=750

The Street. PR Newswire. (2011). *Convenient sports physicals offered at minute clinic walk-in medical clinics inside select CVS/Pharmacy stores for just $39.00.* Woonsacket, RI: Author.

Thomas, K. C., Ellis, A. R., Konrad, T. R., Holzer, C. E., & Morrissey, J. P. (2009). County-level estimates of mental health professional shortage in the United States. *Psychiatric Services (Washington, D.C.), 60*(10), 1323–1328. doi:10.1176/appi.ps.60.10.1323

Thompson, D. W. (1989). Canadian experience in cytology proficiency. *Acta Cytologica, 33,* 484–486.

Toda, Y., Toda, T., Takemura, S., Wada, T., Morimoto, T., & Ogawa, R. (1998). Change in body fat, but not body weight or metabolic correlates of obesity, is related to symptomatic relief of obese patients with knee osteoarthritis after a weight control program. *The Journal of Rheumatology, 25.*

Torre, A., Rodriguez, C. H., & Garcia, L. (2004). Cost analysis in telemedicine: Empirical evidence from sites in Arizona. *Health Services: Telemedicine, 20*(3), 253–257.

Torrence, G. (1996). Measurement of health state utilities for economic appraisal – A review. *Journal of Health Policy, 5,* 1–3.

Travis, J. W. (2008, May 6). Beyond ordinary wellness: A roadmap to high-level wellness. Durack, Australia: National Wellness Institute of Australia Inc. Retrieved June 24, 2012, from http://www.wellnessaustralia.org/NWIA%20Travis%20forum%20may%202008.pdf

Trist, E., & Murray, H. (1993). The social engagement of social science: *Vol. II. The socio-technical perspective*. Philadelphia, PA: University of Pennsylvania Press.

Truscott, A., Rande, G., McQueen, J., & Parston, G. (2011). *Information governance. The Foundation for Effective eHealth*. Accenture Healthcare Systems.

Tsilimigaki, A., Maraka, S., Tsekoura, T., Agelakou, V., Vekiou, A., & Paphitis, C. (2001). Eighteen months' experience with remote diagnosis, management and education in congenital heart disease. *Journal of Telemedicine and Telecare, 7*(4), 239–243. doi:10.1258/1357633011936462

Tudor–Locke, C. E., Ainsworth, B. E., Whitt, M. C., Thompson, R. W., Addy, C. L., & Jones, D. (2001). The relationship between pedometer- determined ambulatory activity and body composition variables. *International Journal of Obesity, 25*(11), 1571–1578. doi:10.1038/sj.ijo.0801783

Tudor-Locke, C., & Basset, D. R. Jr. (2004). How many steps /day are enough? Preliminary pedometers indices, for public health. *Sports Medicine (Auckland, N.Z.), 34*(1), 1–8. doi:10.2165/00007256-200434010-00001

Tudor-Locke, C., & Lutes, L. (2009). Why do pedometers work? A reflection upon the factors related to successfully increasing physical activity. *Sports Medicine (Auckland, N.Z.), 39*, 981–993. doi:10.2165/11319600-000000000-00000

Tufte, E. R. (1997). *The visual display of quantitative information* (15th ed.). Connecticut: Graphics Press.

Turk, E., Karagulle, E., Aydogan, C., Oguz, H., Tarim, A., Karakayali, H., & Haberal, M. (2011). Use of telemedicine and telephone consultation in decision-making and follow-up of burn patients: Initial experience from two burn units. *Burns, 37*(3), 415–419. doi:10.1016/j.burns.2010.10.004

U.S. Food and Drug Administration. (2009). *MedSun: Medical product safety network improving patient safety by reporting problems with medical devices used in the home*. Retrieved from http://www.fda.gov/MedicalDevices/Safety/MedSunMedicalProductSafetyNetwork/ucm205691.htm#transcript

Umefjord, G., Hamberg, K., Malker, H., & Petersson, G. (2006). The use of an Internet-based Ask the Doctor service involving family physicians: Evaluation by a web survey. *Family Practice, 23*, 159–166. doi:10.1093/fampra/cmi117

United Nations, Economic and Social Affairs, Population Division. (2010). *Population ageing and development 2009*. Retrieved from http://www.un.org/esa/population/publication/ageing/ageing2009.html

Valente, P. T., & Schantz, H. D. (1992). Proficiency testing performance in a workshop setting: Implications for implementation of CLIA 88. *Acta Cytologica, 36*, 581.

Van den Brink-Muinen, A., Verhaak, P. F., Bensing, J. M., Bahrs, O., Deveugele, M., & Gask, L. (2000). Doctor patient communication in different European health care systems: Relevance and performance from the patients' perspective. *Patient Education and Counseling, 39*(1), 115–127. doi:10.1016/S0738-3991(99)00098-1

Van Ginneken, A. M. (2002). The computerized patient record: Balancing effort and benefit. *International Journal of Medical Informatics, 65*, 97–119. doi:10.1016/S1386-5056(02)00007-2

Van Mierlo, L. D., Meiland, F. J. M., Van der Roest, H. G., & Dro¨es, R. M. (2012). Personalised caregiver support: Effectiveness of psychosocial interventions in subgroups of caregivers of people with dementia. *International Journal of Geriatric Psychiatry, 27*, 1–14. doi:10.1002/gps.2694

Vaz, C. (2007). *EMR and device integration*. Retrieved from http://charlesconradvaz.wordpress.com/

Velde, R. V., & Degoulet, P. (2003). *Clinical information systems: A component-based approach* (Hannah, K. J., & Ball, M. J., Eds.). 1st ed.). New York, NY: Springer-Verlag Inc.

Venkatesh, V., & Bala, H. (2008). Technology acceptance model 3 and a research agenda on interventions. *Decision Sciences, 39*(2), 273–315. doi:10.1111/j.1540-5915.2008.00192.x

Vespa, P. (2005). Robotic telepresence in the intensive care unit. *Critical Care (London, England), 9*, 319–320. doi:10.1186/cc3743

Vinals, F., Mandujano, L., Vargas, G., & Giuliano, A. (2005). Prenatal diagnosis of congenital heart disease using four-dimensional spatio-temporal image correlation (STIC) telemedicine via an internet link: A pilot study. Ultrasound in Obstetrics & Gynecology . *The Official Journal of the International Society of Ultrasound in Obstetrics and Gynecology, 25*(1), 25–31. doi:10.1002/uog.1796

Voice, X. M. L. (2005). *VoiceXML tutorial*. Retrieved from http://www.vxml.org/

von Lubitz, D. K., Carrasco, B., Gabbrielli, F., Ludwig, T., Levine, H., & Patricelli, F. (2003). Transatlantic medical education: Preliminary data on distance-based high-fidelity human patient simulation training. *Studies in Health Technology and Informatics, 94*, 379–385.

Wai-Chi Chan, S. (2010). Family caregiving in dementia: The Asian perspective of a global problem. *Dementia and Geriatric Cognitive Disorders, 30*, 469–478. doi:10.1159/000322086

Walgreen's Newsroom. (2011). *Walgreens take care health systems, forms alliance with core performance to offer employees access to advanced wellness, fitness, and nutrition programs*. Bentonville, AR: Author.

Wang, Y. (2005). *Human movement tracking using a wearable wireless sensor network*. Unpublished Master dissertation, Iowa State University. Ames, Iowa

Ware, C. (2004). *Information visualization: Perception for design* (Card, S., Grudin, J., & Nielsen, J., Eds.). 2nd ed.). San Francisco, CA: Morgan Kaufman.

Waterman, D. A. (1986). *A guide to expert systems*. Reading, MA: Addison Wesley.

Watson, E. (2008a, January 15). *BioHarness Bluetooth API guide*. Zephyr - Technology ITD.

Watson, E. (2008b, 2 March). *General comms link specification*. Zephyr - Technology ITD.

Weber, W., Rabaey, J. M., & Aarts, E. (2005). *Ambient intelligence*. Berlin, Germany: Springer. doi:10.1007/b138670

Weinstein, L. J., Epstein, J. I., & Edlow, D. (1997). Static image analysis of skin specimens: The application of telepathology to frozen section evaluation. *Human Pathology, 28*, 22–29. doi:10.1016/S0046-8177(97)90274-4

Weinstein, R. S., Graham, A. R., Richte, L. C., Barker, G. P., Krupinski, E. A., & Lopez, A. M. (2009). Overview of telepathology, virtual microscopy, and whole slide imaging: Prospects for the future. *Journal of Human Pathology, 40*(8), 1057–1069. doi:10.1016/j.humpath.2009.04.006

Weinstein, R. S., Lopez, A. M., Krupinski, E. A., Beinar, S. J., Holcomb, M., & McNeely, R. A. (2008). Integrating telemedicine and telehealth: Putting it all together. *Studies in Health Technology and Informatics, 131*, 23–38.

Weiser, M. (1996). Some computer science issues in ubiquitous computing. *Communications of the ACM, 36*(7).

Wellness Inventory: The Whole Person Assessment Program. (2011). Wellness Inventory. Retrieved June 18, 2012, from http://www.wellpeople.com/index_wp.asp?UID=&Id

Whited, J. D. (2001). Teledermatology: Current status and future directions. *American Journal of Clinical Dermatology, 2*(2), 59–64. doi:10.2165/00128071-200102020-00001

Whittaker, R., Merry, S., Dorey, E., & Maddison, R. (2012). A development and evaluation process for mHealth interventions: Examples from New Zealand. *Journal of Health Communication, 17*(Suppl 1), 11–21. doi:10.1080/10810730.2011.649103

Whitten, P. S., & Cook, D. J. (1999). School-based telemedicine: Using technology to bring health care to inner-city children. *Journal of Telemedicine and Telecare, 5*, S23–S25. doi:10.1258/1357633991932423

Whitten, P. S., Mair, F. S., Haycox, A., May, C. R., Williams, T. L., & Hellmich, S. (2002a). Systematic review of cost effectiveness studies of telemedicine interventions. *British Medical Journal, 324*(7351), 1434–1437. doi:10.1136/bmj.324.7351.1434

Whitten, P. S., Mair, F. S., Haycox, A., May, C. R., Williams, T. L., & Hellmich, S. (2002b). Systematic review of cost effectiveness studies of telemedicine interventions. *British Medical Journal, 324*(7351), 1434–1437. doi:10.1136/bmj.324.7351.1434

Whitten, P., & Love, B. (2005). Patient and provider satisfaction with the use of telemedicine: Overview and rationale for cautious enthusiasm. *Journal of Postgraduate Medicine*, *51*(4), 294–300.

WHO. (2006). *WHS: World health statistics 2006*. Retrieved July 20, 2012, from www.who.int/entity/whosis/whostat2006.pdf

Wiener, H. G., Klinkhamer, P., Schenck, U., & Bulten, J. (2007). Laboratory guidelines and quality assurance practices for cytology . In Arbyn, M., Anttila, A., & Jordan, J. (Eds.), *European guidelines for quality assurance in cervical cancer screening*. Luxembourg: Office of Official Publication European Union.

Wilkes, L., Mohan, S., White, K., & Smith, H. (2004). Evaluation of an after hours telephone support service for rural palliative care patients and their families: A pilot study. *The Australian Journal of Rural Health*, *12*, 95–98. doi:10.1111/j.1440-1854.2004.00568.x

Williams, B. H., Mullick, F. G., & Butler, D. R. (2001). Clinical evaluation of an international static image-based telepathology service. *Human Pathology*, *32*, 1309–1317. doi:10.1053/hupa.2001.29649

Williams, D. L., & Denz, M. D. (n.d.). *European Health Telematics Association EHTEL*.

Williams, N. W., Penrose, J. M. T., Caddy, C. M., Barnes, E., Hose, D. R., & Harley, P. (2000). A goniometric glove for clinical hand assessment. *The Journal of Hand Surgery*, *25B*(2), 200–207.

Williams, T., May, C., & Esmail, A. (2001). Limitations of patient satisfaction studies in telehealthcare: A systematic review of the literature. *Telemedicine Journal and e-Health*, *7*(4), 293–316. doi:10.1089/15305620152814700

Wimo, A., Winblad, B., & Jo¨nsson, L. (2010). The worldwide societal costs of dementia: Estimates for 2009. *Alzheimer's & Dementia*, *6*, 98–103. doi:10.1016/j.jalz.2010.01.010

Wise, P. H. (2007). The future pediatrician: The challenge of chronic illness. *The Journal of Pediatrics*, *151*(5Suppl), S6–S10. doi:10.1016/j.jpeds.2007.08.013

WISR. (2006). *World information society report 2006*. International Telecommunications Union. Retrieved July 20, 2012, from http://www.itu.int/osg/spu/publications/worldinformationsociety/2006/wisr-web.pdf

Wong, D., Paciorek, N., & Moore, D. (1999). Java-based mobile agents. *Communications of the ACM*, *42*(3). Retrieved from http://portal.acm.org/citation.cfm?id=2957 17doi:10.1145/295685.295717

Woodhouse, S. L., Schulte, M. A., & Stastny, J. F. (1999). Proficient or deficient—On the razor's edge: Establishing validity in cytology proficiency testing. *Diagnostic Cytopathology*, *20*, 255–256. doi:10.1002/(SICI)1097-0339(199905)20:5<255::AID-DC1>3.0.CO;2-J

Wootton, R., Bloomer, S. E., Corbett, R., Eedy, D. J., Hicks, N., & Lotery, H. E. (2000). Multicentre randomised control trial comparing real time teledermatology with conventional outpatient dermatological care: Societal cost-benefit analysis. *British Medical Journal*, *320*(7244), 1252–1256. doi:10.1136/bmj.320.7244.1252

Wootton, R., Craig, J., & Patterson, V. (Eds.). (2006). *Introduction to telemedicine*. London, UK: Royal Society of Medicine Press Ltd.

Wootton, R., Dimmick, S., & Kvedar, J. (Eds.). (2006). *Home telehealth: Connecting care within the community*. London, UK: Royal Society of Medicine Press Ltd.

Workforce Review Team. (2009). Workforce summary - Paediatric cardiology. Retrieved from http://www.wrt.nhs.uk/index

World Health Organisation. (2003). *Information technology in support of health care*.

World Health Organisation. (2011). *Health topics: Chronic diseases*.

World Health Organization. (2005). *Global report preventing chronic diseases: A vital investment*. Retrieved October 24, 2011, from http://www.who.int/entity/chp/chronic_disease_report/full_report.pdf

World Health Organization. (2008, September 10). *WHOSIS: WHO statistical information system*. Retrieved May 31, 2012, from http://apps.who.int/whosis/data/Search.jsp?indicators=%255bIndicator%255d.Members%253e

World Health Organization. (2009). Preventing hospital visits through telemedicine. *World Health Organization Bulletin, 87*(10), 739–740. doi:10.2471/BLT.09.021009

Wyss, K., & Lorenz, N. (2000). Decentralization and central and regional coordination of health services: The case of Switzerland. *The International Journal of Health Planning and Management, 15*(2), 103–114. doi:10.1002/1099-1751(200004/06)15:2<103::AID-HPM581>3.0.CO;2-S

Yach, D., Hawkes, C., Gould, C. L., & Hofman, K. J. (2004). The global burden of chronic diseases: Overcoming impediments to prevention and control. *Journal of the American Medical Association, 291*, 2616–2622. doi:10.1001/jama.291.21.2616

Yamaguchi, H., Maki, Y., & Yamagami, T. (2010). Overview of non-pharmacological intervention for dementia and principles of brain-activating rehabilitation. *Psychogeriatrics, 10*, 206–213. doi:10.1111/j.1479-8301.2010.00323.x

Yamashiro, K., Kawamura, N., & Matsubayashi, S. (2004). Telecytology in Hokkaido Island, Japan: Results of primary telecytodiagnosis of routine cases. *Cytopathology, 15*(4), 221–227. doi:10.1111/j.1365-2303.2004.00147.x

Young, F. W., Valero-Mora, P. M., & Friendly, M. (2006). *Visual statistics: Seeing data with dynamic interactive graphics*. Hoboken, NJ: Wiley-Interscience. doi:10.1002/9781118165409

Young, K. M. (2000). *Informatics for healthcare professionals* (1st ed.). Philadelphia, PA: F.A. Davis Company.

Young, L. B., Chan, P. S., Lu, X., Nallamothu, B. K., Sasson, C., & Cram, P. M. (2011). Impact of telemedicine intensive care unit coverage on patient outcomes: A systematic review and meta-analysis. *Archives of Internal Medicine, 171*(6), 498–506. doi:10.1001/archinternmed.2011.61

Yueh-Feng Lu, Y., & Guerriero Austrom, M. (2005). Distress responses and self-care behaviors in dementia family caregivers with high and low depressed mood. *Journal of the American Psychiatric Nurses Association, 11*(4), 231–240. doi:10.1177/1078390305281422

Zanaboni, P., & Wootton, R. (2012). Adoption of telemedicine: From pilot stage to routine delivery. *BMC Medical Informatics and Decision Making, 12*(1). doi:10.1186/1472-6947-12-1

Ziegler, P., & Dittrich, K. R. (2004). Three decades of data integration—All problems solved? *18th IFIP World Computer Congress (WCC 2004)*, (p. 12). Toulouse.

Ziegler, P., & Dittrich, K. R. (2007). Data integration—Problems, approaches, perspectives. In J. Krogstie, A. L. Opdahl, & S. Brinkkemper (Eds.), *Conceptual modelling in information systems engineering* (pp. 39-58). Berlin, Germany: Springer. Retrieved from http://www.springerlink.com/content/tu6g43697442742n/

About the Contributors

Vincenzo Gullà graduated in Electronic Engineering at the University of Rome and continued education with several stages in business and marketing in many technology areas such as satellite communications, mobile, wireless, localization and mobile positioning solutions, high definition video, xDSL, Broadband terrestrial networking, innovative telecommunication services and markets, and telemedicine . He has over 25 years of experience in ICT technologies and markets. He started his carrier in the telecommunications industry working for the most important Italian companies and organizations covering positions as Telecoms Marketing Department Director, Vertical Applications Market Director, Telemedicine, Chairman of the European Market Focus Group, Chairman of the DSL-Forum Marketing Committee, Member of the SIT (Italian scientific telemedicine association), Associated Professor at the University of Camerino (Italy) for Master in Telemedicine and electro- medical devices and an independent consultant. Presently, he is the technical Director of ADiTech SRL Italian company for telemedicine solutions.

Angelo Rossi Mori is a researcher on eHealth at the Istituto Tecnologie Biomediche, Consiglio Nazionale delle Ricerche, in Rome. His research is focussed on comparative studies about design principles and evaluation of impact of National and Regional eHealth strategies. He is developing methodologies to deploy ICT-enhanced health policies at National or Regional levels, for a balanced diffusion of ICT across the health sectors. He is currently assisting the Health Regional Authorities of Sicilia, Campania, Calabria about a sustainable approach to eHealth and modern telemedicine. Other research topics involve the semantics of clinical terminologies, clinical datasets, EHR. He was involved in several EU Projects (GALEN, KAVAS, IREP, GALEN-IN-USE, TOMELO, C-CARE, PROREC, WIDENET, EHR-Q-TN, eHealth ERA, RIDE, ANCIEN). He was active in the standardization on health informatics, contributing to the creation of CEN/TC251 and ISO/TC215; in HL7 he was member of the Technical Steering Committee and co-chair of the Templates SIG.

Francesco Gabbrielli was born August 29th, 1965 in Italy and obtained Medicine-Surgery Degree at University of Pisa, Postgraduate Specialization in General Surgery and PhD in Experimental Surgery at University of L'Aquila. He get also TPM Certification by Transplantation Committee, Council of Europe. Beyond the surgical activity in different hospitals in Italy and Spain, he developed his career in the fields of organ transplantation, telemedicine, project, and team management for healthcare organizations. He was responsible for national and international experimental projects at the Italian Transplant Centre, National Health Institute in Rome, holding other public assignments in quality assurance, data security, patients safety. From 2007 at Surgical Sciences Department, Umberto I General Hospital of Rome, he has continued Coordination for National Transplant Network and researches in Telematic Medicine and Surgery becoming Member of the National Executive Board of the Italian Telemedicine Society, General Manager of the National Group for Telematic Surgery.

Pietro Lanzafame earned his Electronic Engineer Master's Degree in April 2003. He earned a PhD in Neurobiological and Clinical Sciences at University of Messina. During his study and post degree training, his research interests have been dedicated to the computer vision, artificial intelligence, and human-machine interaction. He also developed skills in usability and human acceptance of computer systems and technologies. During a year of research stage, with scholarship, at IRCCS Centro Neurolesi "Bonino-Pulejo" of Messina, he developed a computer vision system for eye movement studies in neurological disease. He has been representative of the Italian Space Agency and Sicilian Region joint committee for the Telemedicine Activities in the Sicilian Region from 07/02/200 and Component of technical committee for a "Regional Desk for EU Projects" at Sicilian Region Health Authority from May 2008 to June 2009. During his PhD period at the IRCCS Centro Neurolesi, he created and led Bioengineering and Telemedicine Group, developing several research projects on ICT application in Neurology. He is scientific liable to Telemedicine projects for Multiple Sclerosis, Alzheimer and Stroke patients. He is scientific liable to Sicilian Region Telepathology project. He is liable to Neurorehabilitation, Bioengineering and Telemedicine research line of the IRCCS Centro Neurolesi.

* * *

Roberto Antonicelli got his MD degree (*summa cum laude*) in 1981, the board certification in Internal Medicine (*summa cum laude*) in 1986, and the board certification in Cardiology, from the University of Ancona (*summa cum laude*) in 1990. Since 1998 he is the Director of the Telemedicine Centre at I.N.R.C.A., Ancona; he has been Director of the Hypertension Centre, Director of the Coronary Care Unit, Director of the Dpt. of Cardiology-UTIC at I.N.R.C.A., Ancona. Since 2009 he is the Co-Chief of the Regional Board on "Diagnostic Molecular in Cardiology." He has been member of the Working Group of the European Space Agency (ESA) on Telemedicine for Elderly People. Since 2002 he is the President of the no-profit Association for Cardiopatic patients Alive Heart (Ancona). He is author or co-author of 228 scientific manuscripts in international journals. He holds several memberships to national and international associations in cardiology related fields.

Stavros Archondakis, M.D., Ph.D, is specialized Cytopathologist, Director of 401 General Army Hospital of Athens Cytopathology Department. He is member of the Technical Committee of the Hellenic Accreditation System for the Accreditation of Medical Laboratories. He is an Executive Board Member of the Hellenic Society for Quality & Safety in HealthCare (HSQSH). He holds his PhD in Medicine (National & Kapodistrian University of Athens). He has also served as a scientific researcher in Greek and European research programs. He has participated as author or co-author in more than 15 Greek and 2 English scientific books. He has authored 65 Greek and 45 English scientific papers in international journals and international conferences proceedings. He has more than five years teaching experience in University programs. Research interests are telemedicine and e-health, e-learning, cytopathology, telecytology, and medical laboratories accreditation.

Michelangelo Bartolo was born in Rome in 1964, and is a Medical Doctor, Angiologist. Currently, he directs the Department of Telemedicine of S. Giovanni Hospital in Rome and serves as Director of Telemedicine of the Community of Sant'Egidio. Since 2001 he has made several missions in African countries to open DREAM Center and clinics for care and telemedicine services. He is Coordinator area of the web medical journal Telemeditalia.it www.telemeditalia.it ; Member of the Advisory Committee of the periodical e-Health care http://www.ehealthforum.it/ Chairman of the Board of Auditors of the SIT (Telemedicine Italian society) . It 'the author of some chapters in Telecardiologia, Universo Editions 2010 and in Towards e-Health 2020, successful Italian and international experiences, Group 24 hours Editions. 2012; He is the author of a novel "Our Africa" Gangemi Editions 2012.

Sergio Bella, born in Rome 22 May 1960, graduated in Medicine at the Catholic University of the Sacred Heart. He qualified as a medical professional in the second session of the year 1984. He specialized in Pediatrics at the University of Rome "La Sapienza" on 14/7/88 votes with 70/70 cum laude. Has achieved the second level Master in "telemedicine" at the University of Pisa, July 23, 2003 with grades 50/50 and praise, title of thesis: Application of Telemedicine in home care of chronic diseases: cystic fibrosis. He graduated in Economics and Management of Health Services on 17/7/08 at the Telematic University "Leonardo da Vinci" based in Torrevecchia Teatina (CH) with 101/110 votes, title of thesis: economic and financial assessment of a system of remote monitoring for patients with cystic fibrosis. From January 2011: High degree Responsibilities: "Continuity of care in chronic diseases" in Pediatric Hospital Bambino Gesù in Rome. He attended in March 2011 the course AMIA 10 x 10 with OHSU from the University of Portland (Oregon - USA). He participated to upgrade to more than 100 national and international congresses. He's the author of 67 publications, 4 book chapters, and 250 abstracts and posters at national and international conferences.

Luigi Benedicenti is the Associate Vice President (Academic) of the University of Regina. A full Professor in the Faculty of Engineering at the University of Regina, Benedicenti received his Laurea in Electrical Engineering and Ph.D. in Electrical and Computer Engineering from the University of Genoa, Italy. He is a Professional Engineer licensed in Saskatchewan and a licensed Italian Engineer. His collaborative network extends beyond Saskatchewan with TRLabs and IEEE, and Canada through collaborative work with colleagues in Europe, South East Asia, and North America. Benedicenti's current research is in three areas: software agents, software metrics, and new media technology. He envisions the unification of platform, tools, and optimizations for the provision of persistent distributed digital services, regardless of people's location and delivery device.

Placido Bramanti has research interests entirely dedicated to the clinical and neurorehabilitaion aspects of neurological and neurodegenerative disorders, such as Parkinson and Alzheimer's disease. During his medical school and residency in neurology, he developed an interest in the clinical aspects of epileptic disorders. During his foreign stage period, as researcher neurologist, he developed a special interest and expertise on traumatic brain injury and innovative therapeutic and rehabilitative strategies. Currently, he is the Scientific Director of the IRCCS Centro Neurolesi "Bonino-Pulejo" of Messina, Ordinary Professor at the University of Messina and charter member of the Italian Society of Telemedicine.

Corrado Cancellotti, born in Gubbio on 29/05/1955, graduated at the Università degli Studi di Perugia on 07/28/81, and he's regularly enrolled in the Physicians of the Province of Perugia from 14/1/82. He received on 29/6/84 the Postgraduate Diploma in Anaesthesiology and Intensive Care at the Università degli Studi di Siena, Dir. Prof. G. Bellucci. He holds since 30/10/90 the Postgraduate Diploma in First Aid and Emergency Care at the Università degli Studi "G. D'Annunzio" of Chieti, Dir. Prof. G. Meneghini. From 31 March 2008 to today is Director of the Emergency Department of the Hospital "High Chiascio" of Gubbio. From 11 April 2000 to 31 March 2008, he was Director of the Emergency Department of the Hospital of Gubbio From 08/01/86 to 11/04/2000, he was Doctor of Anesthesiology and Intensive Care, in the USL High Chiascio. He has made about 40 scientific publications regarding anesthesia, resuscitation, and emergency care.

Frank A. Casey is a Consultant Paediatric and Fetal Cardiologist at The Royal Belfast Hospital for Sick Children. He is also an Honorary Senior Lecturer in The Department of Child Health at Queen's University, Belfast. His research interests are in the applications of Telemedicine to Paediatric Cardiology, Fetal Cardiology, and the long-term educational and psychosocial outcome for children after surgery for congenital heart disease. Dr. Casey has more than thirty published papers and has given many presentations at international meetings.

Mariangela Contenti is an Engineer in Computer Science with a PhD in Business Information Systems and a Master's in Interoperability for Public Administration and Networked Enterprises. She currently works for the National Healthcare Agency, AgeNaS, as a Consultant on telemedicine for the Regional Authorities in Southern Italy. She has been a researcher on eHealth at the Luiss Guido Carlo University, at the Campus Bio-Medico University and at the Institute of Biomedical Technology of the Italian National Research Council, and a consultant for the Department of Innovation at the Presidency of the Council of Ministers. Her research activities evolved from distributed computing, to models and technologies for EHR-S, up to conceptual frameworks and metrics for ICT services in healthcare.

S.A. Davis has been with the University of California Merced since 2009 and prior to that was with the University of California Berkeley, Haas School of Business, and teaches in the areas of Entrepreneurship & Innovation, Organization Behavior and Leadership, Marketing & Brand Management Strategies and Global Marketing encompassing Strategies and Cultures. Dr. Davis specializes in building and managing entrepreneurial teams, marketing strategies, integration of knowledge management tools into marketing consumer brands and services and innovation and product launch management. She is President of Churchill International LLC. Dr. Davis is an accomplished executive manager and leader with a marketing driven and technology enhanced background with experience and expertise in international strategic marketing and branding, market segmentation and consumer profiling, customer relationship management and competitive market analysis. Senior Executive Management Expertise includes working with Volvo in Sweden, BMW in Germany, Renault in France, the British Coal Board in the United Kingdom, Agency for International Development in Brazil, Clorox, Johnson & Johnson, Kendall Health Care, California State Automobile Association, Apple Computer, Levi Strauss & Co., Occidental Petroleum, and General Motors in the United States. She is author of books and articles primarily in the area of entrepreneurship and innovation, marketing research, and marketing knowledge based systems.

Aldo Franco Dragoni received a Laurea Degree in Electronics Engineering from the University of Ancona, discussing a thesis in Artificial Intelligence on "Plan Recognition from Visual Information." Currently, he is in charge as Associate Professor at the "Università Politecnica delle Marche," where he teaches "Fundamentals of Computer Sciences," "Artificial Intelligence," and "Operating Systems 2." His scientific interests concerned several aspects of Artificial Intelligence, from classic knowledge-based approaches to more advanced hybrid systems that integrate symbolic reasoning with neural networks. Recently he started a research activity in "Real Time Systems" and opened a new application area for Artificial Intelligence techniques that he called "NetMedicine," which covers every Health-related activity which is carried on through the Internet.

Kldiashvili Ekaterine holds a MSc in Biology (1995) and Ph.D. in Histology, Cytology, and Embryology (2003) from the Tbilisi State University. Ekaterine works as Executive Director in Georgian Telemedicine Union (GTU), managing NATO Networking Infrastructure Project, BSEC tender, telemedicine pilot actions, whole activity of GTU and also creation of eHealth network in Georgia. Prior to joining GTU Ekaterine worked at department of Pathology of Central Clinic of Tbilisi State Medical University, establishing and leading the electron microscopy laboratory. She was trained in cytological diagnosis of malignant tumors at department of Oncology of the Tbilisi State Medical Academy. Ekaterine also acted as Clinical Cytologist at Department of Pathology of Central Clinic of Tbilisi State Medical University and Virologist at Republic Center of AIDS and Clinical Immunology. She participated as Researcher in Neuroscience project funded by Soros foundation. Ekaterine Kldiashvili represented GTU's activity and pilot actions at international conferences and seminars.

Zhang Feng is now a registered physician in the Department of Cardiology of Shanghai Jiao Tong University affiliated First People's Hospital, majoring in cardiac device implantation and invasive electrophysiology. Till now, Dr. Feng has finished 500 cases of catheter ablation including paroxysmal supraventricular tachyacardia, atrial tachycardia, PVC, and atrial fibrillation. In 2008, Dr. Feng was NASPE fellow in S'orsola hospital in Bologna and San Donato hospital in Milan directed by Franco Naccarella and Riccardo Cappato. In fellow training, Dr. Feng widened knowledge in cardiovascular epidemiology and gained more experience in atrial fibrillation ablation aided by CARTO XP. From 2010, as chief of electrocardiogram in Shanghai First People's Hospital. In 2011, Dr. Feng and team established our remote outpatient electrocardiographic monitoring system which is similar to MCOT system.

Giorgio Galanti graduated with top marks and praise in 1972; he is Specialist in Cardiovascular Diseases, Specialist in Internal Medicine, Specialist in Sports Medicine, Director of the School of Specialization of Sports Medicine, Member of the Academic Council of 19 cycle Doctorate in Clinical Pathophysiology and Aging, University of Florence, Member of the Academic Cycle 21 PhD in Physiological Sciences and Nutrition, University of Florence. he is Owner of teaching sports medicine courses Degree of Medicine, Sports Science, Physiotherapy, Nursing and dietary and Advanced Degrees in Science and Technology Sport, Sport Management and Sciences Adaptive and Preventive. Professor Galanti is the director of the Center for Research Support and former athletes CAVREA University Hospital Careggi. He is author of over 200 publications in international journals and national.

Gianpiero Guerrieri, born in Milan (Italy) in 1969, trained as IT Manager, holds a degree in Information Sciences with a Master's degree in Health Economics. He began working in health care in 1996. Currently, he is Director of ICT unit of the hospital "San Giovanni Addolorata" to Rome and Ideator and consulting of telemedicine service, as well as expert in artificial intelligence and privacy. He is a Member of the Advisory Committee of the periodical *e-Health care*.

Victor Vuni Joseph is a Consultant in Public Health with Doncaster Primary Care Trust (England); a Fellow of the Faculty of Public Health (FFPH) of the Royal College of Physicians of the United Kingdom; and a Fellow of the Royal Society of Public Health (FRSPH), UK. He is a final year PhD student at the University of Leeds where he is investigating factors influencing the update of telehealth in routine healthcare setting. He was the Chief Investigator in a study examining the effects of telehealth in patients with long-term conditions. He is Chair of Africa-UK Telemedicine Working Group, part of Africa-UK Diaspora Engagement Programme.

Ricky C. Leung is Assistant Professor at the Department of Health Management and Informatics in the School of Medicine, University of Missouri. His research interests include health information technology, organization theory, organizational economics, research methods, technological innovation, and global health. Dr. Leung received his Ph.D. from the University of Wisconsin-Madison, and postdoctoral training from the University of Minnesota. He was previously a visiting faculty member in Brown University.

Pierluigi Mancini is Head of the Awareness Activities and Feasibility Studies Division in the Directorate of Telecommunciations and Integrated Applications of the European Space Agency.

Alessandro Maolo got his MD degree (*summa cum laude*) in July 2012. During his course of study he developed a particular interest in Cardiology and he attended the department of Medicina Interna and the Clinica di Cardiologia at the Ospedali Riuniti in Ancona. After this experience, he decided to conduct his thesis work in the Clinica di Cardiologia; he took part in a research project aimed to evaluate the possible role of Telemedicine in the management of atrial fibrillation, under the supervision of Dr. Ilaria Mazzanti, Dr. Roberto Antonicelli, and Prof. Alessandro Capucci. At the present time he is attending the Clinica di Cardiologia, still continuing the Telemedicine research project.

Silvia Marino has research interests entirely dedicated to the clinical and neuroimaging aspects of neurological disorders. During her medical school and residency in Neurology, she developed an interest in the clinical aspects of neurodegenerative disorders. During her PhD period at the Quantitative Neuroimaging Laboratory of University of Siena, she worked on the clinical application of magnetic resonance spectroscopy and functional magnetic resonance in brain of patients with neurological disorders. Currently, she is the neurologist leader of the Quantitative NeuroBioImaging Laboratory and Clinical Research at the IRCCS Centro Neurolesi "Bonino-Pulejo" of Messina, working on the clinical application of new neuroimaging techniques by using high field magnetic scanner. Her interest has focused on patients with Alzheimer, Parkinson's disease, and low levels of consciousness.

Gabriele Mascherini has been with the University of Florence since 2009 as PhD student, and he earned his PhD in April 2012. His work was in order to collaborate in the plan of Exercise as Prescription program in Sports Medicine Center in Florence Hospital. His degree in kinesiology allows him to follow the patients in four specialized area of physiological interest. The first area is biomechanics and by specific tools and evaluations established the attitude of every patient for resistance and flexibility training. The endurance is necessary to plan an individualized aerobic program for a better cardio respiratory performance. Regularly, an analysis of body composition and body hydration is carried out to follow any possible adaptation at the physical training. Finally, the life style evaluation is performed with an accelerometer to verify the spontaneous physical activity during the day of each person. Dr. Mascherini is a physical trainer and his work provides both therapeutic training, both for the promotion of health and performance. He is author of books and articles primarily in the area of evaluation of people life style and physical performance.

Ilaria Mazzanti attended the Università Politecnica delle Marche between 2002 and 2008 and got her Medical Doctor's degree in September 2008 (*summa cum laude*). Since 2009 she has taken part in several Telemedicine research projects, starting her experience in this sector at the Telemedicine Center at INRCA (Ancona) directed by Doctor Roberto Antonicelli. Since 2010 she has attended the Residency School in Cardiology and Cardiovascular Diseases at Clinica di Cardiologia, Università Politecnica delle Marche. She is co-author of several manuscripts such us "Impact of home patient telemonitoring on use of β-blockers in congestive heart failure" (Drugs Aging 2010). She was a relator, with the title "Ruolo del Telecontrollo," in the Corso regionale GIMSI 2010 Marche "La gestione della sincope e l'organizzazione della Syncope Unit." She is a Member of the SIEC (Società Italiana di EcoCardiografia).

Brian A. McCrossan is a Specialist Trainee in Paediatric Cardiology at the Royal Belfast Hospital for Sick Children, which is the Regional Paediatric Cardiology Centre for Northern Ireland. His main research interest is in the application of Telemedicine to Paediatric Cardiology. This research has been presented at international scientific meetings and published in major peer-reviewed journals. Dr. Mc-Crossan has been involved in developing telemedicine services and securing national/ European funding.

Roberto Mugavero has a degree in Environmental Engineering at University of Rome "Tor Vergata," is Professor of "Action Planning for Homeland Security" at University of Rome "Tor Vergata"- Faculty of Engineering, Scientific Director of Master of Science "Systems and Electronic Technologies for Security, Defence and Intelligence" at University of Rome "Tor Vergata" – Department of Electronic Engineering, Head of Branch Security, Defence and CBRNe at University of Rome "Tor Vergata" – Department of Electronic Engineering. President of the national "Observatory on Security and CBRNe Defence." He is a Professor in several Fire Prevention, Security and Safety Courses and Conferences Speaker in the fields of Security, Safety, CBRN Risk, Emergency Management, Risk Management, Crime Prevention and Technological-Industrial Risk. He is National CBRN Defense Expert and Italian Representative, as "Coordination Expert CBRN," in the European Civil Protection Task Force, Board Member at the Ministry of the Interior and at the Presidency of the Council of Ministers – National Department of Civil Protection. Volunteer Firefighter Officer, Rank Colonel, at Rome Fire Brigade.Board Member at ISPRO

Institute – Italian Institute for Studies and Research on Security, Civil Protection and Defense. He also collaborates with several organizations, associations, magazines and industry in the field of security and safety. He has participated in many national and international exercises and emergency activities.

Fabrizio Murgia, born in 1948 in Rome, graduated in Medicine at the University "La Sapienza" of Rome in March 23, 1973. He specialized in Pediatrics in July 21, 1976 and in Neonatology in November 30, 1979 at the 'University "La Sapienza" of Rome. He served as Assistant and Help Pediatrician in Hospital of Civitavecchia (Roma) March 1, 1979 – August 30, 1998, and since 1993, held the Functional Form of Pediatric Gastroenterology and Endoscopy. He has achieved the requisite qualification to national head of pediatrics on the exam session 1986. He served as 1st level Director at the Division of Pediatrics Hospital G.B. Grassi (Roma) September1, 1998 – 28 February 2005, from January 1, 2001, head of the outpatient Pediatric medicine Service. Has achieved the second level Master in "Telemedicine" at the University of Pisa, November 6, 2006 with grades 50/50 and praise, title of thesis: Sviluppo e valutazione dell'efficacia di un sistema per il telemonitoraggio di pazienti affetti da Fibrosi Cistica. Since March 2005, he works as Free Professional in health ICT with the Cystic Fibrosis Unit, Bambino Gesù Pediatric Hospital in Rome as part of Telemedicine. Was member of scientific committee of 1st International Conference of e-Health and Telemedicine. Nicosia (North-Cyprus), october 2011.

Franco Naccarella graduated at the University of Bologna in 1976 in Medicine and Surgery. Specializations obtained at the University of Bologna and University of Milan: He was member of CNR Nato for medical research in USA 1980 1982. He did his Cardiology Fellowship at Presbyterian Medical Center of Penn University 1982 1985, earned Joung Investigator Award of the American college of Cardiology 1984, was Chief of Cardiology and Chief of Internal Medicine 1989 Bologna Maggiore Hospital, and Chief of Cardiology Parma University Hospital 1996. He published many books and more than 600 papers in Cardiology including 100 in foreign languages. Actually he works as a noninvasive electro physiologist and Interventional cardiologist at Villa Maria of Cotignola. Italy. He collaborates also with the San Donato Group in Milan, with the Italian Embassy in Beijing, with the PR China Embassy in Rome with National and International Societies of Arrhythmias ECAS HRS Naspe. He is the Governor for Italy of the International Society of Cardiovascular Pharmacotherapy. He is a nucleus member of the European Society of Cardiology Working Group on drugs.

Andrea Nucita is actually Researcher at the Faculty of Computer Science at the University of Messina, Italy. He received a PhD Degree in Computer Science from the University of Milan in 2004. His research interests are related to geographical information systems, query optimization in the context of spatial databases, and medical informatics. He has co-authored publications in international conference proceedings and international journals in the above-mentioned research fields.

Giorgio Parentela is Telemedicine Task Force Manager of the Telecommunications and Integrated Applications Unit of the European Space Agency.

Giovanni Rinaldi is Physics graduate at Bologna University (Italy). His main research areas are about mathematical models in complex systems, artificial vision, telemedicine, and medical records, for which he has taken part in international project and conferences. He is consultant for different national health organizations and software industries and lectures at high learning course at University.

Valentina Sabato has a degree in Environmental Engineering, and is in charge of Technical Secretariat of the Presidency, advisor of the "Observatory on Security and CBRNe Defense – Osdife," Assistant of "Action Planning for Homeland Security" at the University of Rome "Tor Vergata"- Faculty of Engineering, Scenario Coordinator assistant tin NATO project "Multinational Experiment 7." She has collaborated in the planning and management of territorial emergencies and major events such as G8 L'Aquila 2; gap analysis between national and international management of hazardous waste (Sistema di Tracciabilità dei Rifiuti pericolosi SISTRI – GREEN PAPER).

Giovanni Saggio received the Dr. Eng. degree in Electronic Engineering in 1991 and the Ph.D. degree in Microelectronic and Telecommunication Engineering in 1996, from the University "Tor Vergata," Rome, Italy. For his Ph.D. degree he carried out research at the Nanoelectronics Research Centre, University of Glasgow, Scotland, and at the Cavendish Lab, University of Cambridge, England. From 1991 to 1993, he worked with a grant in CNR (Italian Center for Research Counsel), and was a Visiting Scientist at the Rutherford Appleton Lab., Oxford, England. His researches covered the area of nanodevices, SAW devices, noise in electronic devices. He is currently a Researcher at the University "Tor Vergata," Rome, Italy. He teaches courses about Electronics at the Faculty of Engineering and the Faculty of Medicine (Departments of Medicine and Surgery, Orthopedics and Traumatology, Neurophisiopatology, Hearing Aid Practitioner). His current researches regard BCI and biosensors, about which he has got four patents.

Irene Scacciati a degree in Dietetics in 2009 at the University of Florence. Following graduation, she perfected the profession through a post-graduate internship at the service of the hospital dietetic Nuovo San Giovanni di Dio, and joined the same professional activities and collaboration with the department of Sports Medicine of AOU Careggi that the door to specialize in the sports nutrition. She works as a dietitian with the Fiorentina Football Club. In April of 2012, she graduated with a doctor's degree in Human Nutrition Science.

David Lee Scher is a former Cardiac Electrophysiologist and is an independent consultant and owner/director at DLS Healthcare Consulting, LLC, (www.digitalhealthconsultants.com) uniquely concentrating in advising digital health companies and their partnering institutions, providers, and businesses. A pioneer adopter of remote cardiac monitoring, he lectures worldwide promoting the benefits of digital health technologies. Dr. Scher's most recent accomplishment was chairing the Happtique Blue Ribbon Medical App Certification Program Panel which developed standards for the certification of health, fitness, and medical apps. He was cited as one of the ten cardiologists to follow on Twitter and one of the top ten blogs on health care technology. Board Certified in Internal Medicine, Cardiovascular Diseases, and Clinical Cardiac Electrophysiology, he is a Clinical Associate Professor of Medicine at Pennsylvania State University College of Medicine.

Chitsutha Soomlek is a Ph.D. student in Electronic Systems Engineering at the University of Regina, Canada. Soomlek received her MA.Sc. (Master of Applied Science) in Electronic Systems Engineering from the University of Regina, Canada in 2007. She received her B.E. in Computer Engineering from King Mongkut's Institute of Technology Ladkrabang, Bangkok, Thailand in 2004. Soomlek has been a Thai scholar since 2004. Her research interests are in the areas of mobile agents and their applications, eHealth and applications, software engineering, computer network, visualization, distributed computing, computer and network security, and database system. Soomlek's current research involves software agents, visualization systems, and clinical decision-support systems.

Letteria Spadaro is research fellow in IRCCS Centro Neurolesi "Bonino-Pulejo," Messina, Italy. She is a psychologist actively involved in neuropsychological research, aiming at testing innovative methodologies of care for patients with neurodegenerative disease, especially Alzheimer Disease, Parkinson Disease and, Multiple Sclerosis, and their caregivers. Her research focuses on the neuropsychological rehabilitation with a special attention on the improvement of quality of life. During her psychological school at the University "La Sapienza" of Rome (Italy), she gained significant experience in clinical neuropsychology. During her master in Clinical Neuropsychology at the University of Palermo (Italy), she developed a special interest on cognitive rehabilitation. She is currently involved in a postgraduate course in Cognitive-Behavioral Therapy.

Laura Stefani graduated in 1986 with three specializations in Gastroentology, Cardiology, and Sports Medicine with honors. Working at the University of Florence since 1991 was MD in the Internal medicine Unit for infectious diseases and cardiology intensive. From 2002 to 2004, she was involved in the birth and management of the Oncology Unit as medical internist and management. Since 2004 operates in the Sports Medicine department, since 2011 heads the "Physical exercise Prescription" protocols and teaches physical education, science and technology of sport and adapted physical activity. She has more than 100 manuscripts on cardiology, sports medicine, and prescription of exercise in chronic diseases and is a reviewer for international area application and study of the deformation cardiac parameters and some other heart conditions such as bicuspid aortic valve.

Francesca Timpano got her Master's Degree in Clinical Psychology at University of Padua. During this period she developed an interest in the clinical aspects of neurodegenerative disorders. Currently, she is a Psychologist and Research Fellow at IRCCS Centro Neurolesi "Bonino-Pulejo," Messina, Italy, working on the clinical application of ICT solution to neurological and psychological practice. Her research interests deal with validation of neuropsychological tests and implementation of innovative care methodologies delivered, through telemedicine systems, to patients with neurodegenerative and cerebrovascular disease and their caregivers. She is author of several papers related to this research field and she is scientific responsible of different clinical trials. She is currently involved in a postgraduate course in Constructivist Therapy of Padua.

Rita Verbicaro has a degree in Biomedical Engineering at the University of Naples "Federico II." From 2008 to 2010, she worked at the Monaldi Hospital of Naples about issues related to the integration of application systems for the exchange of clinical data, in accordance with healthcare standards. She has been a researcher at National Research Council (CNR), in Rome. Her main activity is analysis and developing of new methodologies to introduce ICT in health care processes, with particular regard to clinical features and management in chronic diseases. She collaborated with Ministry of Health about the definition of an architectural model for the Electronic Health Record (EHR), in accordance to the national guidelines, by the identification of new approaches of improvement, both in the primary and secondary uses. Currently, she is Consultant at Agenas (Agenzia Nazionale per i Servizi Sanitari Regionali) and she is assisting the Health Regional Authorities of Campania and Calabria about a sustainable approach to eHealth and modern telemedicine.

Index

CPSIA information can be obtained at www.ICGtesting.com
Printed in the USA
BVOW051050250113

311436BV00008B/143/P

9 781466 629790